KU-257-910

Oxford Handbook of
Primary Care and Community Nursing

VICTORIA INFIRMARY
MEDICAL STAFF LIBRARY

PUBLISHED AND FORTHCOMING OXFORD HANDBOOKS IN NURSING

Oxford Handbook of
Primary Care and Community Nursing

Edited by

Vari Drennan
Director of the Primary Care Nursing Research Unit,
Department of Primary Care and Population Sciences,
Royal Free & University College London Medical School,
London, UK

Claire Goodman
Professor of Health Care Research,
Centre for Research in Primary and Community Care,
University of Hertfordshire, UK

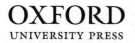
VICTORIA INFIRMARY
MEDICAL STAFF LIBRAR

OXFORD
UNIVERSITY PRESS

OXFORD
UNIVERSITY PRESS

Great Clarendon Street, Oxford OX2 6DP

Oxford University Press is a department of the University of Oxford.
It furthers the University's objective of excellence in research, scholarship,
and education by publishing worldwide in

Oxford New York

Auckland Cape Town Dar es Salaam Hong Kong Karachi
Kuala Lumpur Madrid Melbourne Mexico City Nairobi
New Delhi Shanghai Taipei Toronto

With offices in

Argentina Austria Brazil Chile Czech Republic France Greece
Guatemala Hungary Italy Japan Poland Portugal Singapore
South Korea Switzerland Thailand Turkey Ukraine Vietnam

Oxford is a registered trade mark of Oxford University Press
in the UK and in certain other countries

Published in the United States
by Oxford University Press Inc., New York

© Oxford University Press 2007

The moral rights of the authors have been asserted
Database right Oxford University Press (maker)

First published 2007

All rights reserved. No part of this publication may be reproduced,
stored in a retrieval system, or transmitted, in any form or by any means,
without the prior permission in writing of Oxford University Press,
or as expressly permitted by law, or under terms agreed with the appropriate
reprographics rights organization. Enquiries concerning reproduction
outside the scope of the above should be sent to the Rights Department,
Oxford University Press, at the address above

You must not circulate this book in any other binding or cover
and you must impose the same condition on any acquirer

British Library Cataloguing in Publication Data
Data available

Library of Congress Cataloging in Publication Data
Data available

Typeset by Newgen Imaging Systems (P) Ltd., Chennai, India
Printed in Italy
on acid-free paper by
LegoPrint S.p.A.

ISBN 978–0–19–856890–2 (flexicover: alk. paper)

10 9 8 7 6 5 4 3 2 1

Oxford University Press makes no representation, express or implied, that the drug
dosages in this book are correct. Readers must therefore always check the product
information and clinical procedures with the most up to date published product
information and data sheets provided by the manufacturers and the most recent
codes of conduct and safety regulations. The authors and publishers do not accept
responsibility or legal liability for any errors in the text or for the misuse or
misapplication of material in this work.

Foreword

Primary and community nursing has been through a time, lasting over a decade, of relentless and radical change: the introduction of the NHS and Community Care Act 1991, GP fund holding, the political devolution of health, primary care groups, primary care trusts, walk-in centres, NHS direct as well as numerous reorganizations. The foreseeable future brings new challenges for primary care and community nurses, including practice-based commissioning, new systems of payment by results, and greater patient choice. Throughout the United Kingdom there is a renewed drive to diminish hospital services and bring new and expanded services to the community—under the political rhetoric of care closer to home. The community health agenda has the potential to be overwhelming, making this textbook a wonderful resource for both new and experienced nurses who have chosen to work in the many different community settings.

This book is timely and will without doubt be an essential resource to nurses in health centres, general practices, walk-in centres, and those studying at universities. It will also be of value to those nurses in hospitals who need to acquire knowledge on primary and community health matters. The combination of both the health politics and clinical practice across the lifespan is to be celebrated and the authors need to be congratulated for achieving such an ambitious and worthwhile endeavour. Current and future primary care and community nurses now have the advantage of having access to a most excellent publication to aid them through the diversity and challenges of their daily practice.

Lynn Young
Primary Health Care Adviser,
The Royal College of Nursing,
Cavendish Square, London.
November 2006

Acknowledgements

Our thanks go to those nurses and health visitors in Camden PCT, Islington PCT, and the Primary Care Nursing Research Unit who read some early drafts and commented, to the anonymous reviewers who commented on the final drafts, to Elizabeth Haghirian who tamed the multiplicity of abbreviations, to our contributors, and Nic Ulyatt (our OUP editor) who persevered with us. Most of all our thanks go to our families who lived through the writing, editing, and proofreading of this book—we could not have done it without you.

Preface

Primary Care and community nurses work in a wide range of settings, their work involves addressing the multiple public health, prevention, treatment, and care needs of their patients and local communities. These nurses include: practice nurses, nurse practitioners, district nurses, community staff nurses, health visitors, school nurses, walk-in centre nurses, sexual health and contraceptive service nurses, community paediatric nurses, and occupational health nurses.

Primary Care and community nurses are both generalists and specialists working with individuals and their families and carers at different stages of their life. This book cuts across the traditional service divisions between primary care based specialist nursing practitioners, nurses working in general practice, and those employed by community services. It responds to health policy and professional trends that require a flexible, patient-centred service increasingly provided outside of hospitals. It is a valuable resource for nurses involved in new types of services, nurses in public health, and those with widening responsibilites for health promotion, screening programmes, first contact triage, chronic disease management, care management, and child and adult protection.

This book addresses primary care and community nurses' need to readily access evidence based information for a very broad range of conditions and across an extensive range of preventive care and treatment techniques. It is intended as a quick reference source guide for nurses working in primary care and community health services that supports them in everyday clinical decision-making. As well as evidence based clinical knowledge the book also addresses the organizational knowledge that nurses need to be able to work in primary care and community and across different organizations and the interface of the statutory and voluntary sectors in health, education, and social care. It is written by primary care and community nurses who are directly engaged in current practice, research, education, and policy developments.

Detailed contents

Symbols and abbreviations

↑	increased
↑	decreased
→	leading to
>	greater than
<	less than
♂	male
♀	female
°	degrees
❶	warning
📖	cross reference
🖫	website
ACE	angiotensin-converting enzyme
ADL	activities of daily living
ADR	adverse drug reaction
AF	atrial fibrillation
AIDS	acquired immune deficiency syndrome
AMTS	Abbreviated Mental Test Score
AOB	any other business
ASAP	as soon as possible
ASD	atrioseptal defect
BBV	Blood borne virus
BCG	Bacille Calmette–Guérin vaccine
bd	twice a day
BLS	basic life support
BMD	bone mineral density
BMI	body mass index
BNF	British National Formulary
BP	blood pressure
BST	British Summer time
CAB	Citizen's Advice Bureau
CAMHS	Child and Adolescent Mental Health Services
CBT	cognitive behavioral therapy
CE	Conformité European mark
CF	cystic fibrosis
CHD	coronary heart disease
CIN	cervical intra-epithelial neoplasia
CLDT	community learning difficulties team

CMHT	community mental health team
CMO	chief medical officer
CNO	chief nursing officer
CNS	clinical nurse specialist
c/o	complain of
COC	combined oral contraceptive
COPD	chronic obstructive pulmonary disease
CP	cerebral palsy
CPA	care programme approach
CPD	continuing professional development
CPR	cardiopulmonary resuscitation
CR	creatinine
CVA	cerebrovascular accident
CVD	cardiovascular disease
CXR	chest X-ray
d	day/s
DfES	Department for Education and Skills
DH	Department of Health
DHSSPS	Department of Health Social Services & Public Safety
DLA	disability living allowance
DM	diabetes mellitus
DN	district nurse
DOB	date of birth
DPA	Data Protection Act 1998
DVT	deep vein thrombosis
EC	emergency contraception
ECG	electrocardiogram
ED	emergency department
EEG	electroencephalography
ENT	ear, nose, and throat
EPP	expert patient programme
FBC	full blood count
FH	family history
FI	faecal incontinence
FOI	Freedom of Information Act 2000
GA	general anesthetic
GI	gastrointestinal
GMS	general medical service
GP	general practioner
GPN	general practice nurse
GTN	glyceryl trinitrate
GUM	genitourinary medicine

HFAC4	*Health for all children,* 4th edition
HIV	human immunodeficiency virus
HNA	health needs assessment
HPA	Health Protection Agency
hr	hour
HSC	Health & Safety Commission
HV	health visitor
Hx	history
IBD	inflammatory bowel disease
ICP	intergrated care pathways
IM	intramuscular
INR	international normalized ratio
IS	income support
IV	intravenous/ly
L	litre
LA	local authority
LDP	local delivery plan
LFT	liver function test
LHB	local health board
LMP	last menstrual period
LTC	long-term condition
LTOT	long-term oxygen therapy
LVF	left ventricular function
M, C & S	microscopy, culture and sensitivity
mcg	microgram
MDR	multi-drug resistant
MDT	multi-disciplinary team
mg	milligram
MI	myocardial infarction
min	minute/s
mL	millilitres
mm	millimetre/s
MMR	measles, mumps, and rubella vaccine
MMSE	Mini Mental State Examination
MND	motor neurone disease
mth/s	month/s
MRSA	methicillin-resistant *Staphylococcus aureus*
MS	multiple sclerosis
MSM	men who have sex with men
MSU	mid-stream specimen of urine
NELH	National electronic library for health
nGMS	New General Medical Service contract

NGT	nasogastric tube
NHS	National Health Service
NICE	National Institute for Clinical Excellence
NMC	Nursing and Midwifery Council
NOFTT	non-organic failure to thrive
NP	nurse practitioner
NSAIDs	non-steroidal anti-inflammatory drugs
NSF	National Service Framework
OA	osteoarthritis
od	once a day
OH	occupational health
OOH	out-of-hours
OPD	outpatient department
OT	occupational therapy/occupational therapist
OTC	over-the-counter
pa	per annum
PCO	Primary Care Organization
PCT	Primary Care Trust
PDP	personal development plan
PE	pulmonary embolism
PEFR	peak expiratory flow rate
PEP	post exposure prophylaxis
PHCHR	parent-held child health record
PHCT	primary health care team
PID	pelvic inflammatory disease
PILs	patient information leaflets
PMH	past medical history
PMS	personal medical service
PN	practice nurse
PND	Postnatal depression
PO	per os (by mouth)
POM	prescription-only medicines
POP	progestogen-only pill
POVA	protection of vulnerable adults
PPE	personal protective equipment
PPP	personal professional profile
PREP	Post-Registration Education and Practice Standards
prn	pro re nata (as required)
PSHE	personal, social, and health education
PTSD	post traumatic stress disorder
PTT	prothrombin time
PVD	peripheral vascular disease

QMAS	Quality Management and Analysis System
	quality and outcomes framework
QoL	quality of life
RCC	red cell count
RIDDOR	reporting injuries, diseases, and dangerous occurences
RNCC	registered nursing care contributions
RTA	road traffic accident
Rx	treatment
S	serum
SAP	single assessment process
SC	subcutaneous
SE	side effect
SEHD	Scottish Executive Health Department
SHA	Strategic Health Authority
SHO	Senior House Officer
SIGN	Scottish Intercollegiate Guidelines Network
SLT	speech and language therapist
SN	school nurse
SOB	shortness of breath
SRE	sex and relationship education
SSRIs	selective serotonin reuptake inhibitors
STIs	sexually transmitted infections
SUDI	sudden unexpected death of infant
TC	total cholesterol
TCA	tricyclic antidepressants
tds	three times a day
TENS	transcutaneous electrical nerve stimulation
TFT	thyroid function tests
TIA	transient ischaemic attack
U+Es	urea and electrolytes
UPSI	unprotected sexual intercourse
URTI	upper respiratory tract infection
UTI	urinary tract infection
UV	ultraviolet
VF	ventricular fibrillation
vit.	vitamin
VTE	venous thrombolytic embolism
WCC	white cell count
WHO	World Health Organization
wk/s	week/s
yr/s	year/s
YOT	youth offending team

The health of the UK population

UK health profile

UK population 59,553,800 in 2004 (National Statistics Office see below). Health influenced by a multiplicity of factors as summarized in Fig. 1.1.

Major causes of death
- Circulatory diseases (includes heart disease and stroke) nearly 2 male:1 female.
- Cancers: 4 most common are breast, lung, colorectal, and prostate.
- Respiratory diseases.

Mortality rates by cause of death vary with age and sex
- Young people aged 15 to 29: mortality rates highest for injury and poisoning (41 per 100,000 population for men and 10 per 100,000 for women).
- Adults aged 30 to 44: injury and poisoning leading cause of death for men (45 per 100,000 population) and cancers the leading cause of death for women (32 per 100,000 population).
- Adults aged 45 to 64: cancers were the leading cause of death among both men and women.
- Adults aged 65 to 84: circulatory diseases were the leading cause of death, for both men and women.
- In the 2001 census, 91% of people in private households in England and Wales reported good/fairly good health.

Health inequalities
People are likely to experience worse health than the rest of the population if they experience one or more of: material disadvantage, lower educational attainment, and/or insecure employment. There is also evidence that living in materially deprived neighbourhoods contributes to worse health for individuals and evidence that inequalities are widening.

Average life expectancy at birth is 80.4yrs for females and 75.7yrs for males, however socio-economic gradient and geographic gradient the average for males in some areas is <74yrs.

Infant mortality is 5.6 per 1000 live births in England and Wales but considerable variation by area and socio-economic status of parents. Increased rates in babies with fathers in manual occupations and where only mother registered baby. Highest rates in teenage mothers and lowest where mother 30–34yrs.

Further information
- National Statistics Office www.statistics.gov.uk/default.asp
- Association of Public Health Observatories www.apho.org.uk/apho/

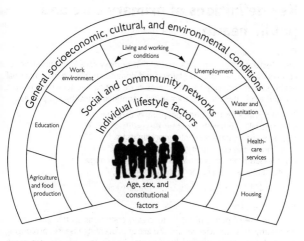

Fig. 1.1 Influences on health. Reproduced with kind permission of the authors Margaret Whitehead and Goran Dahlgren. Dahlgren G. and Whitehead M. (1993). *Tackling inequalities in health: what can we learn from what has been tried?* Working paper prepared for the King's Fund International Seminar on Tackling Inequalities in Health, Ditchley Park, Oxfordshire. London, King's Fund.

Key definitions of primary care and public health

Primary care

The Declaration of Alma Ata[1] stated that primary care is the first level of contact that individuals, the family, and community have with a national health system, bringing health care as close as possible to where people live and work. It is the first element of a continuing health-care process.

The five principles that underpin primary care are:
- Accessibility to health services
- Use of appropriate technology
- Individual and community participation
- Increased health promotion and disease prevention
- Intersectoral cooperation and collaboration.

See also 📖 Overview of services in primary care.

Public health

The purpose of public health is to create conditions so that people can be healthy. It is the science and the art of preventing disease, prolonging life, and promoting physical and mental health through the organized efforts of society. It has a collective rather than an individual view of the health needs and health care of a population.

The aim of public health bodies is to achieve this purpose by:
- Promotion of a safe environment
- Control of community infections
- Health promotion
- The organization of medical and nursing service for the early identification and treatment of ill health and disease
- Health protection.

Underpinning values of public health
- Equity and social inclusion
- Participation, collaboration, and community empowerment
- Social justice where health is a basic human right.

See also 📖 Health needs assessment.

Further information

📖 Health Protection Agency: www.hpa.org.uk
📖 UK Public Health Association: www.ukpha.org.uk
WHO (1998). *Health 21: Health for all in the 21st century*. WHO, Copenhagen.

---

[1] Declaration of Alma Ata (1978). 📖 www.who.int/hpr/NPH/docs/declaration_alma_ata.pdf

Long-term conditions model

Background

>60% of adults report a long-term health problem (DH 2005 see below). This includes diabetes (1.3 million), COPD (600,000), asthma (3.7 million), arthritis (8.5 million), epilepsy (400,000), mental ill health. 8.8 million people have a long-term condition (LTC) that severely limits their day to day ability to cope. Some have multiple conditions, which make care particularly complex and these account for a disproportionate amount of health care (especially hospital care). Different levels of need among people with LTCs can be represented by the 'Kaiser pyramid of care' commonly referred to as the long-term conditions model of care.

The aim is to treat patients:
- Sooner, nearer to home and earlier in the course of disease through: earlier detection, good control to ↓ effects of disease and ↓ complications, effective medicines management, ↓ in number of crises, ↑ independence, and prolonging and extending quality of life.

All patients in health community should be identified and stratified in terms of the 3 levels:
- **Level 3** patients have care managed by a case manager. They will:
  - Identify patients at risk e.g. through numbers of hospital admissions, medical conditions, medicines, GP consultations, falls etc.
  - Have a caseload of about 50 patients, usually for life.
  - Have advanced clinical and prescribing skills.
  - Possess high level decision-making skills, enabling the effective management of interrelated, multiple health problems.
  - Have authority to request investigations and to refer to specialists.
- **Level 2** patients are those with a complex single need or multiple conditions. Needs are met through multi-professional teams based in primary care, with support of specialist advice. Care will be based on agreed standards and protocols and a system of identification, recall and review.
- **Level 1** patients and their carers will be supported to develop knowledge, skills and confidence to care for themselves and their condition effectively. The Expert Patient Programmes or equivalent support this (Expert patients 📖).

Related topics

📖 Individual health needs assessment; 📖 Models of and approaches to health promotion; 📖 Social services.

Further information

DH (2005) Supporting people with long-term conditions: an NHS and social care model to support local innovation and integration

DH (2005) The national service framework for long-term conditions

📑 All available from DH website www.dh.gov.uk

Policies on LTC available on each country's central health department website, see 📖 The NHS in Northern Ireland, Scotland, and Wales

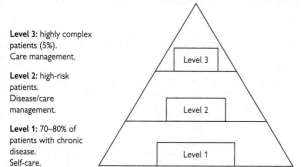

Level 3: highly complex patients (5%). Care management.

Level 2: high-risk patients. Disease/care management.

Level 1: 70–80% of patients with chronic disease. Self-care.

Fig. 1.2 The long-term conditions model of care

The National Health Service (NHS)

The UK NHS was established on 5th July 1948 to provide a comprehensive range of health services to all in need. It is free at the point of delivery and paid through taxation. Some services also incur subsidised charges e.g. NHS prescriptions in primary care. The NHS UK budget was £88,647,000,000 in 2005–6.[1]

The government's key aims for the health and social care system are to:
- Improve the health and well-being of the population
- Improve patients' experience of care
- Reduce inequalities in both the above
- Continue to deliver value for the taxpayer.

Decisions about health policy have been devolved to each of the four countries of the UK. Consequently, structures and policy priorities are slightly different in each country. The Isle of Man and the Channel Islands have independent health service structures.

In each country, there is a senior government minister responsible for health and publicly funded health services. Within government agreed policies, the central NHS administration sets overall priorities and some specific targets. Local NHS bodies (e.g. Primary Care Trusts in England) plan, commission, and monitor services for the residents of a defined area—usually co-terminus with a Local Authority (LA). Each country has its own arrangements for assessing the quality of health care.

[1] www.nhs.uk/thenhsexplained

The NHS in England

The central administration of the NHS

The government sets out its proposed plans for the NHS and other social support services in its election manifesto. These proposals are then detailed in Green Papers (for early stage consultation) and White Papers (firm proposals) and presented to Parliament for debate and translation into legislation. The Secretary of State for Health leads the National Health Service and accounts to Parliament. Public Service Agreements (PSA) are the NHS targets agreed by the Secretary of State with the Treasury in return for the public funds.

The Department of Health (DoH) develops overall policy and guidance for health and social care for adults as well as monitoring NHS performance against the PSA targets. It is led by the Chief Executive, professional advisors include CMO and CNO. DfES leads on policy for children and young people including health. Strategic Health Authorities (StHA)—the link between DoH and the local NHS in ensuring national priorities are integrated into local plans.

Local administration and provider services

The special health authorities: provide health services to the whole population of England and sometimes the other countries e.g. National Patient Safety Agency www.npsa.nhs.uk; NHS Direct (the 24 hour telephone advice line 0845 4647).

Primary Care Trusts (PCTs): responsible for planning and commissioning health services from service providers and improving the health of the local population in conjunction with the LA. They have to demonstrate they meet PSA targets. They control 75% of the NHS budget. PCTs may provide community health service although in some areas, these are being provided by stand alone social enterprise organizations and through practice based commissioning.

NHS Trusts: provide hospital and specialist community services. Services are commissioned by PCTs. Some are Foundation Trusts with greater freedom to control their budgets and determine their services.

Mental Health Trusts: provide both acute and community services for people with mental health problems.

Increasingly local organizations are linking health services and LA services together.

Care Trusts: these provide both health and social care services and have budgets from both the Health Service and LAs.

Children's Trusts: include all education services, childrens social services and acute and community childrens health services. They may also include other services such as Connexions and Youth Offending Teams.

Related topic
📖 Clinical governance.

Further information
🖥 www.dh.gov.uk

The NHS in Northern Ireland, Scotland, and Wales

Northern Ireland

There is a lead minister in the UK parliament while political negotiations continue.

Central administration: the Department of Health, Social Services, and Public Safety (DHSSPS) led by a Permanent Secretary with professional officers including medicine and nursing. Leads on overall policy for health and personal social services, public health, and public safety.

Local administration and providers: four Health and Social Service Boards. They are agents of the DHSSPS in planning, commissioning and purchasing services for the residents in their areas including primary care services. Nineteen Health and Social Service Trusts provide health and social services

Four Health and Social Service Councils take up issues on behalf of the public.

Further information

🖳 www.dhsspsni.gov.uk/index.asp

Scotland

Minster of Health and Community Care is responsible for the NHS to the Scottish Parliament.

Central administration: Scottish Executive Health Department (SEHD). Responsible for health policy and the administration of the National Health Service in Scotland; social work policy and in particular community care. It is lead by a chief executive. Professional advisors include a chief medical officer and chief nursing officer.

Local administration and providers: special NHS Boards have national responsibilities e.g. NHS 24 (the 24hrs telephone advice line). Twenty-four local NHS organization/systems provide acute, mental health and primary care services. Local Health Co-operatives in primary care replaced with Community Health Partnerships involving Local Authorities.

Further information

🖳 www.show.scot.nhs.uk

Wales

The Health and Social Services Minister is responsible to the Welsh Assembly Government for policy direction and for allocating funds to the NHS in Wales.

Central administration: the NHS Directorate and Nursing Division is led by a Director with professional advisors including a CMO and CNO. Three regional National Assembly offices: Mid, North, and South East Wales link and monitor national policy to the local structures.

Local administration and providers: twenty-two Local Health Board (LHBs): co-terminus with local authorities Together they strategically plan health and social care for the people living in their area. LHBs also

commission GP services directly from practices, and community and 2°
care services from NHS Trusts. LHBs are constructed like English PCTs.
Fourteen NHS Trusts manage hospitals and community health services
across Wales; one Trust manages an all-Wales ambulance service.

Twenty-two Community Health Councils take up issues on behalf of the
public.

Further information
www.wales.nhs.uk

Health needs assessment

Health is a subjective concept. Health needs assessment (HNA) wards against value judgement and promotes a strategic and evidence-based approach; it enables evaluation of the effectiveness of interventions and promotes equity. HNA is the essence of public health (Public health 📖). Collating information in a systematic way, HNA makes visible the invisible and enables a targeting of resources where need is greatest. HNA focuses not only on need but on issues of social justice and rights, and informs decision making.

HNA techniques

HNA techniques range from those that are individual to population focused. Increasingly they combine statistical and participatory methods e.g. Participatory Rapid Appraisal using lay participation and multidisciplinary teamwork which takes account of the wider societal determinants of health (UK population health profile 📖). The public health function/departments of PCOs usually undertake population level health needs assessments for strategic planning (Commissioning of services 📖). Also undertaken at a general practice level or a local community level. Practitioners should be cognisant of the ethical dimension of HNA and avoid raising expectations if change/services are not going to be available.

Epidemiological and demographic methods

Statistical data such as mortality rates, use of services, age of population, incidence and prevalence of disease/accidents are collated and analyzed. Increasingly these are plotted using geographical health information systems, which can inform needs assessment at macro level.

Participatory methods

The usefulness of statistical information is enhanced when combined with qualitative data, which explains for example:
- Why people do not attend
- How services might be developed
- The impact of services on health (known as health impact assessment, see below).

Further information

🖳 BMJ Collection on health needs assessment particularly the 1998 series
  http://bmj.bmjjournals.com/cgi/collection/needs_assessment?page=1
🖳 Health Development Agency (2005). *Health Needs Assessment: A Practical Guide.*
  www.publichealth.nice.org.uk
🖳 National Statistics Office www.statistics.gov.uk/
🖳 Nice (2005). Clarifying Approaches to Health Impact Assessment www.publichealth.nice.org.uk/
  page.aspx?o=505665

Commissioning of services

Commissioning is a set of planned activities undertaken with the intended outcome of measurable improvement in the health and well-being of resident populations, involving the implementation of change to secure the most effective and efficient use of resources. It includes:
- The assessment of need and strategy development
- The identification of priorities and investment planning
- Service specification (including quality and development)
- Service contracting, including financial flows
- Service monitoring of activities under the contract for individuals and populations.

Commissioning for secondary and tertiary care services now uses a system of payment by results so that PCOs commission:
- The volume of activity required to deliver service priorities, adjusted for case mix (i.e. the mix of types of patients and/or treatment episodes)
- From a plurality of providers
- On the basis of a standard national price tariff, adjusted for regional variation in wages and other costs of service delivery.

PCOs have a responsibility to work closely with LAs to jointly plan and in some cases commission services for shared populations. Local delivery plans (LDPs) are 3yr plans to deliver and improve services. LDPs based on local health needs assessment, central government priorities, targets and service standards e.g. National Service Frameworks (NSFs).

Practice based commissioning

Practice based commissioning is a new, currently English only, initiative. Practices (or clusters of practices) will hold the budget for their practice(s) population. They will identify the health needs and commission the amount and types of services within the context of agreed LDPs. Applies to GMS (General practice 📖) and PMS (Personal medical services 📖). The budget initially includes outpatients, elective admissions and operations and emergency admissions. Over time will include mental health services, diagnostics, and community services.

Further information

On each UK country's health sections website, see 📖 The NHS in England, 📖 The NHS in Northern Ireland, Scotland, and Wales
🖳 Primary Care Contracting NHS www.primarycarecontracting.nhs.uk

Public health

Public health is focused on *health* as well as disease, and *populations* not individuals. It seeks to protect health and prevent illness by studying health patterns/trends and planning to address health needs. Consequently Health Impact Assessment (HIA) is becoming a defining feature of this work.

Traditional focus used to be the preserve of medicine, focused on the environment and dominated only by disease and quantitative methodology:
* Epidemiology:
  * Patterns of diseases and understanding of causation
  * Control of infectious diseases: management of epidemics (SARS, MRSA, salmonella); vaccination
  * Screening.
* Demography:
  * Population patterns (births, deaths, and migratory trends) to inform public service planning.

Current public health practice uses complementary approaches alongside epidemiology and demography that emphasize:
* Equity: fairness and social justice
* Cross cutting approaches, known as partnership or intersectoral work
* Community participation in the development of services
* Participation in health service commissioning decisions.

Public health policy

In the UK post-devolution, each of the 4 countries has produced a separate public health strategy. Critics argue that devolution poses a threat to the integrity of the welfare state. The European Union (EU), increasingly influences public health governance at national level. Critics argue that this has resulted in a bias towards the traditional disease focus. The growing importance of public health, within policy and practice is reflected in the creation of:
* Public Health Observatories
* Public health specialists working at strategic levels in PCOs
* A voluntary Public Health Register.

All nurses and midwives are expected to contribute to public health. Nurses on the NMC public health register are required to contribute to and influence policies affecting health.

Further information

📖 Association of Public Health Observatories www.apho.org.uk/apho/
Public health policy on each country's central health website, see 📖 The NHS in England, 📖 The NHS in Northern Ireland, Scotland, and Wales
📖 Public Health Electronic Library www.phel.gov.uk/
📖 UK Public Health Alliance www.ukpha.org.uk
📖 UK voluntary register for public health specialists www.publichealthregister.org.uk/

Overview of services in primary care

(See also Key definitions of primary care and public health 📖.)

There are a wide range of NHS services available to the public but some local variation. Different types of services have different relationships to the central NHS:

- Some are directly managed in NHS structures e.g. community health services.
- Some are outside NHS management structures but mainly only provide services under a contract to the NHS e.g. general practitioners.
- Some are independent of the NHS but receive NHS payment for particular activities e.g. community pharmacists.

Core primary care health service elements available to all local populations are:

- 24-hour NHS helpline e.g. NHS Direct, NHS 24.
- General (General practice 📖) or personal (PMS 📖) medical services and their out of hours (OOH) services either provided by the practice or a GP co-operative.
- Dentistry, pharmacy, optometry (Other primary health care services 📖).
- Community health services based in community clinics, health centres, and GP surgeries. Usually includes:
  - Nursing in the home (District nursing 📖)
  - Public health nursing (Health visiting 📖, School nursing 📖)
  - Sexual health and contraceptive services (Nurses in primary care 📖)
  - Chiropody, dentistry, speech and language therapy, physiotherapy for specific vulnerable groups (Other primary health care services 📖).

May also include:

  - Multi-disciplinary specialist teams e.g. palliative care, rehabilitation, intermediate care, rapid response
  - Clinical specialist nurses e.g. continence, diabetes, TB.

The PCOs or their community health services may also have:

- Walk In Centres: assessment and treatment of minor injuries and health problems, usually staffed by nurses.
- Community hospitals: admission and clinical management through GPs and primary care nurse.

Further information

On each UK country's central government health website, see 📖 The NHS in England, 📖 The NHS in Northern Ireland, Scotland, and Wales

🖥 NHS England www.nhs.uk/England

General practice

There are 39,920 GPs in the UK in ↑ 10,000 practices.[1] About 27% are single-handed GPs. Average practice list size between 5–6000 patients. The majority of GPs are independent contractors i.e. not directly employed by the NHS. Most hold General Medical Service (GMS) contracts with the NHS (see below). >40% hold Personal Medical Service (PMS) contracts. GP vocational training includes 2yrs in hospital posts as SHO and 1yr as a GP registrar supervised by GP trainer. GPs with special interests (GPSWIS) are appointed by their local PCO to provide specialist health care in a generalist setting e.g. CHD, child protection, ENT.

The new GMS contract

This is a contract between an individual practice and a PCO. All the partners of the practice (one has to be a GP) have to sign the contract. Its national format is known as 'the Blue Book'. The practice contract states:

- The services that will be provided by that practice.
  - Essential (see below)
  - Additional if not opted out (see below)
  - Out of hours if not opted out
  - Enhanced if not opted out.
- Level of quality of essential and additional services that the practice 'aspires' to (Quality and outcomes framework 📖).
- Support arrangements e.g. IT, premises.
- Total financial resources (includes a global sum + additional monies, and adjustments for the workload and costs incurred by the features of the population served, details on NHS Employers website[2]).

Essential services must be provided by all practices:

- Day to day medical care for the practice patients, includes the management of minor and self-limiting illness, referral to secondary services and other services as appropriate.
- Non-specialist care of people who are terminally ill.
- Chronic disease management.

Additional services

The practice can choose to opt out of these and receive less payment:

- 📖 Cervical cancer screening.
- Provision of contraceptive services (Contraception: general 📖).
- Vaccinations and immunizations, both childhood basic course, those >6yrs, missing the basic course and reinforcing doses (Childhood immunization 📖).
- Child health surveillance excluding the neonatal check (Overview of the child health promotion programme 📖).
  - Maternity services excluding intra-partum care.
  - Minor surgery procedures e.g.: curettage, cautery, cryocautery.

---

[1] 🖳 Royal College of General practitioners Information Sheets www.rcgp.org.uk/information/publications
[2] 🖳 NHS Employers www.nhsemployers.org/PayAndConditions/primary_care_contracting.asp

Out of hours
Defined as from 6.30pm to 8.00am on weekdays, the whole of weekends, Bank holidays, and public holidays. Practices can choose to opt out of this for reduced finance. May be provided by GP cooperative, or local PCO or in combination with NHS Direct.

Enhanced services
These are commissioned by the PCO and attract additional payment. There are 3 types:
- National enhanced services. These have national specifications but the PCO does not have to provide them in primary care e.g. anticoagulation monitoring.
- Local enhanced services: defined and commissioned by the PCO e.g. specific enhanced care for the homeless.
- Directed enhanced services. These have national specifications (specific to each country) and have to be provided by the PCO. Examples include:
  - Childhood immunizations for children <2yrs and pre-school boosters <5yrs. 70% coverage to reach lower payment and 90% coverage to reach higher payment (Childhood immunization schedule 🕮).
  - Influenza immunization for >65yrs and at risk groups (Targeted immunization in adults 🕮).
  - Minor surgery.
  - Access for violent patients removed from practice lists due to aggressive behaviour.

Each practice has to produces a practice leaflet detailing services, practice policies, and route for complaints.

Registration with a practice
People apply to register with a practice by handing in their NHS medical card to the reception or completing an application form. The practice informs the PCO of the registration and it confirms the acceptance with a new medical card to the patient. Temporary registrations can be made if resident >24hrs and <3m.

List closures
Practices can only close their lists after negotiation with the PCO. When a list is closed the practice can only accept new patients who are close family relatives of existing patients.

Removal from practice list
Patients can be removed from practice lists because of violence, or crime and deception to receive treatment, or distance from the surgery.

Patients right to change GP
People can choose to change GP without giving an explanation, giving a period of notice, or informing the GP.

Personal medical services (PMS)

PMS contract is the local alternative to the new national GMS contract (General practice 📖). The PMS contract is made with the PCT. It started as a pilot scheme and is now a permanent option. >40% of GPs in England now work under PMS contracts. Some nurses hold PMS contracts with PCTs. It gives primary care professionals the freedom to innovate, work more closely as a team to improve services for patients, and address inequalities in health-care provision.

The PMS pilots demonstrated: ↑ access for patients to primary care professionals, ↑ delivery of services, ↑ recruitment and retention of nurses and GPs in deprived areas, ↑ team working; ↑ extended roles for nurses; ↓ central bureaucracy; ↑ cash flow.

Elements of the PMS contract

PMS contracts may not contain all the elements of the GMS contract and may contain others. Practices are paid to provide a package of services. How the practice provides those services is up to the practice. Most PMS budgets consist of:

- Core services: usually services patients would expect to receive from any GP (equivalent to GMS contract essential services).
- Additional services: both those usually expected from a GP e.g. maternity, minor surgery, contraception, and those usually provided by community or 2° care services e.g. community nursing, community based specialist services e.g. endoscopy, ultrasound etc. (PMS Plus). Prescribing budget (optional).

QOF

(See Quality and outcomes framework 📖.)

Specialist PMS contracts

This allows new models of primary care delivery for groups poorly served by the current system by removing the need patients to be registered for all 'core' primary care services with that practice. There are three types of Specialist PMS:

- Primary care services for vulnerable groups e.g. the homeless, refugees.
- Specialist services provided in 2° care sector but which could be provided in the community e.g. out-patient older person care; home-based palliative care; dermatology.
- Specific service provision e.g. services for violent patients; OOH care; teenage contraceptive services; sexual health clinics.

Further information

📰 NHS Primary Care Contracting www.primarycarecontracting.nhs.uk/4.php

Other primary health-care services

A range of services and professionals are available in primary care. This provides a summary (alphabetically) of the most commonly used.

Chiropodists

Registered chiropodists (also known as podiatrists) are trained in all aspects of care for the feet and lower limbs. Some are also podiatric surgeons undertaking surgery for conditions such as hammer toes. Services available in consulting rooms, at home and in care homes. Paid for privately. 🔲 Society of Chiropodists www.feetforlife.org

Community chiropody services

NHS funded services for specified vulnerable groups e.g. older people, people with diabetes, rheumatoid arthritis, osteoarthritis. Local referral criteria and pathways, often requiring GP referral.

Dentists

Dental practices take private and NHS patients. NHS dentists have agreements with their local PCO to provide NHS dental services. Patients not eligible for free NHS dental treatment (NHS entitlements 🔲), pay 80% of the cost of the treatment up to a maximum of £384 per course of dental treatment. 🔲 British Dental Association www.bda-dentistry.org.uk

Community dental service (CDS)

Funded by PCOs. Gives dental treatment to people who have difficulties accessing dental care, e.g. people with learning disabilities, housebound people. Usually able to provide a domiciliary service. Local policies on referral process e.g. may only be through GP. CDS usually also provides school oral screening.

Opticians

Provide eye sight tests and examine eyes for abnormalities e.g. glaucoma. Also fit and supply spectacles to a prescription. Dispensing opticians only fit and supply glasses. Free NHS eye tests available to certain groups (NHS entitlements 🔲, Benefits for people with a low income 🔲). PCO funds screening (mostly by orthoptist) as part of child health promotion programme (Overview of the child health promotion programme 🔲). PCO ensures there is a mechanism for a domiciliary service for housebound people. 🔲 General Optical Council www.optical.org

Pharmacists

Community pharmacist (sometimes called chemists) prepare and dispense medicines on prescription (Medicine concordance 🔲) to the general public. May be owners of their business or work for a bigger company. The new contract between local pharmacies and PCOs specifies services in dispensing medicines, waste disposal of medicinal products, and public health activities e.g. smoking cessation, provision of emergency contraception, providing advice about other services and information on self care. Community pharmacists may be involved in new ways of working e.g. facilitating repeat prescribing through electronic transmission of prescriptions, medicine reviews (Principles of medication reviews 📖), supplementary prescribing (Medicines management 📖), home delivery services, OOH. 🖥 Royal Pharmaceutical Society www.rpsgb.org.uk

Primary care pharmacists and prescribing advisors

These pharmacists are employed by PCOs to advise the PCO, general practice, community health service staff, and local community pharmacists on issues related to supply, storage, legislation concerning medicines, formularies, and prescribing budgets.

Physiotherapists

Physiotherapy is concerned with human function and musculo-skeletal movement. Physiotherapists deal with a wide range of issues e.g. sports injuries, incontinence, arthritis, back pain. Work in a range of settings including in private practice. 🖥 College of Chartered Physiotherapists www.physiofirst.org.uk

Community physiotherapists

PCO funded physiotherapists usually work as part of specialist multi-disciplinary teams e.g. stroke rehabilitation, intermediate care teams, children with special needs, providing clinic based and domiciliary services. Local variations in availability and referral pathways.

Occupational therapists

State registered occupational therapists (OTs) work to enhance someone's ability to participate in everyday activities and reduce avoidable dependency through occupation and environmental changes. Available as a private service from OTs working independently. 🖥 British Association of Occupational Therapist www.cot.org.uk/

Community occupational therapists

Usually employed by local authorities to working with specific vulnerable groups e.g. disabled adults, in Community Care processes for aids and adaptions (Aids and equipment: general 📖). Also in PCO commissioned services e.g. community mental health teams or children with special needs teams. Local variation in access and referral routes.

Speech and language therapists (SLTs)

SLTs work with children and adults who have difficulties with communication, or with eating, drinking, and swallowing. Some work in independent practice paid privately. 🖥 Royal College of Speech and Language Therapists www.rcslt.org

Community SLTs

PCO funded SLTs may work as part of specialist teams, e.g. children with special, needs or more broadly across a client group, e.g. children or adults. Local variation in access and referral pathways.

Services to promote hospital discharge and prevent unplanned admission

A range of time limited services for patients and their carers are available in most PCOs to achieve one or more of the following:

- Avoid unplanned hospital admissions triggered by a crisis.
- Facilitate discharge from hospital. NB Community Care (Delayed Discharge etc.) Act 2003 LA has to ensure patients assessed as no longer needing inpatient care can be discharged into the community.
- Respite care for parent/carer to help sustain the caring relationship.
- Provide rehabilitation and support to enable independent living.
- Intensive care at home otherwise provided by 2° care.

NB These services are locally determined; involve a wide range of titles, types of providers and sources of funding. Most services involve partnerships across health and social care and voluntary and private providers. Referral to service is through relevant professional e.g. GP, DN, SW. The following summarizes overlapping approaches to service provision.

Intermediate care

Main focus is older people with the aim of promoting independence by providing enhanced services from the NHS and LA, specifically: intensive time limited support. Care provided by MDT, including therapists, and social workers, with support from care assistants. Provided either at home or in designated care settings (e.g. care homes with designated beds, community hospitals).

Rapid response teams/hospital at home

Allow people who might otherwise be admitted to hospital or have a prolonged in patient stay, to be at home e.g. patients with chest infections, a mild stroke, recovering from elective surgery, or in need of end-of-life care (some areas offer hospice at home). Teams may provide IV antibiotics, blood transfusions, nutritional support, and general health and social care till acute episode of need is over.

Case managers/community matrons for people at risk

(Care/case management models 🕮.) Health or social care professional manages a discrete caseload of people that are considered at risk of unplanned hospital admission and/or vulnerable. PCOs have different criteria for admission to service but often include people with history of unplanned admissions, falls, or multiple health and social care needs.

Partnerships for Older People Projects (POPPs)

Series of cross agency projects across England that aim to reduce demand on 2° care by providing more support for low level community care. Reducing emergency hospital admissions, supporting more people to live at home in sheltered or supported housing e.g. extra care.

Respite care

See 🕮 Carer's assessment and support.

Further information for health-care professionals

🕮 Health and Social Care Change Agent Team: Care Services Improvement Partnership
www.cat.csip.org.uk

Services for children, young people, and families

The UN Convention of the Rights of the Child (1989 🖳 www.unicef. org.crc) is the basis of government policies for children in each country of the UK. These focus on priority outcomes of being healthy, staying safe, enjoying and achieving, making a positive contribution, and achieving economic well-being. The policies emphasize multi-agency planning and provision of publicly funded services for children and families e.g. England under the 'Every Child Matters' policy is introducing children's centres that provide social support, health services, and early year's education provision in one setting.

In any LA area there is a wide range of state funded, voluntary organization and private services for children and families. Sources of information include:
- Local children's information services
- Local public library
- The national ChildcareLink website www.childcarelink.gov.uk and its national information line ☎ Tel: 08000 96 02 96.

Early years—social support and play

This provision ranges from groups to one-to-one support. It can be meetings in community centres organized by a paid worker e.g. parent and toddler groups, one-o'clock clubs, or purely voluntary meeting in each others homes e.g. NCT groups, Meet a Mum. Organizations such as Newpin, Homestart, and some Sure Start services offer one-to-one befriending and practical support schemes for new parents and parents under stress.

Early years—child care, play, and education

Working parents have a range of options, depending on availability and what they can afford, between one-to-one types of care in the home e.g. child minders, au-pairs, nannies, or group care e.g. in nurseries. All child minders and group care for under 8-year-olds have to be registered and meet national standards. Children in need (A child or young person in need 🕮) are usually prioritized for state funded support in day care facilities. Crêches, pre-schools, and playgroups offer sessions focused on play and encouraging early years development. All 3 and 4-year-olds are entitled to a free, part-time place in a nursery school. Sure Start (see below) provides detailed parent leaflets on child care options.

Education

Every child has to receive education from 5–16yrs either at a state school, a private school, or in the home. Every LA provides information on the internet about its schools and entry procedures. Many schools have break-fast clubs and after school clubs. Pupil referral units or home tutoring is provided by each LA for children who need alternative provision e.g. have been excluded from mainstream school or are school phobic. State schools are supported by LA wide services such as education welfare officers or social workers and education psychology services. See also 📖 Children with special educational needs.

Education for 16–18-year-olds is in schools, sixth form colleges, or further education colleges which also provide vocational and access education to >18yrs.

Young people's health services

Many areas provide open access young people's drop-in health clinics. Most of these provide sexual health and contraceptive services. GP services are being encouraged to become more accessible to teenagers.

Leisure activities and sport

Schools, LA services (e.g. education, youth, and leisure), voluntary organizations (e.g. Woodcraft Folk, faith organizations, guides, and scouts) and the private sector may provide a range of different sports and leisure activities in an area. See above for sources of local information.

Careers advice

Connexions in England (see below) provides personal advisors in schools, youth clubs, community centres, and as outreach. Can help with identifying barriers to learning and providing support for young people. 🖥 Careers Scotland www.careers-scotland.org.uk

Social services

See 📖 Social services, also 📖 Looked-after children.

Youth offending team (YOT)

Every LA in England and Wales has a multi-agency YOT to respond to the needs of each young offender and identify suitable programmes to prevent reoffending. 🖥 Further information from: www.youth-justice-board.gov.uk

Related topic

📖 Child health promotion.

Further information for professionals and parents

🖥 Government websites and: www.everychildmatters.gov.uk/
🖥 Sure Start: www.surestart.gov.uk/
🖥 ParentsCentre: www.parentscentre.gov.uk/
🖥 Children in Scotland: www.childreninscotland.org.uk

Further information for children and young people

🖥 Childline www.childline.org.uk/Helpandadvice.asp ☎ Tel: 0800 1111
🖥 Connexions Direct for young people aged 13–19yrs www.connexions.gov.uk/
   ☎ Tel: 080 800 13219
🖥 NSPCC for 12–16yrs olds www.there4me.com

Homes and housing

Office of National Statistics[1] reports:

- 69% of UK households are owner occupied (81% of pensioner households).
- 66% of lone parents with dependent children households are in rented properties.
- In 2003, 137,220 people were statutory homeless (see below).
- About 4% of dwellings were classed as unfit for human habitation. Unfit or in serious disrepair dwellings were most likely to be occupied by people on low incomes, over 75yrs or young people.

CABs and Housing Advice Centres are key resources for advice and help on housing issues (Useful websites 📖).

Help with housing

Not for profit housing

In most areas there is a central waiting list for LA and housing association properties. Each has different systems for accepting applicants and prioritizing people on their waiting lists for housing. Usually includes factors such as poor health made worse by housing conditions, mobility problems, inadequate number of bedrooms for family size, homelessness, length of time in the area. Medical problems are assessed by an independent advisor.

Supported housing

E.g. sheltered housing often run by councils, housing associations or voluntary groups. Available to specific groups of people such as older people or people with physical or mental health problems. May be eligibility criteria and waiting lists. Some supported housing is staffed 24hrs, while in some support is only provided occasionally.

Rented accommodation

Environmental health services inspect rented properties and enforce basic living standards. They assess properties on dampness, disrepair, structural stability, adequate lighting, heating, ventilation food preparation, facilities, sanitary facilities, and drainage. Specific standards for houses of multiple occupation. Failure to tackle basic problems can result in closure of the premises, legal notices served for improvements to be made, or prosecution of the landlord or agent.

Help with house maintenance, heating, and security

Local councils have grant aid schemes for people on low income for repairs, improvements, insulation, and adaptations. Specific schemes may be available for older people e.g. Care and Repair (see below) or linked to home accidents and falls prevention schemes or Keeping Warm in Winter schemes.

Damp

Dampness, condensation, and mould growth. Caused either by water penetration through the fabric of the building or by condensation. Advice for condensation includes increase insulation, reduce moisture production (e.g. don't use paraffin heaters), increase ventilation to remove moisture.

---

[1] www.Statistics.gov.uk

Detailed advice usually available through LA environmental health office (Environmental health services 📖).

Heating

Estimates of 30,000 excess winter deaths related to cold, majority in people over 75. Winter Keep Warm Campaigns include information on local sources of heating and insulation grants for low income families, pensioners and other vulnerable adults.

Security

Many LAs as part of their crime reduction programme have schemes for helping low income households, particularly pensioners, install or improve home security. General advice on home security and defeating burglars who call on vulnerable people then distract them while they are robbed, is available at crime reduction website shown below.

Problems with neighbours

Tacking anti-social behaviour, is a crime reduction partnership activity in all LA areas. Most LAs have information and/or staff dealing with this issue. Issues like noise problems usually dealt with in first instance by environmental health services (Environmental health services 📖).

Help for homelessness

The UK has a legal definition of homeless which includes: no home in the UK or anywhere else in the world; only able to stay in current place on a very temporary basis, have been locked out of home; can't live at home because of violence or threats of violence; it isn't reasonable to stay in that home e.g. home in very poor condition. LAs have a legal duty to provide advice to people who are homeless or threatened with homelessness. They *only* have a responsibility to help with accommodation if people meet all of the criteria:

- Legally eligible for assistance (many groups, e.g. asylum seekers, are excluded).
- Are not intentionally homeless.
- And are in priority need, that is pregnant, or dependent children under 16 or 19 if in full-time education, or through emergency such as flood or aged under 16 (not in Northern Ireland). It may also include people vulnerable through illness or disability, at risk of violence, and homeless after leaving prison, hospital, or the armed forces.

The LA may give temporary accommodation while they investigate. The LA has to help those who qualify but does not have to provide LA properties. Local social services authorities have a duty to provide accommodation for children and young people over 16 leaving care, or in need (A child or young person in need 📖) for other reasons.

Further information

📖 Care and Repair (for older people) England www.careandrepair-england.org.uk/
Wales www.careandrepair.org.uk/ Scotland www.care-repair-scot.org.uk/
📖 Crime Reduction and Home Security www.crimereduction.gov.uk
📖 Shelter www.shelter.org.uk Wales: www.sheltercymru.org.uk
Scotland www.shelterscotland.org.uk Shelter ☎ Free Helpline 0808 800 4444

Environmental health services

Practitioners frequently come across environmental health issues that impact on their patients and clients. Each LA has an environmental health department (sometimes called consumer protection department) employing environmental health officers (EHOs). Their role is to prevent, detect and control environmental hazards which affect human health. The department's core functions are usually:
- Private sector housing
- Food hygiene and safety
- Noise and pollution control
- Pest control
- Occupational health and safety
- Notifiable and reportable diseases control (with NHS public health departments).

It may also include others e.g. waste disposal and cleansing services, animal wardens for stray dogs. EHOs also involved in public health and health promotion campaigns.

Private sector housing (Homes and housing 📖) EHOs can inspect rented properties and enforce basic living standards.

Food hygiene and safety Food premises inspected according to the food safety risk they pose to the public. Premises found to contravene basic food hygiene standards can be closed down and prosecuted.

Noise and pollution control EHOs have powers to deal with noise problems from industry, continual neighbourhood noise e.g. barking dogs, music. Can seize noisy equipment or serve notices to stop. Failure can result in prosecution.

Pest control Advice and action to remove ants, bees, mice, rats, wasps, and other pests from homes and businesses. Fees usually charged unless on low income in receipt of state support or pension.

Occupational health and safety EHOs inspect non-manufacturing premises under the Health and Safety at Work etc. Act 1974 and can stop work activities immediately, require improvements to be made and/or prosecute the businesses. Also investigate workplace accidents.

Infectious diseases and food poisoning EHOs investigate the causes of notifiable and reportable diseases (Infectious disease notification 📖) and food poisoning in conjunction with public health leads for communicable diseases (forming a team for infectious disease outbreak control) as well as other 'reportable diseases'.

Further information for the public and professionals

There is direct access for the public and professionals to these services. Information on the services and how to access them is on every LA website

Social support

Social support is the existence or availability of people on whom you can rely; people who let you know that you are cared about, valued, and loved. The main source of social support comes from family, friends, and involvement in local organizations e.g. clubs, schools, trade unions and churches. It is a concept linked to social capital (Community approaches to health 📖).

Lack of social support

This is associated with:

- ↑ morbidity and mortality.
- Socio-economic classification: those with higher incomes are less likely to report a lack of social support that those with low incomes.
- Gender: ♂ more likely to report a lack of social support than ♀.
- Ethnicity: contrary to popular stereotypes people from a range of ethnic backgrounds often report severe lack of social support.

Questions to assess levels of social support available to clients and patients include

- Is someone available to talk with who will listen?
- Is someone available to help with activities of daily living?
- Is there someone who can provide emotional support?
- What is the frequency of contact with those you feel close to and who you trust confide in?

Sources of social support

- Local community based organizations e.g. community centres, tenants associations, youth clubs, faith organizations, political parties, schools.
- Local support groups for people in the same situation e.g. carers support groups.
- Local branches of national charities and voluntary organizations e.g. Alzheimer's Society, Gingerbread, Family Welfare Association.
- Local volunteer organizations and good neighbour schemes.
- Online and telephone support e.g. Childline, Parentline.
- Health, social work, and other public service professionals.

Every nurse working in primary care needs to know how to provide clients and patients with information about *local* sources of social support. Good starting points for getting local directories are:

- Local library
- LA website
- Local Council for Voluntary Services.

Related topics

📖 Health needs assessment; 📖 Learning to work in primary care.

Social services

Social services departments (England and Wales), social work departments (Scotland), or health and social services board (Northern Ireland) have wide-ranging legal responsibilities to use public funds to provide a range of care, support and protection services for:
• Children, young people, and their families
• Vulnerable adults who, by reason of age or disability, need assistance to live an independent life, and their carers.

They are part of the LA (except in Northern Ireland). They work in partnership with health, education, housing, the police, and the voluntary sector to meet the needs of vulnerable people.

Contacting social services
Social services take direct enquiries from the public as well as take referrals by professionals. People are assessed by a social worker (see below) to determine needs (The assessment of children, young people, and families 📖; Integrated (or single) assessment process 📖; Carers assessment and support 📖). Social workers can provide:
• Information about the care and support services that are available
• An assessment of need
• Practical help and support for some people according to local eligibility criteria
• Information about other organizations that may help.

> **NB Most services are charged for following an individual assessment of ability to pay**

Support for children, young people, and their families includes
• Protection for children and young people from abuse and neglect
• Support to vulnerable families to prevent family breakdown
• Looking after children who cannot live at home
• Support to families with a child who has a permanent and substantial disability
• Work to reduce the likelihood of young people committing offences.

Services likely to be available include
• Safeguarding children (Child protection 📖)
• Family support
• Short-term breaks
• Equipment and adaptations to the home (Aids to daily living 📖)
• Residential care and support for young people leaving care (Looked-after children 📖)
• Youth justice teams.

Support for vulnerable adults include
• Older people with physical and mental frailty
• People with physical and/or sensory disabilities or learning disabilities
• People with mental health needs
• People with problems of substance misuse (drugs, alcohol etc.)
• People who have HIV/AIDS.

Services likely to be available include
- Home care and meals on wheels
- Day centres and group activities
- Short-term breaks
- Equipment and home adaptations (Aids to daily living 📖)
- Registration for disabled people.

The Social Services Directorate may directly provide services or pay for other providers. Some people may have direct payments to purchase their own care with public funds. If locally set cost limits for assistance in the community are exceeded, the person is offered residential or nursing home care (Care homes 📖).

Social work teams can be organized in different ways:
- Cover a geographical area and work generically.
- Be part of a joint service with health, e.g. Community mental health teams.
- Be based in a neighbourhood centre, hospital, or health centre.
- Specialize in:
  - Children and families
  - Adults services
  - Specific groups e.g. people who are blind, deaf, or have dementia.

Most social services have a duty system whereby designated social workers/teams take new enquiries or referrals.

NB Every nurse in primary care needs to identify local referral processes to social services and social workers.

Related topics

📖 Services for children, young people, and families; 📖 Homes and housing; 📖 Environmental services; 📖 Social support

Further information

📱 Commission for Social Care Inspection: www.csci.org.uk
📱 Scottish Social Care Services Council: www.sssc.uk.com

NHS entitlements

The NHS provides health care in the UK. It is paid for through taxation. People living or working in the UK are entitled to free or subsidized (e.g. charges for dentists, opticians, prescriptions unless low income) treatments at the point of care, as are people taken ill whilst in the UK for a short stay. Some countries have a reciprocal agreement where UK residents can get free medical treatment, and residents of that country can get the same in the UK.

People coming from overseas

Treatment always free at the point of care for:
- Accidents and emergency treatment
- Compulsory psychiatric treatment
- Certain communicable diseases, e.g. TB, cholera, food poisoning, malaria, and meningitis, STIs but testing only for the HIV virus not treatment
- Family planning.

Entitlement to NHS treatment depends on the length (>6mths) and purpose of residence in the UK, not nationality. A person who is regarded as ordinarily resident, i.e. stay has some permanence and stability, in the UK is eligible for free treatment by primary medical services. Overseas visitors to the UK are not regarded as ordinarily resident if they do not meet this description except if:
- Asylum seekers and refugees given leave to remain in the UK, or awaiting the results of an application to remain.
- EEA nationals with forms E112 or E128.
- Any person, whether ordinarily resident or not, requiring treatment that a GP regards as emergency or immediately necessary (for <14d).

GPs may offer to accept patients as private and charge if stay <6mths. Entitlements to primary medical services currently under review.

Further information for professionals and public

Detailed policies on each UK country's central website (see The NHS in England 📖, The NHS in Northern Ireland, Scotland, and Wales 📖)
📖 Citizen Advice Bureau www.citizensadvice.org.uk/

Care homes

Four per cent of people >65yrs of age live in care homes and 20% of people >85yrs[1]. Approx 65% are women.

Registered care homes either have on-site nursing care (previously known as nursing homes) or are without on-site nursing care (previously known as residential homes). Care homes are run by not-for-profit voluntary organizations, by private companies or, less frequently, by LAs and the NHS.

Registration and inspection

All care homes are inspected to ensure that they comply with national standards, and are registered by the Commission for Social Care Inspection (CSCI) (the Care Commission in Scotland). Some care homes have specific registration for older mentally infirm (EMI) patients. Local CSCI offices and social service departments provide lists of registered care homes.

Provision

Care homes can provide:
- Long-term care for adults who, through frailty or disability, need help with personal care and/or have nursing care needs
- Long-term care for vulnerable groups in need of special/extra care (e.g. children and adults with learning disabilities)
- Respite and intermediate care
- Continuing NHS care (see below)
- Palliative care (Palliative care in the home 📖).

Personal care

In care homes personal care (i.e. not nursing care) is usually defined as:
- Help with washing, bathing, and showering
- Help with managing continence, including using catheters and stomas
- Assistance with eating and managing special diets
- Help to move around indoors
- Help with simple treatments, e.g. applying creams, lotions, and dressings.

Primary health care

Care home residents are registered with GPs like other citizens (General practice 📖) and receive primary care services in the same way. District nurses (DNs) provide nursing care for residents in care homes.

Public financial assistance for care home fees

Rules for public financial assistance differ in the 4 countries and are linked to national eligibility criteria for NHS continuing care. More than half of residents in care homes have fees paid by LAs. Individuals fund their own fees if their financial resources are above the national threshold (in 2005 these were: England and Northern Ireland, £20,500; Wales, £21,000; Scotland, £19,500). In Scotland, those >65yrs old paying their own fees

---

1 📖 Office of National Statistics www.statistics.gov.uk

receive £145 a week towards personal care fees and a further £65 to nursing care (see below).

The starting point in all countries is the assessment of need by the LA usually by a social worker care manager. Social services have a set ceiling for fees and a list of preferred providers.

Individual's contribution to care fees

The LA financial assessment includes income (e.g. pension), savings, shares, and property (including the individual's own home) when working out an individual's contributions to fees. The value of a home is excluded:
- For the first 12wks after entry into permanent care.
- If the home is shared by spouse, heterosexual partner, relative >60yrs old, incapacitated relative <60yrs old, carer, or child <16yrs old.
- LA discretion, e.g. home of same-sex partner.

The LA must always leave the individual money for personal use, £18.80 a week in England, Scotland, and Northern Ireland; £19.10 in Wales. If the LA is contributing to care home fees and the person chooses a more expensive care home than the LA ceiling amount, a third party, e.g. a relative, has to contract with the LA and care home to pay the top-up amount.

NHS contribution to care home fees

A resident in a care home with nursing may have the nursing care element of their fees paid by the NHS. Primary care organizations will have agreed a system for assessing the need for a registered nursing care contribution (RNCC). Amounts differ in each country, in 2005 (given as general guidance):
- In England there are three bands, high (£129 a week); middle (£80); or low (£40 a week).
- In Wales, a flat rate of £107.63 per week.
- In Northern Ireland, up to £100 a week.
- In Scotland, up to £65 a week (see rules on personal care payment above).

Complaints and concerns

Complaints and concerns not addressed by a care home should be referred to these inspection bodies:
- 🔲 Commission for Social Care Inspection (CSCI): www.csci.org.uk
- 🔲 Scottish Commission Regulation of Care: www.carecommission.com

Related topics

📖 Social services; 📖 People with dementias.

Further information for professionals and patients

🔲 Age Concern: www.ageconcern.org.uk (linked sites for all countries) Age Concern Helpline: ☎ 0800 00 99 66
🔲 Counsel and Care: www.counselandcare.org
Help the Aged Senior Line: ☎ 0808 800 6565, lines are open Mon–Fri 9am–4pm

Nursing in primary care

Nurses in primary care

Primary care services are those services that can be accessed directly by the public without referral from another professional (Overview of services in primary care 📖). Nurses and health visitors (HVs) work in a wide range of primary care settings delivering services that range from public health, preventative, curative, chronic disease management, through to the care of people who are dying. Sometimes the main work roles are categorized as providing first contact services, providing chronic disease management services, and providing public health services. Some groups of nurses focus more on one aspect e.g. HVs on public health roles while others may combine all three aspects e.g. practice nurses. The service can be reactive (in response to people seeking them out or referring to them) or proactive (actively seeking out people or particular populations). Nurses in primary care can be generalists e.g. practice nurses, or specialists (i.e. working with only one type of condition) e.g. people with sickle cell disorders, or only one part of the population e.g. travellers, or providing only one type of service e.g. sexual health or contraceptive services.

In the UK over 68,000 (headcount) nurses and HVs are employed directly by PCOs and over 26,000 (headcount) practice nurses are employed directly by general practices. The numbers are increasing as more health care is delivered in primary health-care settings.

The largest groups of nurses are within:
- District nursing services
- Practice nursing
- Health visiting
- School nursing.

But there are also significant numbers in specialist services such as family planning, sexual health services, community childrens' nursing, walk-in centres, OOH centres, and occupational health services. Some specialist nurses also work in primary care as outreach from the hospital consultant led team e.g. diabetes specialist nurses.

Many services are evolving and changing constantly, sometimes introducing new roles e.g. community matrons in England. Primary care offers a very dynamic environment for career development. Local as well as national advice should always be sought on educational pathways and competencies required of different roles.

Further information

🖳 NHS Nursing Careers: www.nhscareers.nhs.uk/careers/nursing
🖳 NMC Nursing and Midwifery Council: www.nmc-uk.org
See also professional organizations listed (Useful websites 📖)

Learning to work in primary care

Working in primary care and domiciliary settings (Key definitions of primary care and public health 📖) is very different to working in the hospital environment.

❶ Nurses new to primary care, irrespective of prior clinical experience and seniority, become novice practitioners again. This is because:
- The patient is in control of all decisions, the nurse is a guest in the patient's home.
- Patients and their carers undertake most of their own care, the overall nursing contribution is small (Key facts on carers and caring 📖; Expert patient 📖).
- Many systems and infrastructures support the delivery of health and social care and are locally specific and variable; it takes time to familiarize oneself with the full range of available services (e.g. Social services 📖; Homes and housing 📖).
- Clinical decision making and care delivery are often done independently and at a physical distance from other colleagues.
- Nurses in primary care work with uncertainty, changing situations and services; this requires a flexibility in approach and assertiveness to work on the patient's behalf.

Orientation to primary care

Nobody knows how long it will take individual nurses to become oriented to working in primary care. Some adapt rapidly, others take much longer. In addition, the different responsibilities of the range of posts mean that nurses need different preparation. Information about professional preparation programmes are given in each of the topics about the different groups of nurses and services. However, all nurses new to working in primary care should ensure that they have:
- An orientation and induction process from their employer (Clinical supervision and appraisal 📖).
- A mentor to review and discuss work with (Teaching and mentorship 📖).
- Opportunities to work with other nurse role models and to shadow other professionals.
- Access to information (e.g. directories) about the local service environment: the range of local services, referral mechanisms, key contacts, eligibility criteria and funding mechanisms for different services.
- Knowledge of risk assessment processes for both patient and personal safety (Clinical risk management 📖).
- Information on how to get around the area physically.

Related topic

📖 Useful websites—lists all the relevant nursing and professional organizations.

Further information

Drennan, V., Goodman, C. and Leyshon, S. (2005). Supporting nurses new to primary care.
🖳 www.UCL.ac.uk.pcps.research/pcnru/index/htm

General practice nursing

The majority of practice nurses are directly employed by GPs (General practice 🕮; PMS 🕮). They mainly work as self-directing practitioners within the practice organization, often in small nursing teams that may include nurse practitioners and/or HCAs.

Focus of practice nurses' work

- Provide appropriate care/treatment in conjunction with the GP or independently where care has been transferred to the nurse by the GP.
- Assess nursing needs of patients registered with GP practice.
- Document the process of assessment of need and the delivery of care.
- Evaluate the outcome of care, make changes to the care plan, and modify practice with the patient.
- Liaise with other members of PHCT to assure appropriate care.
- Provide counselling and health education.
- Contribute to clinical governance, QOF, and risk management of practice.

In addition those working as NPs (NB the demarcation of roles between NP and practice nurses is fluid) may:

- Receive patients with undifferentiated and undiagnosed problems and makes an assessment of their health-care needs based on advanced level nursing skills and knowledge including physical examination.
- Make differential diagnoses using decision-making and problem-solving skills.
- Provide counselling and health education.
- Work collaboratively with other health-care professionals.
- Provide leadership and consultancy functions as required.

Main areas of responsibility

Require a range of clinical skills developed through experience and training in order to deal with the general nursing care of patients in the surgery according to practice policy and protocols and to refer to the GP as appropriate. These skills include:

- Chronic disease management e.g. diabetes, CHD, hypertension, asthma
- Cervical cytology
- Travel health
- Child and adult immunization
- Wound care
- Ear syringing
- ♀ health i.e. HRT, contraception, well woman
- Health education and promotion
- Triage assessment
- Audit and record keeping, particularly for QOF indicators.

In addition those working as NPs (see above) will have additional skills including:

- Physical examination, investigation, initiate treatment, prescribe medications, referral to another health-care professional in either 1° or 2° care.
- Screen patients for disease risk factors and early signs of illness.

- Order necessary investigations, provide treatment and care, individually, as part of a team, and through referral to other agencies.
- Admit and discharge patients from their caseload, and refer to other health-care providers as appropriate.
- Manage the treatment and care of patients with acute and/or chronic illness.

Education, training, and qualifications

Practice nurses
- A registered nurse usually with some post-registration experience.
- Evidence of ongoing professional and academic education and training.
- Can access degree level education in practice nursing specific degree programmes and modules as well as short courses e.g. diabetes management, COPD management.

Nurse practitioners
- Defined by the RCN as a registered nurse who has undertaken a specific NP course at first degree level (minimum) though currently not regulated or required.
- Changes to NMC regulations will mean that NPs in the future will have to undertake a specific course of masters level study.

Related topics
📖 NHS pay and structure; 📖 Continuing professional development.

Further information for professionals
📲 Nurse Practitioner UK: www.nursepractitioner.org.uk/
📲 Practice Nurse Association: www.practicenurse.org.uk/
📲 RCN: www.rcn.org.uk

School nursing

Focus of work

The main focus of the school nurse (SN) work is enabling children and young people to achieve their potential by staying healthy, staying safe, enjoying and achieving, making a positive contribution and reaching economic well-being (i.e. central government policies for children and young people. Working towards these priority outcomes is based on joint working with school staff, education service staff, social services, other health professionals, and the voluntary sector. SNs in many areas are known as school health advisers to reflect the change in focus of their work in health promotion and public health.

Main areas of responsibility

SNs work with school-aged children and young people and their families to:
- Assess health and social care needs, monitor, and refer as necessary.
- Promote healthy lifestyles through health promoting activities (e.g. sex and relationship education [SRE], personal, social, and health education [PSHE], healthy schools programmes), either in groups or one to one.
- Identify those in need of protection, monitor, refer, and contribute to safeguarding children in accordance with local/national policies.
- Organize and administer immunization programmes in line with DoH guidelines.
- Provide support for those with special/complex needs.
- Provide advice, support and teaching for school staff, parents, carers, children, and young people.

Team and work organization

School health-care services are based mainly in state schools and community settings. It includes school doctors although other health-care professsionals may visit schools as part of their public health work e.g. community dentists. SNs are organized in a variety of ways according to the needs of local state schools e.g.:
- SNs may be named nurses with responsibility for a number of schools (either primary or secondary or both).
- SNs may work in teams with nursery nurses, HCAs, led by a senior SN.
- SNs may work only as part of a school immunization team.

The work of SNs is organized to follow the recommendations from HFAC4 and the child health promotion programme. It may involve specific clinical or health promotion sessions in schools as well as offering open access drop in sessions for school children.

Education and training for school nursing

SNs are qualified nurses mostly employed by the PCOs in the NHS. Independent schools may also employ nurses.

SNs are likely to hold an additional community nursing or public health qualification in the form of:
• Specialist community practitioner public health (school nursing)
• Certificate, diploma in school nursing/public health
• Community practice teacher
• Other specific training in contraceptive and sexual health, health education, mental health, enuresis and counselling or others.

Further information

⌨ CPHVA School Nursing section: www.msfcphva.org/schoolnursing/snhome
⌨ DH & DfES (2006). School Nurse Development Pack: www.teachernet.gov.publications
⌨ RCN School Nurses Forum: www.rcn.org.uk/
⌨ Wired for Health (Health information on the National Curriculum and the National Healthy Schools Programme): www.wiredforhealth.gov.uk

Working in schools

Key principles

Health professionals working in schools are perceived as visitors to the establishment and as such need to negotiate with the school staff on all aspects of their activities with the children and in the school e.g. suitable times for activities in school and booking rooms. The SN needs to develop effective communication processes with key school members including:

- The head/deputy head teacher
- The special educational needs coordinator (SENCO)
  (Childen with SEN 🕮)
- The child protection/safeguarding children coordinator
  (Child protection 🕮)
- Healthy schools coordinator
- PSHE adviser/coordinator (Health promotion in schools 🕮).

A key contact is the school secretary who holds information on both the school organization and details of the children and their families.

SNs identify health needs through school health profiling and plan key health promotion activities with school staff according to local needs and priorities. With the government's modernization agenda and the focus on developing children's centres and extended schools, health provision for children may be delivered in different ways in future e.g. shift working, health assessments on different sites or more work with parents.

The head teacher and school governors are responsible for developing school health related policies e.g. Sex and relationship education (🕮), health and safety.

Year and term planning

School holidays, and most school activities are planned a year in advance. Therefore professionals wanting to get involved in health promotion and curriculum planning need to negotiate with staff in the summer term for the next school year. Some activities/sessions can be organized on a termly basis but it would be wise to do this a term in advance. The school terms in most areas are organized as follows:

- Autumn: September–December
- Spring: January–April
- Summer: May–July.

Children with statements of special education needs

Have yearly reviews with multi-agency input. Dates for these reviews are planned in advance and a list given to the designated medical officer with responsibility for special needs. It is good practice to try and coordinate health reviews to coincide with the educational reviews. School health advisers/doctors should attend these reviews and provide medical or nursing reports as necessary.

School health records

School health records in some areas are kept in locked filing cabinets on school premises, (key access only for SN) in other areas records are kept at the health centre base. Parents and children are encouraged to bring their personal child health record (Client and patient-held records 📖) with them to health assessments in school.

Medicines in schools

There are national and local policies (see below) to help education of staff and health professionals in meeting the needs of children/young people requiring medicines in schools. Responsibility for giving or supervising medicines is usually undertaken by teachers or classroom helpers who are trained by school health advisers, children's community nurses, or specialist nurses to carry out that role. The whole process involves careful planning between the multi-disciplinary team e.g.:
* Proper discharge planning from hospital and suitable drug regimens to facilitate smooth administration.
* GP—for review.
* Training for parents, carers, school staff restorage, administration and disposal.

Working in special schools

Special schools cater for children and young people with complex needs requiring a multi-disciplinary approach (Children with complex health needs and disabilities 📖) involving:
* Allied health professionals—SLTs, OTs, physio-therapists
* Health professionals
* Education staff and parents
* Social services.

Arrangements for nursing cover vary: some areas have nurses on site, while others visit on a regular basis. Nurses will, in most instances, undertake medicine administration, tube feeding, IV, or rectal medicines. Generally nurses working in special schools will perform a wider range of hands-on nursing care compared to those in mainstream schools. Some members of the school staff may also be trained to undertake some tasks such as feeding, emergency medicines, catheter care etc.

Special units

Some children/young people who are excluded from school will attend Pupil Referral units. Some schools also provide for children with hearing/vision impairment or language difficulties in special units. SNs and the medical team support the families and school in meeting their needs.

Related topic

📖 Child health promotion.

Further information

📱 www.teachernet.gov.uk/wholeschool/healthyliving/wholeschoolapproach/—all information about the national healthy schools programme
📱 www.dfes.gov.uk. Managing Medicines in Schools and Early Years Settings. DFES-1448-2005

Health visiting

Focus of work

Health visiting is a public health nursing specialism. The focus of the work is the promotion of health and the prevention of ill health. The main principles in health visiting activity are:

- The search for health needs
- The stimulation of an awareness of health needs
- The facilitation of health-enhancing activities
- The influence on policies affecting health.

This public health focus can be with any group in the population and can be with an individual, a family, group, or community. The search for health needs can be through formalized health needs assessment (Health needs assessment 📖), of a community, a caseload, or an individual. The locus of the activity may be in the client's home, in health centres, surgeries or community settings.

Main areas of responsibility

The majority of HVs are employed to work with families with young children. In addition, some may work with older clients. The HVs will have a caseload of clients, derived either from a GP practice population or a geographical area. HVs use a case management model to inform their practice with individual clients or families. They proactively make contact, offering services, as well as receiving referrals from other services. They work closely with other professionals e.g. GPs and social workers and other agencies e.g. community organizations. Key areas of activity are likely to be:

- Health promotion and support of families expecting, or with new, babies (all new births in an area are notified to the community child health service who in turn informs the named HV).
- Delivering the child health promotion programme and child immunization programme.
- Supporting parents in learning parenting skills, and promoting the development of children <5yrs.
- Identification, protection, and safeguarding of vulnerable children.
- Identification of health (physical, social, emotional and mental) needs of all clients, negotiating and agreeing an action plan with clients, and referral to other services and/or provision of brief counselling/ listening visits by the HV.
- Provision of information about local health, social, education, and community services.

HVs are also employed to work with specific vulnerable groups e.g. children and families, homeless families, travellers, or older people. In some areas they may be employed to specialize in community development or group health promotion activities.

Team and work organization

HVs work collegiately with other HVs either from the same base or working with the same GPs. Some share their caseloads (known as 'corporate caseloads') in order to ensure equity in workloads and improve access and services to clients.

They may be led by a senior HV who also holds clinical responsibilities. Increasingly, HVs are leading teams of other staff such as nursery nurses, staff nurses, and health-care assistants to deliver the public health agenda and the child health promotion programme. HVs may also be part of wider initiatives in multi agency settings e.g. Sure Start, public health departments.

Education and training for health visiting

All HVs are registered nurses or midwives before commencing specialist practitioner training, a 1yr full time or 2yr part-time course at degree level. Usually PCOs provide funding for the course and salary through sponsorship.

The title of registered HV used to be protected in law and have a separate register on the NMC. Since 2005 this has not existed and already qualified and newly qualified HVs are placed on the specialist practitioner public health register of the NMC.

Further information

CPHVA Health visiting section: www.msfcphva.org/health visiting/hvhome

District nursing

Focus of district nursing (DN) work

DN teams will accept direct referrals from, and liaise with, hospitals, health and social care professionals, patients, and carers. They assess, prescribe, monitor, provide, and evaluate nursing care for people in their home, in care homes, and clinics based in primary care settings (e.g. health centres, GP practices). The service provided is dependent on local policies, custom, and practice. The majority of provision is to frail older people in their own homes, adults, and sometimes children, with long-term conditions who require nursing care in the home. DN patients are identified either by being registered with a specific GP practice that the DN team works with (GP attachment) or the locality where they live (geographical working). As well as a 'core' daytime service, many DN services provide 'Out-of-Hours' service which includes evening and night nursing care. DN services are free at the point of delivery and can be contacted through the primary care organization and/or GP practices

Main areas of responsibility assessment and care for people

- Short-term, self care education and support e.g. support and teaching to newly diagnosed diabetic patient.
- Case/care management of people with complex and/or long-term conditions.
- Rehabilitation care and support in recovery.
- Intermediate care and care following discharge from hospital.
- Palliative care.
- Care in collaboration with other clinical nurse specialists (e.g. Macmillan nurses, continence specialists, tissue viability nurses etc.).
- Carer assessment and support.
- Administration and maintenance of technical therapies in the home e.g. IV therapy, PEG feeds, continence care, wound care, diabetic care, some injections.
- Assessment and social support DNs work closely with social care providers and community care agencies.

A DN is a qualified nurse employed by NHS who is likely to be a nurse prescriber (Medicines management 📖) and hold an additional community nursing qualification in district nursing/nursing in the home. Usually works as team leader or member of a skill mixed nursing team (i.e. with community staff nurses and health-care assistants) with responsibility for a specific patient caseload.

Education and training

- William Rathbone established first training school in Liverpool in 1863.
- DN current training (shortened) degree or postgrad diploma. Entry requirement diploma level often with 2yrs post qualification experience. Courses are 1yr FT or 2yr PT, at colleges and universities throughout UK (sponsorship provided through NHS).
- Courses known by a range of titles including Community Health-care Nursing, and Specialist Community Practitioner Award, sometimes

referred to as nursing in the home. Courses combine the theoretical study of subjects such as community practice and public health, counselling and social policy, with practical placements supervised by an experienced DN.
* Work based learning courses for staff nurses entering DN posts/ rotation schemes for flexible entry to primary care.
* Short courses for community nurses in specialist topics e.g. tissue viability, palliative care, case management.

Further information and resources

⌨ Community and District Nursing Associations CDNA: cdna@tvu.ac.uk ☎ Tel: +44 (0) 20 8231 0180
⌨ NHS Careers: www.nhscareers.nhs.uk
⌨ Community Practitioners and Health Visitors Association CPHVA: www.msfcphva.org.uk
⌨ Royal College of Nursing: www.rcn.org.uk

Employment contracts

The contract

In British law a contract comes into existence on starting to work for an employer, irrespective of whether it is verbal or in writing. The contract is formed where there is:
- An offer of work
- An acceptance of that offer
- A promise by the employer to pay the employee in return for the employee's promise to work.

If an offer is withdrawn the employer may be in breach of contract and could be taken to an employment tribunal.

Statement of terms and conditions

There is a legal entitlement to a statement of the terms and conditions of the post within 8wks of start date provided employment lasts for 1mth or more. Must include by law:
- The names of the employer and the employee
- The date when the employment began
- Remuneration and the intervals at which it is to be paid
- Hours of work
- Holiday entitlement
- Entitlement to sick leave, including any entitlement to sick pay
- Pensions and pension schemes
- The entitlement of employer and employee to notice of termination
- Job title or a brief job description
- The date when it is to end if not permanent
- The place of work
- Details of the employer's disciplinary and grievance procedures.

Fixed-term contracts

Legislation exists to ensure people on fixed-term contracts are not treated unfairly. The non-renewal of a fixed-term contract is a dismissal in law and can be contested as unfair dismissal. There is also an entitlement to redundancy payment. There is a statutory limit of 4yrs on the use of successive fixed-term contracts (NB service prior to 2002 does not count towards this statutory limit) then the contract is deemed permanent.

Further information

🖥 Department of Trade and Industry Employment Legislation: www.dti.gov.uk/er/individual. statement-pl700.htm
From all professional and trade union organizations 📖 Useful websites
Nurses employed by GPs RCN Guidance on Good Employment Practice (2005) Publication code 002 435 (includes a specimen employment contract)

NHS pay structure

Agenda for Change is the name of the new UK NHS pay structure and terms and conditions of service to all staff except doctors. Not all general practice employers have adopted this framework (Employment contracts 📖) as non-NHS employers may have different terms and conditions.

Terms and conditions

Standard full-time hours of work are 37.5hrs/wk, excluding breaks. Annual leave entitlement and entitlement to sick leave increase with length of service.

Pay

Each post has a job description and person specification, based on the NHS knowledge and skills framework. Jobs are assigned to an Agenda for Change pay band using the KSF (see Further information). Pay ↑ each year to the next incremental point in that band. A system is being devised for assessing knowledge and skills necessary for pay progress 12mths after appointment and at a point near the top of the pay band. Pay is made up of basic salary then, as applicable, high cost-of-living area supplement, recruitment and retention premium, special duty payments for unsocial hours, and on-call payments. Overtime is paid as time and a half (double on Bank holidays only) or as time off in lieu (TOIL).

NHS occupational pension schemes

All employees of the NHS and general practices can join the NHS occupational pension scheme, which is administered separately in the 4 countries and currently under review.

Travel costs

Employers may have a car lease scheme for staff undertaking domiciliary work. All NHS employers reimburse work-related travel expenses on production of receipts and journey logs.

Further information

🖳 Agenda for Change section of the DoH: www.dh.gov.uk
🖳 NHS Pension Agency England and Wales: www.nhspa.gov.uk/
🖳 NHS Pension Scotland: www.sppa.gov.uk/
🖳 NHS superannuation Scheme N.Ireland: www.dhsspsni.gov.uk/superann/index.asp

Clinical supervision and appraisal

Clinical supervision

Clinical supervision is a practice-focused professional relationship that enables reflection on practice with the support of a skilled supervisor. It is an element of both clinical governance (Clinical governance 📖), and continuing professional development (Continuing professional development 📖). It has some or all of these purposes:

- Normative, i.e. maintaining appropriate standards of practice
- Educative, i.e. developing competence
- Supportive, i.e. providing a mechanism for staff to manage the intense pressures of work and to focus on the emotional resources needed to maintain high-quality care.

Models of clinical supervision

Each work environment and staff group has to develop its own model to fit their needs. Possible models include:

- One to one, using line managers of the same discipline as supervisors
- One to one with another, more experienced nurse or other professional, but excluding line managers as supervisors
- Group supervision, either through peer group or multidisciplinary team case discussions.

It is important to be explicit about:

- The aims of the supervision
- The most appropriate model(s) and skilled supervisor
- Ground rules (including timing, attendance, and confidentiality)
- The mechanism for evaluating the model of supervision.

Appraisal

Appraisal is a formal opportunity for practitioners to review and develop their performance in the context of their organization's goals, their own job description, and the linked KSF. It is a separate process from clinical supervision. It is a formal system to:

- Review past performance, set new objectives, and identify training and development needs in a personal development plan (PDP).
- Highlight individual potential and discuss short, medium, and long-term career development.
- Acknowledge and record employee achievements as well as performance concerns.

In the independent sector it may link to performance-related pay and bonus systems. In the NHS it links to the Agenda for Change gateways in pay bands (NHS pay structure 📖).

Further information

📖 Advisory, Conciliation and Arbitration Service (ACAS) Employee appraisal guidance: www.acas. org.uk/publications/B07.html

Schon, D. (1983). *The reflective practitioner*. Temple Smith, London.

Continuing professional development

Health care and professional practice are continuously changing. All professionals have to maintain and develop competence through a life-long learning process known as continuing professional development (CPD). CPD needs should be identified through everyday reflection on practice, clinical supervision (Clinical supervision and appraisal 📖) and a personal development plan (PDP) developed during induction and appraisal processes.

NMC requirements

The NMC Post-Registration Education and Practice Standards (PREP) for 3-yrs reregistration, state that each nurse must:
• Undertake at least 5d or 35hrs of relevant learning activity during the 3yrs prior to reregistration.
• Maintain a personal professional profile (PPP) of their learning activity.
• Comply with any request from the NMC to audit how they have met these requirements.

Learning may be formal (e.g. through course attendance) or informal (e.g. through reflection on a research paper). The NMC does not accredit courses for PREP and there is no such thing as an 'approved PREP' learning activity. The PPP is used to document the learning activity and how it has influenced practice. A suggested template for the PPP is included in the NMC's PREP handbook.[1]

Sources of support for nurses' CPD

• National level—electronic access to NELH, professional organizations (Useful websites 📖), provision of study days and conferences, as well as financial support opportunities.
• Local level—may include:
  • Access to health-care libraries in local universities and health promotion/public health departments.
  • Practice Professional Development Plans (PPDP) in general practice.
  • PCO-wide general practice and primary care multidisciplinary learning events.
  • In-house PCO and Trust training and development programmes.
  • PCO or Trust learning and development plans that commission places for nurses on formal education courses at universities through strategic health authorities (a slightly different mechanism in each country).
  • Employer paying fees and giving time for higher degrees or specialist courses.
  • PCO or Trust sponsorship (i.e. salary plus fees) for specialist community and primary care qualifications.

Related topic

📖 Clinical supervision and appraisal.

[1] 🖳 NMC handbook on PREP: www.nmc-uk.org/nmc/main/publications/thePREPhandbook2.pdf

Teaching and mentorship

Primary care nurses may provide clinical teaching and mentorship of nursing students undertaking pre- and post-registration courses, sometimes as clinical placements or supervised practice. Many also provide mentorship or preceptorship to qualified nurses new in post, less experienced, or new to primary care (Learning to work in primary care ⬜). Some primary care nurses have designated clinical teaching posts for certain types of students, e.g. practice educators, practice nurse trainers, community practice teachers for DN or HV. These types of posts may attract additional salary (NHS pay structure ⬜) or designated time for teaching. General practices may require payment for practice nurses to act as trainers or provide clinical placements to students. Local higher education institutions provide short courses for clinical teaching roles as well as specific preparation for supporting different types of students.

Principles of effective teaching and mentorship

Adult learners

- Are active in, and respond to, participation in the learning process.
- Have a rich resource of experience to contribute to the process.
- Are aware of their own learning needs linked to work roles and tasks.
- Are competency-based learners wanting to apply or experiment with new knowledge.

Adult learning

Best practice in teaching or mentorship suggests:

- Treat students/mentee with respect.
- Agree:
  - Clear objectives for the teaching/mentorship, based on what they are trying to learn.
  - Learning/mentoring opportunities based on the objectives.
  - Opportunities for reflection on the learning/mentorship process.
- Facilitate independence and active engagement.
- Provide balanced feedback that highlights areas of good practice as well as aspects for development.
- If applicable, use appropriate, objective, fair and relevant assessment tasks for competence.
- Learn from students/mentees—evaluate and improve your teaching/mentorship.

Consent of patients to teaching

The teacher-practitioner should gain the full consent of patients/clients before students 'sit in' on consultations or provide clinical/professional services (Consent ⬜). Statements about the teaching activities of the practice or service and the right of patients/clients to decline to participate are usually in service/practice information leaflets (General practice ⬜) and in waiting rooms.

Related topic

⬜ Professional accountability.

VICTORIA INFIRMARY
MEDICAL STAFF LIBRAR

Research in primary care

Research is the systematic inquiry to develop or contribute to the development of new knowledge that can be generalizable. It is essential for provision of high quality health care. Methodologies may be quantative, qualitative, or mixed as appropriate to the question to be answered. Data collection methods range from clinical drug trials through to surveys, questionnaires, ethnographies, and in depth case studies. All research follows a systematic process (see Fig. 2.1).

Many nurses contribute to research in the NHS. Nurses in primary care often undertake some stages of the research process (see Fig. 2.1) as part of educational programmes. Nurses undertaking higher degrees are required to undertake a research project. The number of academic primary care nurses undertaking and leading funded research is a small but growing group. Recent government polices have placed greater emphasis on research in primary care e.g. England is due to establish a National School for Primary Care Research. NB All country's central health departments have research web pages (Useful websites 📖).

It is important to gain support and advice from more experienced researchers e.g. university supervisors for a particular educational programme or a local research support nurse or mentor identified through local universities or PCO research support.

Ethics

Ethical review of research conducted on patients or staff of the NHS is undertaken by one of a network of committees following the same procedures throughout the UK, using the same electronic forms. All details and guidance on COREC (Central Office for Research Ethics Committees) website: 🖳 www.corec.org.uk.

Research governance

This is concerned with setting standards to improve the quality of research and safeguard patients. All research projects have to gain written permission to proceed from, the NHS organization in which they will take place.

Sources of information

- PCO research offices.
- Opportunities for funding, fellowships, training, research posts, and research conferences:
  - 🖳 RCN Research Coordinating Centre: www.man.ac.uk/rcn/
  - 🖳 Research and Development Information: www.redinfo.org.uk
- 🖳 Ongoing and recently completed NHS research National Research Register: www.nrr.nhs.uk/
- 🖳 Public involvement in research: www.invo.org.uk

- Primary Care Research Networks:
  - ⊞ Primary Care Nursing Research Network: www.man.ac.uk/
    rcn/networks/#PrimaryCare
  - ⊞ UK Federation of Primary Care Research Organizations:
    www.ukf-pcro.org/

Turn the issue or idea into a specific question
↓
Search and review the literature to see what is already known
↓
Write a detailed proposal including:

- The research questions
- Rationale (importance of the question
  and what this study would add)
- Background
- Aim and objectives
- Methods of enquiry
- Ethical and data protection considerations
- Timescale
- Costs and resources required

↓
Obtain funding or resource agreement
↓
Obtain permissions from the health organization
↓
Obtain ethical review
↓
Commence recruitment and data collection
↓
Analyze data
↓
Write report of research and findings
↓
Disseminate findings through publication and presentation

Fig. 2.1 The research process

Teamwork and innovation

Effective teams in organizational settings are characterized by:
- A defined group of individuals who perceive themselves as members of the team.
- Defined roles within the team respected and understood by all team members.
- Regular interaction and communication between team members.
- Clear, shared team goals.
- Equal participation in decision-making by all team members.

A team approach has been shown to improve patient outcomes in a range of settings.

There are many different types of teams, who may have a leader (Leadership in practice 📖) by virtue of a management structure, clinical seniority, or elected by the rest of the team:
- Those that are managed together
- Those that come together with a shared client/patient group
- Those that come together to work on individual issues/events/ problems.

Primary care nurses may be members of many teams, particularly if they work with a number of general practices or provide specialist input. They need to consider how they become an integrated team member, with at the very least face-to-face communication with other professionals also involved with their patients or clients.

Teambuilding initiatives in health and social care have been shown to have some benefits:
- Developing practitioners' awareness of the benefits of team-working
- Improving communication
- Improving shared decision-making
- Improving problem solving
- Improving trust and support.

However, innovations resulting from this may be short lived if no ongoing support from the wider organization (see below).

Innovation and introducing change

Any change process has five parts:
- Precipitating factors
- Team or organization members felt need for change
- Decisions and plans for instigating change
- Implementation
- Outcomes (intended and unintended).

Almost all changes face resistance, most commonly because of a:
- Desire not to lose something of value
- Misunderstanding of the proposed change and its implications
- Belief the change does not make sense
- Low tolerance for change.

Planning for change has to capitalize on the energy and ideas of those supporting the change as well as reduce the resistance to the change. Lewin's force field analysis[1] is one tool to use in planning how to do this in order to consider how to reduce resistance. Strategies include:

• Inviting resisters to help plan and implement.
• Widening dissemination of proposals and consultation processes.
• Demonstrate commitment to modify plans taking in resisters' views.
• Develop alternative plans.
• Start small by piloting the change to learn and adapt as necessary.
• Wear down resistance over time.

A number of change models are used in the NHS e.g. RAID (a variant is Plan-Do-Study-Act (PDSA) cycles):

• Review
• Agree
• Implement
• Demonstrate.

Commonest reasons that innovations fail to be implemented and sustained:

• More time was needed than planned for
• Major problems surfaced that had not been anticipated
• Coordination of important activities was not effective
• Competing activities distract the key members
• Skills and abilities of those involved not sufficient
• Training and support to lower level and support staff inadequate
• Powerful external events interfere.

Detailed planning needs to include time, resources, all staff training and involvement, milestones, feedback mechanisms.

Further information

📖 NHS England Integrated Service Improvement Programme: www.isip.nhs.uk/

---

[1] 📖 Iles, V. and Cranfield, S. (2003). *Developing change management skills. A resource for health care professionals and managers.* www.sdo.lshtm.ac.uk/publications.htm

Principles of successful meetings

Meetings are important as venues for sharing ideas, hearing differing view points and evidence, making decisions, planning, and reviewing actions by a group or team. Meetings are essential to a democratic, efficient organization. Without good planning or forethought they become ineffective both for participants and the organization.

Terms of reference

Groups that are planning to have regular meetings should establish terms of reference to specify:
- The purpose of the meeting
- The participants required to address the purpose
- The frequency of meeting to achieve the purpose
- To name the chair and arrangements for minute taking
- To state who and where the decisions of the meeting will report to
- To state a point in time when the terms of reference will be reviewed.

Groups that only meet once or twice may need to establish these ground rules at the first meeting.

Meeting prerequisites
- An aim—what the meeting aims to achieve
- An agenda—a fleshed-out version of the aim (see below)
- A Chair, who will control the discussion
- A note taker (secretary), who will take notes
- All participants should have the agenda and any supporting documents in enough time to read and think about before the meeting
- An agreed fixed time limit
- A venue that is accessible for all participants.

The agenda

Should include:
- Apologies
- Minutes of last meeting (and agree at this stage that they are accurate. In a formal situation the Chair should sign them to confirm this)
- Matters arising from the last meeting (that are not on the agenda)
- Items listed for discussion
- Items to note for information only
- Any other business (AOB)
- Date and venue of next meeting.

The notes or 'minutes'
- Should have the same headings as the agenda
- Should note who was present
- Should note what was decided
- Should note what actions agreed by who and when
- Not generally necessary to record all the discussion. Edited highlights are usually more useful.

Role of the chair

- Must make sure that the group sticks to the agenda
- Exercise firm but sensitive control of the discussion to ensure one conversation happens that all can participate in (not multiple random conversations)
- In formal meetings, people don't speak to each other and all remarks are addressed to the Chairperson.

Role of participants

- Study agenda and written items before hand to decide what to contribute
- Take an active part
- Make own notes to later check decisions and responsibilities from the meeting.

After a meeting

- Every member (including those absent) should have a copy of the notes or minutes
- Every member should know what actions they have to take before the next meeting
- Every member should know when and where the next meeting will be held and how to place items on the agenda in advance.

Leadership in practice

Leadership is a set of skills, qualities, and behaviours which all nurses and health-care practitioners are expected to demonstrate. Leadership qualities are required throughout an organization and across the NHS and are key to developing modern services that meet individual and population needs. Leadership contributes to the development of continuing professional development (Continuing professional development 📖), appraisal processes (Clinical supervision and appraisal 📖) and clinical supervision.

Principles of leadership

Leadership is a popular topic and much has been written about it—there are now over 3000 texts and references. The NHS Leadership Qualities Framework (used UK wide) has been developed for specific use with NHS staff. There are fifteen qualities arranged in 3 clusters:

• Personal leadership qualities
• Setting direction
• Delivering the service.

The framework describes a set of key characteristics, attitudes, and behaviours to which leaders in the NHS should aspire in delivering modernised services e.g. NHS Plan. It is generally recognized that personal leadership qualities are essential for all leaders, regardless of their position in an organization. It is important to take into account the context in which you work when considering which other qualities apply to you and your service.

Leadership development

There are many opportunities to develop leadership skills. Primary care nurses can access these opportunities by:

• Identifying development needs in annual appraisal
• Getting the support of manager/employer for further development and training
• Contacting PCO's staff development department
• Looking for courses at university/e-based courses
• Undertaking a 360 degree assessment through the NHS Leadership Qualities Framework
• Attending an experiential development programme or leadership workshops, such as those provided by the RCN or other professional organizations.

Further information

📠 NHS Leadership qualities framework is available at: www.nhsleadershipqualities.nhs.uk
📠 NHS general improvement skills booklets available at: www.wise.nhs.uk
📠 RCN Leadership programmes available at: www.rcn.org.uk/pcph

Project planning

Common projects that primary care nurses are involved in include:
- Introducing a new service e.g. new clinic session, specialist team
- Introducing or rolling out new clinical activities
- Reorganizing a team or working practices
- Introducing new clinical or administrative technologies.

Critical to the success of any new project, i.e. any new endeavor, is the planning phase. This involves:
- Detailed planning done by a small group of key people committed to making it happen.
- Consultation on the overall plan or key elements that involves interested and those affected by the change (key stakeholders) to gain their ideas, win their approval, reduce their resistance to the plans.

Project plans

These should include:
- The aim or goal of the project as a broad statement of the problem to be solved or what is to be achieved.
- Objectives derived from the broader aim. They set the realistic targets to achieve during the project. 'SMART' objectives are:
  - **S**pecific—clear about what will be achieved
  - **M**easurable—it's possible to quantify results and measure when they have been achieved
  - **A**chievable—they can be achieved
  - **R**ealistic—attainable with resources or the resources bid for
  - **T**imed—attainable within a specified timescale.
- All projects have an element of risk. A risk analysis addresses the following questions:
  - What could possibly go wrong?
  - What is the likelihood of it happening?
  - How will it affect the project?
  - What can be done about it?
- Roles and responsibilities.
- A breakdown of tasks against timescales deadlines or milestones.
- Resources required and costs.
- Communication mechanisms.
- Review date after completion with all involved.

Costing

These should include:
- Staff salary costs for the time involved in the project activity (NB includes employer's contributions to pensions and national insurance).
- Organizational overheads—usually expressed as a percentage of the salary costs and covers central services that keep the organization functioning. e.g. running and maintenance of premises.
- All materials, equipment, non-staff resources to be used.
- Any additional expenses e.g. hire of rooms, payment for speakers.

Planning tools
- Computer software can be bought to aid project planning.
- Tools such as GANTT (named after developer)—charts with detailed steps and time frames in a diagrammatic way (see below) help identify all tasks, the person responsible for them and monitor progress.
- Other tools include critical pathway analysis which diagrammatically shows when activities can happen in parallel or are dependent on each other.

Task	Person Responsible	Week 1	Week 2	Week 3	Week 4
Collect information	Nurse A	x			
Write draft report	Nurse B		x		
Revise report	Nurse A and B			x	
Present report to general practice meeting	Nurse A to speak. Nurse B to answer questions				x

Fig. 2.2 A GANTT Chart

Common problems in project planning
- Focus is too narrowly on the work of one team and fails to consider how it fits into the larger picture.
- Underestimates the time involved for work.
- Failure to warn others external to the project on whom elements depend.
- Failure to identify all the materials, equipment and staff needed for the project.

The NHS uses a systems approach to planning, scheduling, and controlling high level, high-risk change involving multiple, large scale services. In IT projects the accepted methodology is PRINCE2™. The NHS Integrated Service Improvement Programme (ISIP) is another methodology currently being developed in England.

Further information
The NHS Integrated Service Improvement Programme: www.isip.nhs.uk/

Using information for practice

A key primary care and community nursing activity is to use data to inform and change their practice and activities. This is often called profiling, although other terms may also be used. Three types of profiling activities are used:
- Community profiling
- Caseload profiling
- Workload profiling and resource management.

Nurses working in or closely with general practice may also be using practice patient profiles or (QOF 📖) returns to inform their practice.

Community profiling

This means using local public health data (Public health 📖), to understand the health issues of the community/population they work with, combined with LA and community data on resources to help address those needs. Without having to collect additional information, this informs the nurse what the priority issues to be aware of are, and what she should address her practice to. This links to health needs assessment activities (Health needs assessment 📖).

Caseload profiling

Caseload profiling is a technique for understanding the collated health and social care needs of those within the 'caseload' held by the nurse or team of nurses. The purpose is to assist with planning, prioritizing activities, and identifying particular issues/groups/trends that need addressing either by the team or by alerting others to, or making a business case for, more or different resources. Data should only be included on aspects that address issues of importance to planning. It is usually undertaken on an annual basis as a snapshot. Typically caseload profiles collate (from different sources see below) information on the patients/clients:
- The demographic profile (age, sex, self assigned ethnicity).
- The language profile.
- Presence of morbidity and key health and social issues e.g.:
  - COPD, CHD, DM, CVA, cancer
  - Substance misuse, mental health problems, dementia
  - Carers includes child carers, lone parents
  - Violence or neglect to children, older adults, women
  - Children with special needs
  - Adults in receipt of services under the Community Care Act
  - Indicators of socio-economic status e.g. receipt of state income support
  - In short term or temporary accommodation
  - Asylum seekers and refugees.
- Key public health indicators e.g. breast-feeding rates, influenza vaccination rates, smoking cessation rates.
- The levels of service offered/received from the nursing service e.g.:
  - Many district nursing service have a dependency scale or care objective scale that assigns patients to 1 of 3/4/5 categories that indicate both the objectives of care but also how much nurse time

that involves. Category examples: short-term, self-limiting, intermittent support to long-term condition, weekly support to long-term condition, daily (or near) daily support to unstable and fluctuating long-term condition, palliative care at end stage of life.
  • Health visiting services may also assign clients/families to a grouping that indicates that that family receives more support/home visiting than those receiving the locally determined core service. Categories are likely to include families with children who are or have been on the child protection register, families receiving additional supportive/listening visits (e.g. after detection of post natal depression).
• Any service outcome/performance data in addition to public health indicators e.g. venous leg ulcer healing rates, outcome measures from coding systems such as the OMAHA system, early identification of speech and language problems in children, audit data (Clinical audit 📖).
• The total volume of patients/clients that have been admitted to the caseload in a given period e.g. annual/6mths.
• The total volume of patients/clients that have been discharged/left the caseload through moving or death.

Caseload profile information only becomes meaningful when it is compared to wider information e.g. local teenage pregnancy rates or compared year on year or against a benchmark. Some areas provide proformas with local public health data inserted for instant comparison. It only becomes useful in terms of workload and resource management with other information added and compared to others or accepted benchmarks.

Data from clinical/professional records
The increased use of electronic patient/client records and coding systems (IT and electronic records 📖) will allow easier aggregate data analysis for understanding health issues addressed by nurses, their contribution to service delivery and the outcomes of their interventions. American developed coding systems such as the OMAHA provides additional coding for identification of the problems addressed by nurses and outcomes. Many PCOs in the UK use nurse activity only information systems (e.g. FIP Financial Information Planning) at the nurse (rather than the patient level) to return information to service commissioners and central government statistics. In some areas this is changing so that nurse activity information is derived from computerized patient records held in general practice. In general practice, the implementation of QOF (📖) has made the level of nurse activity in practice outcomes very visible.

Workload profiling and resources
There are no national population to number of nursing staff required guidelines because the number of staff required is dependent on the types of nursing work for different populations that is commissioned (Commissioning of services 📖). Caseload and workload profiling assist practitioners and managers in determining:
• Equitable distribution of staffing to work.
• Increased or decreased demand on the nursing staff resource.

Beyond the aggregate caseload data, workload includes all the other important activities included in the nursing teams responsibilities e.g. nurse education responsibilities, attending GP practice/clinical meetings, liaison sessions to other services, travel distances.

All patients/clients/work activities do not have equal demands on nursing time. In order to determine the impact on nursing resource, weighted scoring systems are applied to the caseload and the extra work activities. In district nursing teams, the weighted scoring system is linked to patient dependency on the nursing team (rather than self-care/informal carers or home carers). In health visiting, the score is linked to issues such as child protection although research has shown that receipt of income support can act as a very accurate proxy for high demands on health visiting team time. In school nursing teams, the weighted score is linked to numbers of children in schools with special needs and child protection needs. Weighted scores are also given to issues such as travel distances, number of GP practices or schools linking with the service.

The weighted scoring results are triangulated with the regular monitoring data of nursing activity levels, outcomes, and quality indicators. Experienced staff and managers then also use their expert knowledge in determining manageable workloads and decisions are made including:
- Shifting or changing team staffing or team activity focus (requires change management planning).
- Discussing increased demand on nursing resource with commissioners in contracting rounds.

Commissioning (contracting) of nursing services

Commissioners are looking to contract, on behalf of the public, nursing services for specified groups of clients, specified activities or specified quality within the NHS reference costs. In the past this has been done by 'block' contracts in most areas e.g. a district nursing service with a range of new contact visits in a year and this level of clients/contacts throughout the 12mths. Many PCO commissioners and practice based commissioners are now looking for greater detail.

Further information

Hurst, K. (2005). *Primary Care Trust Workforce Planning and Development*. Whurr Publishers, London.

Martin, K. (2005). *The Omaha System. A Key to Practice, Documentation, and Information Management*, 2nd edn. Missouri, Elsevier Saunders.

Quality and risk management

Clinical governance

Clinical governance is the term for the quality assurance and continuous quality improvement framework in each health-care organization. In the NHS each country has specific guidance on its implementation. The expectation is that each organization will use nationally available, evidence-based clinical guidelines (e.g. NICE, SIGN), and nationally set quality and service targets (e.g. NSFs) as criteria against which to measure themselves and plan for improvement, through both service change and staff development.

At a PCO and Trust level each organization has a lead clinical professional and provides resources to support an annual clinical governance plan. It has to provide an annual report that is likely to include:
- Evidence of the patients' experiences, and processes for consulting users.
- The use of information about patient safety and outcomes of patient care.
- Quality improvement activities including:
  - Risk management
  - Clinical audit programmes
  - Evidence-based practice and clinical effectiveness
  - Learning from adverse events/incidents
  - Learning from complaints.
- The development of a learning organization e.g. evidence of education and staff development.
- Evidence of leadership and strategic planning in service review and improvement.

In each country, there are mechanisms for PCOs and Trusts to have their performance, patient safety, and quality to be assessed annually. In England this is the role of the Health Care Commission, which uses criteria specified *Standards for Better Health Care*. The annual assessment is concerned with patient safety, clinical and cost effectiveness, governance of the organizations, level of patient focus, accessible and responsive care, the care environment, and public health.

Further information

Department of Health England (updated 2006). *Standards for Better Health Care.*
  www.dh.gov.uk/PublicationsAndStatistics/Publications/
Health Care Commission: www.healthcarecommission.org.uk/Home-page/fs/en
NHS Clinical Governance Resource Team: www.cgsupport.nhs.uk/
NHS Quality Improvement Scotland: www.nhshealthquality.org/

Evidence-based health care

Evidence-based health care refers to the use of all valid, relevant information taken into account when making decisions that affect the care of patients, the provision of health services, and public health. *Evidence-based clinical practice* is when the professional uses the best evidence available, in consultation with the patient or client, to decide upon the option for action.

Critical appraisal is the process of assessing and interpreting evidence by systematically considering its validity, results, and relevance. Evidence is then classified by the source. Results from study type 1 is considered strongest and 4 weakest:

1. Meta-analyses, systematic reviews of RCTs, or RCTs (including cluster RCTs).
2. Systematic reviews of, or individual, non-randomized controlled trials, case-control studies, cohort studies, controlled before-and-after (CBA) studies, interrupted time series (ITS) studies, correlation studies.
3. Non-analytical studies (for example, case reports, case series).
4. Expert opinion, formal consensus.

Guidelines

User-friendly statements to inform decision making, regarding a specific health problem from critically appraised evidence and other information. Increasing numbers produced to reduce harmful, ineffective and expensive variations in health care. NICE and SIGN are NHS funded bodies producing guidelines.

Protocols

Usually refers to specific guidelines on evidence-based professional activities and treatments required for particular conditions and situations. More directive than guidelines.

Integrated care pathways (ICPs)

Statements that amalgamate all the elements of evidence-based care and treatment for a particular patient group, along a patient journey, that includes primary, secondary, and social care inputs. Aim is to improve patient-centered health and social care, making explicit what should happen when, and how communication should happen between different services.

Further information

▦ National Electronic Health Library for databases on guidelines and integrated care pathways, primary care query answering service and access to Clinical Evidence, resource on best evidence: www.nelh.nhs.uk/
▦ National Institute for Health and Clinical Excellence: www.nice.org.uk

Clinical audit

A quality improvement process aimed at improving patient care and outcomes as part of an organization's clinical governance programme (Clinical governance 📖). Systematically reviews current care (i.e. what is happening?) against explicit criteria (i.e. what should be happening?), identifying deficiencies or problems (i.e. what changes are needed?), implements changes at an individual, team, or service level and then monitors to ensure continued improvement in health-care delivery. Often described as the audit cycle or spiral (see Fig. 3.1). Starting points are often significant events, complaints (Complaints procedures 📖), QOF (Quality and outcomes framework 📖) targets, clinical guidelines or protocols (Evidence-based health care 📖), prescribing data, an individual's or teams' observations.

Clinical audit in primary care

- Every PCO and health-care organization has an annual programme of priority areas for audits based on quality standards in service specifications, contracts, QOF, national guidance e.g. NSFs, NICE guidance, Esence of Care Benchmarks (see website below) etc.
- Most organizations are trying to increase the involvement of service users in the audit process.
- Many PCOs have audit officers as part of clinical governance teams who offer training, advice, and sometimes help undertake audits.
- Many professionals find clinical audit very threatening. The organization or team should ensure that audit is undertaken in a culture of supportive development not punishment.

Preparing to undertake an audit: ensure team and organization support the audit, both in the resources, skills to undertake it and the commitment to act on findings. Everyone needs to be clear whether audit is conducted at individual practitioner level and how findings will be reported back.

Choosing a topic for audit: should be important, manageable, clearly defined and preferably have data easily available.

Choosing audit criteria: these should be explicit and evidence-based. Good starting point are statements in national or local clinical guidance. Statements should be made as to what standard is expected i.e. whether the criteria should be fulfilled in 100% or a smaller percentage of cases.

Measuring current performance against the criteria: methods of gathering data depends on criteria trying to measure and available resources. Can include computer records, medical records, data collection sheets, questionnaires. Results should be compared with standards and any other available audit data e.g. published audits from other practices, teams.

Planning for improvement: identifying changes needed requires a team and organizational approach (Teamwork and innovation 📖) as well as plans for continued monitoring of change implementation. May also involve addressing issues in individuals PDPs (Continuing professional development 📖). Following implementation the cycle leads back into re-auditing.

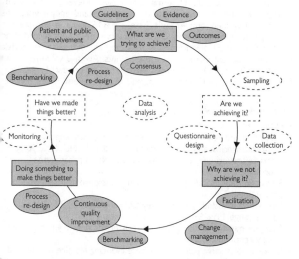

Fig. 3.1 The clinical audit cycle. Reproduced with permission of the National Institute for Health and Clinical Excellence (2002) from *Principles of Best Practice in Clinical Audit*. London: National Institute for Clinical Excellence

Further information

- NHS Clinical Governance Support Team (2005). *Practical Handbook to Clinical Audit*. www.cgsupport.nhs.uk/Resources/Clinical_Audit
- NHS England Essence of Care Benchmarks: www.cgsupport.nhs.uk/Programmes/Essence_of_Care_Programme
- NICE (2002). *Principles for Best Practice in Clinical Audit*. www.nice.org.uk

Quality and outcomes framework (QOF)

The QOF applies to the new GMS and PMS contracts (General practice 📖). Uses a points system linked to financial incentives to encourage high quality care. Determined at a national level but assessed by local PCOs through surgery return of evidence and annual visit. The Quality Management and Analysis System, (QMAS) is a in IT system in England that reports on many QOF indicators from patient record Read codes (IT and electronic records 📖). Some indicators have to reach a minimum % patient coverage to attract points. Average value per point £124.60 (2006/7). QOF and point system indicators reviewed annually in light of evidence and alterations agreed during national GMS contract negotiations.

QOF indicators (as at 2006/2007)

Clinical care

- Secondary prevention of coronary heart disease including practice register, diagnosis, and management of angina and CHD. Max. 96 pts.
- Heart failure including practice register and ongoing management Max. 20 pts.
- Stroke and TIA including practice register and ongoing management Max. 24 pts.
- Hypertension including practice register and record of BP within in normal range. Max. 83 pts.
- Diabetes mellitus including practice register and ongoing management. Max. 93 pts.
- Chronic obstructive pulmonary disease including practice register and ongoing management. Max. 33 pts.
- Epilepsy. Register and ongoing management. Max. 15pts.
- Hypothyroid. Register and record of thyroid tests. Max. 7pts.
- Cancer. Register and case review <6mths of diagnosis. Max. 11 pts.
- Palliative Care. Register and MDT review. Max. 6 pts.
- Mental health including practice register and ongoing management. Max. 39pts.
- Asthma including practice register and ongoing management. Max. 45 pts.
- Dementia—register and review of patients in past 15mths. Max. 20 pts.
- Depression e.g. case finding in people with diabetes or CHD. Max. 33 pts.
- Chronic kidney disease including practice register and ongoing management. Max. 27 pts.
- Atrial fibrillation including practice register and ongoing management. Max. 30 pts.
- Obesity—register >16yrs, BMI >30. 8pts.
- Learning disabilities—register. 4 pts.
- Smoking indicators e.g. recording of smoking status in patients with associated LTC. Max. 68 pts.

Organizational indicators
- Records information about patient e.g. BP >45yrs recorded in previous 5yrs for at least 65% patients. Max. 106 pts.
- Information for patients. e.g. arrangements to speak to GP by phone. Max. 5.5 pts.
- Education and training e.g. The practice has undertaken at least 12 significant event reviews in the past 3yrs. Max. 28 pts.
- Practice management e.g. instrument sterilization complies with national guidelines. Max. 17.5 pts.
- Medicine management: e.g. <72hrs from request for repeat prescription to be available. Max. 40 pts.

Patient experience (max. 78 pts)
- Length of consultations.
- Patient surveys and related action plans.

Additional services (max. 36 pts)
- Cervical screening including policy, recording, and auditing.
- Child health promotion offered in line with national guidelines.
- Antenatal care and screening offered in line with local policy.
- Contraception: a written policy on EC.

Further information

🖳 British Medical Association (2006). Focus on the Quality and Outcomes Framework: www.bma.org.uk/ap.nsf/Content/focusqoffeb06

🖳 Primary Care Contracting NHS: www.primarycarecontracting.nhs.uk

Complaints procedures

All NHS service users who are unhappy with the treatment or service are entitled to make a complaint, have it considered, and receive a response from the NHS organization or primary care practitioner concerned. Each country has an agreed complaints procedures that is also written into the GMS contract. Every organization and general practice has to publicize its complaints procedures to the public. Patient Advice and Liaison Service (PALS) in PCOs can help public identify procedure for complaint. The Independent Complaints Advocacy Service (ICAS see below) is funded by the NHS to support people wishing to make a complaint about their NHS care or treatment.

People who complain generally want:
• Their complaint to be heard and investigated promptly
• To be dealt with courteously and sympathetically
• To receive an apology if mistakes have occurred
• The problem rectified promptly if possible
• To be assured that steps will be taken to prevent a recurrence.

Key principles
• Timescale:
  • A complaint can be made by the affected individual or someone acting on their behalf with their consent.
  • A complaint should be made within 6mths of the event(s) or from time they became aware that they had cause for complaint.
• Form of complaint:
  • Can be to any member of staff who may be able to resolve concerns without the need for a formal complaint.
  • A more formal complaint has to be to the local organization concerned in the first instance.
  • Can be orally, by email or in writing.
• Complaint handling at the local level:
  • Every organization and practice has a designated and publicized complaints manager who receives all complaints and has to respond within 48hrs, also advising of rights to ICAS (and contact number).
  • Complaints manager contacts all involved to investigate facts and actions to be taken.
  • Complaints manager has to respond in writing within 10 working days if GP practice or 20 working days if PCT. Can also report progress in investigation if not completed.
  • Complaints manager has to summarize findings, need for apology, actions taken to rectify situation, actions to prevent recurrence. Response to complainant may be by letter or setting up face to face meeting. Conciliation should also be offered.
  • All attempts should be made to resolve the complaint at local level. Complaints unresolved at GP practice level are referred to PCT complaints manager.

- Failure to resolve complaint at the local level:
  - Complainants have the right to take their complaint to independent review. In England this may mean complaining to the Health Commission. The last level of independent review is the Parliamentary and Health Service Ombudsmen.

All organizations use complaints as part of their clinical governance procedures (Clinical governance 📖) as a way of learning how to improve their services. In the same way they also usually collect positive feedback, such as letters of thanks and appreciation.

Further information

NHS complaints procedures are specified on each country's central health department websites (Useful websites 📖)

📖 Healthcare Commission: www.healthcarecommission.org.uk

📖 The Health Service Ombudsman: www.ombudsman.org.uk

Clinical risk management

It is estimated that 850,000 incidents and errors occur every year in the NHS. All health care and work activities involve risk. Organizations have a duty to manage risks i.e. identify what harm its activities, environments, and working practices *could* do to patients, staff and visitors and assess whether it has taken all possible precautionary measures to reduce the risks to an acceptable level.

Risk management is a key component of clinical governance (Clinical governance 📖) and there are legal responsibilities for some elements (e.g. Health and safety at work 📖). PCOs have to have risk registers that document and grade types of risk in the organization e.g. types of clinical care, hazards to workforce. Clinical risk management aims to:
• Identify what could (and does) go wrong during clinical care
• Understand the factors that contribute to incidents and errors
• Put systems in place to reduce risks
• Minimize the consequences to patients and staff when errors do occur
• Learn lessons from any adverse events and implementing change
• Ensure action is taken to prevent recurrence.

Adverse incidents and events

Adverse incident is any event that could have or did lead to unintended or unexpected harm, loss, or damage. It includes accidents and near misses. These may be identified by complaints (Complaints procedures 📖), audits (Clinical audit 📖) or staff reporting of accidents/incidents (see below). All incidents, errors and adverse events should be accurately documented in patient records (Record keeping 📖).

Reporting incidents and events

There are three types of reporting:
• All organizations have to have systems for centrally reporting incidents and accidents, and investigating so that lessons are learnt. The NHS aims to encourage a 'blame free' culture that acknowledges that most adverse events are part of a systems failure rather than an individual failure. A blame free culture does not override the need for disciplinary or criminal processes in the event of negligent or criminal acts.
• Statutory reporting requirements for different types of incidents to Medical Devices Agency, Health and Safety Executive (i.e. reporting injuries, diseases and dangerous occurrences, RIDDOR) Medicines Control Agency. In England and Wales there is a National Reporting and Learning System (NRLS) for patient safety problems through the NPSA (see below).
• To local level multi-agency bodies e.g. notifying the Local Safeguarding Children Boards (England) Child Protection Committee (Scotland) under local agreed procedures (within 48hrs) when a child dies (or attempts suicide) and child abuse or neglect was known or suspected. This may trigger a multi-agency Case Review as specified in the child protection legislation of each country. (See Child protection processes 📖).

Investigating and learning from incidents and events

NHS makes a distinction between:
* 'Latent conditions'—inadequate organizational policies or inappropriate decisions that mould the environment for an active failure to breech safety defenses.
* 'Active failures'—unsafe acts committed by individuals.

Each organization has policies identifying who has responsibility, and the processes, for internal investigations (or may be stipulated in legislation) or review in the case of 'near misses' and for reporting centrally. The investigation should cover:
* Immediate events:
  * What happened? (Event and those involved.)
  * Where and when did it happen? (Location, date, and time.)
  * What action was taken? (Immediate and longer term.)
* What impact did the event have? (Harm to patient, others, the organization.)
* Why did it happen? (The sequences of events, the work environment, communication processes, levels of supervision, elements of the particular task, availability of guidance, factors related to the individual patient, family or household, factors related to individual members of staff.)
* What factors did, or could have, minimized the impact of the event?

NB Multi-agency investigations e.g. after a child death associated with abuse or neglect, have agreed processes.

Further information

Department of Health, England (2000). *An organization with a memory*. The Stationery Office, London.

National Patient Safety Authority (England): www.npsa.nhs.uk/ provides guidance, tools and reports on patient safety from analysis of incident reporting.

Saferhealthcare: www.saferhealthcare.org.uk provides tools, advice, and research on best practice in patient safety.

Professional conduct

Respect for human rights is the basis for all nursing and health-care practice. Fundamentally, it is about treating people as individuals by enabling them to make choices and having due regard for their wishes. Human rights rest on three key principles:

- Every human has certain rights which are not conferred on him or her but which arise in him or her by virtue of their humanity alone.
- A person cannot be deprived of those rights by another or by their own acts.
- Just laws must be applied consistently, independently, impartially (without fear or favour) and with fair procedures.

Human Rights Act 1998 (HRA): The HRA incorporates into domestic law certain rights from the European Convention for the Protection of Human Rights and Fundamental Freedoms (ECHR) and has three main effects:

- An allegation of a breach of rights can be brought in the UK courts.
- It is unlawful for a public body (including the NHS) to breach rights set out in the Act.
- In situations where the courts find that legislation is incompatible with the rights set out in the Act, Judges can make a 'declaration of incompatibility'. The legislation will then be referred back to Parliament for reconsideration.
- Examples of rights set out in the HRA that relate to health care are shown below.

> Article 2: right to life
> Article 3: prohibition of torture
> Article 8: right to respect for private and family life
> Article 14: prohibition of discrimination (NB this relates to the enjoyment of the rights and freedoms set forth in the HRA)
> Article 17: prohibition of abuse of rights

NMC code of conduct

Beyond practising in ways that respect human rights, the NMC professional code of conduct specifies:

- As a registered nurse, midwife, or HV you must:
  - Protect and support the health of individuals and the health of the wider community
  - Act in such a way that justifies the public's trust and confidence
  - Uphold and enhance the good reputation of the professions.
- As a registered nurse, midwife, or HV, you are personally accountable for your practice. In caring for patients and clients, you must:
  - Respect the patient or client as an individual
  - Obtain consent before you give any treatment or care
  - Protect confidential information
  - Cooperate with others in the team
  - Maintain your professional knowledge and competence
  - Be trustworthy
  - Act to identify and minimize risk to patients and clients.

Further information

- Nursing and Midwifery Council www.nmc-uk.org
- Department of Constitutional Affairs: www.dca.gov.uk
- Liberty: www.yourrights.org.uk

Anti-discriminatory health care

HRA (supported by other legislation, e.g. the Disability Discrimination Act 1995) prohibits discrimination on the grounds of sex, race, disability, sexual orientation, age, religion/faith, or any other status. This applies to all aspects of professional practice, access to and provision of health services, and employment.

All UK countries have NHS programmes to promote equality and diversity in health-care practice, services, and workforce. All policies and guidance have to promote equality and diversity.

Detailed guidance for health-care professionals and good practice examples to increase equality and decrease sexism, racism, ageism, disability discrimination, and sexuality discrimination are available in each country

- ▣ England DoH: Equality and Human Rights:
  www.dh.gov.uk/PolicyAndGuidance/EqualityAndHumanRights/fs/en
- ▣ Northern Ireland DHSSPS: Equality, Diversity and Human Rights:
  www.dhsspsni.gov.uk/equality/race&diversity_links.asp
- ▣ NHS Scotland: Equality and Diversity:
  www.show.scot.nhs.uk/csa/diversity/diversity_soi.htm
- ▣ NHS Wales: Centre for Equality and Human Rights:
  www.wales.nhs.uk/sites/home.cfm?orgid=256

NB Legislation is currently going through parliament to create one statutory body to address human rights, equality and anti-discrimination in relation to age, sexuality, religion, or belief.

Further information for professionals and the public

▣ Commission for Racial Equality (CRE) www.cre.gov.uk (linked pages for Scotland and Wales)
▣ Disability Rights Commission www.drc-gb.org (linked pages for Scotland and Wales)
▣ Equal Opportunities Commission www.eoc.org.uk (linked sites to Scotland and Wales)
▣ RCN (2002). *The role of the nurse and the rights of patients.* www.rcn.org.uk

Also, campaigning groups such as:

▣ Age Concern: www.ageconcern.org.uk
▣ British Council of Disabled People: www.bcodp.org.uk
▣ Stonewall: www.stonewall.org.uk

Consent

This is voluntary agreement with (or refusal of) an action proposed by another. It is fundamental to human rights and professional practice (Professional conduct 📖). It is a continuous process and relates to all aspects of care. Valid consent must have these elements:
- Voluntary, i.e. given without undue pressure or coercion.
- Reasonably informed, i.e. the person must understand:
  - The nature of the act proposed
  - Its associated benefits and risks
  - Alternatives (including doing nothing)
  - The associated benefits and risks of the alternatives.
- Made by a competent person, i.e. someone who has the capacity to understand the information and weigh up the options to reach a decision. Competency is 'function specific': someone may have the capacity to take some health-care decisions but may lack capacity to decide more complex matters. All adults (≥18yrs old in England and Wales, ≥16yrs old in Scotland) are presumed to be competent, but that presumption can be questioned and refuted.

See 📖 Contraception: general, for information on Fraser Guidelines regarding under 16-year-olds and consent.

Format of consent

The professional providing the care, treatment, or investigation should seek consent. It can be:
- Implied consent (e.g. rolling up sleeve for BP measurement)
- Express verbal consent (for minor procedures, such as venepuncture)
- Express written consent (for procedures with ↑ risk, e.g. vaccination).

Consent forms[1] act as a record in case of future disputes. Different types should be used:
- For those consenting for themselves
- Consenting for a child
- Consenting for incapacitated adults (Mental capacity 📖).

Emergencies

Treatment can be provided without consent as long as it is limited to saving life or preventing serious injury and known not to be contrary to previous wishes of a competent patient.

Consent and treatment of patients with mental incapacity

Generally, only treatment for the mental disorder may be given, but may include physical conditions that contribute to the mental condition. New Mental Incapacity Acts in England and Scotland provide a framework for judging mental incapacity in adults, at the same time as protecting their rights and providing health care (Mental capacity 📖).

---

[1] 📖 England and Wales DH Guidance on consent: www.dh.gov.uk/PolicyAndGuidance HealthAndSocialCareTopics/Consent/ConsentGeneralInformation/fs/en

Professional accountability

Accountability means being responsible for someone or something. All nurses are accountable for their professional practice; individually they are answerable for their actions and omissions. Nurses can be called to account via:
- Professional regulation, i.e. the Nursing and Midwifery Council
- Criminal law, e.g. the law of assault
- Civil law, e.g. the tort of negligence (see below)
- Employment law, e.g. through the enforcement of a contract.

Duty of care and negligence
Nurses have a legal and a professional duty of care for patients and clients. A duty of care means taking reasonable care to avoid acts or omissions that can be reasonably foreseen as likely to be injurious to patients and clients. Patients and clients can make complaints (Complaints procedures 📖) to the organization and the NMC about negligent care. They can also sue through the civil court. Any court considering a claim of negligence against a nurse would apply the Bolam Test i.e. that the nurse had acted competently as an ordinary nurse in the view of expert opinion. The Bolitho case amended this to state that the expert opinion had to demonstrate a logical basis. Both the employer and the nurse have a responsibility to ensure the nurse is competent.

Duty of care and new roles
Nurses undertaking roles usually undertaken by other professionally qualified staff would be judged against the ordinary competent other professional performing that role.

Duty of care and students and junior staff
Students and junior staff actions are also judged against the ordinary competent professional and not that of a student or junior. Nurses have a duty to ensure that the care which they delegate to juniors or students is carried out at a reasonably competent standard. This means they remain accountable for the delegation of the work and for ensuring that the person who does the work is able to do it.

Vicarious liability

Employers are vicariously liable for the actions and omissions of their staff, which means that if a patient successfully sues for negligence, the employer will pay the compensation and usually not the nurse. However this *only* includes those activities within the job description and contract (Employment contracts 📖). It does not cover Samaritan acts or acts in roles not specified in the job description. Some employers may seek re-imbursement of compensation paid out from the staff member who committed the negligent act. Most nurses pay for professional indemnity through subscription to a professional or indemnity organization.

Further information
📖 www.nmc-uk.org.uk
📖 NHS indemnity: www.DoH.gov.uk

Chaperones

All consultations, examinations, and investigations are potentially distressing. Patients can find examinations, investigations, or photography involving the breasts, genitalia, or rectum particularly intrusive (these are referred to as 'intimate examinations'). Also consultations involving dimmed lights, the need for patients to undress, or for intensive periods of being touched may make a patient feel vulnerable.

For most patients, respect, explanation, consent, and privacy take precedence over the need for a chaperone (Consent 📖). A chaperone is present as a safeguard for all parties (patient and practitioners) and is a witness to continuing consent of the procedure.

Every health-care organization is expected to have a chaperone policy (Clinical governance 📖).

Good practice principles

The inquiry into how the NHS handled allegations about the misconduct of Dr Clifford Ayling[1] recommended:

- The presence of a chaperone must be the patient's decision, but it should routinely be offered by a health-care professional.
- Trained clinical staff should undertake the chaperone role, rather than unqualified staff (e.g. practice receptionists).
- No family member or friend of a patient should be expected to undertake any formal chaperoning role.

In addition:

- Patients should be made aware of the availability of chaperones through notices and practice leaflets.
- If the patient does not want a chaperone, it should be recorded that the offer was made and declined.
- If a chaperone is present, that should be recorded, including the chaperone's identity.
- If, for justifiable practical reasons, a chaperone cannot be offered, this should be explained to the patient and, if possible, offer to delay the examination to a later date. This discussion and its outcome should be recorded.
- The same principles for offering and use of chaperones should apply in all settings, including home visits and out-of-hours centres.

Further information

📓 Clinical Governance Support Team Model Chaperone Framework: www.cgsupport.nhs.uk
📓 RCN (2002). *The role of the nurse and the rights of patients.* www.rcn.org.uk

---

[1] DH (2004) Committee of Inquiry. Independent Investigation into how the NHS handled alligations about the conduct of Clifford Ayling: www.dh.gov.uk

Whistle blowing

Whistle blowing is when an employee informs on a fellow employee or their employer, who is either breaking the law or in breach of organizational or professional codes of conduct or policy. It is the exposure of:
• Fraud
• Negligent actions
• Abuse by an employee.

It is important for making sure an organization is alert to scandal, danger, malpractice, or corruption.

Protecting practitioners

Practitioners may be too afraid to report something, because of fear of victimization, being shunned by their peers, or losing their job.

The Public Interest Disclosure Act 1998 sets out the mechanisms for promoting whistle blowing and provides legal protection to people who do this. A qualifying disclosure will be 'protected' if the practitioner:
• Makes the disclosure in good faith
• Reasonably believes that the information disclosed is true.

Action to take

If you have a concern, you should:
• Make an immediate note of your concerns, e.g. what was said, date, time and names of people involved
• Convey your suspicions to someone with the appropriate authority and experience. Most PCOs have established policies for whistle blowing (that nurses working in general practice can also access) Human Resource Departments should have details
• Deal with the matter promptly; delay may cause your organization or patients to suffer or increase the risk of harm.

If you have a concern, you should *not*:
• Do nothing
• Forget there may be an innocent or good explanation
• Be afraid of making your concerns known
• Approach or accuse any individuals directly
• Try to investigate the matter yourself
• Convey your suspicions to anyone other than those with the proper authority.

Related topic

📖 Clinical supervision and appraisal.

Further information

Health Care Commission: ☎ 0845 601 3012
🖥 www.healthcarecommission.org.uk/ContatUs/ComplainAboutNHS/Whistleblow
Public Concern at Work: ☎ 020 7404 6609
🖥 www.pcaw.co.uk/legislation/legislation.html

Record keeping

Good record keeping promotes continuity of care (through accurate communication), acts as a means to demonstrate the quality and complexity of nursing, and provides a resource if nurses are called to account at a later date (NB it may be more difficult to convince a court it happened if it wasn't recorded).

What counts as a record?

Any permanent form of data recorded about a client or patient. This includes both paper and information stored electronically.

General principles for good record keeping

Records should be
- Legible
- Written in black permanent ink
- Contemporaneous
- Include the date and time the information was recorded
- Signed and also name printed
- Clear, comprehensive, and focused on the provision of accurate, objective, factual, and relevant information relating to the client's diagnosis/needs and care/treatment
- Written in collaboration with patients.

Records should not
- In general, they should not include anything you are not prepared to say or reveal to the client (Access to records 📖)
- They should not be altered, except to make corrections to inaccurate information (any alterations should be clearly marked as such and signed/dated).

Details to include when making entries to patient records

- Information on which decisions have been based, i.e. problems/needs presented by the patient/client; relevant information on past history (including health, medication, family and social history); observations, test results or examination findings.
- Impressions of the current situation—priorities for care/treatment.
- Action plan—as negotiated with the patient/client (may include referrals made, prescriptions given, tests undertaken).
- Information shared and advice given—concerns/worries of the patient/client or their family/carers; health advice given to the patient; plans for follow-up/next visit.
- Other essential information—including details of correspondence with others.

Storage of records

- When not in use, records should be stored (including laptops and personal digital assistants) under lock and key.
- If the records are patient or parent/child held, then reinforce the need to keep the information secure.

- Electronic records:
  - Do not leave a terminal unattended and signed-in
  - Never share passwords
  - Change passwords regularly
  - Clear the screen of one patient's information before seeing another patient
  - Use password-protected screen-savers.
- Manual records:
  - Store files closed and in a logical order
  - Use a tracking system to monitor the whereabouts of files
  - Return files as soon as they are no longer needed.
- Retention of records: DH suggests the following as minimum retention periods:
  - Children and young people: until their 25th birthday, or 26th if the young person was 17 at the time of conclusion of treatment; or 8yrs after patient's death if death occurred before 18th birthday
  - Maternity (including midwifery and obstetric): 25yrs
  - Mentally disordered patients: 20yrs after no further treatment; or 8yrs after patient's death
  - Oncology: 8yrs after conclusion of treatment
  - General: 8yrs after conclusion of treatment
  - GP records: 10yrs after conclusion of treatment.
- Destruction of records should be through a secure process organized by your employer.

Further information

- Department of Health records management: www.dh.gov.uk/PolicyAndGuidance/ OrganisationPolicy/RecordsManagement/fs/en

Access to records

It is good practice to write records in collaboration with patients in order to promote trust and increase communication. Patients and clients have legal rights to privacy in the processing of personal data and rights of access to those data.

The Data Protection Act 1998 (DPA)

The DPA gives patients/clients (known as 'data subjects') formal rights of access:

- To be informed as to whether personal data are processed.
- To be given a description of the data held, the purposes for which the data are processed, and knowledge of the persons to whom details may be disclosed.
- To be given a copy of the information constituting the data.
- To be given information on the sources of the data.
- To have errors about them corrected in the records.

To gain formal access to records, patients/clients have to write to the organization that holds the records (i.e. PCT or GP practice). The responsible manager has 40d to respond. Access to a record by a data subject is restricted:

- When access would be likely to cause serious harm to the physical or mental health of the data subject.
- When to give access would reveal the identity of a third person (unless consent given to the disclosure). Does not apply if the third person is a health professional, involved in the care of the data subject, unless giving access is likely to cause serious harm to that health professional.

The Freedom of Information Act 2000 (FOI)

This gives a general right of access to information recorded by, or on behalf of, public authorities The Act requires that all public bodies:

- Publish details of classes of recorded information held routinely.
- Permit individuals access to non-personal records of the organization.

Who can seek access to health records?

- Any competent person (including a competent child/young person) can apply for access to their personal records.
- A person with parental responsibility for a child (<18yrs old in England and Wales, <16yrs old in Scotland. NB A competent child/young person has a right to confidentiality (Consent 📖).
- A person appointed by a court on behalf of a person who is incapacitated, in order to discharge their duties (Consent 📖).
- A third party when authorized by the data subject. NB Family, friends and carers don't have right of access unless the patient consents.
- The executor or administrator of a deceased person's estate may apply under the Access to Health Records Act 1990.

Further information

- Department of Health site on patient confidentiality and access to records: www.dh.gov.uk/
  PolicyAndGuidance/InformationPolicy/PatientConfidentialityAndCaldicottGuardians/fs/en
- NHS Freedom of Information site: www.foi.nhs.uk

IT and electronic records

Health-care delivery is based on the use and sharing of information. ↑ use of information technology is central to government strategies for modernizing the NHS.

Resources for professionals

N3 is an NHS intranet, giving access to email and the Internet. It cannot be accessed by anyone outside NHS organizations. All NHS staff should have a work email address and access to the NHSnet. This also gives access to the NHS electronic library online (Evidence-based health care 📖).

NHS electronic patient record

NHS Care Records Service is developing a system by which a patient's electronic NHS record is held centrally online, accessible by any health professional involved in that patient's care, with other detailed information held locally.

NHS clinical classification of conditions and activity

A classification (SNOMED CT[®1]) of clinical terms is being introduced across the UK to enable the easy sharing of information and easy production of patient population summary data (e.g. for audit, HNA). It is replacing Read Codes used in general practice. Codes are given to all types of information: assessment, history (including medical and social), diagnosis, treatment, and professional activities.

General practice

Most general practices are computerized and many are 'paperless', using electronic patient record systems such as EMIS and TOREX. These allow clinical templates, e.g. diabetes review prompt list, to be developed, which can be opened on screen during a patient consultation. General practice also uses electronic methods to:
- Choose and Book: an online method used by GPs and other primary care staff to refer patients and book initial hospital appointments online.
- Electronic transfer of prescriptions: an electronic method by which GPs and primary care staff can issue prescriptions and send them to the pharmacist chosen by the patient.
- Quality Management and Analysis System (QMAS): allows GP practices and PCTs to analyse information they collect against national standards (QOF 📖).

Community health services

Access to computers in community health services is patchy but ↑ Mostly used for administrative purposes (e.g. collection of activity data, sending appointments) rather than being patient-record based. Many PCOs issue community nurses with portable computers to be used in the home. Many GP-attached HVs and DNs record their interactions with patients/clients on the general practice patient electronic record.

---

1 Systemised Nomenclature of Medicine.

Telehealth

A wide range of new technology systems is being explored in all countries of the UK, e.g.:

- For supporting people to remain independently in their own homes.
- For home medical monitoring that relays clinical readings through the telephone to the health professional.
- For video consulting with other remote health professionals.

Further information

▣ National Programme for IT in the NHS: www.connectingforhealth.nhs.uk
▣ NHS Health Informatics community: www.informatics.nhs.uk/index.html

Confidentiality

Confidentiality is when you ensure that information shared by patients/clients is not disclosed to a third party without permission. Preserving confidentiality is:
- Important for maintaining trust between patient and professional.
- Recognized in statue and UK case law (Professional conduct 📖).
- Stated in the NMC Code of Professional Conduct (Professional conduct 📖).
- Stated or implied in your contract of employment.

Although health professionals often routinely share information, this should be with the consent (implied or expressed) of the patient.

Refusal of consent to share information
The patient/client should be made aware of the implications of this decision. Their choice should be documented and, unless the breach falls into categories below, respected.

Circumstances when patient confidentiality can be breached
- When the patient consents (Consent 📖).
- In the best interests of the patient, e.g. in an emergency.
- To protect a child (the Children Act 1989; Child protection 📖).
- Under a court order.
- Where there are statutory duties to disclose, e.g. Public Health (Control of Diseases) Act 1984.
- In the public interest; however, no definition of 'public interest' has been laid down. The risk should be serious and substantially reduced by disclosure.
- The information disclosed should be limited to that which is necessary to protect the patient/client.

Caldicott guardians and principles
Caldicott guardians are senior health and social care staff appointed to ensure Cadlicott principles of disclosure of patient identifiable information are applied:
- Justify the purpose.
- Do not use patient identifiable information unless it is absolutely necessary.
- Use the minimum necessary patient identifiable information.
- Access to patient identifiable information should be on a strict 'need-to-know' basis.
- Everyone with access to patient identifiable information should be aware of their responsibilities.
- Understand and comply with the law.

Further information
📖 Department of Health site on patient confidentiality and access to records: www.dh.gov.uk/PolicyAndGuidance/InformationPolicy/PatientConfidentialityAndCaldicottGuardians/fs/en

Client and patient-held records

Patients and clients increasingly hold their health and social care records in the UK, although they remain the property of the issuing organization. Employers and health and social care partnerships have local policies as to whether duplicates (e.g. carbon copies) or summaries are held by the organization or if the client/patient-held record is the sole record.

Benefits
• Facilitates partnership
• Enables patients/clients ↑ involvement in care
• Ensures all contact with health and social care providers is recorded in one place
• Ensures key information is available to the next professional.

Research studies demonstrate that client/patient-held health records do not get lost. In some countries outside UK client/patient-held records are the norm rather than the exception.

Types most commonly encountered in primary care
• Personal maternity records or cooperation card
• DN home records
• Parent-held child health record
• School child health record
• Personal health records of asylum applicants and refugees
• Local disease-specific patient-held record, e.g. diabetes care.

Further information
🖫 DH England health records for asylum applicants: www.dh.gov.uk/PolicyAndGuidance/International
🖫 National PHCHR: http://shop.healthforallchildren.co.uk

Health and safety at work

Health and Safety at Work Act 1974 provides the main legal framework.

Employers

Employers have a legal duty to ensure staff health, safety and welfare at work. Employers must consult staff or their safety representatives on matters relating to health and safety at work (often through safety committees, set up to monitor systems). Employers must:

- Assess and then address the risks to staff health and safety.
- If there are 5 or more staff, record the risk assessment and plans and draw up a health and safety policy available to all.
- Appoint a competent person responsible for health and safety.
- Set up emergency procedures and provide first-aid facilities.
- Ensure the workplace satisfies health, safety, and welfare requirements, e.g. for temperature, lighting, and sanitary and rest facilities.
- Ensure work equipment is suitable, maintained, and used properly.
- Prevent or control exposure to damaging substances (COSHH legislation) and protect against danger from flammable, electrical, or explosive hazards, noise and radiation.
- Ensure no hazardous manual handling operations and reduce the likelihood of injury.
- Provide health surveillance as appropriate.
- Provide free PPE (Personal protective equipment 📖) when risks are not controlled in other ways.
- Ensure safety signs.
- Report certain occupational diseases, injuries, and dangerous events to authorities (🖥 RIDDOR www.riddor.gov.uk/).

Employees

Employees also have legal duties:

- Taking reasonable care for their own health and safety and that of others.
- Cooperating with employer on health and safety issues.
- Correctly using work items provided by employers, including PPE as trained or in guidance.
- Not interfering with or misuse anything provided for health, safety or welfare.

Safety representatives

Safety representatives are appointed by trade unions to represent their members on health and safety issues, may represent the entire workforce. Entitled to paid time off to carry out their role. Union offers full training and information back up.

Health, safety, and welfare in the NHS

Key areas of attention in the NHS are reducing accidents and musculo-skeletal injuries, reducing stress and violence to staff, providing smoke-free workplaces, tackling bullying and harassment, reducing risk of blood born viruses and latex allergies, ensuring occupational health services offered to all staff including GP staff, ensure sickness absence and opportunities for rehabilitation and redeployment managed well.

Health and safety at work concerns

Concerns should be raised with employer or manager or through the safety representative. If fail to act or respond satisfactorily, employee or safety representative can contact health and safety inspectors of the enforcing authority. Anyone can get health and safety information confidentially from the Health and Safety Executive's (HSE) Information line

Further information

HSE Infoline ☎ 0845 345 0055. www.hse.gov.uk/index.htm

NHS Employers. The Blue Book; *The Management of Health, Safety and Welfare issues for NHS staff* (2006) www.nhsemployers.org/practice/healthy-workplaces.cfm

See also Health and Safety at work web pages of main unions and organizations e.g. RCN, Unison, MSF/CPHVA (Useful websites)

Lone working

Lone working is any situation or location in which someone works without a colleague nearby or when someone is working out of sight or earshot of another colleague. The main factors creating a risk from users/patients to lone workers are impatience, frustration, anxiety, resentment, drink or drugs, and inherent aggression or mental instability. Employers have to assess the risk of violence and put measures in place to avoid or reduce risk to the lowest practicable level (Clinical risk management 📖) e.g. ensure seating arrangements in consultation rooms allows staff to reach door without being blocked, appropriate alarm buzzers.

Wherever possible and legally permissible, health and other public sector providers should share information on individuals and addresses known to be a risk.

All services should have an system for keeping staff details required in an emergency e.g. mobile and home numbers, next of kin, car registration and model, staff photographs.

Good practice guidance for lone working and home visiting

- *Scheduling appointments and reporting movements:*
  - Ensure colleagues are aware of one another's movements including full addresses, details of home visiting, journey details, telephone numbers, and anticipated arrival and departure times. Some areas use texting to let a colleague know when staff member has safely left after each home visit.
  - All staff need to know procedures if colleagues do not return when expected.
- *If the patient, relative or carer has a history of violence or the location is considered unsafe:*
  - Do not visit alone.
  - If possible the contact should take place at a neutral location or within a secure environment, such as within the Violent Patient Scheme in primary care.
- *Key safety equipment to be carried:*
  - ID badge.
  - Mobile phone: keep fully charged and close at hand, emergency contacts on speed dial, check signal before entering lone worker situations, do not use overtly in open spaces.
  - Map of the local area.
  - Personal attack alarm and torch.
  - Emergency telephone numbers.
- *Arriving at and conducting the appointment:*
  - When the front door is opened, carry out a 10 second risk assessment.
  - Have an excuse ready should it be deemed necessary not to enter.
  - Request that animals be secured prior to entry.
  - Shut the front door and be familiar with the door lock.
  - Maintain awareness of entrances and exists.
  - If uncomfortable, do not sit down and do not spread belongings out.
  - If feeling unsafe, make an excuse and leave immediately.

Good practice principles for travelling

- *Lone working and vehicles:*
  - Ensure enough petrol and join a recovery breakdown service.
  - Do not leave valuables visible.
  - Avoid nurse on call badges as may encourage thieves after drugs.
  - Hold keys when leaving premises to avoid looking for them outside.
  - Lock doors/shut windows at slow speed and at traffic lights.
  - Park in well-lit locations, facing the direction you wish to leave.
- *Lone working and public transport:*
  - Use a busy stop or station that is well-lit.
  - Keep a transport timetable.
  - Sit near driver, in an aisle seat and near emergency alarm.
  - Avoid upper decks, empty carriages or carriages occupied by only one other.
- *Lone working and travelling by foot:*
  - Walk briskly and do not stop in unfamiliar areas.
  - If carrying equipment, use bags that do not advertise what is carried.
  - In the event of attempted theft, relinquish property at once without challenge.
  - Keep house keys and mobile phone separately from handbag.
  - Remain aware of location and surrounding people.
  - Avoid waste ground, isolated pathways and subways.

Essential reading

▣ NHS Security Management Service (2005). *Not Alone: A Guide for the Better Protection of Lone Workers in the NHS*: www.cfsms.nhs.uk/doc/lone.worker/not.alone.pdf

Further information

▣ Health and Safety Executive, useful information on different ways of supporting lone workers: www.hse.gov.uk/violence/

▣ The Suzie Lamplugh Trust: www.suzylamplugh.org/home/index.shtml

Patient moving and handling

Moving patients is a major factor in back injury and muscular-skeletal disorders in nursing staff. The manual handling regulations place duties on employers to ensure manual handling is avoided where reasonable and practicable, and if not to carry out an assessment of risk and then minimise risk by implementing measures relating to the working environment such as equipment, uniform, organizational staffing levels, training, written instructions, definition of roles and communication. Employees have a duty to obey reasonable instructions and cooperate with employers in manual handling procedures. Patient handling risk assessments and care plans to minimize risk for each type of moving and handling activity should be documented in patient held notes. All staff involved in patient handling should receive training and regular updating, including equipment use.

Factors which predispose to injury and should be avoided

- Lifting patients.
- Working in an awkward, unstable, or crouched position.
- Undertaking work that requires bending forward, sideways, or twisting.
- Lifting loads at arms length.
- Lifting with a starting or finishing position near the floor.
- Lifting with a starting or finishing position overhead at arms length.
- Lifting an uneven load with the weight mainly on one side.
- Handling an uncooperative or falling patient.

Issues to consider in the handling risk assessment

- The task e.g.:
  - What task needs to be performed e.g. bed to chair?
  - Where is it to be carried out?
  - Number of people required?
  - Equipment required?
- The patient e.g.:
  - Expectations, wishes, willingness to accept equipment
  - Potential for rehabilitation to greater independence
  - Ability to weight bear, history of falls
  - Pain or arthritis
  - Level of cooperation
  - Problems with sight or spatial awareness
  - Body weight and distribution
  - Medication which might affect mobility.
- The handler e.g.:
  - Physical capabilities, health, and fitness
  - Up-to-date in handling training
  - Suitable clothing and footwear
  - Heights of people working together
  - Familiarity with chosen equipment.
- The environment e.g.:
  - Space available
  - Obstacles that might need to be moved
  - Type of floor or surface
  - Gradients or distances involved.

Handling equipment

Patient handling aids should be used whenever they can reduce the risk of injury. Their selection should be based on individual patient assessment. Physiotherapists and/or OT's assessment and advice may be required. Special equipment might be needed for bariatric (i.e. clinically obese) patients. Equipment should be regularly maintained and CE marked as per Medical Devices Regulations. Local policies apply to equipment to aid nursing and to aid independent living (Aids and equipment: general 🕮). Equipment to consider includes:

- Aids for greater patient independent movement:
  - Dutch lifting poles or rope ladders in bed
  - Patient hand blocks
  - Transfer boards
  - Bath boards and rails
  - Raised toilet seats and rails
  - Swivel seats
  - Leg lifters
  - Variable height beds
  - Stair lifts.
- Aids for movement assisted by others:
  - Handling belts and slings
  - Standing turntables
  - Variable height beds
  - Hoists (mobile, freestanding and ceiling mounted) and slings
  - Sliding aids.

If the patient refuses equipment, negotiation skills become important. Staff need to report refusal to line manager as the risk of injury to staff has to weighed up against the risk to the patient if a particular procedure is not carried out.

Essential reading

Smith, J. (ed) (2005). *The Guide to the Handling of People* (5th edn.), Backcare: Teddington.

🖥 RCN (2003) *Manual Handling Assessments in Hospitals and the Community.* www.rcn.org.uk/publications/pdf/
Manual_Handling_Assessments.pdf

Further information

Back in work: www.nhs.uk/backinwork
National Back Exchange: www.home.btconnect.com/nationalbackex/index_files/pages0003.htm

Cleaning, disinfection, and sterilization of equipment

Under the Control of Substances Hazardous to Health (COSHH) regulations (1988), GPs and other community employers are responsible for assessing risks to health in the workplace and implementing effective but safe decontamination practices.

Cleaning

The physical removal of dirt and organic matter (e.g. blood).

- Manual cleaning. Wear gloves, plastic apron, and face and eye protection if splashing a possibility. Use detergent and hot water in a deep, dedicated sink (not hand basin). Dry thoroughly (air or paper towels).
- Automated cleaning. An ultrasonic cleaner is preferred. Change cleaning solution after each sessional use.

Disinfection

↓ the numbers of micro-organisms. Spores are not usually destroyed.

Heat disinfection is preferred to chemical disinfection which is unreliable. Disinfectants should be used for disinfecting heat-sensitive items.

Sterilization

↑ numbers of micro-organisms, including spores. Use autoclaves if possible/practical or single-use disposable instruments. The choice of method depends on conditions and the sterility assurance level required (Table 3.1) Wherever practicable and cost-effective, sterile items should be obtained from a CSSD.

Bench top autoclaves (sterilizers)

Appropriate for use in clinics and GP practices. Must comply with European Safety and Medical Device Regulations (93/42 EEC 1998). They must be validated before use by a 'Test Person'; have their performance monitored on a daily, weekly, quarterly, and annual basis by the owner and be regularly maintained in accordance with the manufacturer's programme. All results must be documented in a log book, available for periodic inspection. There are two types:

- Benchtop steam sterilizers: use for sterilization of unwrapped, solid instruments for immediate use.
- Benchtop vacuum steam sterilizers: (preferred type): use for sterilizing bagged instruments (for future use) and items with narrow lumens and cavities. Packaging must conform to BS/EN 868 Parts 1 and 2.

General principles

- Clean instruments (as above) first.
- Ensure there is sufficient water (distilled or water for irrigation) in the sterilizer chamber.
- Open hinged/ratchet instruments to allow steam penetration. Place items in bag with handle nearest the closure.
- Label bag with contents, date, and sterilizer.
- Arrange items on tray/in basket to allow steam to circulate freely. Invert bowls and gallipots.
- Use an appropriate process indicator.

Table 3.1 Risk categories of decontamination

Risk Category	Indication	Examples	Decontamination level	Method
Low	Items used on intact skin	Wash bowls, commodes, ear syringe nozzles	Clean	Detergent and hot water; dry
Medium	Items that have contact with mucous membranes or are contaminated with micro-organisms that are easily transmitted	Vaginal specula	Disinfected or sterile	Autoclave or single-use
High	Items that penetrate skin or mucous membranes or that enter sterile sites	Surgical instruments, needles, syringes	Sterile	Hospital CSSD; bench top autoclave and use sterile; purchase of single-use disposables

- Close door, select, and start cycle. Enter date, time, cycle details etc. in the log book.
- Examine cycle printout to ensure satisfactory cycle and keep record.
- Unpackaged items—use immediately or keep clean and dry and covered with a sterile field until needed.
- Packaged items—check integrity of packaging; store clean and dry.
- Ensure stock rotation.

Decontamination prior to inspection, service, and repair

All medical equipment must be decontaminated before being sent for inspection, service, or repair. A certificate must be completed detailing the method of decontamination prior to work being carried out.

Equipment loan stores

Loan stores are responsible for collection, decontamination, maintenance, calibration, storage, and dispatch of loan equipment. Should be equipped with manual and automated cleaning, disinfection, and sterilization facilities. Thermal decontamination preferred but disinfectants sometimes required for bulky or heat-sensitive items.

Single-use items must not be re-processed unless the reprocessor can ensure the integrity and safety of the item.

Related topic

📖 Use of chemical disinfectants.

Further information for health professionals

DoH (2000). *HSC 2000/032. Decontamination of Medical Devices.* DoH, London.
Medical Devices Agency (2000). *Guidance on the Purchase, Operation and Maintenance of Vacuum Benchtop Steam Sterilizers.* MDA DB 2000(05). DoH, London.
NHS Estates (1994/95). *Sterilization. Health Technical Memorandum 2010.* HMSO, London.
NHS Management Executive Health Service Guidelines HSG (93) 26 (1993). *Decontamination of Equipment Prior to Inspection, Service or Repair.* DoH, London.

Personal protective equipment (PPE)

Personal protective equipment (PPE) is worn to protect nurses' clothing, skin, and mucous membranes from contamination with the patient's blood, body fluids, secretions or excretions and to reduce the transmission of micro-organisms between patients and staff. All must be provided by the employer, includes; aprons, gloves, masks, eye visors/goggles

Use: based on an assessment of the risk of contamination.

Plastic aprons

Plastic aprons must be worn when assisting patients with toileting, bathing, or any activity that could disperse pathogens and/or procedures which cause splashing of blood or body fluids.

Gloves

Never a substitute for appropriate hand washing. Gloves must be worn for invasive procedures, contact with sterile sites and non-intact skin or mucous membranes, and all activities that have been assessed as carrying a risk of exposure to blood, body fluids, secretions or excretions, or to sharp or contaminated instruments. Used correctly, they can:
- Prevent gross contamination of nurses' hands.
- Reduce transmission of micro-organisms to patients during invasive or other patient care (e.g. wound care).
- Protect the skin against hazardous substances, e.g. chemicals.

Types of gloves: rubber, latex, nitrile neoprene, vinyl, sterile, and unsterile. Powdered gloves and polythene gloves should not be used for health-care activities. Double-gloving is recommended for procedures associated with a high risk of glove tear or percutaneous injury.

Latex: some resistance to puncture and resealing properties, more appropriate for procedures involving the handling of sharp instruments. NB Latex allergy is on the increase.

After gloves removed: hands must be washed because:
- They do not eliminate hand contamination completely.
- They may be punctured.
- Hands are easily contaminated as gloves are taken off.

Medical gloves must comply with British Standard EN455 and European Community (CE) standards.

Disposal of aprons and gloves
- Aprons and gloves are single-use items that must be disposed of at the end of individual patient care.
- Depending on the procedures being performed, may need to be changed inbetween care activities on the same patient.
- Gloves and aprons must be discarded as clinical waste.
- Gloves must never be washed or disinfected and reused as the soap solution can cause glove damage.

Tabards

If these are used as aprons they are not water repellent and, when wet, micro-organisms pass through them easily. If worn, they must be laundered to prevent cross-infection (see Work clothes/uniforms below 📖).

Fluid repellent gowns: full-length, fluid repellent gowns must be worn where there is a risk of extensive splashing of blood, body fluids, secretions or excretions onto the skin.

Face masks and eye visors/goggles

Should be worn when there is a risk of blood, body fluids, secretions or excretions splashing into the face and eyes, e.g. respiratory suction, if excessive secretions are present; obstetric procedures. Eyewear should conform to British Standard BS7028.

Respiratory protective equipment

A particulate filter mask must be used when clinically indicated, e.g. caring for a patient with highly infectious respiratory disease.
• High-efficiency respirator masks are occasionally needed when caring for patients with infections transmitted by droplet nuclei in the air, e.g. multi-drug resistant tuberculosis (MDRTB). (Severe acute respiratory syndrome (SARS) 📖.)

Work clothes/uniforms

• During patient procedures clothes/uniforms become contaminated by organisms such as MRSA, *Clostridium difficile*, and glycopeptide-resistant enterococci (GRE). Even if not visibly soiled, contact transfer of bacteria from clothes/uniforms to patients is possible.
• To minimize risks of cross-infection, uniforms and own clothes should be washed at temperatures to achieve thermal disinfection in the laundering process, i.e. 65°C for the first part of wash cycle. Lycra or polyester fabrics may not withstand such temperatures. Dry quickly and iron. NB If the employer does not provide a free laundry service for uniforms, nurse can claim tax relief for cleaning costs.
• Shoes should envelop the feet, be non-slip, and provide support. Sandals and clogs may be inadequate protection against sharp objects.

Related topic
📖 MRSA

Further information for health professionals and patients

Health and Safety at Work Act (1974). HMSO, London.
▣ NICE (2003). *Infection Control. Prevention of Healthcare-Associated Infection in Primary and Community Care*. Clinical Guideline 2. NICE, London. www.nice.org.uk
Personal Protective Equipment at Work Regulations (1992), and Workplace (Health and Safety and Welfare) Regulations (1992), Health and Safety Executive Series, HMSO, London.
▣ Royal College of Nursing. *Guidance On Uniforms And Clothing Worn In The Delivery Of Patient Care*. RCN, London. www.rcn.org
Wilson, J. (2006). *Infection Control in Clinical Practice* (3rd edn.) Elsevier, London.

Occupational exposure to blood-borne viruses

Occupational exposure to blood born viruses (BBVs) is unnecessarily common. Many exposures result from a failure to follow recommended procedures, including safe handling and disposal of needles and syringes, or wearing personal protective eyewear where indicated (Personal protective equipment 📖). Risk for HIV transmission after exposure to HIV-infected blood in health-care settings is about 3 per 1000 injuries for percutaneous exposure and 1 in 1000 after mucotaneous exposure. There is no risk of HIV transmission where intact skin is exposed to HIV-infected blood. Every employer should have a policy on the management of occupational exposures to BBV such as HIV, HBV, and HCV. All nurses must have immediate, 24-hrs access to advice through either:

- An occupational health service
- Out-of-hours cover provided by accident and emergency departments.

Increased risk of BBV exposure associated with:

- Deep injury
- Visible blood on the device which caused the injury
- Injury with a needle which had been placed in the source patient's artery or vein
- Terminal HIV-related illness in the source patient.

Any person significantly exposed to risk of occupationally acquired HIV infection, should be assessed and managed according to the guidance issued by the Expert Advisory Group on AIDS (EAGA). This includes relatives and friends providing care in the home, as well as nurses. If a child is exposed, specialist advice from a paediatrician with experience in the HIV field should be sought.

The following types of exposure are associated with significant risk:

- Percutaneous injury (from needles, instruments, bone fragments, significant bites which break the skin)
- Exposure of broken skin abrasions, cuts, eczema etc.
- Exposure of mucous membrane including the eye.

Post-exposure prophylaxis (PEP)

PEP following exposure to HIV consists of a combination of antiretroviral drugs which, if necessary, should be started within the hour and should normally be continued for 4wks. PEP may still be considered even if up to 2wks have elapsed since the exposure. Exposed nurses should be encouraged to:

- Provide a baseline blood sample for storage up to 2yrs and a follow-up sample for testing.
- Seek psychological support.
- Report any sickness absence associated with adverse effects of PEP drugs following an occupational exposure does not contribute to an individual's sickness absence record.

Nurses who have acquired HIV infection because of exposure to HIV-infected material in the workplace may be able to claim Industrial Injuries Disablement Benefit.

PEP for patients may be required:
- Following an exposure-prone procedure performed by nurse unaware of his/her HIV status.
- In the unlikely event that an invasive device or product contaminated by use on one patient is accidentally re-used on another patient.

Where either of the above incidents occurs, the following should be performed:
- The procedure should be stopped as soon as reasonably practicable.
- If relevant, wash and dress the wound and stem the bleeding.
- Report the incident to the clinical supervisor or line manager or according to local policies.
- Ensure that, in accordance with local policy the occupational health department, infection control officer or other nominated individuals are informed without delay and appropriate treatment offered.
- Complete an accident/incident form.

Related topics
📖 HIV; 📖 Sharps injuries; 📖 Hepatitis.

Further information for health professionals and public
UK Health Departments. (1998). *Guidance for Clinical Health Care Workers: Protection Against Infection with Blood-borne Viruses. Recommendations of the Expert Advisory Group on AIDS and the Advisory Group on Hepatitis.* (HSC 1998/063). TSO, London.

UK Health Departments. (1998). *AIDS/HIV Infected Health Care Workers: Guidance on the Management of the Infected Health Care Workers and Patient Notification.* (HSC 1998/226). TSO, London. Revised guidance currently out for consultation.

🖥 UK Health Departments. (2004). *HIV Post-Exposure Prophylaxis. Guidance from the UK Chief Medical Officers' Expert Advisory Group on AIDS.* TSO, London. www.advisory bodies.doh. gov.uk/eaga/publications.htm

Use of chemical disinfectants

Chemical disinfection is an unreliable process. Most are not active against all micro-organisms, should only be used when heat disinfection is not possible and cleaning with hot, soapy water is insufficient (Cleaning, disinfection, and sterilisation of equipment 📖). Chemicals should always be used with reference to the COSHH regulations (Health and safety at work 📖)

Rules for chemical disinfection

- First clean article with hot, soapy water, rinse, and dry.
- Measure the dilution and immerse the article completely in the solution, expel all air bubbles.
- Soak the article for specified length of time.
- Ensure aqueous disinfectants e.g. chlorhexidene 0.05 are sterile.
- Where possible use single dose sachets.
- Discard containers of aqueous solutions within 24hrs of opening/use.

Some chemical disinfectants and use

- *Alcohol:* ethanol (industrial methylated spirit, IMS), isopropanol (ISP).
  - Does not penetrate protein-based organic matter, only use on clean surfaces and clean, intact skin.
  - Hand disinfection (see Hand hygiene 📖).
  - Prior to injections. Alcohol impregnated wipes. Allow alcohol to evaporate before injecting.
- *Chlorhexidene.* Good spectrum of activity against *Staphylococci spp.*
  - Umbilicus of newborns. Ster-zac powder chlorhexidene acetate 1% powder used to reduce staphylococcal colonization and infection.
- *Hypochlorites* (and other chlorine-based disinfectants) e.g. bleach, Milton.
  - Easily inactivated by organic matter; corrosive; harmful chlorine gas is released if mixed with large volumes of acidic substances, e.g. urine.
  - *Blood spillages (<30ml).* Treat with chlorine-releasing agent e.g. dichlorocyanurate (NaDCC 1%,) 10 000 parts per million available. Sprinkle granules on spill (do not use on fabrics or carpets), leave for 3min, absorb into paper towel, discard in yellow plastic bag as infectious waste, wipe the surface area with fresh hypochlorite 0.1%, 1000 ppm av. Cl., rinse with clean water, dry.
  - *Blood spillages (>30ml).* Absorb into paper towels then proceed as above.
  - *Spills on carpets:* absorb into paper towels then wash area with hot, soapy water.
  - *Home deliveries:* protect carpet and furnishings with a fluid-repellent, disposable covering.
  - *Babies' bottles* (Bottle feeding and weaning 📖) wash with hot soapy water and rinse, heat disinfection by boiling best, otherwise immerse in hypochlorite 0.0125% 125ppm av.Cl 1h, make up fresh solution daily (NB Milton disinfects it does not sterilize).

Decontamination of the environment, e.g. floors, furniture

Rarely indicated. May be necessary to help control outbreaks of Noro-virus in schools and nursing homes. Use hypochlorite 0.1%, 1000 ppm av Cl. Do not use on carpets and soft furnishings.

Chemical disinfection of heat sensitive equipment

E.g. endoscopes: Peracetic Acid. This peroxygen compound kills bacteria, fungi, and viruses rapidly and bacterial spores within 10 min, e.g. Nu-Cidex, Steris®. Strong smell, irritant to skin and mucous membrane. Only use in area with exhaust ventilation.

Equipment used on patients with vCJD

No attempt should be made to disinfect or sterilize reusable instruments or protective clothing. Quarantine pending incineration. Single-use items must be used where possible.

Related topic

📖 Hand hygiene.

Further information for health professionals

▨ Health & Safety Executive (2002). *Control of Substances Hazardous to Health Regulations. Approved Code of Practice and Guidance.* 4th edn. HSE Books, London. www.hsebooks.co.uk

Hoffman, P., Bradley, C., Ayliffe, GAJ. (2004). *Disinfection in Healthcare* (3rd edn.) Blackwell Publishing, Oxford.

Hand hygiene

Hand washing is the single, most important practice to prevent health care-associated infection.

Risk assessment

To help decisions about when to wash your hands and what to use before patient contact. Assess:
- Risk of infection to the patient
- The susceptibility of the site to infection
- The nature of the activity.

After patient contact. Assess:
- The risk of infection to self, to others e.g. family members
- The extent and type of contamination resulting from the activity.

Types of hand washing

Social handwash: use soap to remove transient micro-organisms, dirt, and organic matter. Apply to wet hands. Essential before preparing/food and drink and after using toilet facilities.

Aseptic handwash: use antiseptic detergent solution e.g. chlorhexidine gluconate 4%; triclosan 2% to remove most transient micro-organisms and most resident micro-organisms. Apply to wet hands. Essential before invasive procedures.

Hand rub: use alcohol rubs, gels, foams etc. to disinfect *clean hands*. Rub hands together vigorously, covering all surfaces, until all the alcohol has evaporated. Useful during aseptic technique and in the patient's home where hand washing facilities may be limited. Alcohol hand rubs do not reliably remove spores from the hands. *Do not* use when caring for patients with *Clostridium difficile* or after handling faeces or faecally contaminated equipment.

Additional factors to reduce cross infection

- Finger nails: short and no false nails.
- Rings: staff who wear rings have higher numbers of organisms on their hands than those who do not. Ensure wash under ring as often heavily colonised with Gram negative organisms.
- Cuts and abrasions: cover with waterproof dressings.
- Staff with skin infections e.g. boils and exfoliative skin conditions (e.g. psoriasis, eczema) should seek advice from OH.
- Hair: wear so that it does not need readjustment as this contaminates hands.
- Carers/relatives: remind them to wash their hands on completion of care and after contact with a patient with an infection.

Further information for professionals

National Institute for Clinical Excellence. (2003). *Infection Control. Prevention of Healthcare-Associated Infection in Primary and Community Care*. Clinical Guideline 2. NICE, London. www.nice.org.uk

Wilson, J. (2006). Infection Control in Clinical Practice (3rd edn.) Elsevier, London.

Infectious disease notifications

Since the beginning of the 19th century certain infectious diseases have been notifiable. The statutory process aims to ensure:
- Speed in identifying possible outbreaks and epidemics
- Prevention of spread of infectious disease.

The specific diseases are selected for notification because they are:
- Potentially life threatening
- Spread rapidly
- Cannot be easily treated.

Occasionally notification is used to monitor success of immunization programmes and the development of localized outbreaks.

If a GP becomes aware/suspects that a patient has a notifiable disease or is suffering from food poisoning (📖) there is a statutory duty in England and Wales to notify the 'Proper Officer' (usually the Medical Consultant for environmental health or Consultant in communicable disease control): for local contact details Health Protection Agency www.hpa.org.uk

The information must include (form available from LA PCO, HA, if urgent action required information should be phoned/faxed):
- Name, age and sex of patient.
- Address where patient is.
- Details of disease or poisoning and date of onset.
- Other relevant information (e.g. if individual has been abroad).

Table 3.2 Notifiable diseases

• Acute encephalitis	• Meningitis	• Scarlet fever
• Acute poliomyelitis	• Meningococcal	• Smallpox
• Anthrax	• Pneumococcal	• Tetanus
• Cholera	• Haemophilus influenzae	• Tuberculosis
• Diphtheria	• Viral	• Typhoid fever
• Dysentery	• Other specified	• Typhus fever
• Food poisoning	• Unspecified	• Viral haemorrhagic fever
• Leptospirosis	• Meningococcal septicaemia (without meningitis)	• Viral hepatitis
• Malaria	• Mumps	• Hepatitis A
• Measles	• Ophthalmia neonatorum	• Hepatitis B
	• Paratyphoid fever	• Hepatitis C
	• Plague	• Whooping cough
	• Rabies	• Yellow fever
	• Relapsing fever	*Leprosy is also notifiable, but directly to the Health Protection Agency
	• Rubella	

In Scotland, health-care providers and other agencies should report to NHS organizations who are required to notify the Common Services Agency who inform Health Protection Scotland (see below).

Schools

Ofsted inspectorate for children and learners in England, should be notified of:

- Any food poisoning affecting 2 or more children.
- Any child having meningitis or the outbreak on the premises of any notifiable disease identified as such in the Public Health (Control of Disease) Act 1984 or because the notification requirement has been applied to them by regulations (the relevant regulations are the Public Health (Infectious Diseases) Regulations 1988).

Related topic

📖 Infectious disease exclusion times.

Further information for health-care professionals

▣ Health Protection Agency: www.hpa.org.uk
▣ Health Protection Scotland: www.hps.scot.nhs.uk

Managing health-care waste

Disposal of clinical waste

Part of an employer's overall health and safety management system. Staff training is essential. The organization should have access to a dedicated qualified waste manager.

The following represents 'best practice'. If not followed should demonstrate that equivalent steps are being taken to comply with legislation.

Key changes

'The Unified Approach' is a new methodology for identifying and classifying infectious and medicinal wastes that complies with health and safety, carriage, and waste regulations.

- Clinical waste is classified as 'hazardous waste' and should be transported as an infectious substance.
- An 'offensive' waste stream describes non-infectious wastes.
- A revised colour-coded waste segregation and packaging system enables standardization across the UK.
- Use of European Waste Catalogue (EWC) codes to classify waste which are now mandatory for all waste transfer documentation.

The following types of waste are considered here: domestic waste, infectious waste (2 types); offensive waste, sharps (see Table 3.3).

Identification of infectious waste

Only waste generated from health-care practice undertaken by a suitably qualified health professional will be considered infectious waste. Soiled waste e.g. sanitary products, plasters are not considered to be infectious.

- Bodily fluids that may be infectious: blood, semen, vaginal secretions.
- Non-infectious bodily fluids: faeces, nasal secretions, sputum, tears, urine, vomit. NB These may be considered infectious if they contain visible blood or the source patient has been assessed as having an infection that might be transmitted via the waste i.e. an infection pathway exists, e.g. faeces known/suspected of contamination with enteric pathogens such as *Salmonella spp.* or *Shigella spp.* or vomit from patient with acute vomiting virus.

Collection of waste

- Frequency of collection:
    - Infectious waste: weekly.
    - Sharps bins: no less than 3mths.
- Waste transfer note. Required to keep track of the waste.
- Producer notification. All sites producing hazardous waste including health-care centres and GP practices, are required to notify the Environment Agency. Can be done through the PCO.
- Registered waste carriers. Community nurses and those working in home health care; health-care providers' vehicles carrying waste generated by them are exempt from registration procedures.

Table 3.3 Waste categories, colour coding, and disposal required

Waste category	Receptacle/ colour coding	Examples of contents	Minimum treatment/disposal required
Domestic waste	Bag Black or clear	General refuse incl. newspapers, flowers etc.	Landfill
Infectious waste	Bag Orange	Infectious and potentially infectious waste e.g. soiled dressings. Autoclaved laboratory waste.	Licensed/permitted treatment facility
Infectious waste	Bag Yellow	Infectious waste including theatre and anatomical waste.	Hazardous waste incineration
Offensive waste	Bag Yellow with black stripes	Incontinence pads, nappy bins, sanitary wastes etc. from human hygiene; animal faeces; non-infectious disposable equipment, bedding, gowns, plaster casts.	Landfill
Sharps	Bin	Not contaminated with cytotoxic products. Sharps from phlebotomy.	Licensed/permitted treatment facility
Sharps	Bin	Contaminated with cytotoxic and/or cytostatic medicinal products	Hazardous waste incineration

EU policy promotes the following
- Waste reduction and prevention.
- Reusable/recyclable products.
- Reduction of disposal of waste to landfills.
- The use of cleaner technologies.
- Energy recovery.
- An integrated network of waste management facilities.

Think Green. What can you do to minimize waste?

Further information

Department of Food & Rural Affairs (DEFRA). *Waste Management, The Duty of Care: A Code of Practice.* London. TSO: www.defra.gov.uk

▣ Environment Agency (EA): www.environment-agency.gov.uk

▣ Health & Safety Executive (HSE): www.hse.gov.uk

Health Services Advisory Committee. (1999). *Safe Disposal of Clinical Waste.* Health & Safety Commission, London.

Lawrence, J., and May, D. (2003). *Infection Control in the Community.* Churchill Livingstone, London.

▣ National Institute for Clinical Excellence. (2003). *Infection Control. Prevention of Healthcare-Associated Infection in Primary and Community Care.* Clinical Guideline 2. NICE, London. www.nice.org.uk

Sharps injuries

Sharps include needles, blades, suture cutters, broken glass. Sharps injuries are a major cause of transmission of BBVs and should be treated as a serious event however many go unreported.

> ❶ All staff at risk of sharps injuries should have up to date hepatitis B vaccination

Prevention of sharps injuries

- Needle safety devices (devices built into the needle manufacture to reduce risk of needlestick injuries e.g. by creating a barrier between needle and user's hand) must be provided where there are clear indications that they will provide safer systems of working for nurses.
- Sharps containers that conform to UN3291 and BS 7320 standards must be used.
- Sharps must not be passed directly from hand to hand.
- Handling should be kept to a minimum.
- Needles must not be recapped, bent or broken or disassembled after use or disposal.
- Containers in public areas must be located in a safe position, and must not be placed on the floor.
- Used sharps must be disposed of into a sharps container at the point of use by the user.
- Containers must not be filled above the mark that indicates that they are full.
- Where a patient uses sharps as part of their self treatment they are responsible for safe disposal. They can arrange for LA to collect sharps bins for disposal.

Carriage of sharps containers in cars by Community Staff

No specific guidance available but practice should conform to the requirements of the Carriage of Dangerous Goods Regulations (1996). The employer should agree practice with the infection control committee. The car should be securely locked when unoccupied and the sharps container kept out of site.

Disposal: containers must be disposed of by the licensed route in accordance with local policy.

Sharps injuries

Immediately following ANY exposure—whether or not the source is known to pose a risk of infection:

- The site of exposure, e.g. wound or non-intact skin should be washed liberally with soap and water, but without scrubbing.
- Free bleeding of puncture wounds should be encouraged gently but wounds should not be sucked.
- If there has been a splash into mucous membranes, including conjunctivae, these should be irrigated copiously with water, before and after removing contact lenses.

- The nurse must know how to access urgent advice about occupational exposure and PEP for HIV. (See Occupational exposure to blood-borne viruses 📖.)
- Accidental exposure to blood or body fluids must be reported through the employers incident/accident reporting system (Health and safety at work 📖).

Related topics

📖 Occupational exposure to blood-borne viruses; 📖 HIV and AIDs; 📖 Hepatitis.

Further information

Lawrence, J., and May, D. (2003). *Infection Control in the Community*. Churchill Livingstone, London.
📖 National Institute for Clinical Excellence. (2003). Infection Control. Prevention of Healthcare-Associated Infection in Primary and Community Care. Clinical Guideline 2. NICE, London.
www.nice.org.uk

Approaches to individual health needs assessment

See also 📖 The assessment of children, young people, and families

Individual health needs assessment

Systematic assessment of need is one of the core skills of primary care and community nurses, and has the potential to substantially affect a person's quality of life. The purpose of assessment at an individual level is to create an agreed care/action plan. In addition, aggregated data informs population Health needs assessment (🕮) and Commissioning of services (🕮). High quality comprehensive assessment is the means by which individual's access care and services are tailored to their needs. Assessment strategies are influenced by:

- The problem-solving framework of the nursing process
  (i.e. assessment, planning, implementation, evaluation).
- Nursing models, theories, and values (e.g. focus on ADLs, self-care, health promotion).
- Specialism (e.g. HV, DN, GPN, SN) and client group (older people, adult, children).
- National and local policy e.g. Single Assessment Process for assessing older people, Common Assessment Frameworks for assessing a child and family in need.
- Electronic patient/client records and databases often dictate how assessment data is collected, recorded and shared.

Principles

- Assessment is one part of case/care management (Case/care management models 🕮).
- Assessment should incorporate a sense of a person's own rating of health status and focus on the needs of the individual and their carers. What is available from the service should *not* limit the assessment.
- Objective, quantifiable plus subjective, client-focused data are both important for a rounded assessment.
- Assessment includes the extent and ways identified needs/problems are already addressed, plus the factors that ameliorate or reduce the impact of problems/needs.
- It should lead to the identification of agreed needs/problems for which an action/care plan is agreed with the patient/client.
- Assessment and needs/problems identification provides the basis for selection of nursing interventions and referrals to other professionals/organizations.
- Taking a nursing health history depends on highly developed communication and interpersonal skills (Principles of good communication 🕮).
- After implementation of the care/action plan, further assessment serves to evaluate outcome and effect as well as identify new problems/needs.

Most individual health needs assessment will include biographical profile, physiological, psychological, sociocultural, developmental, and spiritual domains.

Values models and in assessment

At an individual level, theories of need have largely provided the basis for primary care nurses to understand how patients respond. These include:

- Maslow's[1] hierarchy of needs suggest lower level needs must be met before higher. Physiological → safety → belonging → esteem → self-actualization.
- Bradshaw's[1] typology of the perceptions of need. Identified as 1. normative (that accepted as the 'norm' in society) needs, 2. felt (as stated by the individual) needs, 3. expressed (felt and acted upon in some way be the individual) needs and comparative (compared with others) needs.

Models for directing assessments by nurses in primary care include:

- Activities of Daily Living Model[2] uses the 12 activities of living as units of assessment to encourages a focus on health, rather than ill health.
- Self-care model[2]—widely used in areas of disease prevention and health promotion. Assessment based on self-care requisites and self-care deficits.
- Biomedical or diagnostic[2] model comprises history taking, physical examination and requesting clinical investigations to arrive at a clinical judgment about disease/illness and an individual's response to that. More commonly used in advanced and first-contact roles.
- Models and approaches to health promotion (📖)
- Child and family assessment frameworks (The assessment of children, young people, and families 📖).

Standardized assessment tools

Standardized assessment tools are often used for identification of specific problems e.g. mini-mental state examination for dementia.

[1] Detailed information on Maslow and Bradshaw in Harris, A. (ed). *Needs to know: Guide to Needs Assessment in Primary Care.* (1997). Churchill Livingstone, London.

[2] Detailed information on nursing models in Pearson, A., Vaughan, B., FitzGerald, M. (2005). *Nursing models for practice* (3rd edn.) Butterworth Heinemann, Edinburgh.

Care/case management models

A systematic, proactive, and cyclical care approach to caring for people who have highly complex care needs (Long-term conditions model 📖).

Approach characterized by one person (e.g. nurse, social worker, key worker) having the designated responsibility to coordinate and oversee care to ensure care is actively managed and 'joined up'.

The concept originated in USA and developed in UK in the contexts of:
- Community Care—under the NHS & Community Care Act 1990 case managers (later referred to as care managers by DH) coordinated the care of individuals with complex, multi agency needs.
- Care Programme Approach and the Mental Health Act 1983—where a mental health worker (mental health nurse or social worker) acted as case manager or key worker for patients leaving inpatient care and needing monitoring and support.
- Management of Long-term Conditions—the government's proposed framework includes the appointment of case managers/community matrons to case manage those with the most complex needs. People identified as likely to benefit include:
  - People suffering with chronic disease and/or long-term conditions.
  - People with learning disabilities or enduring mental illness.
  - Older people with high health service use and/or co morbidity and polypharmacy.
  - Older people at risk of hospitalization.

A case/care management approach involves:
- Targeting/case finding—based on pro-active outreach and set referral criteria that identifies individuals likely to benefit from case management.
- Assessment of the individual's problems and need for services using information from patient, carers, and other services involved in care. May include physical assessment and diagnosis.
- Care planning and securing care—to address the agreed needs and formation of an action plan involves coordinating interventions, making referrals, may have a clinical input.
- Implementation of plan (either by direct care or by coordinating care).
- Monitoring and review of plan, regular review, monitoring and consequent adaptation of the care plan leading to either discharge from care or continuing care.

Models of case management
- Brokerage model—where the case manager is an independent client advocate, linking services to needs. Largely confined to USA.
- Cultural tradition and focus of a discipline and/or clinical speciality e.g. district nursing, rehabilitation.
- Social entrepreneurship model—where the case manager is agency based and holds a budget for purchasing tailored packages of care for clients. Emerged as a social care model.

- Clinical and/or care coordination model—where the case manager is a member (or members) of an existing multidisciplinary team and assumes responsibility for arranging and monitoring care for specific clients. Often a preferred health model.
- In legislatively agreed systems led by social services/social work.
- As specialist posts for the case management of people with multiple conditions e.g. community matrons.
- As clinical specialists with dedicated case loads that support people with particular diseases and/or conditions e.g. diabetes, MS.

Nurses assuming a case management/community matron role

Additional preparation and mentoring may be needed in:
- Advanced clinical and diagnostic skills
- Independent/supplementary prescribing and medicines management
- Management of exacerbations of illness
- Information management
- Coordination across primary and 2°
- Management of cognitive impairment
- Management of care at end of life
- Health promotion and patient empowerment.

DH/Skills for Health have produced competency statements for case managers and community matrons available on the DH (England) web site in the long-term conditions section (Useful websites 📖).

Related topic

📖 Integrated (or single) assessment processes.

Further information

📓 NSF for long-term conditions: www.dh.gov.uk/PolicyAndGuidance/HealthAndSocialCareTopics/LongTermConditions

Integrated (or single) assessment processes

For child and family assessment, see 📖 The assessment of children, young people, and families.

Assessment of need for social care

Under the provision of the NHS and Community Care Act 1990, assessment of need for community care is the duty of local authorities and specifically social services (📖). NB there is not an equivalent duty to *provide* services. Locally determined finite resources determine availability of public funding for services. The purpose of the assessment is to establish needs for the provision of means tested services according to eligibility criteria (which may be provided by a range of LA, voluntary and/or private providers). Provision of services may include:

- Support to people in their home: by providing domiciliary care (e.g. social home carers), day care (e.g. day centres) and respite care.
- Services for carers (Carers assessment and support 📖).
- Provide adaptations to housing (Homes and housing 📖).
- Assessment for long-term care and related funding (Care homes 📖).

Integrated health and social care assessment processes

Integrated health and social care assessment processes for adults in need are being promoted by all UK countries i.e. integrated between disciplines, agencies and organizations. The procedures are similar to England where it is called the Single Assessment Process (SAP), first outlined in NSF for Older People (see below). The purpose of a SAP is:

- To ensure that older people receive appropriate, effective, and timely responses to health and social needs.
- The scale and depth of the assessment is kept in proportion to older people's needs.
- To ensure that agencies do not duplicate each other's assessments.
- Ensure professionals contribute to the assessment in the most effective way.

Many areas are developing shared electronic records between health services and social services for the SAP.

Four types of assessment

- **Contact** (where significant needs are first identified or suspected, a simple/or single need is addressed).
- **Overview** (if a more rounded assessment is required).
- **In-depth or specialist** (specific problems explored in detail).
- **Comprehensive** (exploration of most or all domains (Individual health needs assessment 📖) and level of support required will be intensive or complex).

Nurse's role—may contribute to all 4 types of assessment. May have an important role in coordinating assessment and care planning, where a number of agencies are involved. Nurses may also be a named case/care manager (see Case/care management models 📖).

Assessment tools and accreditation

Organizations are free to develop their own shared assessment tools. The domains will include the user perspective, clinical background, disease prevention, activities of daily living, relationships, housing and environment, physical well-being and senses, mental health, safety, and current resources. There are 6 accredited tools that can be used for assessment although NHS and Social Care in England:

- CAT: Cambridgeshire Assessment Tool
- EASY Care: University of Sheffield
- FACE: Functional Assessment of the Care Environment of Older People
- MDS: Minimum Data Set for Home Care
- NOAT: Northamptonshire Overview Assessment Tool
- STEP: Standardized Assessment of Elderly in Primary Care.

These assessment tools may incorporate or add on specialized assessment tools. All assessment processes lead to a statement of agreed needs/problems and statements about the agreed care plan/action plan, with review dates (see Case/care management models 📖).

Each LA (and PCO) publishes information about services and eligibility for services.

Related topic

📖 Long-term conditions model; 📖 IT and electronic records.

Further information

📘 Centre for Policy on Ageing Professional Development and Learning Materials for SAP: www.cpa.org.uk/sap/sap

📘 Single Assessment Process website includes links to accredited tools and examples of best practice: www.dh.gov.uk/PolicyAndGuidance/HealthAndSocialCareTopics/SocialCare/Single AssessmentProcess

Standardized assessment tools for adults

A range of tools, scales, and interview schedules can complement clinical practice. Standardized assessment tools for specific problems can:
- Help identify their severity, associated risk, and the need for health and social care services, aiding equitable allocation of resources.
- More accurately inform the commissioning of services.
- Ensure problems and conditions can not be missed e.g. depression and early onset of dementia, diabetes, hypertension, carer stress etc.

Standardized assessment tools can be used as part of an integrated (or single) assessment process, in nursing assessments (see Models of individual health assessment 📖) and used in health promotion consultations (Healthy ageing 📖). NB many specific assessment tools are given in relevant topics e.g. impact of caring (see Carers assessment and support 📖), pressure sore assessment.

Other useful standardized adult assessment tools
Mental health assessment
- Depression (People with depression 📖). 🖳 15-item Geriatric depression scale (GDS). 🖳 Geriatric Depression Scale is available at: www.jr2.ox.ac.uk/geratol/GDSdoc.htm
    - Easy to administer, well validated in home and clinical environments and for evaluating the clinical severity of depression, and therefore for monitoring treatment.
- Dementia (People with dementias 📖). 🖳 Mini-mental State Examination (MMSE) available at www.aaaonline.org.uk
    - Screening test for cognitive impairment that estimates severity of cognitive impairment at a given point.
    - Useful in following the course of cognitive changes in an individual over time.
    - Documents an individual's response to treatment.

Assessment of ADLs and physical dependency
Barthel index measure of physical ability originally developed in hospital but widely used to assess physical disability and ability to perform ADL (NB underestimates impact of cognitive impairment). Scored out of 20 where 14 indicates some disability. An example can be found on www.strokecenter.org/trials/scales/barthel.pdf

Further information for professionals, patients, and carers
🖳 Alzheimer's society: www.alzheimers.org.uk Information sheets for people and their carers
🖳 Social Care Institute for Excellence has information on relevant mental health standardized tools for older people: www.scie.org.uk

Principles of good communication

Communicating is a fundamental social need, important in developing and maintaining patient trust and confidence. Patient-centred care and shared decision-making are key NHS objectives and the following principles help achieve them:

• Know the subject
• Know the audience
• Get the message across effectively
• Look for and act on responses.

The following are important:

• The way in which you greet the patient and introduce yourself sets the level at which your relationship will continue.
• Maintain reasonable eye contact and sit comfortably towards your patient.
• People differ in the ways that they communicate. Some may need more time from you than others.
• Read and acknowledge both the verbal and non-verbal cues the patient sends.
• People sometimes find it hard to face facts or to hear clearly what you are saying. It may be necessary to say clearly what the situation is and what needs to be done.
• People remember most accurately the first thing that you say, and 20% of what they hear overall. If you have something particularly important to say, this may need to be highlighted.
• It may be helpful to offer a leaflet to illustrate what you are saying, or to illustrate your message with a diagram.
• Sharing your thoughts with the patient is one of the skills that can be helpful in a shared decision-making process.

With children

• Adjust how you communicate to take account of child's age, ability and maturity.
• Open ended communication works best with the young—more information is elicited by asking 'tell me about…' rather than asking direct questions like 'what did you …?'.
• Prompt, nod, smile, and encourage as necessary.

Written information for patients and their carers

Written information for patients and their carers falls into two broad categories:

• Information about services provided and how to access them.
• Clinical information about conditions, illnesses, and treatment.

Patients should be offered a copy of any letter/report written about them by clinicians. Printed material is not however a substitute for discussion between staff and patients.

PCOs and Trust communication units may have standards to which information should comply and may even have an accessible information policy.

Written information can:
- Reinforce the information given in consultations and help people remember it.
- Give more details than can be given verbally.
- Be kept for future reference.
- Be shown to others, helping patients to share the information.

Consider
- Who the target audience is (age, sex, disability, ethnic and cultural background).
- How it fits in with other information being provided.
- The formats in which it should be offered e.g. Braille, large print, translated.
- How the information will be distributed.
- Make sure that the factual content is accurate, up-to-date, and unambiguous.
- Prioritize information—include the essentials and not unnecessary or confusing details.
- Involve patients in developing information e.g. some organizations have 'Patient Reading Groups' who will consider the suitability of information produced for public use.

Further information
- The DH (England) Toolkit for producing patient information: www.dh.gov.uk/assetRoot/04/06/84/62/04068462.pdf
- The DH (England) Patient Information Bank contains over 100 patient information leaflets and factsheets. Covers common health conditions and available in 12 other languages: Punjabi, Urdu, Bengali, French, Gujariti, Somali, Arabic, Turkish, Spanish, Portuguese, Korean, and Polish: www.patientinformationbank.nhs.uk/Default.aspx
- Clinical Knowledge Summaries (PRODIGY) Patient Information Leaflets on the management of conditions: www.cks.library.nhs.uk/ClinicalGuidance/
- The 'Plain English Campaign': www.plainenglish.co.uk/ It has introduced a seal of approval—the Crystal Mark—to encourage organizations to communicate clearly with the public
- www.uwm.edu/Dept/CUTS/bench/commun.htm for principles of good communication, oral, written, and visual
- www.HealthcareSkills.nhs.uk/ offers educational opportunities to address essential learning needs of health-care professionals

Communicating with people and children with additional communication needs

Information is a crucial part of any patient journey and central to their experience of care. The way in which information is communicated takes many forms and needs to be varied depending on the patient's needs and preferences. Information includes verbal, written, signed, Braille, taped, pictorial, drama, translated etc. It is good practice to reinforce verbal communication with another method e.g. a leaflet.

PCOs and Trust communication units may proof read and provide advice on layout and design of information.

Communicating with people and children with additional communication needs

This encompasses a very broad range of patients and it is important not to make assumptions about how best to communicate with them. The need will probably be individual to each patient.

Identify with them what, if any, communication support is needed and book e.g. induction loops, palantypists (speech-to-text reporting for hearing impaired readers), Makaton (using gestures/signs with language), signers (for hearing impaired) touch signers (deafblind patients), lipspeakers (deaf person who lip reads), Braille (read by touch).

Remember
- Find a suitable place to talk, with good lighting and away from noise and distractions.
- Speak at a moderate pace, directly to the patient, even when using communication support. Don't shout.
- Use natural facial expressions and gestures.
- Use clear, simple language, avoiding jargon, ambiguity and medical terminology.
- Check throughout that you are being understood.
- Use illustrations/pictures where suitable. www.photosymbols.com/index.jsp is a useful resource.
- If the patient needs to do something, make this obvious.
- Ask whether they want to be copied reports and letters about them and in what format.

Children
In addition to the above:
- Address them as individuals
- Use plenty of illustrations
- Try to adjust your language to their age
- Do not talk down to them.

Communicating with people with a learning disability

Plan what needs to be said. Keep the client group in mind and consider whether they will be able to understand you.

Many people with learning disabilities can understand written information if they have support, especially if it is written with pictures, symbols and photos e.g. www.photosymbols.com/index.jsp Local Speech & Language Therapy services and/or the Learning Disabilities Services are useful sources of support.

- Keep sentences short. Use one clause per sentence. Try not to use conjunctions such as: but, because. Use 'and' only if you are writing a short-list e.g. pyjama, dressing gown, and towel. For longer lists, use bullet points.
- Use plain English. Avoid jargon, abbreviations or difficult words. Try to replace long words with short ones e.g. hard not difficult.
- Information should be succinct. Omit anything that is not needed or is ambiguous.
- If the patient needs to do something, make this obvious. Stress the instruction or use bold text.
- Be consistent. Use the same words and phrases even if this seems repetitive.

Written communication for people with learning disabilities

- Use figures: 5, 10, 12, for numbers, rather than words.
- Lay the text out clearly, with plenty of space.
- Use the Arial typeface and larger print—at least 14 point.
- Whole words in capitals, underlined or in italics are more difficult to read, so avoid doing this. Highlight important words in bold.
- If written information is hard to understand, consider other formats e.g. audiotapes or CDs. Meetings, where clients can ask questions, might also be appropriate.

Useful sources of information

Local interpreting/advocacy services.
- The RNIB: www.rnib.org.uk/ ☎ 020 7388 1266
- The RNID: www.rnid.org.uk/ ☎ 020 7296 8000
- British Institute of Learning Disabilities (BILD): www.bild.org.uk/

Communicating with people who have English as an additional language

This is a broad category of patients and can include people:
- Without any knowledge of English.
- Who apparently speak it well but may understand comparatively little.
- Who understand a great deal, but may be unable to speak much English.

A well-designed, legible sign system can benefit everyone by increasing people's awareness of their surroundings and helping them to get around. Videos, tapes, electronic text can also be effective ways of communicating.

In verbal communication:
- Try to ascertain how much English the patient actually understands, and consider using an interpreter or an advocate.
- Use clear, simple language.
- Address the patient directly.
- Check whether concepts and terminology, if used, can be directly translated into another language.
- Ask whether there are cultural/religious factors that need to be considered.

Interpreters translate without adding, changing or omitting anything, and:
- Will intervene and ask for clarification when needed.
- Will point out when a patient may have misunderstood something.
- Will not enter into discussion, give advice or express opinions.
- Will not take on additional work on behalf of staff/patients.

Advocates provide advice and support, and:
- Facilitate linguistic and cultural communication.
- Voice patients' concerns and expectations.
- Advise how to access health care.
- Enable patients to become informed of their rights and to make informed choices.

Best practice suggests that 'official' interpreters are most appropriate.

Remember
- Some patients e.g. political refugees may take time to trust 'official' interpreters, preferring initially to use informal interpreters. While this has limitations, not least because the person is probably not trained to interpret, the benefits to the patient might outweigh them in the short term.
- Some parents may prefer to use their children as interpreters, desiring family privacy. In general this should be discouraged because the burden of responsibility may be too great for children. Additionally they may be unequipped or too young to undertake the expected role.
- Some people may prefer a person of a particular gender to interpret for them. This should be accommodated, where possible.

It is important to reassure patients that 'official' interpreters are bound by the same confidentiality rules as other health professionals, and that the service is free to them.

Telephone interpreting can be useful in emergency situations and your organization may have a contract with one e.g. Language Line. This provides a confidential telephone interpretation service available in over 150 languages, 24hrs a day, every day of the year. (🖥 www.languageline.co.uk/).

Further sources of information

🖳 The DH Patient Information Bank contains over 100 patient information leaflets and factsheets. They cover common health conditions and are available in 12 other languages: Punjabi, Urdu, Bengali, French, Gujariti, Somali, Arabic, Turkish, Spanish, Portuguese, Korean, and Polish. www.patientinformationbank.nhs.uk/Default.aspx (for NHS net users)

Counselling skills

Counselling provides an opportunity to talk about any matter which may be causing concern. The aim of the process is to help an individual understand their situation to the point where they can see for themselves the most appropriate course of action.

Many nurses and HVs in primary care use the skills of counselling (see below) in their consultations. Some (usually with additional training/support) actively use brief counselling interventions over a number of contacts e.g. 'listening visits' with women identified with postnatal depression, solution focused brief interventions with couples with relationship problems, bereavement visits.

Model of counselling

Two main models are used by nurses and HV:

- Client centred or non-directive counselling, associated with the writings of Carl Rogers.[1] Emphasis on:
  - Unconditionally acceptance of the person.
  - Being a genuine person in the relationship.
  - Having empathic understanding of the person.
  - Being able to communicate acceptance, genuineness, and empathy in such a way that the other person can receive them.
- Problem management models associated with writings of Gerard Egan.[2] Emphasis on helping the person answer 3 main questions:
  - What is going on? (What's the story? Where are the blind spots?)
  - What do I want instead? (Preferred scenario? Realistic goals?)
  - How might I get to what I want? (What will work for you and how to get there?)

Skills in counselling

These include:

- The acceptance of individuals in a non-judgemental manner.
- Treat the person with genuine respect.
- Active listening (includes positive non-verbal body language, checking for understanding).
- Paraphrasing and summarizing.
- Reflecting and ensuring concreteness.
- Able to allow silence.
- Able to deal with the others distress.
- Able to help individual plan actions.
- Awareness of own abilities and limitations, when to refer on to others.
- Strategies for dealing with own stress.

Related topic

📖 Talking therapies.

---

[1] Rogers, C. (2003). *Person Centred Therapy*. Constable and Robinson, London.

[2] Egan, G. (2001). The Skilled Helper - a problem management approach to helping. Belmont, Calif. Wadsworth.

Further information

🖳 British Association of Counselling and Psychotherapy: www.bacp.co.uk/

Medicine management and nurse prescribing

Medicines management

The legislation for the prescription, dispensing, safe custody, and administration of medicines applies across the UK but each country's central health department determines the extent of NHS implementation for some aspects e.g. non-medical prescribing.

Non-medical prescribing

A non-medical prescriber is a health-care professional other than a doctor, who holds a registered first level qualification with their regulatory body e.g. NMC and a recordable prescribing qualification with the same body. Five types in UK:

- Nurse Independent Prescribers: from May 2006 Nurse Independent Prescribers are able to prescribe any licensed drug which lays within their field of competency from anywhere in the BNF including some controlled drugs. Those previously known as extended Formulary Nurse Prescribers have been known as Nurse Independent Prescribers from April 2006.
- Community Practitioner Nurse Prescribers: Nurses who hold a Community Specialist Practice Qualification with additional NMC recorded prescribing qualification able to prescribe from a limited formulary.
- Supplementary Prescribers: nurses, pharmacists, and designated allied health professionals with recordable qualification able to prescribe with GP or dentist (as independent prescriber) to a patient specific clinical management plan (CMP). See 🖳 Clinical management plans online www.cmponline.info/.
- Supplementary prescribers can prescribe Controlled Drugs and unlicensed medicines in partnership with a doctor, where the doctor agrees within a patient's CMP. From July 2006 chiropodists/podiatrists, physiotherapists, radiographers, and optometrists are also able to prescribe Controlled Drugs as supplementary prescribers, but only where there is a patient need and the doctor has agreed in a patient's CMP. DH (2006) Medicines Matters: see further information.
- Pharmacists independent prescribers cannot at present prescribe any Controlled Drugs independently.

All NHS employers have to keep a list and specimen signatures of their non-medical prescribers. Good practice for private sector employers to do the same. Non-medical prescribers not employed by a general practice are issued prescription pads by their employers.

Prescriptions

NHS prescriptions are made on FP10 (GP10 in Scotland) forms or computer generated and are completed giving the nurse's NMC number, and the patient's general practice code. NHS Business Services Authority (NHSBSA) records the costs from each prescription by practice and prescriber. It provides regular analysis to each practice (ePFIP) and prescriber (ePACT) for monitoring and auditing prescribing patterns. See also 📖 Prescribing.

Dispensing medication

Medicines are usually supplied (dispensed) by local pharmacists (or a dispensing GP) to the prescription and are the property of the patient.

Nurses working in specialist services may also supply medicines provided by the PCO e.g. family planning clinics, STI clinics. All dispensed medicines must be labelled with patient's name and accompanied by patient information leaflet. Local policies apply.

Administration of medicines

- In primary care most people administer their own medicines.
- Anyone can legally administer a prescribed medicine including controlled drugs to another person with their consent.
- Vulnerable and frail adults at home may be assisted in taking medicines by both nursing and home care services. Local guidance applies on division of responsibilities and mechanisms for shared record keeping.
- See also 📖 School nursing for administration of medicine in schools.
- Directions for administration by nursing staff are given in 1 of 2 ways:
  - A written patient specific direction (PSD) for a named patient. Either as directed on the patient's pharmacy supplied medicine label or through a written direction by an independent prescriber e.g. GP request. See also 📖 Controlled drugs.
  - Patient group directions (PGD) provide a legal mechanism for medicines to be supplied and/or administered by named nurses to groups of patients without prescriptions having to be written. There is specific guidance on the authorization process by a senior doctor and pharmacist. Common examples in primary care are for childhood immunizations, travel vaccines, contraceptives. 🖥 For PGD templates and examples please see www.portal.nelm.nhs.uk/PGD/default.aspx

Prescribed, supplied/administered medicines and appliances should be recorded in clinical and any personally held records.

Errors in medication dispensing or administration

- Report to prescriber.
- Consult doctor with responsibility for clinical care e.g. GP if not the prescriber.
- Report incident to line manager, complete incident and accident form in line with local policies for opportunity to learn from error and improve systems (See also Clinical risk management 📖).

The monitoring of adverse drug reactions

Any prescribers or patients can report suspected ADRs to any drug, including those self-medicated by the patient, reactions to blood products, vaccines, radiographic contrast media, and herbal products to the Medicines and Health Care products Regulatory Agency online 🖥 www.mhra.gov.uk or ☎ freephone (0800 731 6789) or yellow card in BNF.

Further information

Beckwith, S. and Franklin, P. (2006). *The Oxford Handbook of Nurse Prescribing*. Oxford University Press, Oxford.

Department of Health (2006). Medicines Matters: A guide to mechanisms for the prescribing, supply, and administration of medicines. The Stationery Office, London.

🖥 National Prescribing Centre: www.npc.co.uk

🖥 NHS Electronic Library for medicines: www.nelm.nhs.uk

🖥 NHSBSA: www.nhsbsa.nhs.uk

Medicine concordance

NHS prescriptions cost >£6 billion/yr. Estimated that people take medicines as directed to reach therapeutic effect less than ½ the time. Reasons include:
- Lack of information about their condition and the importance of treatment.
- Beliefs about medicines e.g. unnatural, should be able to manage without.
- Unwilling to tolerate side effects.
- Practical difficulties, such as getting the prescription filled, remembering to take medicines, opening containers.
- Costs of filling prescriptions.

Concordance

Concordance is defined as a partnership process between professional and patient that addresses the beliefs, experiences, and wishes of the patient as well as other factors to reach successful prescribing and medicine taking. Patients are more likely to take medicines as prescribed when they:
- Have had their condition explained so they understand and accept it, and recognize the consequences of not treating it.
- Agree with course of action and the proposed treatment.
- Have had any concerns or questions about the medicines answered.
- Have the simplest regimen e.g. od or bd that can fit with their routine.
- Have clear verbal instructions, reinforced with written instructions they can read (e.g. appropriate font size and language).
- Have an opportunity for a follow-up discussion with a professional in 2–3wks if a long-term regimen or difficult technique e.g. inhalers.
- Have an opportunity for medication review if long-term use.

Help with costs of medicines

Some medicines are cheaper bought OTC than with the prescription charge. Information on these circulated in Drugs and Therapeutics Bulleting periodically. There is also help with the cost of prescription items for people on low incomes, particular conditions and multiple medication costs.

Free prescription entitlement

Information on NHS leaflet HC11.
- Box ticked on reverse of prescription for
  - Contraception
  - >60yr, <16yr, or 16–18yr if in full-time education
  - Patient or family receiving income support or income based job seeker allowance.

Payment exemption certificates

- MatEx certificate for pregnant women, for 12 months after the EDD or women who gave birth <12mths ago.
- Medical Exemption Certificates (Medex) certificate for certain conditions, using form FP92A signed by doctor (or authorized member of practice staff). The conditions are:
  - Diabetes insipidus or other forms of hypopituitarism
  - Forms of hypoadrenalism (for example Addison's disease) for which specific substitution therapy is essential
  - A permanent fistula (for example caecostomy, colostomy, laryngostomy, or ileostomy) requiring continuous surgical dressing or requiring an appliance
  - Diabetes mellitus except where treatment is by diet alone
  - Hypoparathyroidism
  - Myasthenia gravis
  - Myxoedema
  - Epilepsy requiring continuous anticonvulsants
  - A continuing physical disability so that the person cannot go out without the help of another person. Temporary disabilities do not count even if they last for several months.

Pre-payment certificate (PPC)

May be cheaper for patients who have to pay for >5 prescription items in 4mths or 14 items in 12mths to buy PCC.
- Can only be used by applicant for own prescriptions
- Cost of PCC (2007) £26.85 for 3mths, £98.70 for 12mths
- Apply to Prescription Pricing Authority by phone 0845 850 0030 or online (see below).

Further information and support

🖻 Medicines Partnership: information and help to promote methods of concordance: www.medicines-partnership.org/

🖻 NHS Prescription Pricing Authority Help with health costs including PPC and MedEx certificates: www.ppa.org.uk/ppa/hwhc.htm

Prescribing

Prescribing a product or medicine is a complex process and has considerable impact on patients, colleagues, and the NHS in general. The NHS National Prescribing Centre (NPC) (see below) has a 7-step model for prescribing considerations:

1. Examine the holistic needs of the patient
- A thorough assessment may show that a non-drug therapy is indicated.
- A full medical, including allergies, social history and drug history including prescribed items, OTC items, homely remedies, homeopathic and herbal remedies and any ADRs.

2. Consider the appropriate strategy
- Is the diagnosis established or a GP referral indicated?
- Is a prescription needed at all or is patient expectation a factor?

3. Consider the choice of product
- Critically appraise evidence to assess a product's effectiveness.
- Consider appropriateness. Check BNF for ADRs, contraindications, special precautions, or drug interactions.
- Consider dose, formulation, and the duration of treatment.
- Does the patient require specialist consideration?
- Is there a non-proprietary (generic) named suitable product?

4. Negotiating a contract and concordance
Shared decision making between the patient and health-care professional is known as concordance. The patient needs to understand:
- What the prescription is for, how to take it, at what dose and for how long, how long it will take to work, and any side effects.
- How and who to contact if they have any concerns.

5. Reviewing the patient—consider
- Is treatment is still needed, working and still the best choice?
- Is any adjustment in the treatment needed?
- Have there been any adverse effects?
- Is the patient taking any treatment you were unaware of?
- Does the patient understand their treatment and are they taking it correctly and is the next review planned?

To avoid ADRs the NPC recommend you:
- Use as few concurrent drugs as possible and the lowest effective dose.
- Check if the patient is breast feeding or of either extreme of age.
- Know all the medication being used by the patient including OTCs and family remedies.
- Check for contraindications such as renal or hepatic impairment.
- Check if the patient has experienced a previous ADR.

6. Accurate, up-to-date records

7. Reflecting on your prescribing
Reviewing and reflecting on prescribing decisions and PACT (prescribing analysis and cost) data and SPA Scottish Prescribing Analysis (available through PCOs and practices) will help prescribing practice and knowledge base.

Prescription writing

Prescriptions should be completed as per specimen given on the inside cover of this book ensuring unused space is deleted with Z. Each prescription requires nurses NMC PIN number (to ensure correct registration) and patient's GP code (for costing to NHS prescribing budget).

Hand written prescriptions

- Write legibly, sign in ink.
- State patient's full name, address, preferably include their age and DOB (legal requirement for a child <12yrs) and date.
- The BNF recommends:
  - Avoidance of unnecessary decimal point e.g. 3mg not 3.0mg, put zero in front of unavoidable decimal point e.g. 0.5ml. Use units that give whole numbers where possible e.g. paracetamol 500mg rather than paracetamol 0.5g.
  - Units, micrograms and nanograms should not be abbreviated.
  - Use the term millilitre (ml or mL) not cubic centimetre cc or cm^3.

Computer generated prescriptions

- Must print the date of issue, the patient's surname, one forename, any other fore names as initials, address, age of those <12yrs or >60yrs.
- The prescriber's name, surgery address, telephone contact number and reference number should be printed.
- Signed in ink.

Security of NHS prescriptions

- Kept in locked drawer, not left in cars or unattended, nor signed blank.
- Any loss or suspected theft reported immediately to line manager and police.

Record serial numbers of prescriptions held so that these can be circulated if a pad is stolen.

Further information

The NHS National Prescribing Centre: www.npc.co.uk

Prescribing for special groups

Particular consideration needs to be given to the altered pharmacokinetics and pharmacodynamics of the old, very young, pregnant and breastfeeding ♀, people with reduced renal function, and people with liver disease.

Older people

- Important to recognize the diversity and individuality of older people.
- Important to assess not only the presenting problem but also:
  - Altered pharmacodynamics and kinetics (natural ageing process see below).
  - Any underlying pathologies and/or polypharmacy (4 or more medicines) ↑ the risk of drug interaction and ADRs, implicated in 5–17% of hospital admissions of people >65yrs.
  - The use of herbal remedies, 'homely remedies', and OTC medication.
  - Check for possible drug interactions and food–drug interactions.
- Common to initially prescribe at the lower end of a range of adult doses.
- Consider issues such as cognitive impairment, physical dexterity to undo containers medication is dispensed in, need for large print labels on containers, ability to swallow sold dosage forms, etc.

Altered pharmacokinetics i.e. altered ways the body processes the drug
- **Altered elimination:**
  - It is recommended to assume at least mild renal impairment (see below) when prescribing for older people. ↓ renal clearance results in slower drugs excretion and ↑ susceptibility to nephrotoxic preparations.
  - ↓ in renal clearance exacerbated by routine illnesses, such as UTI. Results in adverse effects or overdose in a patient previously stabilized on a drug with a narrow therapeutic margin (e.g. digoxin).
- **Altered absorption:**
  - Total body water ↓ = ↑ plasma levels of water soluble drugs.
  - ↓ body mass, ↓ saliva production, atrophy of intestinal epithelium, slower gastric emptying.
- **Altered distribution:**
  - ↓ reduced cardiac output, ↓ renal mass, ↓ renal blood flow.
  - ↓ plasma proteins = ↑ in 'active' free protein binding drugs.
- **Altered metabolism:**
  - ↓ hepatic blood flow decreases, first pass metabolism ↓.
  - Liver size ↓, blood flow ↓, enzyme production ↓, ↑ likelihood of toxicity with repeated doses.

Altered pharmacodynamics: i.e. altered number, specificity, and responsiveness of receptors to the drug.
- ↑ sensitivity to drugs due to changes in the responsiveness of target organs, commonly increased sensitivity to: opioid analgesics, benzo diazepines, antipsychotics, antihypotensives, and NSAIDs.
- Common adverse reactions affecting older people are gastrointestinal and haematological in nature.

Infants and children

Pharmacokinetics and pharmacodynamics are often different for children.
Key points:

- Always refer to the latest edition of the *BNF for Children*. Consult with senior clinician or specialist if in doubt. Many drugs are not licensed for children and cannot be prescribed by nurses unless as part of a clinical management plan.
- Doses are generally calculated using the child's body weight in kilograms.
- Prescribe sugar-free solutions.
- Legal requirement to write the child's age if <12yrs.
- Advise parents not to add the drug to the child's feed (there may be an interaction or the child may not complete their feed).

Pregnant women

Key points:

- Only prescribe for pregnant women when it is essential.
- Where possible, avoid prescribing for pregnant women during the first trimester.
- Prescribe drugs which have been tried and tested as safe in pregnancy.
- Appendix 4 of the BNF (latest edition) lists drugs to be avoided at which trimester during pregnancy. The absence of an entry here does not mean it is safe; it means the answer is not known.

Breast-feeding women

Key points:

- Only absolutely necessary drugs should be taken when breast feeding as may harm infant or inhibit sucking reflex or suppress lactation.
- See Appendix 5 BNF for breast feeding and drug information.

People with renal disease

Reduced renal function effects ability to excrete drugs, increase sensitivity reduce effectiveness of drug.
Key points:

- Problems can be avoided by reducing dose or using different drugs.
- Dose adjustment depends on grade of renal failure (mild, moderate, severe) measured by creatine clearance.
- Appendix 3 current BNF for a table of drugs to be avoided or used with caution/dose reduction.

People with liver disease

Liver disease may impair drug metabolism, and alter the body's response to drugs e.g. increase toxicity, and increase sensitivity. Drug prescribing kept to a minimum in severe liver disease. See Appendix 2 current BNF.

Related topic

📖 Prescribing.

Further information

- BNF & BNF for Children: www.bnf.org/bnf/children
- DoH (2001). *Medicines and Older people*. NSF, The Stationary Office, London. www.doh.gov.uk/ nsf/medicinesop
- National Prescribing Centre (2000). *Prescribing for the older person*. MeReC Bulletin vol 11 no 10. www.npc.co.uk

Principles of medication reviews

Prescribing medication is the most common medical intervention in the UK and 80% of drugs prescribed are repeat prescriptions. NSF for older people states people >75yrs should have medicines reviewed at least annually and those taking 4 plus should be reviewed 6-monthly.

A medication review is:
'a structured, critical examination of patient's medicines with the objective of optimizing the impact of therapy, minimizing the number of medication related problems and reducing waste.'

(National Medicines Management Collaboration)

There are 4 levels of medicine review

Level 0: an **ad hoc** opportunist meeting done by anyone without access to patient's notes and without the patient. Perhaps to verify name or dose of medication or as a triage to indicate patients requiring prioritisation for higher level review.

Level 1: **prescription review.** Either a *prescription intervention*, patient not present and no access to their notes, or *medicines use* here the patient is present but with no access to their notes. These may be undertaken by a community pharmacist, practice technician, or practice nurse.

Level 2: **full medication review**. Full access to the notes but the patient is not present. Undertaken by a doctor, practice assistant, nurse prescriber or specialist nurse.

Level 3: **clinical medication review**. Full access to patient's notes, patient present and consulted, all medications and all conditions reviewed. Undertaken by a doctor, practice assistant, nurse prescriber or specialist nurse.

(Only levels 2 and 3 count in QOF for reviews of repeat medication.)

Principles of medication review

- Seeks to optimize the treatment for an individual patient.
- Is undertaken in a systematic way, by a competent person.
- Any changes resulting from the review are agreed with the patient.
- The clinical medication review gives patients an opportunity to ask questions and highlight problems regarding their medicines.
- Review is documented in the patient's notes (READ codes Medication Review–8B3S or Medication review done–8B3V).
- Impact of any change is reviewed.

NO TEARS tool[1]

First principle: do no harm

N—Need and indication of the medicine. (Why prescribed? Are they still needed?)

O—Open questions (gain patients' views on how medicines used, side effects and intended effects).

T—Testing and monitoring. (Are doses at the appropriate level?)

E—Evidence and guidelines. (Any changes in EB since prescription started?)

[1] Lewis, T. (2004). No Tears Tool *studentBMJ*, **12**, 349–92.

A—Adverse events (check for interactions, duplications, or contraindications).

R—Risk reduction and prevention (update opportunistic screening e.g. risk of falls, blood pressure).

S—Simplification and switches. (Can bd or tds be replaced with od?)

Setting up a medication review system

- May be local guidance for the conduct of a medication review.
- Medicines Partnership Room for Review (see below) provides templates and checklists.
- Review systems may start with targeted population e.g. >75yrs.
- Documentation important for auditing for:
  - Clinical outcomes
  - Patient views
  - Cost effectiveness indicators
  - Quantitative data e.g. number reviewed.

Further information

DoH (2001). Medicines for Older People: *Implementing medicines-related aspects of the NSF for older people*. DoH, London.

Managing Medicines Resource Centre: www.managingmedicines.com/

Medicines Partnership—Room for Review. www.doh.gov.uk/nsf/pdfs/medicinesbooklet.pdf

www.medicines-partnership.org/medication-review

Controlled Drugs (CDs)

Under the Misuse of Drugs Regulations (2001) and subsequent amendments CDs are divided into 5 categories or schedules depending upon their potential use and misuse:

- Schedule 1. Have no medicinal use and contain hallucinogens e.g. coca leaf, mescaline.
- Schedule 2. Includes major stimulants, opiates e.g. secobarbital and amphetamine.
- Schedule 3. Minor stimulants and drugs less likely to be misused than those in schedule 2 (some can be stored on open dispensary shelves).
- Schedule 4. Split into 2 parts:
  - Part 1. Benzodiazepines plus eight other substances.
  - Part 2. Anabolic steroids.
- Schedule 5. Preparation of CDs such as morphine and codeine at lower strengths.

Following the trial of Harold Shipman in the UK, the Independent Shipman Inquiry recommended changes to current systems for prescribing dispensing, collecting and delivering CDs.

All GP practices and PCT provider organizations must have Standard Operating Procedures for ordering, storing, prescribing etc CDs.

CDs dispensed to patients are their property and responsibility. They should be advised specifically on safe, secure storage.

CD registers

- All GP practices and primary care premises where controlled drugs are stocked for dispensing or used in 'Doctors Bag' are required to maintain CD registers. This register is inspected regularly by governing bodies acting as inspecting agencies.
- It is recommended to have a CD register as good practice in care homes. It is obligatory for care homes providing nursing services if the nurse in charge of the home requisitions stock.
- Community nursing services do not hold CDs registers.

Prescribing CDs

'Nurse independent prescribers are able to prescribe the following list o CDs, solely for the medical conditions indicated:

- Diamorphine, morphine, diazepam, lorazepam, midazolam, or oxycodone for use in palliative care.
- Buprenorphine or fentanyl for transdermal use in palliative care.
- Diazepam, lorazepam, midazolam (oral, parenteral or rectal) for the treatment of tonic-clonic seizures.
- Diamorphine or morphine (oral or parenteral) for pain relief in respect of suspected myocardial infarction, or for relief of acute or severe pain after trauma including in either case post-operative pain relief.
- Chlordiazepoxide hydrochloride or diazepam (orally) for treatment of initial or acute withdrawal symptoms, caused by the withdrawal of alcohol from persons habituated to it.
- Codeine phosphate (orally), dihydrocodeine tartrate or co-pheno trope (orally)'.

DH (2006). Annex G–Controlled Drugs.
NB This list is under consultation to widen

Supplementary prescribers (SPs)

SPs can prescribe CDs providing they are prescribing within the legal parameters of an agreed clinical management plan and within the limitations of their competencies.

Writing a prescription for CDs

NB Follow the guidelines in a current BNF.

- Must always state:
  - Name and address of patient
  - The form and strength of preparation
  - Total quantity or number of dose units in words and figures
  - The dose and frequencies in full; ensure clarity of dosage instructions particularly when using syringe drivers.
- Prescription now legally limited to 30d unless exceptional circumstances which should be recorded in patient's notes. If prescription is for instalment dispensing, limited to 14d on the FP10MDA form.
- Anticipate the amount of drugs needed over a set period of time to avoid excess amounts in home.
- Prescriptions for CDs for substance misusers are written on FP10 (MDA) forms. Nurses can only do this as SPs or as independent prescribers for alcohol withdrawal.

Administration of CDs

- CDs only administered by nursing staff under specific written not verbal directions of an independent prescriber.
- Nurse independent prescribers, or nurses acting under their direction, can only administer CDs as listed opposite.
- Always record in patients' records.
- There is no legal requirement for administration to be witnessed by a second person unless as part of stock control procedures for CD register.

See also 📖 Syringe drivers.

The disposal and destruction of CDs

Patients, or their representative, should be advised to return unused/expired CDs to the local pharmacist for destruction. Care homes providing nursing care cannot at present return unused CDs to a pharmacist, but must make arrangements with a licensed waste contractor.

The transport of CDs

- Legally, nurses can transport prescribed CDs from pharmacy (requires ID and signature) to a named patient if unable to collect or return unwanted prescribed medicines. Should only be done if no alternative.
- If it is necessary to transport CDs should be in locked bag/box and kept out of sight.

Essential reading

National Prescribing Centre (2007). *A Guide to Good Practice in the Management of Controlled Drugs in Primary Care in England* 2nd edn. NPC, Liverpool.

Further information

Department of Health (2006). *Improving Patients' Access to Medicines: A Guide to Implementing Nurse and Pharmacist Independent Prescribing within the NHS in England.* DH, London.

Storage, transportation, and disposal of medicines

In the course of using medicines for therapeutic benefit it is important to comply with current legislation, follow guidance issued by the Health Departments and other Government Departments e.g. Home Office and manage the risks to patients and staff arising from the use of medicines. PCO prescribing advisors provide up to date local guidance.

Storage on community sites and general practice

Key principles:
- Each service should have standard operating procedures (including designated responsible person) for the safety and security of medicines used in it.
- Medicines which are not required for the treatment of anaphylaxis or resuscitation should always be kept locked in a cupboard or refrigerator (designated for the storage of medicines) as applicable.
- The cupboard or refrigerator must conform to British Standards (BS) 2881 (1989) NHS Estates and Building note No. 29.
- Maximum/minimum thermometers should be used to monitor the temperature of the refrigerator (usually 2°–8°C). These temperatures should be recorded each working day and records kept for 6mths.
- Medicines held for clinical emergencies should be in packs labelled as such and available in those clinical sessions, otherwise securely stored.
- CDs held as stock e.g. GP practice, legally require CD register, and to be held in fixed, locked cupboard sited away from the public. The key should be secured, never left in the cupboard door.

Storage in the patient's home

Patients' medicines are their property. Key messages to promote:
- Keep medicines in cool, dark place away from light, heat (including steam) or as directed on instructions e.g. fridge.
- Always read medicine information leaflets for storage instructions.
- Keep in original container as it has instructions, expiry date etc. If choose to use compliance devices should label contents. Some drugs are unsuitable for compliance devices if affected by light, moisture, or temperature.
- Keep out of reach and sight of children.
- Return unused drugs to pharmacy for destruction rather than domestic disposal as may harm the environment.

Administering home stored medicines
- Nursing staff should be aware of individual medicine storage requirements. If drug potency compromised by poor storage, new supplies need to be obtained for administration or prompting.
- Local guidelines apply to involvement of nursing staff in filling and prompting from medicine reminder devices. Many types available but widespread safety concerns re: labelling, opportunities for mix-ups particularly if person has cognitive problems or multiple carers helping with medication. Many areas now have schemes for pharmacist to dispense into sealed monitored dosage systems e.g. blister packs.

Transportation

See also ▢ Controlled drugs.
Key principles:

- Do not leave medicines in the car overnight or for long periods.
- Consider safety issues.
- Ensure temperature sensitive preparations are transported in conditions to maintain the appropriate temperature range (i.e. preserve the cold chain).
- Cool boxes and bags should be monitored and maintained at the correct temperature e.g. for vaccines between 2°–8°C.
- Wherever possible the patient, their carer or agent should collect any prescribed items from the pharmacy. Some local pharmacists have delivery systems.

Disposal

Disposal into the sewerage system an environmental hazard. Key principles:
- Patients/carers/agents should be encouraged to return any unwanted and out of date medicines to their supplying pharmacy for safe disposal. CDs can be returned to any pharmacy, but should be separated from any non CDs
- Local guidelines should be followed on the disposal of out of date or unwanted medicines or medicinal products for clinic/surgery held stocks. This includes records of disposal.

See also ▢ Managing health-care waste.

Further information for professionals

▣ Royal Pharmaceutical Society of Great Britain (RPSGB) (2005). *The safe and secure handling of medicines: a team approach.* (revised on 1988 Duthie Report).
www.rpsgb.org/pdfs/safsechandmeds.pdf
▣ RPSGB (2003). The Administration and Control of Medicines in Care Homes and Children's Services: www.rpsgb.org.uk/pdfs/adminmedguid.pdf

Further information for patients

▣ NHS Direct. Medicines (General) Section: www.nhsdirect.nhs.uk/chq/chq.aspx?Classid=24
▣ Patient Medicines Guides and latest Patient Information Leaflets for each medicine available at: www.medicines.org.uk

Child health promotion

Child health promotion

The UK ratified the UN Convention on the Rights of the Child in 1989. This includes:
- Participation rights including an active role in their communities and nations.
- Provision rights including basic needs such as food, shelter, and access to health care. Those with disabilities to receive special services.
- Developmental rights including to achieve their full potential through education, play, freedom of thought, conscience, and religion.
- Protection rights against all forms of abuse, neglect, exploitation, and discrimination.

Children in the UK

There are 14.8 million children in UK. Some key statistics from the Office of National Statistics (🖳 www.statistics.org.uk) and *Health for All Children*:[1]
- 3.5 million live in households with income poverty.
- Infant mortality rate 70% higher in social class 5 than social class 1 in 1993–5.
- Approximately 400 babies die each year in the UK from SUDI.
- International comparisons show the UK has some of the highest rates of children 2–15yrs diagnosed with asthma (21%), eczema (24%), hay fever (9%).
- Approximately 36,000 children are on child protection registers.
- 11% boys/young men and 5% girls/young women <20yrs have a severe disability. Disabilities are more frequent in children from families with lower incomes.
- Boys and young men age 11–20yrs are the group at highest risk of committing suicide.

National child health promotion programmes

These emphasize preventive health care and promotion of good health for children and young people in the context of their families and communities. In each UK country, the programme is based on the evidence in *Health for All Children 4*[2] and country-specific policies e.g. NSF for children, young people and maternity services England[3]. The programme:
- Acknowledges the social as well as biological determinants of health.
- Emphasizes the importance of community based services for families such as Sure Start (Community approaches to health 📖 and Public health 📖) approaches to improving child health.
- Is delivered in partnership with parents to help them make healthy choices for their children and families.
- Is an additional service under the GMS contract (General practice 📖).
- HVs, public health nurses, and SNs are key health service providers.

---

[1] Hall, D.M.B. and Elliman, D. (eds) (2003). *Health for all children* (4th edn.). Oxford University Press, Oxford.
[2] 🖳 HFAC4 www.health-for-all-children.co.uk
[3] 🖳 NSF children, young people and maternity services:
England www.doh.gov.uk/policyandguidance
Scotland www.childreninscotland.org.uk

The main elements of the programmes are:
- Every child and parent should have access to a universal or core programme of preventative pre-school care (Overview of the child health promotion programme 📖) based on:
  - The delivery of agreed screening procedures
  - The delivery of health promotion and support for parenting programmes
  - The need to establish which families have more complex needs and respond appropriately to those following full assessment.
- Formal screening is confined to those activities agreed by the National Screening Committee (UK screening programmes 📖).
- Formal universal screening for speech and language delay, global development delay. Autism, and postnatal depression is not recommended but professionals should elicit and respond to all parental concerns with appropriate assessment and action.
- Health promotion (Models and approaches to health promotion 📖) activities should include:
  - Prevention of infectious diseases (Childhood immunization 📖)
  - Reducing the risk of sudden infant death (Sudden unexpected death of an infant 📖)
  - Supporting breast feeding (Breast feeding 📖)
  - Encouraging better dental care (Development and care of teeth 📖)
  - Encouraging good nutrition and prevention of obesity (Nutrition and healthy eating 📖).
- The personal child health record should be used (Client- and patient-held records 📖).
- There are clear care pathways for children with health or development problems.
- Statutory responsibilities are fulfilled in respect of child protection (Child protection 📖), looked-after children, adoption procedures (Looked-after children 📖), and children with special educational needs (📖).
- Health professionals working with adult patients should recognize the impact of adult problems on children (Children in special circumstances 📖) and also enquire about them.
- Health care for children and young people in school should include:
  - Support of children with problems and special needs
  - Participation in Healthy Schools programmes
  - Promotion of personal, social, and sexual health including emotional literacy (Sex and relationship education 📖)
  - Provision of agreed screening and immunization programmes.

Overview of the child health promotion programme

Table 6.1 opposite provides an overview of the currently recommended programme.

Table 6.1 Overview of the currently recommended child health promotion programme

Age	Intervention
Soon after birth <72hrs	General physical examination including inspection of the eyes and red reflex, Ortolani and Barlow tests for developmental dysplasia of the hips (DDH), examination of the heart, and testes
About 6d	Newborn bloodspot screening
Usually around 12d	New birth visit to assess child and family needs. Information/support to parents on key health issues
Within first month of life	Semi automated hearing screening
6–8wks	General physical examination including inspection of the eyes and red reflex, Ortolani and Barlow tests for DDH, examination of the heart and testes
	Review of general progress and delivery of key health promotion messages. Usually at the same time as the first set of immunizations
3mths	Review of general progress and delivery of key health
4mths	promotion messages at the same as the second and third set of primary immunization
8mths	Hearing testing (if not done at birth)
By the 1st birthday	Overall review of the child and family
12mths	First MMR vaccine
2–3yrs	Review of child and family (not necessarily a face-to-face contact)
3–4yrs	Pre-school booster and second MMR vaccine. Review of child's progress and delivery of key health promotion messages
4–5yrs	Assessment of visual acuity
School entry	General review
	Hearing screening
	Height and weight measurement
Throughout school years	Ongoing support by the school health service—no further routine screening procedures recommended. Where there are vision screening programmes in place, in the absence of good evidence, those apart from vision screening at 7yrs old may continue as long as they are properly evaluated
13–18yrs	School leaver's booster vaccine

The assessment of children, young people, and families

The promotion of children's and young people's health involves consideration of:
• Their developmental needs
• The quality of parental care
• The circumstances in which they grow up in.

Each of these three dimensions has a number of elements as shown in Fig 6.1.

These dimensions form the basis for structuring and recording in PHCHR, assessments of children in routine practice as part of the child health promotion programme (📖). The dimensions are also essential in determining whether a child or young person is 'in need or suffering significant harm' (A child or young person in need 📖).

All assessments should be carried out in partnership with parents and young people to identify strengths, problems, and opportunities for health promotion. HFA4 emphasizes that child health promotion has to assess and address the needs of the parents as well as the children. Having jointly agreed problems and areas for health promotion, the next step is to plan to provide as necessary, information, advice, supporting resources, practical help and referral to other services as appropriate. Like all individual health needs assessments (📖) the plan and its outcome should be jointly reviewed and amended as the child develops.

Further information

▣ England Common Assessment Framework: www.everychildmatters.gov.uk/
   deliveringservices/caf/
▣ HFAC4: www.health-for-all-children.co.uk
▣ Scotland: www.childreninscotland.org.uk

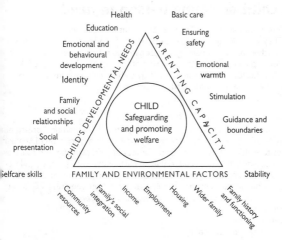

Fig. 6.1 The assessment framework (Reproduced with permission from the *Framework for the assessment of children in need and their families*. Department of Health, Department of Education and Employment, Home Office (2000). The Stationery Office, London).

A child or young person in need

Under the Children Act 1989 a child is considered in need if:
- They are unlikely to achieve or maintain, or to have the opportunity of achieving or maintaining, a reasonable standard of health or development without the provision of services for them by the LA.
- Their health or development is likely to be significantly impaired, or further impaired, without such provision.
- They are disabled.

Integrated assessment frameworks

All UK countries are developing integrated or common assessment frameworks (and records) for use by staff of all agencies providing services to children. It is emphasized that assessment, planning, and monitoring processes should be undertaken in partnership with parents, children and young people. England has developed a pre-assessment checklist to help professionals determine vulnerable children requiring full assessment. It asks whether the child or young person appears:
- Healthy?
- Safe from harm?
- Learning and developing?
- To have a positive impact on others?
- Free from the negative impact of poverty?

Children identified as vulnerable and in need are referred to specialist and targeted services (Social services 📖; Children with special educational needs 📖). Local child protection procedures are followed if there is risk of harm (Child protection 📖).

Full common assessment frameworks cover:
- General health
- Physical development
- Speech, language, and communications development
- Emotional and social development
- Behavioural development
- Self-esteem, self-image, and identity
- Family and social relationships
- Self-care skills and independence
- Understanding, reasoning, and problem solving
- Participation in learning, education, and employment
- Progress and achievement in learning
- Aspirations
- Basic care, ensuring safety and protection
- Emotional warmth and stability
- Guidance, boundaries, and stimulation
- Family history, functioning, and well-being
- Parents' health, ill health, or disability and impact on child
- Wider family
- Housing, employment, and financial considerations
- Social and community elements and resources, including education.

Impact of adult health problems on children

HFA4 emphasizes that professionals should assess the impact and needs of children and young people when working with adults with health problems particularly if they are:

- Parents with mental health problems
- Parents with long-term conditions and disabilities
- Parents with addictions.

Care planning, management, monitoring, and evaluation

Assessment should be part of a care management process with an identified lead professional, key worker, or care manager who will work closely with the family to help coordinate:

- A plan to address the identified and agreed needs
- The delivery of services and support
- The monitoring and review of the plan.

Related topics

📖 Services for children, young people, and families; 📖 Children with special educational needs; 📖 Child protection; 📖 Support for parenting programmes.

Further information

📖 England Common Assessment Framework: www.everychildmatters.gov.uk/
    deliveringservices/caf/
📖 HFAC4: www.health-for-all-children.co.uk
📖 Scotland: www.childreninscotland.org.uk

Child screening tests

Nationally agreed child screening tests are carried out on the whole population. Where there is professional or parental concern additional interventions may be appropriate. Children who are at high risk of a condition may need extra investigations despite a normal screening test. Other topics have been considered at one time or another for inclusion in screening programmes but have not satisfied the criteria. These include screening tests for developmental and behavioural problems.

Throughout the 4 countries of the UK, there are different policies on screening for dental disease with surveillance and screening overlapping. The policy is under review.

Fully informed consent (Consent 📖) should be sought from a person with parental responsibility before any screening test or immunization is undertaken.

Further information
📖 UK National Screening Committee: www.nsc.nhs.uk/index.htm

Physical examination
What
- Eyes (Eyes and vision screening 📖).
- Hearts: congenital heart disease (600 per 100,000 moderate or severe).
- Hips: developmental dysplasia (DDH)—dislocated/dislocatable (120 per 100,000).
- Testes: undescended (6000 per 100,000).
- Growth.

Why
Early treatment can reduce disability:
- Surgery for congenital heart disease before symptoms develop is beneficial.
- Early treatment (splinting) of DDH reduces the need for surgical intervention.
- Early surgery (referral by 1yr of age) for undescended testes may improve fertility and facilitate the early diagnosis of malignancy.
- Birthweight and head circumference at birth act as a baseline for future measurements.
- At 6–8wks weight can provide reassurance that a baby is growing appropriately during a period of rapid growth.

How and by whom
All form part of routine physical examination carried out by a competent practitioner, this might be a nurse or a doctor. Weight should be measured using appropriately calibrated scales, head circumference using a tape measure around the occipito-frontal.

When
By 72hrs old and again between 6–8wks old.

Further information
◪ National Service Framework for Children: www.dh.gov.uk/assetRoot/04/08/92/20/04089220.pdf

Neonatal blood spot screening

What
- Phenylketonuria (1 in 10,000 births).
- Congenital hypothyroidism (1 in 3500).
- Sickle cell disease (depending on ethnicity: overall 1 in 2400, West African 1 in 80 live births, West Indian 1 in 200 live births) by the end of 2005 in all areas.
- Cystic fibrosis (1 in 2500 live births) in some areas at present, in all areas in the future.
- Introduction of medium-chain acylCoA dehydrogenase deficiency (MCADD) (1 in 10,000 live births) is planned in England and being considered elsewhere.

Why
Preventive treatment reduces the risk of disability.

How and by whom
Heel prick blood sample usually by midwife.

When
At 6d. Standards for performance have been agreed nationally and are available on the website. All results from laboratories are sent to child health record departments who are responsible for monitoring coverage and informing HV/GP. HVs are responsible for informing parents of negative results and recording them in PHCR. Positive results are reported to hospital paediatrician and GP by laboratory for follow-up and copied to Child Health Records Department.

Further information
◪ NHS Haemoglobinopathy Screening Programme: www.kcl-phs.org.uk/haemscreening
◪ The UK Newborn Screening Programme: www.newbornscreening-bloodspot.org.uk/

Eyes and vision screening (children)

This is the currently agreed UK screening programme. See 📖 Child screening tests for background information on UK screening test policies for children.

Congenital ocular opacities
What and why
Looking for cataracts (incidence 30 per 100,000 live births), retinoblastoma (40–50 cases in UK per year) and congenital glaucoma (1 in 10,000 births per year). Early treatment leads to improved prognosis.

How and by whom
Inspection, including red reflex, as part of the neonatal and 6–8wks physical examinations. Carried out by a health-care professional trained to do this.

When
Within 72hrs of birth and again at 6–8wks.

Impaired visual acuity
What and why
Amblyopia—suppression of vision in a healthy eye due to different images falling on the two retinae—and other causes of impaired visual acuity. Early intervention with glasses and/or patching may lead to improved visual function.

How and by whom
• Visual acuity of both eyes assessed separately using standard charts in an appropriately lit environment.
• Carried out by trained personnel, ideally an orthoptist or as part of an orthoptic-led service.

When
Usually at primary school entry. Policy moving towards 4–5yrs old, so that performed by the time of 5th birthday.

Related topic
📖 Overview of the child health programme.

Further information
📖 National Electronic Library for Health, Screening Specialist Library:
   http://libraries.nelh.nhs.uk/screening/
📖 NSC: www.nsc.nhs.uk/library/lib_ind.htm

Hearing screening

This is the currently agreed UK screening programme. See 📖 Child screening tests for background information on UK screening test policies for children.

Neonatal

What and why

Congenital sensorineural hearing impairment (100 per 100,000). Early detection allows implementation of optimal management (hearing aids and parental interaction) with improvement of language development.

How and by whom

Semi automated techniques. Oto-acoustic emissions (OAE) and auditory brain responses (AABR), by specially trained personnel.

When

Either in first days in hospital or by a trained person in the first month of life.

Targeted ongoing surveillance

Irrespective of newborn screen outcome if:
- Parental or professional concern.
- Meningitis, chronic middle ear effusion and cranio-facial abnormalities (CFA).
- High levels of ototoxic drugs.
- Other specific risk factors for late-onset, progressive or acquired deafness.

Neonatal programme currently being adopted in all areas. The 6–8mths distraction hearing test programme organized by health visiting teams remains in place for 12mths after introduction to ensure all infants are screened. Protocols for distraction hearing test are available (see websites below). Tests require:
- The infant to be able to sit independently.
- Two trained people, a distractor and an assistant, working in unison.
- A suitable quiet room, ↓ visual and olfactory stimuli.

Positive results require infant's full head turn to stimulus at 40–50db presented at both sides at high and low frequencies e.g. high frequency rattle, 's' and low frequency hum.

School entry

What and why

Acquired hearing impairment and some cases of congenital sensorineural hearing loss not already identified. A further 50–90 per 100,000 cases of sensorineural deafness will be identified and many more cases of conductive loss. Most commonly acquired conductive loss due to secretory otitis media (glue ear). Hearing loss may contribute to problems with learning, appropriate management can minimize this.

How and by whom

Pure tone audiometry by trained personal, usually audiometricians or SNs. Involves using a regularly tested and calibrated audiometer in a quietened room and presenting tones (usually at each octave between 125 Hz and 8 kHz) through headphones at amplitudes related to expected thresholds for a normal hearing person. The child indicates when they can hear the tones and this is charted. Local protocols specify referral pathways for identified hearing loss. ▣ British Society of Audiology produces recommended procedures at www.thebsa.org.uk/

When

Primary school entry.

Further information

▣ NHS Newborn Hearing Screening Programme:
England: www.nhsp.info/index.php
Northern Ireland: www.dhsspni.gov.uk/index/phealth
Scotland: www.show.scot.nhs.uk/nsd/services/hearing/
Wales: www.wales.nhs.uk/sites3/home.cfm?orgid=34

Childhood immunization

Childhood immunization is important for both the individual and public health (see HPA website[1]). It is an essential part of the child health promotion programme (Overview of the child health promotion programme 🕮).

Information (including leaflets) about immunization programmes is usually given to parents at new birth visits and opportunities offered for parents to discuss any issues or concerns.

Fully informed (i.e. including process, benefits and risks) consent (Consent 🕮) should be sought from a person with parental responsibility before immunization is undertaken.

Each PCO should have a named person who has oversight of the programme. This person should act as a source of expert advice and, if they cannot answer clinical queries, be able to call on a local clinician.

There are national targets for immunization uptake.

PCO child health record departments act as a repository for immunization data, recording consent or refusal to be considered for a course, and administration of immunizations. In some areas they also provide parent and professional reminder systems, although this is done independently by many GP practices. The primary course of immunization is part of nGMS contract global sum (General practice 🕮), but may also form enhanced services or PMS contracts for areas or populations with particular challenges in reaching coverage targets.

Immunization should be offered as per UK immunization schedule (Childhood immunization schedule (UK) 🕮).

Vaccines
- Community pharmacists in PCOs support the supply of vaccines. Information on suppliers of vaccines also available on the 'Green Book' website.[2]
- Vaccine must be stored at 2–8°C and must not be frozen. The cold chain must be preserved if transported to other sites or on domiciliary visits.

Addressing parents concerns
- Safety and side effects:
  - All vaccines are carefully tested, both for their efficacy and safety, before being introduced.
  - Each batch of vaccine is tested and close post-marketing surveillance is initiated. Part of this is the 'Yellow Card' system.[3]

---

[1] 🖳 Health Protection Agency (HPA): www.hpa.org.uk/default.htm Protecting the health of the Nation's children: the benefit of vaccines HPA Publications on Training: www.hpa.org.uk/ infections/topics_az/vaccination/training

[2] 🖳 *Immunization against infectious diseases* (The Green Book): www.dh.gov.uk/PolicyAnd Guidance/HealthAndSocialCareTopics/GreenBook/GreenBookGeneralInformation

[3] 🖳 Yellow Card Scheme Medicines and Healthcare Products Regulatory Agency: www.mhra.org.uk

- MMR: much research has been conducted on the vaccine and it has been shown to have a good safety profile with no evidence of a link with autism or chronic bowel disease.
- Thiomersal: some vaccines used to contain thiomersal, a mercury-containing preservative. No research has shown it to be toxic in the doses contained in vaccines but, based on the 'precautionary principle', it is being phased out and none of the routine childhood vaccines contain any.

Homeopathy

Increasing numbers of people are turning to alternative forms of health care. There is no evidence that any of these are effective in preventing the diseases against which vaccines are used.

Further information for parents and professionals

- Great Ormond Street Hospital/Institute of Child Health Immunization: www.ich.ucl.ac.uk/immunization/
- Health Protection Scotland, Scottish Centre for Infection and Environmental Health (SCIEH): www.show.scot.nhs.uk/scieh/
- National Public Health Service for Wales: www.wales.nhs.uk/sites/page.cfm?orgid=368&pid=3334
- NHS immunization information: www.immunization.nhs.uk www.mmrthefacts.nhs.uk/ http://80.168.38.66/files/thiomersalfsht.pdf
- Royal College of Paediatrics and Child Health. *Immunization of the Immunocompromised Child.* www.rcpch.ac.uk/

Childhood immunization schedule (UK)

Table 6.2 The UK childhood immunization schedule—Autumn 2006

Age	Vaccine	Mode of delivery	Site
8wks	Diphtheria/tetanus/acellular pertussis/inactivated Polio vaccine/*Haemophilus influenzae* type b/ (DTaP/IPV/Hib), and	One injection	IM thigh
			Same time different site (2.5cm apart) or limb
	Pneumonoccocal conjugate vaccine (PCV)	One injection	
12wks	DTaP/Hib/IPV and	One injection	IM thigh
			Injections guidance as 8wks
	Meningococcal group C (MenC)	One injection	
16wks	DTaP/Hib/IPV and	One injection	IM thigh
	MenC and	One injection	Injections guidance as 8wks
	PCV	One injection	
12mths	Hib/menC	One injection	IM upper arm or thigh
13mths	MMR and	One injection	IM upper arm or thigh
	PCV	One injection	Injections guidance as 8wks
Pre-school	DTaP/IPV or dTaP/IPV (Pre-school booster)	One injection	IM upper arm
	MMR (second dose)	One injection	Injections guidance as 8wks
13–18yrs	Tetanus/low dose diphtheria/ IPV (Td/IPV) (school leavers' booster)	One injection	IM upper arm

Other vaccines may be indicated for high-risk individuals. These include: pneumococcal vaccine, influenza vaccine, hepatitis B vaccine and BCG (TB 📖).

New targeted BCG neonatal and 'other at risk' based programme replaces the current schools' programme for older children. Recommended that BCG offered to:

- Infants in areas where TB ≥ 40/100,000.
- Infants and children <6yrs old whose parents or grandparents were born in a country with a TB incidence ≥ 40/100,000.
- Previously unvaccinated new immigrants from high TB prevalence countries.
- Children and young people who are going to stay, or have stayed in close contact with the indigenous population in high TB prevalence countries for at least a month.

NB Infants i.e. those under 12mths old do not need Mantoux test prior to BCG. For older groups, consult the Green Book.

Where and by whom

Routine vaccines for young children are usually given in primary care and for older children by the school health service. Given by someone trained in the administration of vaccines and a high level of knowledge about vaccines and immunization. Nurses and HVs often administer vaccines under PGDs (Prescribing 📖). Anyone administering vaccines should be competent in CPR and dealing with anaphylaxis according to local policies.

Contraindications

- Anaphylaxis to a previous dose of the vaccine or a component of the vaccine.
- In children who are moderately or severely systemically unwell with a fever, vaccination should be delayed.
- In addition, live vaccines such as MMR may be contraindicated in some immunosuppressed individuals.

Travel vaccines

(See Travel vaccinations 📖.)

Essential reference

Immunization against infectious diseases (The Green Book):
www.dh.gov.uk/PolicyAndGuidance/HealthAndSocialCareTopics/GreenBook/
GreenBookGeneralInformation/

Further information for parents

📖 NHS immunization information:
www.immunization.nhs.uk/
www.mmrthefacts.nhs.uk/

Further information for professionals

📖 Health Protection Agency (HPA): www.hpa.org.uk/default.htm
📖 Protecting the health of the Nation's children: the benefit of vaccines: www.hpa.org.uk/
hpa/publications/HPA_protect_health_children/protect_health_children.htm

Children in special circumstances

Children who live in special circumstances may need particular attention to ensure they receive the full child health promotion programme and any particular and exceptional needs are addressed.

Children as young carers

See also ☐ Carers assessment and support. 6% of children in need are registered because of parental illness or disability. Young carers often miss time from school, have little time for peers and friendship, and may experience stigma by association e.g. parent has mental health problems. Young carers have the right to a full assessment of their needs and support in their caring role (The assessment of children, young people, and families ☐). Some areas have specialist projects and groups to support young carers.

Unaccompanied asylum seekers and refugees

See also ☐ Asylum seekers and refugees. Unaccompanied children <18yrs have the right to be 'looked after' (Looked-after children ☐), to have somewhere to live, and to education and health care. They are identified as children in need (A child or young person in need ☐) and should have a full integrated assessment to develop a specialized care plan that includes emotional needs. Their health problems will reflect those of the region they come from e.g. malaria is endemic in parts of Africa. In addition, they may come from an area with no child surveillance programme and have missed immunizations (Childhood immunization schedule (UK) ☐). Psychological distress may be related to separation from family but also from experiences e.g. war and some may need referral to child and adolescent mental health services (☐).

Homelessness

See also ☐ Homeless people. Children and young people may be part of a family that is homeless or may be homeless as a single person. They are often placed in temporary accommodation such as hostels and bed and breakfast accommodation. This is often unsuitable with limited opportunities for play, shared and cramped space for cooking and food storage, and shared toilet and bathroom facilities. Accidents, behaviour problems and minor infections are common. In some areas close liaison with housing departments, designated HVs and primary care teams ensure that families and young people are identified soon after moving in. Priorities are to ensure:

- They have information as to registering with a GP.
- They have information about local health, early years, education, social and community support services.
- The child promotion programme is up-to-date and a plan to address any problems is made.
- Immunization is up-to-date.
- The PHCHR is used for all contacts or the young person is given a record of all contact and referrals.

Children, young people, and prison

All children and young people whose lives are touched by prison have special needs. The circumstances may be:

- Baby born in prison and may stay with mother. However there are few Mother and Baby Units (only 4 in England and Wales). Babies can stay until 9mths or 18mths dependent on unit. Local HVs provide the child health promotion programme to these units. When mothers and babies cannot stay together early opportunities for bonding and psychological attachment are lost (Emotional development in babies and children 📖).
- A parent may be imprisoned. The children are separated and experience significant loss. This is particularly painful if the mother is imprisoned as not only is there separation but many children have to live with relatives or end up looked after by local authorities. Visiting may be difficult as there are few women's prisons so they can be at a great distance. There are emotional and psychological consequences for children and young people of all ages.
- Young people detained in their own right. These are vulnerable young people. The prison health service is currently transferring to local primary care organizations and identifies health needs at an entry assessment.

Related topics

📖 Services for children, young people, and families; 📖 Child protection.

Accident prevention

Every year in UK over 2 million children are taken to an ED with injuries caused by accidents and about 300 children die. It is the most common cause of death age in children aged 1–14yrs. Accidental injury is more common in children from lower social classes e.g. children in poorest households are 16 times more likely to die in a household fire. Other consequences are permanent disfigurement and/or disability, sometimes behavioural and psychological problems. Some parents carry lifelong guilt.

Types of accidents

- Road traffic accidents (RTAs) are the most common cause of accidental death (single biggest cause of accidental death in children aged 12–16yrs) including:
  - Child pedestrian. Most common in boys aged 5–9yrs.
  - Child passengers in vehicles, particularly if unrestrained.
  - Bicycle accidents. 1 in 80 boys have a chance of admission to hosptial through a cycling accident.
- Head injuries. Minor head injuries common with little long-term effect but 1 in 800 of these develop serious problems.
- Burns and scalds, 2nd most common cause of death from accidents (includes from house fires).
- Drowning, 3rd most common cause of accidental death. Most victims are young children, 3 times more common in boys than girls.
- Choking, suffocation, strangulation:
  - Babies and small children choke on small toys, food, or vomit.
  - Accidental strangulation on curtain cords, bedding, and necklaces.
- Dog bites. 1 in 100 children present in ED with dog bites.
- Poisoning: peak age 30mths, ingesting medicines, household cleaning products, eating plants.

Action for prevention

- Accident prevention is most successful at a public health (Public health 📖) and legislative level e.g. traffic calming measures, child resistant medication containers, compulsory use of seat belts in all parts of car.
- Individual parents also need to be aware of:
  - Risks at different child developmental stages and preventative action.
  - Use of home safety equipment and schemes that loan equipment e.g. stair gates, or provide for free e.g. smoke detectors (particularly for low income families). Often run by LA, Sure Start, or in the case of smoke detectors, the local fire brigade.
  - Risks associated with different leisure and sport activities and preventative action e.g. cycling and the use of helmets.
- There are also opportunities for education for children and young people on safety e.g. crossing the road, learning to swim from an early age, cycling proficiency courses. These types of learning opportunities may be provided by parents, local leisure organizations, early years education, PSHE in schools.

Related topic
📖 Child health promotion.

Further information for professionals and parents
▣ Child Accident Prevention Trust: www.capt.org.uk/
▣ Royal Society for the Prevention of Accidents: www.rospa.org.uk
▣ Road Safety Education for 14–18yrs olds: www.noaccident.org/
▣ ROSPA website on child car sea safety: www.childcareseats.org.uk
▣ Think Road Safety: www.thinkroadsafety.gov.uk/ includes links for children's websites on green cross code, be safe be seen, cycle safely etc.

Working with parents

This might involve parents expecting a first child or those living with adolescents. Work might be preventative or in response to significant problems defined by the parents, school or the wider society; and all points between, such as sleep problems, aggression towards other children and theft.

Overall aim

The aim is to work with parents to achieve 'good enough parenting', protecting the child and promoting physical, intellectual, emotional, and social development. Different approaches exist which may have various theoretical underpinnings:

- Behavioural modification, which concentrates on the behaviour to be changed for instance attention seeking or bed wetting by rewarding acceptable behaviour.
- Parent advisory models, these seek to understand the individual context in which child and parent live. The helper–parent relationship is seen as central, with the helper an active listener which is followed by a negotiated plan to meet the individual family's needs.
- Brief interventions, a short-term interaction focused on a particular issue.
- Child development programme, which sees the developmental achievements of the child as central. Considering what the child can do, the parents develop ideas for care and stimulation, including health factors such as diet.

Many draw from different perspectives, humanistic, counselling, social learning, and active listening. Integrating these views can lead to an approach specific for the family.

Current and most effective approaches include

Relationship Building

Central to this is the spirit of partnership based on informal interactions, respect, mutual esteem, and recognition. Health workers need to demonstrate genuineness, humility, empathy, qualified enthusiasm, and confidence building as they seek to empower the parent. Shared records are likely to part of this. Parents and professionals need to make clear what they can contribute to the relationship, the frequency and duration of the interaction, if the focus is to be the individual, group or community, and if meetings will take place in the home or a health centre.

Two way sharing of knowledge experience and responsibility

The health worker draws on their expertise in child development, health promotion or adolescent health. The parents know the child, family circumstances, and the socio-cultural context in which the family lives. Both contributions are valued as neither can 'solve' the problem alone. Interactions will lead to the development of skills of both parent and professional. Reflection on the situation clarifies the issues and establishes the priorities for action.

Getting parent (and child or young person) to set own goals and together working out a strategy

The family need to 'own' the issue and define what they want to achieve and what is manageable, this may be different from the professional or others parents' views. Professionals will advocate for the parents and often lobby with them, supporting them to provide the best opportunities for their children.

Recognizing and celebrating success

Small positive developments need to be noted and celebrated, this builds up the confidence of all involved, develops self-esteem, and increases expectations of success.

Accessing other parenting support if necessary

This may include early year's provision, regular attendance at school, after school facilities and the activities of the community or the extended school.

Parents may have issues that impact on parenting. Interventions in terms of domestic violence (📖), family breakdown, mental illness (see people with depression 📖; People with schizophrenia 📖), and overuse of alcohol (Alcohol 📖), substance misuse (📖) health issues, housing (Homes and housing 📖), and income support (Benefits for people on low income 📖) may be appropriate.

Parenting may be linked with child mental health work. SNs, HVs, GPs, nursery nurses, teachers, and youth workers should be involved at the first level, promoting sound parenting and child mental health. Entrenched difficulties may need the involvement of mental health teams and specialist multidisciplinary teams. Working with parents needs to begin early. Personal social and health education and citizenship in schools is one area together with youth organizations, pre-conceptual care and early antenatal interventions (Health promotion in schools 📖).

Related topic

📖 Antenatal education and preparation for parenthood.

Further information for parents and professionals

▣ A site set up By Parenting Education & Support Forum focusing on parenthood preparation in schools: www.parenthood.org.uk/

▣ Positive Parenting: www.parenting.org.uk/

▣ The Parenting Education & Support Forum: www.parenting-forum.org.uk/

Support for parenting programmes

All national polices on children have support for parenting as a key standard e.g. NSF for Children. 'Good enough parenting' providing love, care, and commitment, can act as a buffer against adversity e.g. poverty. It contributes to emotional well-being reducing the need for later reactive intervention. Good parenting will include:
- Provision of resources to facilitate growth and development.
- Meeting the child's needs for love and security.
- Realistic expectations of the child linked to their development and maturity.
- Provision of appropriate stimulation and opportunities for social development.

A quality environment, providing appropriate accommodation and nutrition, good nursery provision, playspaces, maternity/paternity leave, family friendly working patterns, and financial support, supports parenting.

Support for parenting

Traditionally extended families provided practical and emotional encouragement. This still exists with some groups but when families are spread throughout the country/world, support may come from community links and faith/cultural groups. Those without support may not be obvious and may include lone parents, father or mother, and those whose previous focus was on career development.

Home visits by health workers or volunteers are effective in developing parenting skills, promoting the child's development, improving breast-feeding rates, and reducing unintentional injury.

Support is available in groups facilitated by HVs and SNs such as postnatal support groups, parent drop-ins and parenting groups. These seek to build parental confidence and local networks. Mother and Toddler groups and local branches of organizations such as the National Childbirth Trust and Meet a Mum may have similar aims.

A variety of programmes to groups and communities seek to support parenting, some are local, some nationally based. They include:
- *First parenting programmes* for new mothers and fathers as they make the transition to parenthood.
- *Homestart* a voluntary organization providing informal support for families with young children in their own home. Friendship and practical support is given with reassurance and encouragement, as they try to get the fun back into family life.
- *Newpin* another voluntary organization working through a network of centres to break the cycle of destructive family behaviour by raising self-esteem and empowering families. Centres offer befriending, group work, and play programmes.

These and other groups may include play and space for children, peer support for parents, talking and listening, valuing of parents, help with setting boundaries and what ever the parents find useful.

Sure Start a government programme aimed at delivering the best start in life for every child, bringing together early education, childcare, health and family support. It is committed to early intervention, increasing parenting skills, improving the quality of child interaction, and reducing abuse and neglect. It is a multi-disciplinary strategy and involves partnership with parents, carers and the community.

Teenage parents may draw on any of the above but may need further support to continue or re-enter education or employment. Regeneration officers, specialist programmes, and extra childcare may all facilitate this.

The programmes listed above, as well as others will generally aim to:

- Take a partnership approach
- Raise parents' self-esteem
- Build up parent support networks
- Take a positive approach to discipline, setting clear boundaries
- Understand how families see issues.
- Recognize there are different parenting styles.

Setting up such programmes should involve partnership with parents in the planning, development, and monitoring of services. They might be involved in the writing of the mission statement, recruitment and appraisal of staff, design and evaluation of the service, contributing to new ways of working for both staff and users.

Related topics

📖 Antenatal education and preparation for parenthood; 📖 Working with parents.

Further information for parents and professionals

- Homestart is an organization that supports families in local communities across the UK: www.home-start.org.uk
- Newpin a voluntary organization working with families to help break the cycle of destructive family behaviour: www.newpin.org.uk/
- Parentline Plus registered charity which offers support to anyone parenting a child: www.parentlineplus.co.uk/
- Sure Start website showing Sure Start news and development from round the country: www.surestart.gov.uk/

New birth visits

A new birth visit is the first contact (usually at home) with a family with a new baby made by the health visiting service 10–14d after birth. Usually by the HV (rather than other members of team). The HV may already know the mother from antenatal contacts, classes, or from contacts with previous children.

Information about a new birth

Every maternity unit provides the details of all births to the child health department in the PCO where the mother resides. The child health department informs the health visiting service which covers that mother's home address or the GP that the mother is registered with. This is currently done by paper records but increasingly electronic systems are being developed. Any change of address is logged in the child health system and on moving out of the area, the child's records are forwarded to the next child health department and/or appropriate HV or SN.

Handover from community midwife

The community midwife will usually contact the HV and pass on a summary of the delivery and midwifery care, highlighting any particular problems and maternal or baby needs.

Key principles of the new birth visit

These include:
- To introduce themselves, the health visiting and the child health promotion services to the family, particularly the mother.
- To begin to establish a relationship of trust with the mother and family so that the client feels safe to raise issues or problems they are experiencing, and be prepared to receive information and support in dealing with them.
- To encourage and support all aspects of learning to nurture the baby, and being a parent.
- To encourage and support all aspects of ensuring good physical and emotional health in the mother (see also Postnatal depression).
- To encourage and support all aspects of ensuring good physical and emotional health in the baby, including establishing infant feeding (especially Breast feeding).
- To identify any maternal, baby or family health (physical, mental and emotional) or social problems and offer advice and agree steps to addressing the problems, such as onward referral to another service.
- To identify children in need (A child or young person in need) and plan with the parent appropriate action.
- To provide information on the child health promotion programme ( ), particularly child immunization (Childhood immunization schedule (UK)) and seek written consent to the inclusion of the child in the computerized call and recall system for immunization and child health screening by the child health department.
- To provide information about local services, local parent and child networks, including Sure Start provision, birth registration, child benefit, state support for families and children as required.
- To agree a pattern of future contact and provide information about how to contact the health visiting service.

Local PCOs have guidelines and standards on this important contact informed by NICE guidance (see below).

Style of contact

HVs usually conduct the visit conversationally, with open ended questions, inviting the parents to raise the issues that concern them. HVs often start by asking what the birth was like as a way into understanding what the experience has been like so far (see NICE guidance below). Many PCOs or PHCHRs provide specific checklists e.g. for assessing the baby including items such as assessing umbilical stump healing, checking neonatal blood spot undertaken, all doses of vit. K given but most HVs use these as an aide memoire in their conversations rather than as a yes/no checklist.

Records

All local PCOs have record keeping (Client and patient held records 📖) guidance. PHCHR may be given out by HV or midwife according to local guidance. All contacts are usually recorded in PHCHR, with duplicates held in HV-held child health record in base office. These may be carbon copies or written out again on separate records or on GP practice electronic records. In addition HVs may keep separate family health records for contact specifically about adults health issues. Local policies apply. Integrated child health e-records and systems are being developed.

Related topics

📖 Postnatal care; 📖 Postnatal depression; 📖 Working with parents; 📖 Support for parenting programmes; 📖 Birth injuries.

Further information for professionals

📱 NICE (July 2006). Postnatal Care: routine postnatal care of women and their babies. Professional version: www.nice.org.uk

📱 The Directory of Community Nursing is published annually by Professional, Managerial and Health Care Publications Ltd admin@pmh.co.uk providing full contact details of all child health departments and health visiting services in the UK

Further information for parents

Department of Health England (2005). *Birth to Five Guide: guide to parenthood and the first five years of a child's life.* DH, London. Distributed to all first-time parents.

📱 NICE (July 2006). *Postnatal Care: routine postnatal care of women and their babies.* Public version: www.nice.org.uk

Child development 0–1 years

Child development is the interaction between heredity and the environment (Overview of the child health promotion programme 📖). In assessing development as part of the common assessment framework (📖) it is often subdivided into 4 areas:

- Gross motor
- Fine motor and vision
- Speech, language, and hearing
- Social, emotional, and behaviour.

Developmental progress is about the sequential acquisition of skills. It is important to remember:

- There is a wide timescale within normal range e.g. children walking unaided 25% by 11mths, 90% by 15mths, 97.5% by 18mths.
- Median ages indicate when ½ a standard population should have acquired the skill (see Table 6.3 for children 0–1yrs).
- Pre-term babies are assessed from EDD up until 2yrs of age.

Referral for more in-depth assessment if:

- Failure to meet acquisition by upper limits of age need more detailed assessment and investigation often through referral to community or hospital paediatrician e.g.:
  - No responsive smile by 8wks
  - Not achieved good eye contact by 3mths
  - Not sitting unsupported by 9mths.
- Also refer if:
  - Parents concerned
  - Discordant levels of development between areas
  - Regression of previously acquired skills
  - Development plateaus.

Development can be delayed or sub optimal

- Indirectly from adverse environmental factors or ill-health.
- Directly from neurological or neuro-developmental problems.

Further information

Sheridan, M. *From birth to five years: children's development progress.* Revised and updated Frost, M. and Sharma, A. (1997). Routledge, London.

Table 6.3 Overview of median age of development in children 0–1 years

	Newborn	6–8wks	3–4mths	6–7mths	8–10mths	11–12mths
Gross motor	Limbs flexed, symmetrical postures; marked head lag on pulling up; primitive reflex Moro and stepping	Raises head to 45°	3mths: holds head up while lying prone	Sits without support 6mths, with rounded back; 8mths straight back	8mths crawling, 10mths furniture walking	Walking unsteadily, broad gait, hands apart
Fine motor and vision	Reflex grasp; follows face in midline	6wks: follows moving object by turning head	4mths: reaches out for objects	6mths: palmar grasp; transfers objects from one hand to other	Pincer grip	
Language, speech, and hearing	Startles and blinks to loud noises	4–6wks gurgles in response; notices sudden sounds and pauses to listen	Vocalizes alone, or when spoken to; laughs, squeals, blows between lips; quietens or smiles to voice of parent	Coos and babbles uses syllables—da, ba, ka; 7mths: turns immediately to parent's voice; turns to soft sounds out of sight if not preoccupied	Two-syllable babble; sounds used discriminately, e.g. dada, mama	At least one word with meaning and understands some words
Social, emotional, and behaviour	Soon after birth flickers eyes when spoken to; after 2wks recognizes parent	Smiles responsively, responds to conversation through movements	Responds in conversations with smiles, gurgles, movements; finger feeds from 6mths	Curious about all sights, sounds, people; 6mths: puts arms out to be picked up; may be shy of strangers; 7mths: looks for dropped items	8mths: separation anxiety; familiar with routines; 10mths waves bye-bye, plays peek-a-boo; looks for hidden items	Drinks from cup; gives kisses

Pre-term infants

Pre-term describes infants born <37wks. Estimated that 42,500 pre-term babies born annually in UK. Infants born at 23–26wks gestation have 17–50% chance of survival. They have many problems (e.g. respiratory distress, hypotension, metabolic problems), require many weeks in intensive and special care, and have high levels of mortality. Very low birth weight (<1500g) babies ↑ risk of neuro-developmental problems (5–10% have severe problems) including visual impairment, hearing loss, cerebral palsy, and learning difficulties. Those born after 32wks have good prognosis with few problems.

On returning home from hospital

- Parents may need extra reassurance and support.
- Very premature and low birth weight babies ↑ risk of hospital readmission in first year.

Key areas of support and advice from primary care professionals may be:

Bonding: may have been difficult while in hospital and added to by fear of baby dying (Child development 0–1yrs 📖).

Feeding: pre-term babies are suck and swallow' poor so need frequent feeding (Breast feeding 📖). Breast milk (sometimes with calorie supplements) or special low birth weight formula is used. Vitamin and iron supplements are routine. Weaning advice for each baby will be different so parents should ask for advice from paediatric team.

Clothes that fit very small babies: advice from BLISS see below.

Temperature control: may be poor at first. Needs a controlled temperature and adequate insulation with clothes and blanket.

Respiratory problems: sometimes sent home on oxygen via nasal cannulae (Oxygen therapy in the community 📖). ↑ risk from respiratory infections. Sometimes advised to use apnoea monitor at home.

Vision problems: as a result of ↑ partial pressures of oxygen in special care. May need follow-up in primary care.

Hearing: ↑ risk of hearing problems. Should have neonatal screening and follow-up.

Sudden infant death: pre-term babies have ↑ risk. See 📖 Sudden unexpected death of an infant for prevention advice.

Further information and support for parents

🖥 BLISS (the Premature Baby Charity): www.bliss.org.uk
☎ Parent support helpline Freephone 0500 618140

New babies

Many parents, particularly first-time parents, need reassurance and advice about the changes and minor problems that arise in their new baby.

Head

May appear elongated or mishapen as a result of the bones moving during the birth process. Resolves spontaneously during the first weeks.

The umbilicus

After birth the umbilicus dries, becomes black, and separates at about 1wk of age. Problems:
- Stump can become infected—offensive odour, pus, malaise—refer to GP for antibiotics;
- Sometimes a granuloma forms—refer to GP for silver nitrate cautery;
- Hernia—weak abdominal wall allows intestines to bulge out. This is common and usually resolves by 1yr.

Skin

The vernix protects against minor skin problems such as peeling and flaking. Peeling is best dealt with by a non-irritant moisturizer, e.g. olive or baby oil, aqueous cream (Baby hygiene and skin care 📖). Skin may be blotchy as blood vessels are unstable. Babies of black parents are often light skinned at birth, then produce melanin and reach permanent skin colour by 6mths.

Birth marks
- Strawberry (stork) marks: pink areas, may grow, but fade. Sometimes raised bumps that shrivel and go by 2nd year.
- Spider naevi: network of dilated vessels, usually go by 2nd year.
- Port wine stains: found anywhere; can be treated with lasers or camouflaged.
- Mongolian blue spots: dark-skinned children often have harmless bluish black areas on back or base of spine. These fade by 2yrs.

Common skin problems
- Milia: tiny pearly white papules on the nose and face, blocked sebaceous ducts. Disappear spontaneously.
- Neonatal urticaria: red blotches with a central, white vesicle. Common in first week. Disappear spontaneously.
- Heat rash: small, red spots on face. Encourage not to overwrap or overheat rooms.
- Harlequin colour change. One side of the body flushes red while the other stays pale; harmless vasomotor effect.

Hair

The baby may be bald or have full head of hair. Hair colour may change. Lanugo (downy hair on body) will fall off soon after birth.

Eyes
- May have broken blood vessels following birth; this is harmless and resolves within a couple of weeks.

- Sticky eyes: this is common, usually due to a blocked tear duct. Treated by swabbing with boiled water at each nappy change. Purulent discharge requires referral to GP and swabs for M, C, & S (<21d to exclude ophthalmic neonatorum caused by *N. gonorrhoeae*).

Nose

Sneezing and snuffling are very common to clear amniotic fluid. Reassure parents.

Genitals

Many babies, male and female, may appear to have enlarged genitals and swollen 'breasts' shortly after birth, due to maternal hormones in their bloodstream. Advise to leave alone as this will subside spontaneously.

First nappies

- Bowel movements: meconium (blackish-green) is the first bowel movement passed within 24hrs. Stools then change to greenish brown then yellow semi-solid. Stools of bottle-fed babies often resemble scrambled eggs. Most babies have bowel movements soon after feeding (Baby hygiene and skin care 📖).
- Red-stained nappy: common usually due to urinary urates, but may be due to blood from vagina through oestrogen withdrawal. Reassure parents.

Feeding

See 📖 Breast feeding; 📖 Bottle feeding and weaning.

Weight gain

See 📖 Growth 0–1yrs.

Related topics

📖 Overview of the child health promotion programme.

Further information for parents

Department of Health England (2005). *Birth to Five Guide: guide to parenthood and the first five years of a child's life.* DoH, London. Distributed to all first-time mothers.

Twins and multiple births

Twins occur in 1:80 pregnancies, triplets 1:8000, quadruplets in 1:73,000. Multiple pregnancies most common in ♀ treated for problems with fertility (📖). Identical (monozygotic or uniovular) twins come from splitting of the same fertilized egg. Non-identical or fraternal (dizygotic or binovular) result from two sperm fertilizing two eggs.

Special considerations

- Pregnancy can be more tiring, anaemia and fluid retention more common and may need extra prenatal care and monitoring.
- Babies are often born earlier, or smaller than singleton babies, and are therefore more vulnerable (Pre-term infants 📖). Some multiple births result in the death of one or more babies (Bereavement, grief, and coping with loss 📖).
- Coping with two or more newborn babies can seem an overwhelming task, and parents may need support with caring for the babies.
- Multiples may experience language delay, behavioural disorders, excessive rivalry or dependency.

Extra help

Extra help is usually needed at first not just to cope with physical demands but also to give time to each baby individually and to the parents' own needs. There is no state funded support for help with twins unless the children have been assessed as vulnerable and in need (Assessment of children, young people, and families 📖). During pregnancy parents need information and advice to work out their options outside of family and friends for extra help. HVs are able to provide local information on child care support (Services for children, young people, and families 📖). Sometimes local nursery nurse courses are looking for placements for students but these can only help with child care under direct supervision.

Feeding

Breast feeding (Breast feeding 📖) should be encouraged particularly in premature babies and because two babies can be fed and held close at once. Bottle feeding allows others to help. Developing a routine or carrying on the one from the Special Unit is important.

Sleeping

Twins, particularly premature twins, placed in the same cot are often more contented then when alone. Usual advice on sleeping (Babies and sleeping 📖).

Equipment

TAMBA (see below) provides advice on equipment such as buggies and sources of second hand equipment.

Development and treating each baby and child as an individual

Parents should be encouraged to remember that each baby has their own needs and to create time to spend with each. Identical twins need to be treated as individuals rather than merged and will have different developmental progress (Child development 0–1yrs 📖). Elements to help treating them as individuals are different clothes, feeding equipment, bed clothes etc.

Related topic

📖 Overview of the child health promotion programme.

Further information for professionals and parents

▣ Multiple Births Foundation. Works primarily health professionals providing information, books, and educational events: www.multiplebirths.org.uk

▣ Twins and Multiple Birth Association: www.tamba.org.uk/html/home.htm

Has a helpline for parents ☎ Tel. 0800 138 0509 and a network of Twin Clubs.

Has links with a range of specialists in multiple births who can be contacted for referral about specific problems.

Produces leaflets for parents and professionals.

Breast feeding

Breast feeding is the optimum method for at least first 6mth of life. Levels of acceptability differ between social classes and cultures in the UK. While $^2/_3$ of mothers initiate breast feeding, this rapidly drops off. Nearly 90% of mothers in social class I start breast-feeding compared to <50% from social class V. Many PCOs have breast-feeding support co-coordinators. Unicef Baby Friendly UK initiatives promote environments and the training of professionals to support breast feeding.

Benefits:

- Provides the right nutrients for a growing baby (baby >6mths advise to give vitamin drops).
- Convenient, at the right temperature, and needs no preparation.
- Helps develop intimate, loving relationship between mother and baby.
- ↓ GI in babies and ↓ inflammatory bowel disease, diabetes mellitus in later life.
- Breast feeding promotes mother's uterus and pelvis to return to pre-pregnant state.
- Some protective effect against premenopausal breast cancer in the mother.

Issues to be aware of

- Certain diseases can be transferred in breast milk e.g. hepatitis B, HIV. NB HIV+ mothers should not breast feed as it is a route of viral transfer. See 📖 HIV for more information on preventing mother-to-child transfer.
- Some drugs/medicines can pass from mother through breast milk to baby or inhibit sucking reflex. Full list in BNF Appendix 5. COC contraindicated in breast-feeding mothers (Contraception: missed rules COC 📖).

Establishing breast feeding

Every woman and baby needs to learn how to breast feed together, it is not completely instinctive:

- First 72hrs breasts produce colostrum: ↑ protein and immunoglobulin. ↓ in volume but no supplement formula feeds or water required. Supplements interferes with milk let-down reflex (see below). Milk comes in 3rd or 4th day.
- Let-down reflex: sucking action on breast stimulates pituitary gland to release prolactin, for milk manufacture, and oxytocin lets down milk from glands to the reservoirs behind the areola.
- Latching-on: use the rooting reflex to ensure baby opens mouth wide enough to take large part of areola as well as nipple in mouth (see positions below).
- Baby needs frequent small feeds to start with, usually about every 2hrs including night, then as weight increases spacing widens. Let-down reflex means that the breasts produce milk as demanded. By about 6wks night feeds are reduced.
- Breast feeding mothers are advised to have a good diet and take vitamin D (10mcg/d)[1].

Positions for breast feeding

- Mother should be comfortable seated or lying down.
- National Child Birth Trust uses saying 'tummy to mummy/chest to chest/nose to nipple/chin to breast' to remind women of right position for baby to latch-on well.
- Three positions:
  - Traditional—sitting up, cradling baby in front. Support baby on pillows so high enough to face breast.
  - Underarm—baby on pillow at side with legs pointing behind mother. Right hand cradles head while at right breast. Often a good position for women starting to breast feed for the first time, for feeding twins, and those who have had Caesarians.
  - Lying down—on side facing baby. May need pillow behind to prevent backache and towel under rib to support breast.

Common problems

- Sore/cracked/bleeding nipples: caused by poor positioning. Check baby latching-on correctly, check position, try different one. Feed from least sore side first.
- Full, hard, lumpy breasts: engorgement when milk first comes in or when baby drops a feed later on. Use warm flannels, shower or bath before feeding to help milk flow. Express by hand first so baby can latch-on.
- Small tender lump in breast: blocked duct may be because bra too tight or slept awkwardly. Hand massage and warm flannels etc. as above to help milk flow.
- Red, inflamed areas on breast and flu-like symptoms: mastitis, needs rest, pain killers, fluids, warm massage as above, continue breast feeding, offer sore side first, and advise to see GP if continues, as may need antibiotics.

Expressing milk

Expressing milk allows someone else to feed breast milk by bottle. Can be expressed by hand or by commercially available hand pumps (information through NCT see below). Electric pumps also available often through NCT or if baby in special care units often have electric pumps to help mothers maintain supply. Breast milk can be frozen (special bags are available) and defrosted as required. Bottles and milk should be treated as for bottle feeding (Bottle feeding and weaning 📖).

Further information for professionals and parents

- 🖳 Association of Breastfeeding Mothers: www.abm.me.uk/
- 🖳 www.breastfeeding.nhs.uk
- ☎ Breastfeeding Helpline Line 0870 444 8708
- 🖳 La leche League: www.laleche.org.uk/
- 🖳 National Child Birth Trust: www.nctpregnancyandbabycare.com
- ☎ Parent helpline: 0845 120 2918
- 🖳 UK Unicef Baby Friendly Initiative (information, training, accreditation): www.babyfriendly.org.uk/home.asp

1 Scientific Advisory Committee on Nutrition (2007). *Update on Vitamin D*. The Stationery Office, London.

Bottle feeding and weaning

Bottle feeding

Feeding a baby with a bottle is an opportunity for close, intimate relationships to develop. The parent should be in a comfortable position with the baby well supported in his or her arms.

If not breast fed, infants require a formula milk modified to approximate the composition of human milk, with added iron and vitamins. A formula based on cows' milk that has the casein to non-casein ration modified by addition of demineralized whey, provides an amino acid profile more like breast milk. There is no evidence that any one brand is superior to another. Families on low incomes may be entitled to free formula milk for their babies (Benefits for people on low income 📖). Formula-fed babies do not need additional vitamins.

Preparing bottles

Advise parents to make up formula exactly to the manufacturer's instructions and not to add extra powder.

- Formula milk is available ready-made in cartons (↑ expensive) and in powder form.
- Prepared bottles can be stored in a fridge for up to 24hrs. Unfinished feeds should be thrown away.
- Bottles should be warmed by standing them in a bowl of warm water and the milk heat tested (neither too hot or too cold) on the inside of the parent's wrist before offering it to the baby.
- Feeding bottles and teats should be well washed and, until >6mths of age, sterilized (sterilizing tablets or steam units).

Soya-based and other types of formula milk

- Concerns that if babies drinking soya-based formula they may absorb high levels of phytoestrogens (shown to affect rats reproductive systems).
- Other artificial formulas are available for babies intolerant of cows' milk. Such babies are usually under the care of a paediatric consultant and formula milk is prescribed as advised.
- Modified goats' milk is not approved for use in Europe.

Introduction of whole, pasteurized cows' milk

Not recommended until the baby is >1yr old as this is less digestible and deficient in vitamins A, C, D, and in iron. Breast or first formula milk should be used until 1yr and then switched to whole cows' milk. A 'follow-on' formula is not necessary.

Weaning

The gradual shift from a milk-based diet to family food. WHO and UK DoHs recommend that milk only is sufficient until 6mths. However, some younger babies are hungry soon after their last feed and start waking during the night. Advise not to start solids before 4mths.

- Start with 1 flavour of finely puréed food, e.g. baby rice, potato, yam at one feed. Most food will flow out of the baby's mouth to start with. Babies only take 2–3 teaspoonfuls initially.
- If baby is <6mths old, sterilize bowls and spoons.
- Gradually increase amounts, try new foods one at a time. Gradually move on to mashed foods.
- Foods to avoid:
  - Salt should not be added to any food
  - Sugar should not be added to foods; try naturally sweet foods, e.g. bananas
  - Avoid honey until >1yr, as some contains bacteria that causes illness in babies
  - Avoid raw eggs
  - Avoid nuts until >5yrs
  - Low fat foods are not suitable until 2yrs
  - Introduce foods that commonly cause allergies, e.g. wheat, eggs, seeds, one at a time after age 6mths, to check for reactions.
- Introduce lumpier foods gradually and 'finger foods', e.g. pieces of fruit, toast (at 6mths+).
- Encourage babies to get involved in feeding themselves—use bibs and newspapers, etc. under chairs to catch the mess.
- By 9mths the baby should be eating 3 meals a day, which include protein, carbohydrates, and fruit and vegetables (vitamin C is important for absorption of iron).
- Intake of milk is reduced as solid food increases, but the child still needs at least 600mL/day of milk.

Further information for professionals

📖 DoH England (2004). *HIV and infant feeding*: www.dh.gov.uk/PublicationsAndStatistics
📖 DoH (England) Infant feeding recommendation: www.breastfeeding.nhs.uk
📖 Food Standards Agency: www.food.gov.uk/healthiereating/

Further information for parents

Health Departments in each country produce specific leaflets, e.g. DoH (England) (2005). *Weaning*. DoH, London.
Health Departments Northern Ireland, England, Wales: *Birth to five*. DoH, London. Scotland: *Ready, Steady, Baby*.

Growth 0–1 years

Growth starts *in utero* and ends after puberty.

Infantile growth

- Dependent on nutrition, good health, happiness, and a normal thyroid.
- Definitions:
  - Low birth weight: <2.5kg; and very low birth weight: <1.5kg
  - Small for dates: birth weight <2nd or 3rd centile
  - Large for gestational age: birth weight >90th centile.
- Patterns of weight growth are different for breast fed and bottle-fed babies.
- Babies are likely to at least double their weight in the first 6mths.
- 50% cross at least one centile band, and 5% cross two bands on the weight chart by 12–18mths.
- Growth monitoring:
  - Detects disorders, e.g. hypothyroidism (Growth disorders 📖)
  - Is valued by parents
  - Is the focus of health promotion advice.

Weight monitoring

- Weigh baby at each child health promotion programme (📖) routine visit for review or immunization (i.e. at a minimum: birth, 2mths, 3mths, 4mths, and 12–15mths) plus if requested by parent or if a professional is concerned.
- Remove baby's clothes and weigh on a modern, metric, self-zeroing, and properly maintained device, as far as possible at same time of day and consistently before or after food. Weighing in sling devices is no longer acceptable.
- Record on a nine-centile chart (see Fig. 6.2) and parent-held record
- Record on centile charts for infants born <37wks, correction for gestational age up to 2yrs is essential (Pre-term infants 📖).

Interpretation

- A single measurement is difficult to interpret unless on a markedly different centile to height.
- Slow weight gain, or the weight graph crossing centile lines downwards, may be that baby's normal trajectory. Referral and review by community clinic doctor or GP may be appropriate.
- If <2nd centile, refer to GP/clinic doctor for assessment.
- The term 'faltering weight gain' is used when a slow weight gain occurs that is abnormal for that baby, or when weight crosses 2 centiles downwards. Prolonged failure to gain weight or continuing weight loss may indicate more serious implications, but other signs and symptoms usually present, e.g. coeliac disease (Gastrointestinal problems in children 📖). Needs review and assessment by GP/clinic doctor.
- When psychosocial factors are directly linked to poor growth, this is known as non-organic failure to thrive (NOFTT).
- Organic causes e.g. coeliac disease.
- Weight crossing a centile upwardly may cause concern, but it is difficult to assess the long-term impact.

Length monitoring

- Measured with the baby supine, most easily on a measuring mat, and plotted on a 9-centile chart and PHCHR. Correct for pre-term babies as above.
- Best practice:
  - Soon after birth if premature or small for dates baby
  - At 6–8wks for low birthweight babies, if any disorder suspected, or any cause for concern
  - Thereafter only if cause for concern.
- Refer to doctor if any measurement is below the 0.4 centile.

Occipito-frontal head circumference

Soon after birth and at 6–8wks with plastic or fibre-glass insertion tape. Plotted on a 9-centile chart and PHCHR. Correct for pre-term as above. Referred and reviewed by GP if concerns or growth line crosses a centile upwards.

Key reading

Hall, D.M.B. and Eliman, D. (eds.) (2003). *Health for all children* (4th edn.). Oxford University Press, Oxford.

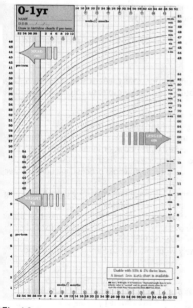

Fig. 6.2 Diagram of growth chart (0–1yrs) (reproduced with kind permission of the Child Growth Foundation)

Baby hygiene and skin care

Many new parents need reassurance and advice about hygiene and skin care. Parents can be reminded that these activities create good opportunities for talking and playing with the baby.

Key principles
Skin cleaning
- A daily bath is not necessary although with an older baby it is helpful as part of an evening routine (see below).
- Face, hands, and neck creases need washing as necessary but at least once a day.
- Eyes should be washed in the new born with wet cotton wool balls, avoid poking around in ears and nostrils.
- Skin in nappy area needs protecting at every nappy change by:
  - Washing (can be with a wipe)
  - Applying a waterproof barrier e.g. petroleum jelly or zinc and castor oil cream. Talcum powder should not be used.
- Nappy changing should happen at least after every feed and more frequently as necessary.
- In girls, nappy area cleaning should be from front to back i.e. towards the anus, without opening vulva. In boys, it is not necessary to pull back foreskin.
- Skin care products should be non-perfumed to avoid irritation and dryness.

Bathing babies
Key principles involve concern for safety (Accident prevention 📖), maintaining body temperature, and having a pleasurably interactive time together.
- Bath in warm room with no draughts.
- Make sure all equipment is to hand before starting.
- Cold then hot water to shallow depth (5–8cm for new baby), temperature should always be checked with elbow, or inner wrist, or bath thermometer. Bath lotion in water easiest cleanser to use.
- Talk, smile, and reassure baby through whole process, introduce water toys as gets older.
- Wrap baby in towel, wash and dry face before placing in bath. In young babies also wash and dry hair/top of head before lowering baby in.
- Always support a young baby in water, with adult's arm under its back grasping furthest away baby's arm. Bath seats are available for older babies but babies should never be left alone in them.
- On lifting out, immediately wrap in towel and dry to maintain body heat.

Hair care
- Hair washing is easiest as part of bath routine using the bath lotion water.
- After about 3–4mths, hair is thicker and a small amount of baby shampoo (i.e. non-stinging if gets in eyes) is better at cleaning.

- Soft baby hair brushes are available.
- Cradle cap (a form of seborrhoeic dermatitis) common in young babies with thick, yellow scales over scalp. Daily gentle shampooing may help. Also rubbing olive oil into scalp, leave overnight to soften scales, then shampooing out and rubbing scales off with fingers. If becomes inflamed may need antibiotic or steroid treatment.

Nail care

- Best trimmed after a bath when soft.
- Blunt-ended baby scissors are available.
- Some parents find it so unnerving to use scissors on a small baby, they prefer to bite off nails.

Nappies

- Parents choose disposable or cloth nappies according to their circumstances and available information.
- LAs and Real Nappy Campaign (see WEN below) provide detailed comparative information on types of nappies. New types of cloth nappies are both cheaper and more environmentally friendly than disposables. Some local authorities are providing financial incentive not to use disposable nappies.
- Cloth nappies now come in much easier designs e.g. using Velcro™ that use disposable or washable liners. They do not need soaking if washed in machines at 60°C. Some areas have nappy laundering services.
- Principles in preventing nappy rash:
  - Good skin care (see above), regular and prompt changing of nappies
  - Correct washing of nappies in non-irritant powder if washables.
- Managing nappy rash:
  - More frequent changing and cleaning
  - Exposure to air
  - Different barrier cream (see BNF 13.2.2)
  - If associated with fungal infection e.g. candida albicans, an antifungal should be prescribed (see BNF 13.10.2).

Further information

Womens Environmental Network (WEN): www.wen.org.uk/ ☎ UK Nappy Helpline details of local cloth nappy contacts: 0845 850 850

Development and care of teeth

The age at which teeth cut through the gum and appear varies enormously. Most start around 6mths but very occasionally babies are born with a tooth (sometimes removed if lose or badly positioned) and some don't cut teeth until after 12mths. Primary teeth are important as they guide adult teeth into the correct position. Erosion and loss of primary teeth affect placement of adult teeth.

20 primary teeth cut through gum in the same order:
• The lower then upper 2 incisors (6–12mths)
• The lower then upper canines (6–18mths)
• The 1st molars (12–20mths)
• The 2nd molars (18–24mths).

Teething

Signs of teething are:
• Dribbling
• Wanting to chew or gnaw
• Often irritable, grizzling and/or fretful
• Red cheeked.

Discomfort may be relieved by:
• Giving something hard to gnaw on e.g. carrot, teething ring
• Use of OTC teething gels (see BNF 12.3.1).

Teeth care: prevention of caries and misalignment
• Teeth need to be cleaned twice a day as soon as they appear with a smear of fluoride baby toothpaste on the finger and massaged over tooth/teeth and gum.
• For <7yrs British Dental Association recommends toothpaste with low dose fluoride formulations (around 500ppmF but not less).
• A soft baby tooth brush should be introduced as they get older. Encourage tooth brushing as a game/copy cat activity to avoid struggles.
• Children need help and supervision in teeth cleaning until about 8yrs:
  • Easiest to clean babies teeth with them on lap or in chair and head slightly tilted for a good view inside mouth
  • Adults need to stand behind older children to clean
  • Children should spit out water after teeth cleaning with fluoride toothpaste. Advise *not* to rinse so the fluoride remains around teeth.
• Encourage:
  • Water and milk-only drinks
  • Savoury and calcium-rich diet
  • Use of cup rather than bottle when weaning to promote good alignment of teeth
  • Sugar-free medications.
• Discourage:
  • Sweetened drinks
  • Dummies and sucking on thumb to avoid misalignment of teeth
  • Use of bottle for drinks other than water and milk to avoid sugary liquid held in mouth.

- Babies should be registered with dentist from birth if possible. First appointment with a dentist should be when first teeth break thorough. NICE guidance recommends dental check up between 3mth and 12mths in <18yrs according to individual assessment. <18yrs exempt from payment for NHS dental check-ups and treatment.

The use of fluoride supplements

- Each PCO area will have a policy on the need for fluoride supplements in view of the levels of fluoride in the drinking water.
- PCO community dental service provides advice.
- Use of fluoride supplements should only be on the advice of a dentist and at the recommended dosage (see BNF 9.5.3).
- Dental fluorosis can occur when too much fluoride is taken e.g. when the water supply is already fluoridated and supplements are taken, or when children 'eat' toothpaste. Fluorosis can lead to the pitting, flecking of the tooth enamel.

Related topic
📖 Care of teeth in older children.

Further information
British Dental Health Foundation: www.dentalhealth.org.uk/

Crying babies

All babies cry and some babies cry a great deal. Some parents need support to recognize that this is the baby's way of alerting adults of a need for attention. A crying baby can be exhausting and stressful. When they cry during the night it can be particularly stressful. Parents, particularly first time, may need help recognizing the causes and developing strategies that work for them and the baby. Dealing with babies that cry a lot can be very frustrating and parents and carers need to be aware that shaking a baby is particularly dangerous.

Soothing babies

As a general rule, most babies are soothed by movement, contact, and sound e.g. rocking, mobile over cot, cuddling and walking, holding them at the same time as talking or crooning. Having babies in baby slings or closely wrapped on the parents back creates contact and movement. Some babies are more 'sucky' than others and might calm with a feed, or thumb in mouth or dummy.

Parents learn to recognize signs in their own babies of the causes and address them:
- Hunger or thirst—offer a feed or boiled water, check for problems with feeding (Breast feeding 📖).
- Tiredness but fighting sleep—lay them down either in quiet darkened place or in buggy to go out for a walk.
- Discomfort with wet or dirty nappy—change it (Baby hygiene and skin care 📖).
- Discomfort as too hot or cold—remove or add clothes or covering.
- Lack of contact—lift and cuddle, stroke, talk to.
- Pain—through a physical cause e.g. wind after feeding, colic (see below), teething (Development and care of teeth 📖).

Parents need to be alert that the crying and associated behaviour may be unusual for their baby and it is a sign of illness or infection that requires medical attention.

Colic

Affects about 1 in 4 babies in first 3–4mths. Inconsolable crying, drawing up of knees can last for hours and occurs mostly in the evenings. Cause is unknown, it is benign but distressing for parents. No evidence that gripe water, herbal remedies, changing mother's diet are of benefit. Reassure parents, work through possible list of causes above, and suggest soothing strategies.

As babies get older, the causes change, can include;
- Boredom—needs company and distractions such as rattles, toys, talking to, playing with.
- Frustration—as they start to crawl and cruise, items have to be put out of the way (Accident prevention 📖) leading to great frustration, distraction tactics become important.
- Fear of separation and strangers—usually between 6–8mths—lots of reassurance, cuddling, comfort, gradual periods of separation, gradual familiarity with new surroundings help.

When the crying becomes too much

Sometimes, parents feel overwhelmed and frustrated by a baby who will not stop crying. Any health professional working with parents who say their babies cry a lot should help them work through coping strategies to ensure they don't overreact, lose their tempers, or become rough with the baby. These include:

- Getting help from other adults.
- Having someone else look after the baby for an hour or so.
- Creating time to think through the other causes and strategies to stop the baby crying by putting the baby down safely and leaving the room.
- Putting the baby down safely and leaving the room if they feel it is all too much and getting another adult or using a helpline.
- Talking to someone about how you feel, such as the HV or a helpline (see below).
- Remembering this difficult time won't last forever, it is only for a short time.

Further information for professionals and parents

Cry-sis for support to families with excessively crying, sleepless, and demanding babies. www.cry-sis.org.uk ☎ 08451 228 669

Babies and sleeping

A new born baby's sleep pattern is determined by their weight and feeding requirements. When not feeding most babies are asleep although some are active and alert for long periods. As a rough guide (but may be very different in individual babies/breast-fed babies):

• 2kg baby awake for 7–8 feeds
• 3kg baby awake for 5–6 feeds
• 4.5kg baby awake for 4–5 feeds.

Most babies are able to sleep for longer periods through the night without feeds by 6wks. The periods of wakefulness during the day extend as they get older. Most older babies need morning and afternoon naps during the first year.

Safe sleeping

The safest place for a baby to sleep is in a cot beside the parents' bed for the first 6mths. To reduce the incidence of SUDI (Sudden unexpected death of an infant 📖) the baby put down to sleep should:

• Be on their back.
• Have their head uncovered.
• Feet to foot of the cot.
• Not get too hot or too cold. Advice includes:
  ◦ Cotton sheets and blankets not duvets, baby nests, or sheepskins.
  ◦ No pillows, wedges, or cot bumpers.
  ◦ Never placed with hot water bottles, electric blankets, or next to radiators, fires, or in direct sunshine.
  ◦ Ideal room temperature is about 18°C (65F).
  ◦ Only need to wear nappy, vest, and sleep suit.

Other advice to prevent SUDI includes parents to stop smoking and no smoking in same room as baby.

Co-sleeping

While there are many advocates of sharing there are real risks to the baby (Accident prevention 📖, Sudden unexpected death of an infant 📖) and potential for disrupted sleep patterns for both parents.

Parents should never share a bed or bring the baby into the bed if:

• Either parent smokes (risk of sudden unexpected death of an infant (📖)).
• They have been drinking or taking illegal drugs or medication that increases drowsiness.
• Are unwell or extra tired so it might affect their ability to arouse or respond to the baby.

❶ Parents or carers should never fall asleep with a baby on an armchair or sofa as there are real dangers of the person shifting and suffocating the baby.

Sleeping and settling routines

Bed time sleep routines help babies and parents establish good patterns of separating to sleep. Around 6wks is a good time to start and they are usually established by 3–6mths. Most routines tend to include some or most of the following:

• A bath
• A feed

- A quiet time
- Placing in bed, lullaby, later story
- Cuddle and kiss goodnight
- Leaving them in a darkened room, with a night light, baby listener switched on, and gentle music e.g. part of a mobile
- Parents not to go back at first whimper or crying.

Night waking babies 0–6mths

- Any night feeds still required should be very low key with little eye contact or words; all signals that this is not the time to be awake.
- Check for all causes of crying (Crying babies 📖) and settle.

Night waking babies 6–12mths

Babies who wake at night or only go back to sleep with lots of parent attention/feeds can usually be persuaded to change their behaviour by the checking routine (also used for older children). Over a 2wks period when the baby wakes:
- Leave to cry for 5min
- Parent goes in checks him, tucks in, and leaves
- Parent does not cuddle, give drink, or 'reward' in any way
- This process is repeated often with increasing intervals until baby recognizes night time waking produces no results and stays or quickly returns to sleep.

Parents need to be convinced of the value of this process and not undermine their own efforts by re-starting to 'reward' night waking.

Further information for professionals and parents

📖 Cry-sis for support to families with excessively crying, sleepless, and demanding babies. www.cry-sis.org.uk ☎ 08451 228 669
📖 Department of Health /FSID 2004 Reducing the risk of cot death an easy guide. www.Dh.gov.uk
📖 Foundation for sudden Infant Death and UNICEF's Baby Friendly Initiative. *Sharing a bed with your baby–advice for breast-feeding parents.* www.sids.org.uk/

Promoting baby development safely 0–1 years

Health professionals, particularly HV teams are in a good position to advise parents on how to help their babies develop (Child development 0–1yrs 📖), at the same time providing health promotion advice on accident prevention (📖) particularly as they become mobile.

Key principles to promote with parents and carers

- Babies are learning from the first day and their abilities quickly develop.
- New parents often need to learn to play and talk to their babies.
- Interacting with the baby in every activity promotes attachment or bonding, learning and speech development:
  - Talking to them with eye-to-eye contact, with face up close when new born, and responding to their noises at every opportunity.
  - Holding them to feed, holding on lap, carrying, cuddling, singing nursery rhymes, games like peek-a-boo.
- Help babies find out about the world around them e.g.:
  - From 6wks babies can be propped up against pillows or in bouncing chairs (always on floor not tables).
  - Out and about to parks, friends' houses, shops in buggies.
- To have realistic expectations of the developmental stage e.g. babies explore through their mouths so don't try to stop them just make sure the things they take to their mouths are clean, safe, and can't be swallowed or are small enough to cause a blockage.
- Simple toys are the best: people are better than toys early on.
- Encouraging movement safely:
  - Learning to crawl: needs opportunities on tummy on the floor, once able to roll never leave alone accept on floor in clear space without objects that could hurt or be swallowed.
  - Once independently moving by rolling, crawling, furniture cruising— remove poisonous substances from reach level, fit safety gates, remove glass topped items, protect sharp edged furniture (Accidents prevention 📖).
  - Discourage parents from using baby walkers—they cause more accidents than any other baby equipment.

Resources to support development

- Many HV and Sure Start teams have produced resource packs or have drop-in sessions to support parents in helping the development of their babies (see below).
- HV teams in many areas distribute book bags under the Bookstart scheme (see below) at 7–9mths.
- Toy libraries often provide packs and ideas for 0–1yrs (Services for children, young people, and families 📖).

Promoting accident prevention

All baby equipment should be to British Standard or European Standards. ❶ Baby car seats—new babies should be in rear facing car seats and never placed in the front seat if the car has air bags.

Accident prevention for babies includes:

- Falls. e.g. rolling off changing mats etc. Promote strapping in buggies, placing on floors and safe places.
- Burns and scalds e.g. too hot bath water, spilt hot drinks. Promote cold water then hot water in bath, testing bath water, not having hot drinks near baby.
- Fires in the home e.g. distracted parent leaves chip pan over heat. Promote smoke alarms.
- Drowning e.g. in bath. Highlight danger in leaving baby alone in, or near, water.
- Choking. Highlight danger of prop feeding and small items sticking in trachea.

Many Sure Start, HV teams or local children's services provide first aid classes for parents (see Accident prevention 📖),

Further information for professionals and parents

📖 Bookstart: www.bookstart.co.uk
📖 British Association for Early Childhood Education: www.early-education.org.uk
📖 British Literacy Association Talk to Your Baby: www.literacytrust.org.uk/talktoyourbaby
📖 Sure Start: www.surestart.gov.uk/

Accident prevention

📖 Child Accident Prevention Trust: www.capt.org.uk
📖 Royal Society for the Prevention of Accidents dedicated site on child car seats: www.childcarseats.org.uk/

Child development 1–5 years

Child development is the interaction between heredity and the environment (Child health promotion 📖). Development is assessed as part of the child assessment framework (The assessment of children, young people, and families 📖).

Developmental progress

This is about the sequential acquisition of skills. It is important to remember that:
- There is a wide time scale within the normal range, e.g. children walking unaided: 25% by 11mths, 90% by 15mths, 97.5% by 18mths
- Median ages indicate when half a standard population should have acquired the skill (see Table 6.4 for children aged 1–5yrs)
- Pre-term babies are assessed from EDD up until 2yrs of age only.

Referral for more in-depth assessment

Failure to meet acquisition by upper limits of age need more detailed assessment and investigation, often through referral to community or hospital paediatricians, e.g.
- Not walking unaided by 18mths
- No pincer grip by 18mths
- Not saying single words with meaning by 18mths
- No 2- or 3-word sentences by 30mths.

More detailed and in-depth assessment is also required if:
- Parents concerned about an aspect of development
- Discordant levels of development between areas
- Regression of previously acquired skills
- Development plateaus.

Development can be delayed or suboptimal
- Indirectly from adverse environmental factors or ill-health
- Directly from neurological or neuro-developmental problems.

Related topics

📖 Overview of the child health promotion programme.

Further information

Frost, M., and Sharma, A. (1997). From birth to 5 years: children's development progress. *Revised and updated version of Mary Sheridan's work.* Routledge, London.

Table 6.4 Overview of median age of development in children 1–5 years

	15mths	18mths	2yrs	3yrs	4–5yrs
Gross motor	Walks alone steadily	Bends to pick up without toppling	Kicks a ball without toppling; runs; $2\frac{1}{2}$: jumps with both feet off the ground	Up and down stairs without holding on; pedals trikes	Hops, skips, catches ball
Fine motor and vision	Scribbles with pencil	Turns pages in books; feeds himself with spoon; able to put on some clothes; builds tower of 3 bricks	Builds tower of 6 bricks; able to take off most clothes and put some on	Builds bridge with 3 bricks; draws O (copies 6mths earlier); does up buttons	Builds copy of 6 bricks in steps; draws x at 4; at $4\frac{1}{2}$yrs, △; at 5yrs uses scissors
Language, speech, and hearing	Shows 2 parts of body; follows simple instructions, single words	10–20 words, usually nouns, hums	Uses 2 or more phrases to make simple sentences; $2\frac{1}{2}$: talks constantly in 3–4-word phrases	Vocab 200–300 words; starts asking 'why?' frequently; begins to grasp concept of numbers; knows age and a few colours	Talks a great deal, boasts, tells stories
Social, emotional, and behaviour	Imagination appears in doll play	Symbolic play; imitates adults; plays alongside (parallel) others	Learning to play with others but often rivalries; dry by day and bowel control, later; starts saying 'no' often	Interactive play with other children; takes turns; dry by night, later	Expanding sense of self, growing confidence, wants to be grown up

Growth 1–5 years

Growth starts *in utero* and ends after puberty. It is good practice to record height and weight in any child about whom there is concern, who has chronic ill-health, or requires prolonged follow-up for any reason. Growth charts are available in PHCHR, in Lloyd George size for GP practices, and for special conditions, e.g. Down's syndrome.

Growth

- Dependent on nutrition (Food and the under fives 📖), good health, happiness, and normal thyroid function.
- Growth monitoring:
  - Detects disorders, e.g. hypothyroidism (Growth disorders 📖)
  - Is valued by parents
  - Is the focus of health promotion advice.

Weight monitoring

- Weigh the child at each routine visit for review or immunization (i.e. at a minimum: 12–15mths, 24mths, between 3 and 4yrs and at 5yrs (Overview of the child health promotion programme 📖), plus if requested by a parent or if a professional is concerned.
- Weigh toddlers in vest and pants, older children in light clothing on a modern, metric, self-zeroing, and properly maintained device.
- Record on a 9-centile chart (see Fig. 6.3) and parent-held record.
- Correction for gestational age up to age 2yrs is essential (Pre-term babies 📖).

Interpretation

- It is difficult to interpret a single measurement unless on a markedly different centile from height.
- If <2nd centile or >99.6 centile, refer to GP for assessment.
- The term 'faltering weight gain' is used when there is a slow weight gain or when the weight crosses 2 centiles. Prolonged failure to gain weight or continuing weight loss may indicate more serious implications, but other signs and symptoms usually present (e.g. coeliac disease (📖)). Needs review and assessment by doctor.
- <5% faltering weight due to organic causes. When psychosocial factors are directly linked to poor growth, this is known as non-organic failure to thrive (NOFTT). A full assessment and care plan will address more than just improved nutrition (The assessment of children, young people and families 📖).
- Concern about overweight between 2–18yrs: measure height (see below) then assess on British BMI charts for children: >98 centile overweight, >99.6 obese and cause for concern.

Height monitoring

- Only recommended at school entry, unless there is a concern about health or growth, and is measured at the same time as weight.
- Measured standing as soon as child can stand. The most accurate devices are the Minimeter or Leicester height measures.
- Recorded on growth chart (see Fig. 6.3) and PHCHR. Correct for pre-term babies to 2yrs only.

- Any child with a height <0.4 centile or >99.6 should be referred to the doctor.

Related topic

📖 The assessment of children, young people and families

Further information

Hall, D.M.B. and Eliman, D. (eds.) (2003). *Health for all children* (4th edn.). Oxford University Press, Oxford.

📓 Information to support *Health for all children* and supplies of all growth-monitoring charts, equipment, BMI for children and equipment: www.healthforallchildren.co.uk/

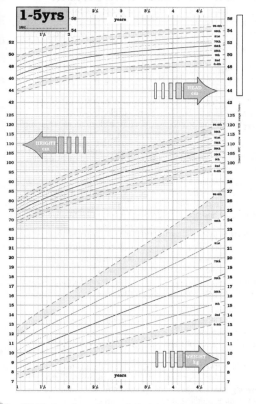

Fig. 6.3 Diagram of growth chart (1–5yrs) (reproduced with kind permission of the Child Growth Foundation)

Promoting development in the under fives

Health professionals, particularly HV teams are in a good position to advise parents on how to help their young children develop (Child development 1–5yrs 📖), at the same time providing health promotion advice (Models and approaches to health promotion 📖) on accident prevention (📖).

Key principles to promote with parents and carers

- Young children are curious and learning about life, their family, and their home all the time.
- They learn by being part of everyday life in their family life, playing, and asking questions.
- Parents, family, and carers help children develop by:
  - Encouraging and rewarding all efforts, attempts, new achievements and good behaviour with touching, smiling, words of praise, listening, cuddles.
  - Including them in daily activities e.g. shopping and family events.
  - Talking to them, singing with them, reading together.
  - Playing games and providing opportunities for different types of games e.g. outdoor running games, wet play in the bath, imaginative play with dressing up clothes, manipulation games with puzzles.
- Social skills are developed through opportunities to meet other children and adults e.g. drop-ins, play groups (Services for children, young people, and families 📖).
- Children need the opportunity to be outside, to run about, let off steam and get fresh air every day.
- Most of all relax and enjoy children—they won't be this age long.

Resources to support development

- Many HV and Sure Start teams have produced resource packs or have drop-in sessions to support parents (see below).
- Libraries and toy libraries often provide packs and ideas for under 5s.
- Local children's or early years services may provide a range of resources about play groups, drop-ins etc.

Promoting accident prevention 1–5yrs

- Many Sure Start, HV teams, or local children's services provide first aid classes for parents.
- Young children need constant supervision as very curious.
- ↑ increased mobility ↑ risk of:
  - Falls: think about window safety catches, safety gates.
  - Burns and scalds: keep hot drinks and saucepans out of reach.
  - Drowning: never leave <4yrs in bath alone, fill in or fence off ponds, empty paddling pools.
  - Poisoning: keep household cleaners, medicines in locked cabinets out of reach.
  - Cuts and bruises: protect sharp edges in home, fit safety glass, use door guards to prevent trapped fingers.

- Out and about: teach the green cross code to children (see Rospa below), use age appropriate car seats, think sun safety (Skin cancer prevention 📖).

Related topics

📖 Working with parents; 📖 Support for parenting programmes.

Further information for professionals and parents

▣ British Association for Early Childhood Education: www.early-education.org.uk
▣ British Literacy Association Talk to Your Baby: www.literacy-trust.org.uk/talktoyourbaby
▣ Sure Start: www.surestart.gov.uk/ information on early education, childcare, health, and family support

Accident prevention

▣ Child Accident Prevention Trust: www.capt.org.uk
▣ Royal Society for the Prevention of Accidents dedicated site on child car seats: www.childcarseats.org.uk/

Emotional development in babies and children

General

Significant and critical brain and intelligence development occurs during the first 3yrs of life. It is influenced by nutritional and health status, also by interactions developed with people and objects. Key points:

- Highly dependent upon adequate nutrition, stimulation, and optimal care.
- During first years, key brain pathways for lifelong capabilities are established. Once developed, the brain is much harder to modify.
- Adequate attention to the first months and years (including prenatally) of a child's life are crucial in determining lifelong outcome.
- Duet relationship created by caregiver and baby builds and strengthens brain architecture and creates relationship in which a baby's experiences are affirmed and new abilities nurtured.
- By school age, a lot of key language abilities, physical capabilities, and cognitive foundations have been set in place.
- While a focus on primary education is important, 8yrs is too late to start paying attention to children's emotional development needs.
- Sensitive and responsive parent–child relationships is also associated with stronger cognitive skills in young children and enhanced social competence and work skills later in school.

Developmental guideline

- Think in terms of stages not ages. Below ages are *guidelines only*.
- 1mth: voice recognition, express interest: attend to pictures, visual focus.
- 6mths: senses pleasure: smiling, mouthing objects important, different communication methods: pointing, vocalizing, crying; also words and pictures.
- 9mths: facial expressions reflecting emotions e.g. fear, comfort objects.
- <2yrs: attachment vital, self-centred, gaining personal identity, change resistant.
- 3yrs: conforms, more secure, adventuresome, enjoys music, imaginative play, regulation of emotion and self-distraction beginning.
- 4yrs: sure of self, tests self, often negative, needs controlled freedom.
- 5yrs: self-assured, stable, self-adjusted, enjoys responsibilities, capable of self-criticism, likes to follow rules.
- By 6yrs: learnt which emotions are socially (un)acceptable.
- Middle childhood: aware actions lead to (dis)approval, internalize standards of conduct.

Basics for positive emotional health

- Unconditional love from family: praise, firm but realistic goals, honesty, encouragement.
- Safe and secure surroundings.

- Supportive caregivers, encouraging teachers.
- Self-confidence and self-esteem.
- Appropriate discipline.
- Make time for play.
- Set good example/role model.
- Opportunity to play with other children.

Key principles for parents

- Think of stages not ages, social and emotional milestones harder to pinpoint than signs of physical development.
- Early support and intervention may prevent damaging patterns being established within families.
- Significant events in adult carer and family life impact on children too e.g. deaths of grandparents, birth/illness of siblings, family break up.

Related topics

📖 Emotional problems in children; 📖 Behavioural disorders in children.

Further information for professionals and parents

🖳 Association of Infant Mental Health: www.aimh.org.uk
🖳 Child Psychotherapy Trust: www.childpsychotherapytrust.org.uk
🖳 Young Minds: www.youngminds.org.uk
🖳 Zero to Three: www.zerotothree.org

Food and the under fives

Good nutrition in pre-school children is important because it:
- Ensures optimum growth and functional development.
- Encourages a taste for healthy foods in preference to fatty, salty, and sugary foods.

By 5yrs children should be eating family food that is a balanced healthy diet (Nutrition and healthy eating 📖).

Nutritional requirements

1–5-yr olds have high energy and nutrient requirements relative to their size and need nutritious snacks between meals as part of a fixed routine (not constant snacking). Estimated average requirements (EAR) for energy:
- Boys 1–3yrs 1230 kcal/day, 4–6yrs 1715 kcal/day.
- Girls 1–3yrs 1165 kcal/day, 4–6yrs 1545 kcal/day.

The developing body, in particular bones and teeth, need a good supply of protein, calcium, iron, and vitamins A and D. Parents should be encouraged to offer children the family meals not a different menu.

Diets of pre-school children

Should include:
- A variety of foods each day from 4 food groups (1. cereals; 2. fruit and vegetable; 3. meat, egg, pulses; 4. milk and milk products).
- Contain full fat cows' milk until 2yrs when semi-skimmed can be substituted provided the diet is otherwise nutritionally adequate. Skimmed milk not suitable <5yrs.
- Plenty of fluids, preferably plain tap water, to prevent constipation.
- Contain no more than 10% of dietary energy in sugars.
- Be low in salt, avoiding salty foods and the addition of salt at the table.
- Avoid excessive fibre intake which compromise energy and mineral intake.
- Avoid tea and coffee to ensure mineral (especially iron) bioavailability.
- Promote dental health by keeping sugary foods and drinks to meal times only.
- Be supplemented with vitamins A, C, and D, from 6mths, unless adequate vitamins assured through diverse diet and moderate exposure to sunlight.

Vegetarians and vegans

Children need to be offered a mixture of plant proteins (e.g. cereals, pulses, seeds, ground-up nuts) to ensure the combinations complement each other in forming high quality protein ≥animal protein. Iron from plant sources is better absorbed with vitamin C e.g. fruit juice. Children on vegan diets may need supplements of fortified foods to achieve enough calcium, vitamins D and B12, and riboflavin.

State nutrition support for children

- Vitamin drops and l pint of whole milk a day are free to children <5yr in families receiving benefits (📖) or income based job seekers allowance (currently being reviewed).
- Children attending nursery sessions >2hrs are eligible to receive $^1/_3$ pt free milk each day they attend through the Nursery Milk Scheme.
- School fruit and vegetable scheme.

Eating: a social skill

Food and eating offers opportunities for learning and interaction with adults such as helping to shop, cooking, laying the table, washing up. Specific skills include:

- How to feed themselves more skillfully in accordance with family practices, including using utensils.
- How to participate in a social occasion that requires certain ways of behaving.

Children have to be given opportunities to feed themselves, to sit at a table to eat with others and to enjoy mealtimes. Parents need to be:

- Prepared for messy mealtimes with toddlers.
- Consistent about the expected behaviour at the meal table and realistic in what is manageable for the child's age,

Food problems

Food preferences and refusal are common <5yrs and are part of growing up and asserting independence. Often a source of great tension at meal times. Parents may need advice on positive behaviour management. Key advice for parents;

- Children will not harm themselves if they do not eat for a short while.
- No one food is essential but don't allow the child to stop eating an entire food group e.g. fruit and vegetables.
- If a food is rejected try:
  - Another in the same food group
  - Presenting it cooked in a different way
  - Presenting it in a more fun way.
- If the child refuses to eat, don't insist, and don't substitute with snacking.

Food allergies

See 📖 Allergies.

Foods for children to avoid

- Whole nuts in case of choking.
- Shark, swordfish, and marlin because levels of mercury may affect development of nervous system.
- Raw shellfish to avoid risk of food poisoning.
- Infants and toddlers: raw or runny eggs to avoid risk of food poisoning.

Further information for professionals and parents

- British Nutrition Foundation: www.nutrition.org.uk
- DoH England 5 a day web site with resources and information for professionals and public on increasing fruit and vegetable consumption: www.5aday.nhs.uk/
- Vegetarian Society Information section on food and pre-school children: www.vegsoc.org/index.html

Further information for parents

Health Departments Northern Ireland, England, Wales *Birth to five.*

Toilet training

Most children can do without nappies by day from 2–3yrs and by night from 2–5yrs. How to approach toilet training will vary from child to child.

General principles

- *Wait until the child is ready*: this usually means that the child can indicate to the parent that they are going to the toilet and has shown an interest in using the potty or toilet. It is helpful to have a potty or child's toilet seat to put on the normal toilet for the child to become familiar with before starting toilet training.
- *Pick a good time*: when the child can have a few days at home without nappies in an environment where accidents don't matter. Make sure the child has plenty of spare clothes available.
- *Keep the potty handy or stay within easy reach of the toilet*: when the child says they wish to go, sit them immediately on the toilet. Reward any result with praise. Don't punish the child for any accidents—advise the parent to ask the child to help clear up any mess and reinforce that it would be better to use the potty/toilet next time.
- *Until the child (and parent) are confident in the child's ability to use the toilet continue using nappies when out and at night*: take the child to the toilet at night before bed time. When dry nappies are consistently noted in the mornings, try the child without nappies at night—a plastic sheet on the mattress is a good idea. Even when a child has been dry day and night for some time, accidents are common if the child is tired, unwell or unsettled—whether excited or unhappy.

❶ If the child does not succeed within a few days, either try training pants or revert to nappies and try again at a later date.

Toilet training for children with developmental delay

The same basic principles apply only at a later chronological age. Parents usually advised to watch for signs of child becoming aware of need to go to toilet e.g. fidgeting, and for signs of physical readiness e.g. dry for an hour or two and during naps. Parents may be advised to institute a toileting programme i.e. a structured daily programme around that child's toileting habits, supported by visual signs to indicate each activity e.g. take down pants, flush toilet, and reinforced with rewards.

Related topics

📖 Constipation and encopresis; 📖 Enuresis.

Further information for professionals and parents

- 🖥 Education and Resources for Improving Childhood Continence Leaflet on potty training: www.eric.org.uk
- 🖥 National Child Birth Trust Advice on Potty Training: www.nctpregnancyandbabycare.com
- 🖥 The National Autistic Society web pages on toileting training: www.nas.org.uk

Understanding behaviour 1–5 years

Developing from a helpless baby to a relatively independent 4yr-old is a time of great learning and emotion that can often feel very difficult for parents and carers. Toddlers and children are at an egocentric stage in their development, seeing themselves at the centre of the world, ready to be involved in everything but often overwhelmed with feelings that they can't manage yet. Children react individually and very differently to the triumphs and set backs of each day, needing different types of support and understanding from parents and carers.

Children may become:
- Bossy: it's one way of covering up that they are still small and there are things they can't do. Often irritating to other children and adults but they still need love and support.
- Fussy: e.g. fads and rituals: it's one way of asserting independence against adults. Adults need to demonstrate how to give in gracefully over things that are less important e.g. wearing odd clothes. Sometimes, child is anxious or worried but unable to talk about it so it's easier to control what goes on the plate than control the anxious feeling. These feelings come and go but if behaviour becomes particularly difficult consider if there is a particular stress and address that.
- Clingy and fearful: it's one way of saying they still feel small but can be trying to parents and carers. Like all children they need support, love, encouragement, but also more time to take those steps to independence. Important to take new things slowly e.g. settling into play group, meeting new people.

Key principles for parents
- Give positive attention (e.g. active listening, smiling, talking to, hugging) to the child in daily activities so they feel encouraged, supported, loved (Promoting development in the under fives 📖).
- Reward efforts, attempts, and good behaviour with smiles, words of praise, cuddles etc.
- Help build self-esteem by letting children have a go at things.
- Relax and enjoy your children, do fun activities together.
- Reduce your own stress e.g. create time away.
- When things get tense over behaviour:
  - Don't reward misbehaviour and encourage its continuation with lots of attention.
  - Make sure you stay in control of your own behaviour, leave the room if you are not.

See also 📖 Working with parents and 📖 Support for parenting programmes.

Temper tantrums
Children are coping with strong feelings all day. A temper tantrum is a display of how it feels on the inside at a point when they can no longer cope, are feeling exhausted, and haven't got the words to describe or deal with the feelings. In dealing with a tantrum parents should be advised to:
- Count to 10 before doing anything, unless the child is putting themselves in danger.

- Stay calm, acknowledge the child's feelings.
- Recognize the child is beyond reasoning and not get into an argument.
- Don't ask more of them than they can manage.
- Try to avoid saying hurtful things that you don't mean.
- Trying to hold or hug the child may make it worse. After it subsides cuddling may help reassure while explaining it was not acceptable behaviour.

New siblings

More than one child brings additional complexities to family life. A new baby is the choice of the parents not the siblings. Key principles of advice for parents:

- Prepare the other child(ren) during the pregnancy.
- Recognize that the older child may feel sad, angry, or upset as they are no longer the centre of attention.
- The older child needs attention, reassurance, expressions of love, and time alone with parents.
- Find small, manageable ways for the older child to help with the new baby.

Further information for professionals and parents

- Child Pyschotherapy Trust Information Series of Leaflets on understanding childhood: www.understandingchildhood.net/
- Parents' website of the National Family and Parents Institute: www.e-parents.org/
- Parentline: www.parentlineplus.org.uk/

Speech and language acquisition

Children follow a systematic path to the effective use of language and communication skills (see Child development 0–1 yrs; and 1–5yrs 📖). Speech and language development is multidimensional including speech, vocabulary, syntax, expression, and verbal comprehension. Speech, language and communication difficulties can affect future learning and achievement, literacy, behaviour and social emotional functioning, confidence and independence.

Speech and language is developed through parents and carers talking and listening to babies and young children. Primary care nurses and HV teams promote good interactive practice by advising parents to:
- Talk to the child when playing or doing things together.
- Have fun with nursery rhymes and songs, especially those with actions.
- Encourage the child to listen to different sounds, such as birds, animals.
- Gain the child's attention when you want to talk together.
- Encourage the child to communicate in any way, not just through words.
- Increase vocabulary by giving choices, e.g. 'Do you want an apple or banana?'.
- Talk about things as they happen, e.g. when bathing, shopping.
- Listen carefully and give the child time to finish talking. Take turns to speak.
- Always respond in some way when the child says something.
- Help child to use more words by adding to what is said, e.g. if they said 'car' adult responds 'Yes, it's a red car driving down the road'.
- If child says something incorrectly, repeat it correctly e.g. 'Goggy bited it'. 'Yes, the dog bit it, didn't he?'.
- Try and have a special time with the child each day to play with toys and look at picture books together.

(Adapted from *Help Your Child To Talk*, Royal College of Speech and Language Therapists, 2002.)

HV teams in most parts of UK are also involved in distributing free Bookstart packs of books to babies with guidance materials for parents and carers:
- First Bookstart pack usually delivered to families at baby's 7–9mth health check with their HV.
- In England two additional packs—Bookstart Plus for 18-month-olds, and My Bookstart Treasure Chest, aimed at 3-yr-olds.

Interactive practice skills are also promoted in parenting skills programmes e.g. Sure Start as well as in other types of group settings for parents and babies e.g. mother and baby groups, postnatal groups, infant massage groups.

Babies and young children in bilingual families should be encouraged to speak both family languages and English. Bilingualism does not delay speech and language acquisition.

Speech and language delay

Primary speech and language delays are those not attributed to other conditions such as hearing loss (Hearing screening 📖) or other more general developmental disabilities. Difficulties may arise with receptive language, expressive language, social communication, speech, fluency or voice. Estimated at 6% but higher in some areas. Such delays are important as:

- Cause concern to parents.
- Often associated with behavioural and other difficulties in the pre-school period.
- Constitute a risk factor for subsequent poor school performance, and for a wide range of personal and social difficulties.
- More common in ♂ than ♀.

Up to 60% of speech or language delays may resolve without treatment between the ages of 2 and 3yrs. However, unable to predict which children will spontaneously resolve at time of identification.

Identification and action

- No universal screening test (Child screening tests 📖) but nurses and HV teams should be alert to parental concerns and observe children's communication behaviours for evidence of delay (see also Overview of the child health promotion programme 📖).
- On identification of speech or language delay nurses and HVs:
  - Check no other related problem e.g. hearing.
  - Refer to speech and language therapy services according to local policy.
  - Offer advice on improving interactive communication. In some areas nursery nurses in HV teams run learning to play sessions for parents and children.
  - Suggest or introduce parent/carer and child to socializing and play opportunities e.g. one o'clock club, play group, mother and children group, childminder group.
- Some PCOs are using early identification of risk of delay to target some parents and children into structured SLT-led programmes e.g. WILSTAAR (Ward Infant Language Screening Test Acceleration and Remediation programme).

Further information for professionals and parents

📖 Bookstart: www.bookstart.org.uk/bookstart/index.php4
📖 Talking Point (Information on communication development and disabilities): www.ican.org.uk/sitecore/content/TalkingPoint/Frontpage.aspx
📖 Talk to Your Baby Campaign with resources: www.literacytrust.org.uk/talktoyourbaby/index.html

Child development 5–11 years

Child development is the interaction between heredity and the environment (Child health promotion 📖). Development is assessed as part of the child assessment framework (The assessment of children, young people, and families 📖). Developmental progress is about the sequential acquisition of skills, and there is a range of time within which children acquire the skills indicated in the table opposite.

Children are expected to achieve nationally defined skills and knowledge in a range of subjects specified in the national curriculums for state schools. In England and Wales: Key Stage 1 by age 7 and Key Stage 2 by age 11. Standard Assessment Tests (SATS) are taken in reading, writing, and mathematics in school year 2 (age 6–7) and school year 6 (age 10–11). In Scotland each subject is described at 6 levels, starting at Level A. The majority of children are expected to reach Level B by the end of Primary year 4.

Puberty follows a well defined set of stages starting between 8.5 and 12.5yrs in girls and between 10 and 14yrs in boys. The first stage is breast development in girls and testicular development in boys (see Young people and adolescence 📖). Girls with early onset of puberty while in primary school may need particular support in dealing with their difference from their peers.

Further information for professionals and parents

📖 Department for Education and Skills England: www.dfes.gov.uk/
📖 Learning and Teaching Scotland: www.ltscotland.org.uk
📖 Learning Wales: www.learning.wales.gov.uk.

Table 6.5 Overview of median age of development in children 5–11yrs

	5–7yrs	7–11yrs
Gross motor	Increasing strength e.g. running faster, jumping higher. Increasing agility e.g. stand on one leg longer, walk a narrow beam. Increasing coordination e.g. learns to ride a 2-wheel bike, learns to swim.	Strength, agility, stamina and coordination continue to develop. Increasingly able to play in team sports.
Fine motor and vision	Fine motor skills further developed in manipulating smaller objects with more precision. Able to dress and undress.	Fine motor skills increasingly developed. Dressing, undressing and self-care skills much more developed.
Cognitive development	Increased linguistic skills. Conversations more complicated. Learning to read, write, and problem-solve. Dominant mode of thought is tied to immediate circumstances and specific experiences. Beginning to grasp more abstract ideas, like numbers, time, and distance.	Abilities described in 5–7yrs continue to develop. Egocentrism reduces— greater ability with language leads to greater socialisation. More objective view of world and causes of physical events and their relationships.
Social, emotional, and behavioural	Increasing independence from adults and personal confidence. Able to wash and bath with less supervision. Still needs help in brushing teeth properly. Plays games with simple rules and many fantasy games. Identifies with same-sex friends. Peer acceptance and approval begins to become important.	Increased desire for independence at the same time as a continued need for parental support. Friends still primarily of the same gender, but interest in opposite gender beginning. Increasing joining into groups and sometimes cliques. Exclusion can feel devastating. Increasingly competitive and self-conscious. Peer approval and acceptance continues to grow in importance.

Growth and nutrition 5–11 years

2–12yrs contributes about 40% of adult height, often in rapid growth spurts. Growth is dependent on nutrition, good health, happiness, pituitary growth hormone, thyroid hormone and vitamin D. Estimated average requirements for energy: boys 7–10yrs 1970 kcal/day, girls 7–10yrs 1740 kcal/day. See also 📖 Nutrition and healthy eating.

Nutrition: all children should be eating family food in a balanced healthy diet i.e. 47–50% carbohydrates (preferably complex), 15% protein, 5+ portions of fruit and vegetables a day, some fats, and low in salty and sugary foods. Vegetarian diets need to ensure adequate protein, iron, and selenium, as well as adequate B12 for vegans.

Monitoring

Routine monitoring of weight and height at school entry (reception years 4–5yrs) recommended and national policies then apply e.g. England requires monitoring in year 6 (10–11yrs) as part of public health monitoring of childhood obesity.

Good practice to record height and weight in any child over whom there is a concern, has chronic ill health, or requires prolonged follow-up for any reason and plot on growth chart.

Weight monitoring

- Weigh in light clothing on a modern, metric, self-zeroing, and properly maintained device.
- Record on 9 centile chart (see further information).

Interpretation

- Difficult to interpret single measurement unless on markedly different centile from height.
- <2nd centile or >99.6 centile refer to doctor for assessment.
- Term 'faltering weight gain' used when slow weight gain or when weight crosses 2 centiles. Prolonged failure to gain weight or continuing weight loss may indicate more serious implications but other signs and symptoms usually present (e.g. Coeliac disease 📖). Needs review and assessment by doctor.
- <5% faltering weight due to organic causes. When psychosocial factors are directly linked to poor growth is known as NOFTT. Full assessment and care plan will address more than just improved nutrition (The assessment of children, young people, and families 📖).
- Concern about overweight 2–18yrs needs height measurement (see below) then assessed on British BMI charts for children. >98 centile overweight, >99.6 obese and cause for concern.

Overweight

Despite a need for high energy intake, about 1 in 5 boys and 1 in 4 girls are overweight. These children should not be expected to lose weight. They should be encouraged to remain at a constant or slow increase while their height increases through healthy eating and increased exercise.

Height monitoring
- Only recommended at school entry unless there is a concern about health or growth and done at the same time as weight.
- Measured standing. Minimeter or Leicester height measure most accurate devices.
- Recorded on a 9 centile chart.
- Any child with a height <0.4 centile or >99.6 should be referred to the doctor.

Food in schools

Parents can buy reduced cost 250mL milk daily for children in primary schools via the EU school milk subsidy scheme. Children whose parents receive Income support or Income based Jobseekers Allowance are eligible for free school meals. There is increased focus on good nutrition in school dinners with government set standards in all countries of the UK. Many schools now have whole school food policies, incorporating a range of activities throughout the curriculum and school day as well as guidance on healthy packed lunches for parents (see toolkit below).

Food allergies
See 📖 Allergies.

Foods for children to avoid
- Shark, swordfish, and marlin because levels of mercury may affect development of nervous system.[1]
- Girls should limit the portions of oily fish to 2 a week because of the potential build up of dioxins and PCBs that may affect the development of any fetus in later life.[2]

Essential reading
Hall, D.M.B. and Eliman, D. (eds.) (2003). *Health for All Children*. (4th edn.). Oxford University Press, Oxford.

Further information
📖 British Nutrition Foundation: www.nutrition.org.uk
Royal College of Paediatrics and Child Health, Guidance (2004). *An approach to weight management in children and adolescents (2–18) in primary care*. RCPCH, London.
📖 DH (England) (2006). *Measuring childhood obesity*. DH website. 📖 Useful websites.
📖 Food in Schools Toolkit: http://foodinschools.datacenta.uk.net
📖 Information to support Health for All children and supplies of all growth monitoring charts, equipment, BMI for children and equipment: www.healthforallchildren.co.uk/

---

[1] Food Standards Agency 2002 Nutritional Essentials: www.eatwell.gov.uk
[2] Food Standards Agency: www.food.gov.uk one portion = 140g

Communication and learning problems

Around a fifth of school children require extra help at some point in their schooling, ♂>♀. Poor progress at school can be caused by a range of physical, social, and emotional problems, as well as problems in the school or home environment. Children may also have specific communication and learning problems that require individual assessment, and support, that may include special education needs statements (Children with special educational needs 📖).

Dyslexia

Dyslexia is a combination of abilities and difficulties that affect the learning process in one or more of reading, spelling, and writing. Term often used interchangeably with 'specific learning difficulties' (SpLDs). Affects 3–5% of population, ♂>♀. It is a persistent condition, affecting children across the ability range. Accompanying difficulties often in areas of:
- Spoken language and motor skills.
- Speed of processing information and short-term memory;
- Organization and sequencing items.

If suspected, teachers consider specific educational support and involve SENCO (Special Educational Needs Co-ordinator). May requires assessment and recommendations for educational support by educational or chartered educational psychologist.

Dyscalculia

Dyscalculia is the mathematical equivalent of dyslexia i.e. difficulty in conceptualizing numbers, number relationships, outcomes of numerical operations, and estimation. If suspected, teachers consider specific educational support and involve SENCO. May require assessment and recommendations for educational support by educational or chartered educational psychologist. May require speech and language therapy.

Dyspraxia

Dyspraxia is the impairment of the organization of movement, may be associated with other problems of language, perception, and thought. Used to be known as clumsy child syndrome, or developmental coordination disorder, or motor learning difficulties. Affects <2%, ♂>♀. Common features include:
- Pre-school was late in reaching milestones e.g. rolling over, sitting, standing, walking, and speaking.
- Clumsiness, poor body awareness, poor posture, awkward gait.
- Difficulty hopping, skipping, riding bike, catching things.
- Reading and writing difficulties.
- Unable to remember or follow instructions, poorly organized.
- Better in one-to-one than group teaching situation.
- Speech production difficulties (developmental verbal dyspraxia).

If suspected, teachers consider specific educational support and involve SENCO. May require assessment and recommendations for educational support by educational or chartered educational psychologist. May require speech and language therapy, physiotherapy, occuaptional therapy support.

Dysfluency (stammering)

About 5% of all children will have some difficulty with their fluency during the development of their speech. About 80% of these will achieve normal fluency. Causes are multi-factorial. The problem can fluctuate from mild to severe depending on the situation, the time of day, or for some other unidentifiable reason. Often embarrassing or distressing to speaker so child will often adopt strategies to minimize or hide problems e.g. not speaking in class or avoiding words that they stammer on. General advice for adults:

- Don't say the word or finish the sentence for the child.
- Be patient, don't ask multiple questions, give time for child to talk.
- Don't tell the child to slow down or take a deep breath (becomes part of the struggle to speak).
- Praise the child for the things that they are doing well.

General advice for child/young person:

- Take time rather than rushing, speak a bit more slowly.
- Pause for a moment before starting to speak.
- Remember to think well done for having a go.

If parent and child agree there is a cause for concern then refer to speech and language therapist according to local policy.

Further information and support

- Afasic Information and resources for unlocking speech and language: www.afasic.org.uk/speechlang.htm
- British Dyslexia Association: www.bdadyslexia.org.uk/index.html
- Dyspraxia Foundation: www.dyspraxiafoundation.org.uk/
- The Michael Palin Centre for Stammering Children: www.stammeringcentre.org/s-index

Dental health in older children

Most children start to lose their primary teeth and gain their adult teeth at about 6yrs. By 12yrs most children will have 28 adult teeth. The 4 molars or wisdom teeth usually appear 16–22yrs.

Surveys show that caries levels in 5-yr-old children show a marked geographic gradient with caries prevalence lowest in England, rising in Wales then Scotland, and highest in Northern Ireland. In each country children from disadvantaged groups have the poorest dental health and are more likely to have dental caries.

Caries prevention
See 📖 Development and care of teeth.

Orthodontic treatment

Common dental problems include protruding upper front teeth, crowding assymetrical alignment, bite problems, impacted teeth. Children are referred by their dentist to a specialist for orthodontic treatment. This may start in primary school years but more commonly in teenagers. Treatment:
• May include removable braces, fixed braces, functional braces, removal of teeth, use of orthodontic headgear, retainers (for ensuring teeth remain in place after treatment).
• Usually takes between 18–24mths but can be much longer with appointments every 4–6wks.

Day-to-day management
• Orthodontists give advice on managing discomfort when appliances altered (painkillers and soft diet for a day or two) and on dental hygiene (special toothbrushes and mouthwash).
• It is recommended that removable appliances are removed for contact sports, and that mouthguards should be worn over fixed appliances.
• Teenagers often feel very self-conscious about having to wear an appliance. Adults need to be very supportive and encouraging not to become shy or withdrawn. Also be alert to signs of excessive teasing or bullying.

Further information for professionals and parents

🖥 British Dental Health Foundation: www.dentalhealth.org.uk/
🖥 British Orthodontic Society: http://new.bos.org.uk/

Young people and adolescence

Adolescence

The period between childhood and adulthood broadly corresponds with the teenage years, a time of rapid physical development and deep emotional changes. These are exciting times but also can be confusing and uncomfortable for child and parents. Young people:

- Become more independent, learn how to get on with other people, and gain a sense of identity that is distinct from that of the family.
- Make close relationships outside the family, with friends of their own age. Friends and peer group identity very important to most.
- Parents become less important in their children's eyes as their life outside the family develops. Develop views of their own that are often not shared by their parents.

Puberty

The period when secondary sexual characteristics develop and the sexual organs mature. Starts ♂: 10–14yrs, ♀: 8.5–12.5yrs.

Girls

Oestrogens stimulate the growth and development of the reproductive organs, the deposition of fat (to produce narrow shoulders, broad hips, breasts, external genitalia), body hair, softer texture skin. The sequence of changes:

- Breast development is the first sign. Breast buds are the initial phase followed by breast growth with smooth contoured areola, then areola projects above the breast and breast tissue grows to adult shape.
- Pubic hair growth and rapid height spurt (Growth and nutrition 12–18yrs 📖) occur almost immediately after breast buds appear. Then axillary hair.
- Menarche (first menstruation) occurs on average 2.5yrs after the start of puberty and signals the end of growing (on average another 5cm height remain).

Boys

Androgens, primarily testosterone, stimulate the growth and development of the reproductive organs, body hair pattern, enlargement of the larynx, and muscles. Boys will begin to experience erections as soon as they start to mature sexually, often unconsciously. The sequence of changes:

- The first sign is testicular enlargement.
- Pubic hair growth follows testicular growth.
- Testicular enlargement accompanied by growth in length then circumference of penis, darkening of scrotal skin.
- Husky voice often first indicator of larynx enlargement that lowers pitch of voice by an octave.
- Sequence of hair growth is pubic, axillary, facial, thoracic, scapular, pinnal, nasal.
- Height spurt occurs later and of greater magnitude than in girls (Growth and nutrition 12–18yrs 📖).

Up to a $^1/_3$ of boys around 12–14yrs will start to develop breasts that disappears later on. Caused by lag in production of testosterone allowing female hormones to act. As soon as testosterone increases, the breast growth goes. Causes great worry and embarrassment.

Most experience unconscious erections and ejaculation during their sleep ('wet dreams'). For the first time, sexual feelings become strong urges which require conscious control.

Both sexes
Development of body odour, acne, and mood changes.

Body odour
Two types of sweat glands:
- Eccrine glands produce sweat used to control body temperature.
- Apocrine glands only start working at puberty. Secrete a different type of odourless sweat in response to stress, excitement, and sexual excitement. When bacteria start decomposing it, it releases a strong distinct smell causing body odour.

Sleep
- Sleep patterns changed by both behaviour and hormonal changes.
- Enough sleep essential as during sleep hormone released to stimulate growth spurt.
- Lack of sleep contributes to moodiness, impulsivity, and depression.

Spots
- 80% of teens suffer to some degree. Boys more than girls because testosterone increases spots, whereas oestrogen prevents them.
- The face most common area but can appear on the neck, upper back, shoulders, and chest.
- Cause is overactive sebaceous glands (Acne vulgaris 📖).

Mood changes
Teenagers experience mood swings. Could be the effect of raging hormones (particularly for girls in premenstrual hormone fluctuations) but also response to physical and emotional changes that leave them feeling uncertain and self-conscious. Moodiness changes as become more confident.

Early or delayed puberty
See 📖 Growth disorders.

Further information for parents and young people
📖 BBC Science and Nature, Body and Mind Information on Puberty:
　　www.bbc.co.uk/science/humanbody
📖 Connexions (all teenagers): www.connexions-direct.com
📖 Lifebytes for 11–14-yrs-olds: www.lifebytes.gov.uk
📖 Royal College of Psychiatrists Leaflet Surviving Adolescence—a toolkit for parents:
　　www.rcpsych.ac.uk/info/help/adol/index.asp

Health promotion in schools

Health promotion is part of the school curriculum in each country of the UK although it may have slightly different emphasis. In addition, the science curriculum also includes a range of issues such as reproduction, and the effect on the body of different substances e.g. tobacco. Each country also has a programme for encouraging whole system approaches to healthy schools (see websites below). Many SNs are involved in a range of activities (Working in schools 📖) for achieving healthy school standards.

Personal, social and health education (PSHE) programme (in England but other countries have similar) aims to give children the knowledge, skills, and understanding to take responsibility for themselves, show respect for others, and to develop the self awareness and confidence needed for life. The school is responsible for the delivery of the PSHE appropriate for the age and cultural identity of their pupils. There are specific statutory requirements for sex and relationship education (📖) and drug education.

SNs (school health advisors) are often involved with teachers in delivering parts of the PSHE as requested by the school. The DH and DfES jointly run a professional development programme for teachers and community nurses supporting and teaching PSHE. Nurses may also be involved in a range of innovative health promotion activities e.g. supporting a peer educator programmes, Baby Simulator programmes, anti-bullying awareness programmes.

The PSHE health objectives for children 5–7yrs include
- How to make simple choices that improve their health and well-being.
- To maintain personal hygiene.
- About the process of growing from young to old and how people's needs change.
- The names of the main parts of the body.
- That all household products, including medicines, can be harmful.
- Rules for, and ways of, keeping safe, including basic road safety, and about people who can help them to stay safe.

The PSHE health objectives for children 7–11yrs include
- The components of a healthy lifestyle, including the benefits of exercise and healthy eating.
- The importance of hygiene in stopping the spread of diseases.
- How the body changes approaching puberty.
- Substances and drugs that are legal and illegal, their effects and risks.
- To recognize the different risks in different situations and then decide how to behave responsibly, including sensible road use.
- How to recognize and resist pressures to behave in an unacceptable or risky way and how to ask for help.
- Basic emergency aid procedures.

The PSHE health objectives for children 11–14yrs include

- To recognize and manage the physical and emotional changes that take place at puberty.
- How to keep healthy and what influences health, including the media.
- That good relationships and a balance between work, leisure, and exercise can promote physical and mental health.
- Basic facts and laws about alcohol, tobacco (by 15yrs, 24% are regular smokers), illegal substances (experimentation starts around 13–14yrs) and the risks of misusing prescribed drugs.
- SRE (see Sex and relationship education 🕮) links with strategies to reduce teenage conceptions.
- To recognize and manage risk and make safer choices about healthy lifestyles, different environments, and travel.
- How to recognize and resist pressures to behave in an unacceptable or risky way and how to ask for help.
- Basic emergency aid procedures.

The PSHE health objectives for children 14–16yrs include

- To think about the alternatives, long- and short-term consequences when making decisions about personal health.
- The causes, symptoms, and treatments for stress and depression, and to identify strategies for prevention and management.
- About the link between eating patterns and self-image, including eating disorders.
- About the health risks of alcohol (of 15-yr-olds drinking alcohol—average intake is 9 units a weeks), tobacco and other drug use (24% of 15-yr-olds have tried illegal substances), early sexual activity and pregnancy, different food choices and sunbathing, and about safer choices they can make.
- SRE links with strategies to reduce teenage conceptions.
- To seek professional advice confidently and find information about health.
- Develop the skills to cope with emergency situations that require basic aid procedures, including resuscitation techniques.

Further information

- 🖳 Drug Education Forum: www.drugeducationforum.com/
- 🖳 England PSHE resources: www.teachernet.gov.uk/pshe/index.cfm?sectionId=72
- 🖳 England The National Healthy School Programme (England): www.wiredforhealth.gov.uk/home.php?catid=872
- 🖳 England Teenage pregnancy unit resources: www.dfes.gov.uk/teenagepregnancy/dsp_content.cfm?pageid=112
- 🖳 Scotland Health promoting schools: www.healthpromotingschools.co.uk/
- 🖳 Welsh Network of Healthy School Schemes (WNHSS): www.cmo.wales.gov.uk/content/work/schools/wnhss-e.htm

Working with teenagers

Teenagers are coping with the ambiguity of not being a child or an adult. Professionals need to assess their biological, psychological, and social development so they interact relevantly and give appropriate responsibility without unacceptable risk. This is reflected in what they can do at particular ages:

- Be held criminally responsible   age 10
- Buy cigarettes   age 16
- Drive a moped   age 16
- Join the armed forces   age 16
- Drive a light motorcycle or car   age 17
- Vote in an election   age 18
- Order alcohol in a public house   age 18

Teenage health care

Significant because:
- Health indicators for the age group have improved very little in past 20yrs.
- Patterns of behaviour and use of services acquired at this point carry on into adult life.
- Teenagers are represented in key target areas of sexually transmitted disease and teenage pregnancy.
- Adolescents assess risk differently from health professionals, peer pressure is more significant than long-term consequences.

Services

Should be age appropriate, responsive to their needs. Teenagers use general services in hospitals, surgeries, and health centres and those designed specifically for them, SN drop ins, child and adolescent mental health services, and young people's sexual health clinics. Encouraging teenagers to take responsibility for their own health, professionals face the challenge of encouraging teenagers to use mainstream services—peer educators, teenagers who work along side those of a similar age and background may facilitate this. Ideally they appreciate different health services in one relaxed setting without appointment systems.

Any contact needs to

- Foster a spirit of partnership identifying the needs of the young person (e.g. stress, body piercing and menstruation) as well other high profile issues (nutrition, sexual health, mental health and substance misuse).
- Have confidentiality explained and guaranteed except in the case of child protection issues when it might be broken.
- Let the young person increasingly take decisions appropriate to his/her age and development. Consenting to health interventions (Fraser competencies) is dependent on age and understanding of the issues. See also 📖 Consent also in 📖 Contraception: general.
- Focus on communication, establishing rapport and an honest open relationship by listening, questioning, understanding, responding, explaining and summarizing. Teenagers value staff being approachable and positive in attitude.
- Empower young people to set and achieve their own goals.

Individual contact with teenagers needs to go alongside national and community approaches. This might include banning of smoking in public places, the wider availability of contraception, and whole school approaches impacting on nutrition in the school canteen.

Further information.

⊠ A site aimed at teenagers but relevant for health and youth workers:
www.teenagehealthfreak.org

⊠ The connexions site that gives information and advice to help young people make decisions and choices: www.connexions-direct.com/

Viner, R. (2002). *ABC of Adolescence*. BMJ Books, London.

Growth and nutrition 12–18 years

The pubertal growth spurt is the 4th phase of human growth. Sex hormones cause the back to lengthen, adding 15% to final height, and fuse the epiphyseal growth plates. If puberty is early (not uncommon in girls) the final height is reduced because of early fusion of epiphyses.

Nutrition

All young people should be eating a balanced healthy diet. In the short term this helps appearance (shiny hair, healthy skin) and in the long term protects against cardiovascular disease and osteoporosis. Energy requirements ↑:
- Boys 11–14yrs 2220kcal/day; 15–18yrs 2755kcal/day.
- Girls 11–14yrs 1845kcal/day; 15–18yrs 2110kcal/day.

Protein requirements ↑ by approximately 50%. Calcium requirements higher than adults: ♂ 1000mg; ♀ 800mg a day as skeletal development is rapid. Once menstruation starts girls need 14.8mg of iron a day compared to boys 8.7mg.

Key issues in teenagers
- About 60% regularly skip breakfast (breakfast cereals and breads are fortified with vitamins and minerals).
- Inadequate nutrients (particularly vitamins and minerals) in diet, and fats feature highly for energy sources. About 50% ♀ 15–18yr do not have adequate nutrients (especially iron and calcium) in diet.
- 46% ♂ and 69% ♀ 15–18yrs spending less than recommended 1hr a day in activites of moderate intensity.
- Increasing use of unsuitable methods control weight e.g. skipping meals, very low energy dieting, and smoking.
- Vegetarianism more common among teenagers (more ♀) but with a poor understanding of how to achieve a balanced diet with adequate protein, iron, selenium.

Monitoring
Routine monitoring of weight and height beyond reception class entry (4–5yrs) and year 6 (England only) not recommended. Good practice to record height and weight in any young person over whom there is a concern, or has chronic ill health and plot on 9 centile growth chart.

Key messages
Best delivered through media that reach young people, in peer settings, through PSHE curriculum and healthy schools initiatives.
- Base your meals on starchy foods
- Eat lots of fruit and vegetables
- Eat moderate amounts of protein, iron rich foods, low fat diary produce, more fish
- Don't skip breakfast
- Get active
- Cut down on saturated fat and sugar
- Try to eat less salt—no more than 6g a day
- Drink plenty of water.

Weight management

Food in schools

- <16yrs whose parents receive Income support or Income based Jobseekers Allowance are eligible for free school meals.
- Many schools now have whole school food policies, incorporating a range of activities throughout the curriculum and school day (see toolkit below).

Food allergies

See 📖 Allergies.

Eating disorders

See 📖 People with eating disorders.

Foods for young people to avoid

- Shark, swordfish, and marlin because levels of mercury may affect development of nervous system,
- Girls should limit the portions of oily fish to 2 a week because of the potential build up of dioxins and PCBs that may affect the development of any fetus in later life.[1]

Further information for professionals and teenagers

- British Nutrition Foundation: www.nutrition.org.uk
- Connexions (all teenagers): www.connexions-direct.com
- Food in Schools Toolkit: http://foodinschools.datacenta.uk.net
- Food Standards Agency: www.food.gov.uk/healthiereating/
- Lifebytes for 11–14-year-olds: www.lifebytes.gov.uk
- Vegetarian Society: www.vegsoc.org/index.html

---

[1] Food Standards Agency: www.food.gov.uk

Sex and relationship education (SRE)

Much SRE takes place in schools and may involve health professionals, particularly SNs and sexual health outreach nurses. Given that some children are not in school because of exclusion or truancy, or are withdrawn by parents from this potentially sensitive subject, educational input in other settings, whether home, youth group, or a community group is to be encouraged. Government guidance states SRE should be part of PSHE and citizenship. All schools (primary and secondary) must have a written policy on sex education developed with parents and agreed by the school governors. Opinions are often strongly held as to how SRE should be taught or if it should be taught at all. Any SRE has to be as stated within the school policy. Most agree that SRE should begin before children reach puberty. Discussion of relationships in its widest sense is appropriate from school entry and before.

SRE seeks to help and support young people through their physical, emotional, and moral development. SRE is about the importance of stable and loving relationships, respect, love, and care as well as teaching about sex, sexuality, and sexual health. SRE is seen as important in contributing to a reduction in the number of teenage conceptions.

Elements of SRE
- Attitudes and values including:
  - Issues of individual conscience
  - Value of family life
  - Nurturing of children.
- Personal and social skills including:
  - How to manage emotion
  - Developing respect for self and others
  - Realizing the consequences of own choices
  - Recognizing and avoiding exploitation and abuse.
- Knowledge and understanding including:
  - Physical development at particular stages
  - Understanding human sexuality, reproduction, sexual health, emotion, and relationships
  - Contraception, avoidance of pregnancy, and protection from sexually transmitted diseases
  - Reasons for choosing to delay or to commence a sexual relationship.

Delivery of SRE
Whoever is involved in SRE, the following contribute to positive evaluations:
- Established skills in facilitating groups.
- Relevant and up-to-date knowledge in relation to sexual health and supporting resources.
- Motivation to lead the session.

- Positive attitudes and values in relation to sexual behaviour.
- The use of discussion as a teaching strategy. Young people do not like the emphasis on physical aspects of reproduction, preferring the opportunity to discuss feelings, relationships, and values.
- A safe environment facilitated by agreed ground rules and depersonalization of the issues.

Issues to consider

- Single sex groups. Single sex groups more appropriate for some issues at some points.
- Confidentiality (Confidentiality 📖). A statement of confidentiality needs to be discussed with the whole class, exhibited and adhered to by all involved.
- Age of Consent. Sexual activity with <16yrs is illegal yet the average age of onset of sexual activity is now about 17 with 20% commencing before 16. Anxieties will be raised by sexual activity involving a young person <13yrs or a significantly older partner.
- Sexual orientation. Some teaching staff have been concerned they will be accused of promoting homosexuality. Good practice requires that questions are dealt with honestly and sensitively but there should not be direct promotion of any sexual orientation.

CPD

SN and HV education programmes will have prepared staff to work with groups of young people. The PHSE certification for community nurses programme provides applied professional development by portfolio. 📖 See www.wiredforhealth.gov.uk/

Further information for professionals

📖 DEfS (England) Guidance on sex and relationship education in schools:
www.dfes.gov.uk/sreguidance/sexeducation.pdf
📖 Sex Education in Scottish Schools: www.scotland.gov.uk/library3/education/natadvice.pdf
📖 Sex Education Forum at the National Children's Bureau, is the national authority on sex and relationship education: www.ncb.org.uk/sef/
📖 TeacherNet, provides material for teachers: www.teachernet.gov.uk/
📖 Wired for Health joint health information website between DoH England and DEfS for teachers, health professionals, and young people: www.wiredforhealth.gov.uk/

Further information for young people

📖 RU thinking about it enough? For <18yrs on sex, relationships, and contraception:
www.ruthinking.co.uk
📖 Wired for Health: www.wiredforhealth.gov.uk/

Children with complex health needs and disabilities

The National Statistics Office (www.statistics.org.uk) reports about 770,000 (7%) of UK children are disabled and the prevalence of severe disability is increasing. Up to 6000 children living at home are dependent on assistive technology. A number of issues have still to be addressed to ensure these young people reach their full potential e.g. 29% of disabled children live in poverty, educational achievements are lower than their peers, only 4% of disabled children are supported by social services. The term disabled children is used here to include children and young people with learning disabilities, autistic spectrum disorders, sensory impairments, physical impairments, and emotional/behavioural disorders. The aim as specified in policies such as *Every Child Matters* (see below) is to ensure children with disabilities and complex health needs and their families:

- Are supported to participate fully in family and community life.
- Receive integrated multi-agency assessments, leading to timely, responsive care plans and interventions that support the child to reach their full potential.
- Children, young people, and their families are actively involved in those decisions.

Integrated assessment and care planning

Increasingly local areas have integrated health, education, and social care services e.g. specialist children services (community based involving a variety of LA and health teams), child development centres (multi-disciplinary assessment and treatment centres often in hospital premises), and child development teams (community based multi-disciplinary teams). The rationale is to provide a coordinated assessment and care plan. Child development teams commonly include:

- Community paediatricians specializing in child development
- Specialist HVs
- SLTs, OTs, and physiotherapists
- Home-based learning support teachers and nursery nurses e.g. Portage
- Orthoptist
- Educational psychologist
- Social worker.

Key principles for working with children and families

- Early identification through antenatal screening (📖), child health promotion programme (📖), response to parental concern, follow-up of high-risk newborn babies.
- Integrated diagnosis and assessment processes.
- Early interventions through Portage, home-based learning services, as well as interventions to support optimal physical and cognitive development, while promoting the child and family's inclusion in the community.

- Coordination between primary, secondary, and tertiary health care.
- Provision of a key worker/care manager recognized by others in multi-disciplinary service environment to ensure delivery of services is coordinated, family has access to all services, and becomes first point of contact if problems arise.
- Supporting parents and families as carers (Carers assessment and support 📖).
- Promote social inclusion by:
  - Ensuring family have knowledge about all benefits (Benefits for disability and illness 📖), and charities that can help e.g. the Family Fund.
  - Access to mainstream public services and children services including social services, therapy services, and CAMHS as these children are more vulnerable to mental health problems than others.
  - Reduce impact of multiple health-care appointments on school and family life.
  - Access to suitable housing, equipment, and assistive technology.
  - Access to play, sport, leisure, and holiday facilities.
- Offer expert patient programme (EPP) to parents and carers.
- Access to appropriate educational opportunities.

In addition:
- All professionals need to be aware that these children are at greater risk of abuse than other children, particularly if they live away from home (Child protection 📖).
- Transition from child to adult services needs particular care in planning as in many cases it is poorly coordinated resulting in a decline in support and deterioration in health and social inclusion.

For some children their condition may require adequate consideration of palliative care needs (Palliative care in the home 📖) and additional support to family and carers through this period and on a child's death (Bereavement, grief, and coping with loss 📖).

Planning for children and families
Under the Children Act 1989, Social Services must keep a register of all children with disabilities in that area. However, it is a voluntary decision whether the child or young persons details are added.

Further information
📓 Contact a Family UK Charity Fact Sheets: www.cafamily.org.uk/
📓 DH (England) NSF Children, Young People and Maternity Services: Disabled children and young people and those with complex health needs 2004. Available at: www.everychildmatters.gov.uk/socialcare/disabledchildren/
📓 Family Fund Charity for disabled children and their families: www.familyfundtrust.org.uk/

Children with special educational needs (SEN)

Children with SEN are defined as having considerably greater difficulty in learning than others of the same age, as well as children who cannot use the educational facilities their peer group use because of their disability. Children under school age who fall into either category without extra help are also included.

Codes of practice (UK)

Each country sets out the key principles for identifying, assessing, and reviewing children with SEN and the role of different agencies. Codes of practice are slightly different in each country but all follow similar principles (taken from England Children with SEN code) as below:
- All emphasize working in partnership with parents and child/pupil involvement.
- Emphasis on early identification (but full assessments <2yrs rare).
- Places emphasis on inclusion of children with SEN in mainstream schools.

Involvement of health services

- In early years: the child health services must alert the parents and the LEA to the child's potential difficulties. A child development centre or team may provide a multi-professional view at an early stage.
- All education settings need to know how, with parental consent, to obtain information and advice on health related matters, using the school health service, GP, or a relevant member of the child development centre or team.
- Each PCO has to designate a medical officer to work with the LEA on behalf of children with SEN and to lead the PCO's contribution to the statutory assessment process.

Graduated educational assessments for children >2 years

3 levels:
- *Early years and school action*: early years staff or teachers identify child who needs extra support. Parents and SENCO (SEN co-ordinator) consulted, agree a plan for extra support. Written in individual Education plan (IEP), reviewed x2 a year with parents.
- *Early years and school action plus*: this level involves outside support services or more specialist advice being sought to help a child's development or additional needs. Requested after meeting with parents.
- *Requests for a statutory assessment:* if the levels above not adequate to additional needs. The education provider, with the parents and anyone else involved with the child, should consider a request to the LEA for a statement. Request can be made by a parent. LEA may consider request and decide not to proceed. Parents have right of appeal.

Statutory assessment

A detailed multi-professional examination includes educational, medical and psychological advice, and advice from social services and from other agencies. Parents are also asked to give a report and given a named LEA officer to help record their views and information. An assessment also includes, where possible, the views of the child.

Statement of SEN and provision

If a child needs extra provision to meet his/her SEN, a proposed statement is made and sent to parents. Statement includes: proposed educational provision (e.g. extra help, school placement, extra equipment) and non-educational provision (e.g. speech and language therapy and social services). Parents have the right to negotiate, put their views forward, and appeal if they disagree. Once the proposed statement is agreed the LEA issues a final statement which the LEAs must provide from the date of the statement. The Special Educational Needs and Disability Tribunal (SENDIST) is an independent tribunal which hears parents' appeals against LEA decisions affecting children with SEN and disabilities.

Annual review

All statements must be reviewed at least annually (>5yrs every 6mths), involving parents and the child or young person. The LEA requests the review, usually coordinated by SENCO. A medical advice form has to be completed by designated medical officer, specialist doctors, CAMHS if involved. Two reviews are of particular note:
- Year 6 timed so parents know by February which secondary school their child will attend.
- Year 9 annual review is used to develop transition plan for moving into further education, training or employment. It is multi agency, including services such as Connexions Service and other agencies with a major role in the young person's post-school life, such as health and social services.

Further information and support

🖵 Department of Education Northern Ireland Special Educational Needs:
www.deni.gov.uk/index.htm
🖵 DES England TeacherNet Special Educational Needs and Disabilities:
www.teachernet.gov.uk/wholeschool/sen/
🖵 Learning and Teaching Scotland Supporting Inclusive Education Executive:
www.ltscotland.org.uk/inclusiveeducation/index.asp
🖵 Learning Wales Special Education: www.learning.wales.gov.uk/index.asp
🖵 Parents Centre information on SEN: www.parentscentre.gov.uk/educationandlearning

People with learning difficulties (LD)

Definition of terms

A learning disability or LD is not an illness or a disease. All types of LD are lifelong, and occur before the age of 18. They can affect people's ability to learn, communicate, or do everyday tasks, such as getting dressed. Types of LD:

- Mild
- Moderate
- Severe
- Profound.

People with severe and profound LD require significant help, and those with mild/moderate LD will usually be able to live independently with support. Government policies (see below) outline a vision with 4 key principles of: 1. Rights, 2. Independence, 3. Choice, and 4. Inclusion at the heart of strategy for the 21st century.

Prevalence in the UK

Approximately 1.5 million people in the UK have a LD. Approximately 200 babies are born with a learning disability every week. The majority of children and adults with LD live with their family. The remainder of individuals live in a wide range of settings in the community either independently, or in supported housing providing 24hr support.

Health profile

Children and adults with learning disabilities have significantly worse health in comparison to the general population, in particular, respiratory problems, diabetes, gastrointestinal problems, heart disease, epilepsy, depression, schizophrenia, hypothyroidism, and sensory impairments. Mortality rates are ↑ for all causes compared with the general population.

Access to health services

There is an inverse relationship between the high level of health needs and the low use of health services. Contributory factors:

- Attitudinal barriers by professionals
- Communication difficulties
- Diagnostic overshadowing (i.e. the disability masks the illness)
- Lack of accessible information
- Confusion about law regarding consent to treatment (Consent 📖, Mental capacity 📖, and see below).

Good practice guidance

- Never make assumptions
- Speak clearly and not too fast
- Avoid medical jargon—use simple everyday language
- Photographs and objects to accompany information may help
- Use concrete terms
- Try to avoid negative words such as don't
- Use key events in the persons life such as Christmas, birthdays, to help recall

- Use open-ended questions
- Use active language e.g. Jane will give you a blood test
- Use health action plans or personal hand held records
- Use Makaton or British sign language when required.

Specialist support for children and adults

General Health care is provided through primary care services.

Multi-professional specialist teams are in most areas providing specialist support to children and adults with learning disabilities.

For children these services may be located at Child Development Centres (Children with complex needs and disabilites 📖), some areas may have specialists staff working in mainstream services such as CAMHs.

For adults these services are usually called Community Teams for Learning Disabilities (CLDT). These are made up of staff from health and social care professionals such as LD nurses, social workers, physiotherapists, OTs, psychologists, speech and language therapists and psychiatrists. CLDT have an open referral system.

These services can help with finding a home, benefits, occupation, education, leisure, bereavement, respite care, relationships, health access, communication, mobility, aids, appliances, and dealing with behaviour difficulties.

Adolescence to adulthood is a vital transitional point, and it's crucial that services work in partnership with the young person to ensure that they are actively involved in the choices, and decisions about their future.

Growing older. Adults with learning disabilities are living longer and require service supports to be robust, as they often do not have close family support.

Family carers. Play a critical role, often providing lifelong support to their relative. They need access to information, training and support, and can also make valuable contributions to staff and service development Services need to work sensitively, and help families plan for the future.

Challenging Behaviour. This is a term used to describe a wide range of behaviours that puts themselves/others at risk of harm. Much behaviour can be attributable to environmental stresses, lack of occupation and opportunities. Physical complaints should always be considered as a cause of change in behaviour, and then a psychiatric assessment to exclude a mental health disorder.

Adult protection. People with learning disabilities are often at risk of abuse, this may be physical, verbal or psychological. Local adult protection guidance should be available. See 📖 Abuse of vulnerable adults.

Further information for professionals and families

- Challenging Behaviour Foundation: www.thecbforg.uk
- Down's Syndrome: Health Issues: www.ds-health.com
- Easy Info (how to make accessible information): www.easyinfo.org.uk
- Foundation for People with Learning Disabilities: www.learningdisabilities.org.uk
- Intellectual Disability Health Information: www.intellectualdisability.info

- Mencap: www.mencap.org.uk
- People First: www.peoplefirstltd.com
- Turner's syndrome UK: www.tss.org.uk

Further information on government policies

- DoH England Valuing People 2001 Valuing People Support Team: www.valuingpeople.gov.uk
- DoH Northern Ireland Equal Lives 2004: www.rmhldni.gov.uk
- English Law on consent and people with learning disabilities: www.dh.gov.uk/PolicyAndGuidance/HealthAndSocialCareTopics/Consent
- Scottish Executive Same as You 2000: www.scotland.gov.uk/library3/social/tsay.pdf
- Welsh Office Fulfilling the Promises 2001: www.wales.gov.uk/subisocialpolicy/content/learning/letter_e.htm

Child and adolescent mental health services

Psychological well-being in children and young people is well recognized as essential for healthy emotional, social, physical, cognitive, and educational development. Mental health problems can be observed in difficulties in capacity for play and learning, personal relationships, psychological development, and in distress and maladaptive behaviour. They are relatively common and may or may not persist. When they persist, are severe and affect functioning they are defined as mental health disorders. Approximately 10–15% of 15-yrs-olds have a diagnosable mental health disorder, the most severe described as mental illness e.g. psychotic disorders (People with schizophrenia 🕮). Similar numbers are thought to have less serious mental health problems. Important to be especially aware of 3 groups:

- Looked-after children (5 times more likely to have mental health disorder than peers).
- Children and young people with significant learning disabilities.
- About 40% of young offenders found to have a diagnosable mental health disorder.

It is recognized that everyone has a role in ensuring the environment in which children grow up promotes their mental health. Policies particularly promote health, education and public services to:

- Tackle bullying and racism.
- Increase awareness of mental health issues.
- Improve the recognition of childrens' emerging needs.
- Provide support for those children with particular needs.

Current estimates that 40% of children with a mental health disorder do not receive any specialist service. Polices such as the NSF for Children explicitly addresses how services can be improved and the standards they should meet linking primary care services to specialist services.

UK 4 tier CAMHS framework

- Tier 1: primary level of care. Includes all services contributing to mental health care of children and young people e.g. GPs, HVs, SNs, social workers, teachers, juvenile justice workers, voluntary agencies. Focus on the initial assessment and identification of difficulties, may include advice or the provision of therapeutic help not requiring specialist training.
- Tier 2: specialist individual professionals relating to workers in primary care. May include clinical child psychologists, community paediatricians, specialist community nurses, child and adolescent psychotherapists.
- Tier 3: specialised multi-disciplinary service for more severe, complex, or persistent disorders. Likely to include child and adolescent psychiatrists, clinical psychologists, nurses, psychotherapists, OTs, SLTs, art, music and drama therapists, family therapists.

[1] 🕮 NSF Children, Young People and Maternity Services (England) (2004). Available on DH publications website www.dh.gov.uk/Home/fs/en

- Tier 4: tertiary level services e.g. day units, in-patient units and out-patient teams provided by teams in tier 3.

All policies emphasize the need for clear, coordinated care pathways for referrals as well training and support to primary care and front line professionals.

Further information

- Anti-bullying Network (Scotland) Resources and links for public and professionals across UK: www.antibullying.net/
- Young Minds Charity provides information for public and professionals on mental health and mental problems of children and young people: www.youngminds.org.uk/

Child protection

In the UK, inquiries into child deaths from abuse and neglect show that:

- Most occur in what is perceived to be a context of low-level need (The assessment of children, young people, and families 📖).
- The agency most likely to be involved is the health service.
- Common professional failings include:
  - Inadequate sharing of information
  - Poor assessment processes
  - Lack of clarity about roles and responsibilities
  - Poor recording of information
  - Failure to keep the child in focus.

National frameworks

Working Together to Safeguard Children—England, sets out the parameters of good practice:

- Be alert to indicators of abuse or neglect (Identifying the child in need of protection 📖).
- Be alert to the risks that individuals may pose to children.
- Share information that relates to concerns about child safety and welfare (Confidentiality 📖).

❶ Familiarize yourself with:

- The government guidance, e.g. 'what do you do if you are worried that a child is being abused' (England).
- The local child protection procedures agreed through the local Safeguarding Children Board (England) or Area Child Protection Committee.

These detail exactly what individuals and agencies must do when abuse is suspected.

Sources of advice and support

Every Trust and PCO has specialist nurses and designated child protection doctors responsible for providing advice and support to any member of staff who has concerns about a child.

❶ Find out the names of the specialist nurse and designated doctor for child protection and how to contact them.

What nurses should do in cases where abuse is suspected

- **Discuss** with senior colleagues as appropriate.
- **Decide** whether the child needs:
  - Immediate protection and/or
  - Urgent medical attention.

If the answer is yes:

- Contact social services or the police and the relevant medical service.
- Discuss the concern with parent/carer and child, unless it is unsafe to do so. In some cases it could ↑ risk to child.
- Record all relevant information and action taken.

If the answer is no:
- Discuss the concern with the parent/carer.
- Listen carefully to the child.
- Consult colleagues who know the child/family, such as the social worker, GP, HV, or teacher. There may be earlier or ongoing concerns.
- Record suspicions and evidence that supports them.
- Decide whether to refer to social services.
- Seek advice if necessary from one of the named or designated professionals (see sources of advice below) or other experienced colleague.

Referral to social services

Social services have the statutory responsibility for making enquiries into child protection referrals and coordinating the inter-agency response (Child protection processes 📖).

When making a referral to social services
- Discuss concerns with a social worker and confirm the referral in writing within 48hrs.
- Record whether the parent has been informed and, if not, why.
- Follow-up outcome to referral to establish that it has been understood and responded to appropriately.

Further information

Barker, J. and Hodes, D. (2004). *A Child in Mind, A Child Protection Handbook.* Routledge, London.
📓 NSPCC online child protection resource: www.nspcc.org.uk/inform/
See central government health departments' websites on child protection guidance. 📖 Useful
websites

Identifying the child in need of protection

Sustained abuse or neglect can have a major impact on all aspects of a child's health, well-being, and development. Assessment should be made within the child assessment framework (A child or young person in need 📖).

Factors that ↑ risk of abuse or neglect

- If parent/carer has a history of any of the following:
  - Drug and/or alcohol misuse
  - Domestic violence
  - Mental health problems
  - Learning difficulties
  - Abuse in their own childhood.
- The risk is further ↑ if:
  - Poor attachment to child, e.g. intolerant and/or indifferent
  - Non-compliance, e.g. parent denies there is a problem and/or refuses to engage with the professional network.
- If child is:
  - A premature or low birth weight infant
  - A multiple birth (e.g. twins) or <18mths between siblings
  - A child with a disability
  - Born unwanted and/or unplanned
  - A child not attending school.
  - A looked after child.

Evidence of harm

Harm means ill-treatment or the impairment of health or development. Ill-treatment is classified under 4 categories of abuse and neglect (see below).

Evidence that a child is being harmed (see below) is obtained by:
- *Observation* of signs in child, e.g.
  - Unexplained bruising or bruising in unusual places
  - Injuries with inconsistent explanations or inappropriate to developmental age
  - Appears afraid, quiet, withdrawn
  - Appears constantly tired, hungry, or dirty.
- *Observation* of perpetrator acting aggressively, violently, or in a sexual manner to child or young person.
- *Allegation* from a child or another person.
- *Disclosure* from a child or someone who says they are harming a child.

Ill-treatment

Physical abuse

Violence directed towards children, including hitting, shaking, suffocating burning, poisoning. Points to remember:
- The younger the child the ↑ risk from physical abuse.
- Sometimes minor injuries signal something more serious.
- Domestic violence (📖) and child abuse coexist in most cases and can begin in pregnancy.

Child sexual abuse

Sexual molestation of children by adults or older children. It involves forcing or enticing a child or young person to take part in activities that lead to the sexual arousal of the perpetrator. Points to remember:

- It is an abuse of power which often relates to the age difference.
- The perpetrator is usually known to the child, probably a family member.
- Most perpetrators deny the abuse and refuse treatment programmes.

Emotional abuse

A relationship between a child and parent that is characterized by harmful interactions that convey to the child that they are worthless or unloved. Integral to all forms of abuse and neglect, but also occurs alone. Points to remember:

- This is under-reported despite easily identifiable negative parent/child interactions.
- Sustained abuse has an impact on long-term mental health, self-esteem, and behaviour.

Neglect

The persistent failure to meet a child's basic physical and emotional needs (Child health promotion 📖) and the failure to provide or respond to the changing needs of a growing child. Points to remember:

- Neglect is the most prevalent form of child maltreatment.
- Neglect is usually chronic and rarely a single incident.
- Mental health problems, learning difficulties, and substance misuse are common in the histories of the parents (Children in special circumstances 📖).

Further information

📖 NSPCC online child protection resource: www.nspcc.org.uk/inform

Information and advice for children

☎ ChildLine: freephone 0800 1111

Information and advice for adults

☎ NSPCC helpline: 0808 800 5000 📖 www.nspcc.org.uk
☎ Parentline Plus: freephone 0808 800 2222

Child protection processes

All countries have legislation and agreed frameworks for these processes. Following a referral reporting a concern about a child, social services will:
- Carry out an initial enquiry and assessment.
- Decide whether to hold a child protection conference.

The child protection conference

Convened by social services, it is a confidential meeting of parents, social workers, health and other professionals involved with the family, and the police. Its purpose is:
- To share information and assess the risk to the child.
- To decide whether to place the child's name on the child protection register. If the decision is 'yes', then a review conference has to be held within 6mths.
- To draw up a protection plan to safeguard the child, including:
  - The support and services to be provided to child and family
  - The changes required to ↓ risk
  - How social services will monitor the child's welfare.

Information sharing and confidentiality

Sharing confidential information is essential (Confidentiality 📖). In many cases it is only when information is shared that it becomes clear that a child is at risk. Points to remember:
- Disclose information relevant to safeguarding the child. This will be about:
  - The health and development of a child and her/his exposure to harm
  - A parent/carer who is unable to care adequately for a child
  - Other individuals who may present a risk to the child.
- Share information on a 'need-to-know' basis.
- If in doubt, consult one of the named or designated nurses or other experienced colleague.

Advice and information for parents and children

☎ ChildLine: freephone 0800 1111
☎ NSPCC helpline: 0808 800 5000; 🖥 www.nspcc.org.uk

Looked-after children

Children in the care of LAs are described as 'looked-after children'. They are among the most vulnerable children in the UK. The National Statistics Office (🖳 www.statistics.org.uk) report approximately 78,000 children in the care of UK LAs at any one time. Main reasons:

- 65% are children subject to a care order under section 31 of the Children Act 1989. Court has been satisfied a child is suffering or would suffer 'significant harm' without one.
- About $\frac{1}{3}$ are accommodated on a voluntary basis under section 20 of the Children Act 1989.

Children may be placed in residential children's homes (some in secure units), in foster homes or with members of their extended families. The system aims to support children back into care of families where that is possible. About 40% return home within 6mths but 60% are looked after for longer.

Recent substantial criticism that public authorities are failing these children. Current policy aims to:

- Improve the stability of placements and continuity of at least 1 carer.
- Increase adoption orders (see below) and special guardianship orders.
- Improve educational attainments of those looked after longer >6mths.
- Improve health and access to health care, particularly CAMHS.

Health needs

Many of these children have increased health needs in comparison to those with their families from comparable socio-economic backgrounds. These may arise from:

- Living in families affected by alcohol, domestic violence, or drugs.
- A disability or special needs.
- Having a highly mobile family.
- Poorer access to universal services such as dental services, immunizations, routine child health surveillance, and health promotion.
- Grief and loss through the experience of leaving family and being placed in care.

Improving health care

Each LA area has to notify PCO of each child moving in or leaving area. Each PCO has a designated community paediatrician(s) and designated nurse (s) for looked-after children, as well as specific access to CAMHS. They are responsible for ensuring:

- A holistic health assessment (including health promotion) by a doctor as soon as practicable after a child starts to be looked after.
- The health assessment is recorded, a health plan is included in the care plan for the child, the child and/or carer holds a personal health record.
- Subsequent health reviews undertaken by nurse, 2–5yrs at least every 6mths, >5yrs at least annually.

- Children/carers are able to access universal health (e.g. GP) and health promotion services and records are 'fast tracked' if moving placement.
- Issues of particular risk in this group i.e. unsafe sex, self-harming, substance and alcohol misuse, are addressed for each young person.

Each health professional who comes into contact with children or young people in this situation is expected to consider the widest range of health and health promotion needs of the young person.

Adoption

Up to 5000 children are waiting for permanent new families at anytime. Fostering is a temporary arrangement, though sometimes it may be the plan until the child grows up. An Adoption Order severs all legal ties with birth family and confers parental rights and responsibilities on the new adoptive family (can be married, single, unmarried couple of any sexuality). Adoption is through an adoption agency, usually social services, but also voluntary agencies e.g. Barnardos. Applicants:
- Are screened for suitability (including requesting information from GP).
- Then matched to children (via the Adoption Register in England and Wales).

Proposed matches:
- Presented to an adoption panel, who decides whether to proceed with the placement.
- The child moves to live with their new parent/s after a planned period of introductions, with support of social worker.
- A court cannot make an adoption order until the child has lived with the adopters for at least 13wks (19wks if newborn).
- A number of organizations provide support for new adoptive parents and children (see below).

All adopted children receive the usual Child health promotion programme (▢) and any additional services in response to particular needs.

NB International adoption has different regulations (see website below).

Further information and support

▢ British Association of Fostering and Adoption: www.baaf.org.uk/
▢ DfES Intercountry adoption: www.dfes.gov.uk/intercountryadoption/index.shtml
▢ Looked-after children policies in central government health departments (Useful websites ▢).
▢ National Children's Bureau Supporting improved health care for looked-after children: www.ncb.org.uk/Page.asp?sve=783

Child and adolescent common health problems

The sick baby and child

Minor illnesses e.g. viral URTI, are commonplace. Most <5yrs have at least 5 viral URTI a year. Parents need to be reassured as well as informed on how to manage minor illness and recognize the signs for seeking medical attention. Ill babies and children become pale, listless, and do not want to eat.

Advice for parents on managing minor illness

- Ensure plenty of fluids, wake babies to offer feeds if sleeping a lot.
- Ensure does not overheat, particularly babies, remove clothing and tepid sponge if necessary.
- Use paediatric liquid paracetamol (BNF 4.7.1) to address discomfort and keep temperature down.
- Use a temporal thermometer to monitor temperature (37°C normal).
- Keep monitoring how they look, their breathing, how much they are drinking and how much fluid they lose e.g. how often they vomit, or have wet nappies.

Ill babies <6mths may deteriorate rapidly. Parents should be encouraged to seek medical advice promptly.

Advice for parents on when to seek medical attention promptly for a baby

- High pitched or weak cry
- Much less active or more floppy than usual
- Looks very pale all over
- Grunts with each breath or has dips in upper tummy or between ribs when breathes
- Takes less than $^1/_3$ of usual fluids
- Has less wet nappies than usual
- Vomits bile (green fluid)
- Passes blood in stool
- High fever or sweating a lot
- Fontanelles bulging or sunken.

Any practitioner consulted about a sick baby or child should refer for medical opinion if significant signs as above.

Advice for parents on when to seek urgent medical attention i.e. ring 999 for an ambulance

- Stops breathing or goes blue
- Is unresponsive
- Has glazed eyes and does not focus on anything
- Cannot be woken
- Has a fit, even if recovers without medical attention (Febrile convulsions and epilepsy 🕮).

Any practitioner consulted or first on scene when a baby or child has these symptoms should request an ambulance is called, if in surgery or clinic call for medical help, and then assess and commence CPR if required (Child BLS 🕮).

Further information for parents

⊠ NHS Direct (England Wales) www.nhsdirect.nhs.uk

☎ NHS Direct helpline is open 24hrs: 0845 4647 for nurse advice and health information

☎ Scotland. NHS 24 is a free 24hrs helpline offering advice on personal health care: 0141 225 0099

Acne vulgaris

A disease of the pilo-sebaceous units that can occur on the face, chest, or back. Most commonly occurs between 13–16yrs. Everyone gets some acne. May continue into the 20s or 30s and occasionally into later life. Often has an emotional impact on confidence and self-esteem.

Causes

- Genetic factors are important in the severity, duration, and clinical pattern.
- Rarer causes include endocrine problems, chemicals, steroids.

Factors

There are 4 primary pathogenic factors in the development of acne:
- Increased sebum production
- The presence of proprionibacteriumacnes
- Abnormal keratinization
- Inflammation.

Stress, heavy sweating, and premenstrual hormonal changes may have an impact. Some beauty products e.g. pomades, de-frizzing agents, suntan oils may also impact. Misconceptions that diet or poor hygiene has impact on the development or severity of acne.

Clinical features

- Comedones (or blackheads): plug of keration and sebum extrudes from pilo-sebaceous orifice.
- Whiteheads, papules, pustules, nodules, cysts, and scars may also be present.

General advice on management

- Skin care: wash x2 a day with soap and water.
- Squeezing: don't squeeze red pustules (traffic light guide on squeezing for teenagers on StopSpots website below).
- OTC preparations (BNF 13.6.1): use lowest concentrations and consult health professional if no improvement within 2mths.
- Make-up: avoid using thick, oil-based types.

Treatment (BNF 13.6)

Treatment should be commenced early to prevent scarring.
- Comedonal acne: azelaic acid or benzoyl peroxide (OTC).
- Mild inflammatory acne: topical retinoid and topical antibiotic or benzoyl peroxide plus topical antibiotic.
- Moderate inflammatory acne: long-term tetracycline plus topical retinoid or other antibiotic (doxycycline, erythromycin, lymecycline, minocycline). For females oral antiandrogen plus topical retinoid.
- Severe inflammatory acne: referred to dermatology specialist. Treated with oral isotretinoin or high dose oral antibiotic plus topical retinoid.

Referred to dermatology specialist if severe, any scarring or associated with fever, arthritis or no improvements to treatments.

Related topics

📖 Growth and nutrition 12–18yrs; 📖 Bacterial skin infections.

Further information for professionals and patients

▢ Acne Support Group www.m2w3.com/acne/
▢ Acne Support Group Teenage site www.stopspots.org ☎ 0870 870 2263
▢ Clinical Knowledge Summaries (Prodigy) guidance on acne vulgaris (includes patient information sheets): www.cks.library.nhs.uk

Asthma in children

Asthma is a lung disease, with intermittent narrowing of the bronchi, causing shortness of breath, wheezing, and cough. During an asthma attack the muscles in the bronchi contract and the lining swells, becomes inflamed, and produces excess mucus.

National Statistics Office (🖥 www.statistics.org.uk) reports it as one of the most common chronic conditions in children. Ratio 2♂:1♀ in childhood, but equal numbers in adolescence. Breast feeding (📖) has preventative effect for wheezing. The majority of children presenting aged <2y are free of symptoms by age 6–11yrs. Accounts for 10–20% of acute hospital admissions. Although detection and treatment is improved, it is still a major cause of school absenteeism, major anxiety in children and families and 15–20 children die from asthma in the UK each year.

Predisposing factors

Both genetic predisposition and environmental:
- Family history of atopy (i.e. allergies, eczema, rhinitis, hayfever)
- Co-existence of atopic disease
- Bronchiolitis in infancy
- Parental smoking
- Prematurity.

Common precipitating factors

- Infection, exercise, emotion
- Household allergens including house mites, fur and feathered pets
- Weather (fog, cold air, thunderstorms), air pollutants (smoke and dust).

Symptoms

- Recurrent wheeze
- Noisy breathing
- Dry cough particularly at night
- Breathlessness.

Diagnosis

On history and clinical examination. Often referred for skin allergy testing also. >5yrs: bronchodilator responsiveness, peak flow variability or bronchial hyper-reactivity tests are used to confirm diagnosis as for adults (Measuring lung function 📖). Height of children is the only determinant of PEFR (see predicted PEFR table Normal spirometry and peak flow values 📖). Often referred to specialists for diagnosis and establishment of treatment.

Management and treatment

Aims:
- To let the child lead as normal life as possible
- To minimize the need for reliever medication
- To prevent severe attacks or exacerbations.

Treatment is by stepwise approach (BNF 3.1, Asthma in adults 📖) that includes short-acting inhaled bronchodilator therapy (relievers) e.g. salbutamol or tetrabutaline and prophylactic therapy (preventers) e.g. regular inhaled steroids. As the severity and frequency of symptoms increase so do the addition of therapies until good control reached then treatment is stepped down. Advice on other measures also given e.g. parental smoking cessation, restricting access to fur or feathered animals, reducing house mites.

Types of chronic asthma and management

- Infrequent episodic i.e. <4 episodes/yr (75% of asthmatic children), need no regular treatment only inhaled bronchodilators as required.
- Frequent episodic i.e. symptoms every 2–4wks (20%), need regular inhaled prophylactic therapy, initially with low dose steroid, plus an inhaled bronchodilator as required.
- Persistent asthma (<5%) need prophylaxis with inhaled steroids, also may need long-acting bronchodilator and oral steroids. Usually treated and monitored in specialists clinics.
- Exercise induced asthma. Mild symptoms controlled by bronchodilator before exercise. Warm up exercises important.

Structured proactive review and monitoring

Regular, structured patient review of symptoms, level of symptom control and use of medications should be organized and delivered by nurse or doctor in primary care with asthma management training. Review should include asthma education, parent/child self-management and action plans as well as use of symptom diaries. Adolescents in particular are high users of emergency departments (EDs) with acute asthma. Encourage parents and young people to seek review if:

- Needing more and more reliever treatment
- Waking at night coughing, wheezing, SOB
- Non-attendance at day care, nursery/school because of asthma
- Unable to do usual physical activities, sports.

Inhalers

Inadequate technique may be mistaken for drug failure. Children <15yrs should have a pressurized metered-dose inhaler and spacer device. <5yrs with face mask if necessary, if not effective nebulized therapy is considered. Advice on inhalers and spacers includes:

- Shake inhaler well before fitting to spacer, press inhaler once and without delay allow child to take 5 slow breaths in and out of the spacer (tidal breathing).
- Remove inhaler, shake well, and repeat as prescribed.
- Spacers should be cleaned monthly in mild detergent as per manufacturers instructions, replaced every 12mths (BNF 3.1.5).

See also ⚏ Asthma attacks.

Essential reference

⚏ British Thoracic Society/SIGN British guideline on the management of asthma (revised 2004) www.brit-thoracic.org.uk/

Further information

⚏ Asthma UK: www.asthma.org.uk ☎ 08457 01 02 03

Autistic spectrum disorder

Autistic spectrum disorder is a behavioural syndrome with no known cause or underlying condition. It is rare: 3/10,000 children, commoner in boys than girls. It presents in early childhood, usually <3yrs but is a life-long condition. Only about 15% live independently in adulthood.

Children with developmental difficulties associated with autistic spectrum disorders are identified during the child health promotion programme. Key areas are failure of social interaction skills e.g. no gestures like waving 'bye' by 12mths, and lack of speech skills e.g. no babbling by 12mths. Some professionals use the Checklist for Autism in Toddlers (CHAT from the National Autistic Society see below) to assess gaze monitoring, pretend play and proto-declarative pointing. The absence of these is strongly associated with an autistic disorder.

Autistic children have a triad of difficulties:
- A severe language disorder. About half never speak at all.
- A profound difficulty in relating to other people e.g. extreme indifference to others and failure to meet gaze.
- Marked routines and rituals associated with poverty of imagination e.g. insistence on the same foods, sameness of environment. Imposing change often precipitates violent temper tantrums.

In addition, odd physical patterns such as flapping hands and walking on tiptoe are common. Some children have hypersensitivity e.g. to noise or light. About $^2/_3$ have a general learning disability. About $^1/_4$ have epilepsy (📖). Many children with autism have very challenging behaviour.

Management
No specific treatment available. Referred to specialist services and will need assessment for special educational needs (Children with special educational needs 📖). Parents need a great deal of support as with all families with children with disabilities (Children with complex health needs and disabilities 📖). Behaviour modification techniques are often used to teach social skills and reduce difficult behaviour. Education usually within special school environments.

Key advice for parents on communication with child with autism includes
- Have their full attention when speaking to them, reduce background noise.
- Keep language simple, direct, specific and literal (e.g. no 'frog in the throat' type phrases).
- Use pictures to reinforce words if possible.
- Provide thinking time to process words.
- Use positive rather than negative language e.g. what to do rather than what not to do.

Key advice for parents on behaviour management includes
- Be consistent and keep your word.
- Try to develop routines through the day and help your child understand what will happen next e.g. through pictures.
- Try to recognize patterns or events that are upsetting for child and trigger tantrums and move in early to distract from or remove these.
- Encourage child to go somewhere safe when they become upset or angry.
- Find ways of positive encouragement for good behaviour.

The National Autistic Society (see below) provide a range of information leaflets to help parents with particular issues e.g. toilet training.

Aspergers syndrome

A mild form of the social impairments of autism in the presence of near-normal speech development. Difficulties in social encounters, stilted language, narrow interests often not shared with others.

Related topic

People with learning difficulties.

Further information for professionals and families

National Autistic Society: www.nas.org.uk/ Helpline: 0845 070 4004 (Mon–Fri, 10am–4pm)

Behavioural disorders in children

Also known as 'externalizing' disorders. Includes oppositional defiant disorder (ODD), attention deficit/hyperactivity disorder (ADHD), and conduct disorder (CD). Behaviours are usually noticeable by others: aggression, hyperactivity, distractibility, and defiant behaviours.

Attention deficit/hyperactivity disorder

Prevalence suggested by Royal College of Psychiatrists (see below)
- Affects 3–5% school-age children
- Ratio of boys to girls 4–9♂:1♀

Presentation

All children can be overactive and behave impulsively, find it hard to concentrate sometimes. With ADHD, this behaviour is persistent, occurs wherever the child is, not just in one place, e.g. school or at home. Varying degrees of severity, sometimes found together with other conditions, e.g. dyslexia. ADHD is a distinct condition, part of make up of child Presentation must be >6mths old and includes:
- Associated with impairment in social and/or academic functioning compared to individuals at a comparative level of development
- Developmentally inappropriate degrees of inattention
- Impulsivity
- Hyperactivity
- Present before 7yrs
- Present in 2 or more settings
- Not better accounted for by another disorder.

Need to ensure behaviors not due to other problems e.g. hearing loss, epilepsy, Tourette syndrome, etc.

Aetiology
- Strong evidence of genetic contribution
- High maternal consumption of alcohol during pregnancy.

Treatment/management
- Early identification important, often by teachers
- Identify and address any other medical or social problems
- Important that all involved with child work together to assess and agree on ways of managing
- Referral to specialists or CAMHS for:
  - Medication frequently used, e.g. methylphenidate (Ritalin®)
  - Parental education
  - Behavioural management
  - Parenting skills work.

Outcome
- Family disturbance contributes to continuity of childhood ADHD into adolescence, 50–80% cases.
- $^1/_3$ hyperactivity decreases after adolescence; $^1/_3$ mildly impaired as adults; $^1/_3$ persist into adult ADHD with worsening of functions.

Associated problems

Difficult interaction with peers; delayed social and educational development; more psychological problems, low self-esteem; evokes cycle of 'negative parenting'.

Conduct disorders

Characterized by excessive levels of fighting, bullying, cruelty, destructiveness, stealing, lying, truancy, temper tantrums, disobedience. Severe and persistent (>6mths). Delinquency: antisocial law-breaking behaviour.

Prevalence

About 5% with an excess of boys.

Aetiology

* Adverse psychosocial environments
* Child's temperament, poor physical health.

Treatment/management

* Referral to specialists or CAMHS for:
  * Problem-solving skills training
  * Family therapy: parent management training.

Outcome if not 'treated'

* Delinquency, offending and criminality
* Emotional disorders
* Substance misuse
* Teenage pregnancy
* Early violent deaths.

NB Most antisocial disorders do not progress to adulthood but many aggressive antisocial adults had pattern in childhood.

Related topics

📖 Understanding behaviour 1–5yrs; 📖 Working with teenagers.

Further information

🖳 Mental Health Foundation: www.mentalhealth.org.uk
🖳 National Mental Health Association: www.nmha.org
🖳 Royal College of Psychiatrists: www.rcpsych.ac.uk/info/mhgu/index.htm
🖳 The National Attention Deficit Disorder Information and Support Service: www.addiss.co.uk/
🖳 Young Minds: www.youngminds.org.uk

Birth injuries

Babies may be injured at birth if they are too large for the pelvic outlet or malpositioned. More rare are injuries from assisted vaginal deliveries e.g. using forceps.

Soft tissue injuries

- Bruising and swelling to face, after face delivery, or to buttocks after breech delivery. Resolves in a few days.
- Caput succedaneum: bruising and oedema of the presenting part of the body. Resolves in a few days.
- Cephalhaematoma: rare. Haemorrhage beneath the periosteum. Resolves over a few weeks.

Parents need reassurance as can look very alarming.

Nerve injuries

Can occur during breech deliveries or with shoulder dystocia (shoulder trapped behind pelvic bone) during birth. Damage to cervical nerve roots in brachial plexus. Palsy (loss of control of muscles) according to which cervical nerve damaged. Most common types:

- Erbs palsy—upper nerve root injury. One arm abducted, rotated in and fingers flexed.
- Klumpkes palsy—lower nerve root injury causing hand weakness and fingers don't move.
- Complete brachial plexus palsy—entire arm is paralysed with sensory loss.
- Facial palsy causes facial asymmetry.

Most offered paediatric physiotherapy and followed up by paediatricians. Most resolve within a few weeks. In some care cases injury may not resolve, referred to paediatric neurologist. Nerve or tendon release surgery may be considered. Parents need support and reassurance.

Bone injuries

- Clavicle fracture occurs in some births from shoulder dystocia. Heals rapidly without treatment.
- Humerus or femur fractures can occur in breech deliveries requires immobilization and heals rapidly.
- Parents need support, reassurance and advice on care of baby while limb immobilized.

Related topics

📖 New birth visits; 📖 New babies; 📖 Complicated labour.

Information and support for parents

🖳 The Erbs Palsy Group: www.erbspalsygroup.co.uk/

Bone and joint problems

Variations of normal posture

These are common and most resolve without any treatment but any that are severe, painful, or asysmetrical are referred for specialist opinion. This includes:

- Bow legs (genu varum): bowing of tibiae. Common up to age 3 and resolves spontaneously. Other causes include rickets (usually caused by vit. D and calcium deficiency and treatable with oral supplements or injections).
- Knock knees: seen in children 2–7yrs, usually resolves spontaneously.
- Flat feet (pes planum): all babies and toddlers have flat feet. The arch develops after 2–3yrs. of walking. Persistent flat feet may be familial or due to joint laxity. If painful referred for specialist advice.

Disorders of the hip, knee, and foot

Development dysplasia of the hip (previously congenital dislocation of the hip). Describes a spectrum of disorders from dysplasia through to dislocation of the hip. 6–10 per 1000 live births. Detected at routine neonatal and 6wk screening (Child screening tests 🕮). Most resolve spontaneously. Referred for specialist opinion. Treatment depends on when the condition is diagnosed:

- Young babies: splinting—the hips are held in partial abduction using slings under each thigh attached to a body harness—e.g. von Rosen splint. Usually babies wear a splint for ~3mths. Parents need specific advice on handling and hygiene.
- Older babies, toddlers: surgery is required.

Irritable hip: most common cause of acute hip pain 2–12yrs. Cause is unknown, usually resolves in 7d.

Talipes (clubfoot)

- Positional talipes from intrauterine compression is common and resolves with passive manipulation usually demonstrated by physiotherapists.
- True talipes. The foot is inverted, supinated and the forefoot abducted. Refered to orthopaedics. Treatment: physiotherapy, splints ± surgery at 6–9mths.

Disorders of the back and spine

Back pain: uncommon pre-adolescent. A young child with back pain should be medically assessed. In adolescents common causes are muscle spasm often from sports related injuries and poor posture.

Scolioisis: lateral curvature of the spine, may lead to pain and limitation of activities, respiratory restriction. Causes can be idiopathic, congenital or secondary to another disorder e.g. cerebral palsy (🕮). Early onset idiopathic usually resolves. Late onset idiopathic scoliosis (most common 85%) mainly affects girls at pubertal growth spurt (Growth and nutrition 12–18yrs 🕮). Treatment of severe scoliois is with spinal braces and sometimes surgery.

Torticollis (wry neck) sudden restriction of head turning due to a mobile, nodule in muscle in first weeks of life (and later). Resolves in 2–6mths.

Painful limb

Growing pains (also nocturnal idiopathic pain) common in pre-school children. Children with hypermobility in joints often also complain of pain in limbs. Cause unknown. Often wakes child at night and settles with massage and comforting.

Arthritis: rare in children. Presents with well-localized joint pains ± hot, tender, swollen joints. Two types:

- Septic arthritis: a serious infection of the joint space that can lead to bone destruction. Most common <2yrs. The child is usually systemically unwell and the joint may be swollen, hot, and tender. Requires urgent medical assessment, admission to hospital, and IV antibiotics.
- Juvenile idiopathic (chronic) arthritis (Arthritis 📖): a group of conditions which last >6wks. Includes Still's disease: acute illness, fever, weight loss, salmon pink rash, pains in joints and muscles. Referred to specialist, requires physiotherapy, pain control and suppression of inflammation by NSAIDs. Child may be identified as having special needs according to severity and effect (A child or young person in need 📖).

Genetic

Osteogenesis imperfecta: autosomal dominant inheritance. Group of disorders of collagen metabolism resulting in fragile bones which fracture easily. Other features include lax joints, thin skin, blue sclerae, hypoplastic teeth and deafness. Severe forms present with fractures at birth (many still born). Less severe cases present later and may be mistaken for non-accidental injury. Treatment is supportive with treatment of fractures as occur. Child may be identified as having special needs according to severity and effect.

Osteopetrosis (marble bone disease) rare, bones dense but brittle. Autosomal dominant presents presents in childhood with fractures, osteomyelitis ± facial paralysis. Recessive form is more severe causing bone marrow failure, (bone marrow transplantation can be curative) and death.

Marfan's disease: autosomal dominant disorder of connective tissue associated with altered body proportions, tall stature, hyperextensible joints, long thin digits, scolioisis, cardiovascular problems and disclocation of the eye lenses and sever myopia.

Related topics

📖 Children with special educational needs and disabilities; 📖 Children with complex health needs.

Further information for families

📑 Brittle Bone Society: www.brittlebone.org ☎ 08000 282 459
📑 Great Ormond St. Hospital Factsheets: www.gosh.nhs.uk/factsheets/
📑 Scoliosis Association (UK): www.sauk.org.uk ☎ 020 8964 1166
📑 The Childrens Chronic Arthritis Association: www.ccaa.org.uk/

Cerebral palsy

Cerebral palsy is the most common cause of physical disability in childhood characterized by impaired movement and posture. It is due to non-progressive lesion of the motor pathways in the developing brain. It affects about 2 per 1000 live births, ↑ in premature babies/babies small for dates.

Causes

- Antenatal (80%): cerebral malformation, infections e.g. rubella, cyto-megalovirus
- Intrapartum (10%): birth asphyxia/trauma
- Postnatal (10%): head trauma, brain infections e.g. meningitis, hydrocephalus.

Associated problems

- Intellectual impairment (60%)
- Epilepsy (40%)
- Visual impairment (20%) and squints (30%)
- Hearing loss (20%)
- Speech and language disorders.

Classification

Three main types—but mixed forms are common:

Spastic CP: 70–80%. Damage to upper motor neurone pathway. Affects motor function and may → hemiplegia, quadriplediga, or diplegia. Affected limbs are underdeveloped and have ↑ tone, weakness, and a tendency toward contractures. A scissors gait and toe walking are characteristic.

Ataxic CP: 5–10%. Damage to the cerebellum. Poor coordination, low muscle tone, poor balance, unsteady gait, tremor, and difficulty with and fine movements.

Athetoid and dyskinetic syndromes: 10–20%. Damage to basal ganglia. Constant involuntary movements, poor postural control, and unsteadiness in walking and sitting.

Diagnosis Often abnormalities in tone, reflexes and posture are noted during routine developmental screening. Referred for paediatric assessment if suspected. Formal diagnosis is usually made by 2yrs.

Care management

There is no cure. Physiotherapy, OT, and speech therapy can all improve the effects of CP especially if introduced as early as possible. The overall goal is to enable children to develop maximum independence and support the family in achieving this. The range of health and social care problems have to be individually identified and addressed through coordinated care plans in a multidisciplinary team approach involving physiotherapists, OTs, speech therapists, community paediatricians, GPs, HV, social workers, early years care staff and teachers, in liaison with the child and his parents.

Related topics

📖 Children with complex health needs and disabilities; 📖 Children with special education needs.

Further information for professionals and parents

SCOPE (cerebral palsy): www.scope.org.uk Free Helpline:. ☎ 0808 800 3333

Cancer in childhood

Cancer in children is not common: 120–140 new cases per million children aged <15yrs.[1] Most cancers occur as a result of mutations in cellular genes which may be inherited or sporadic. Most children with cancer in UK are initially treated in 1 of 22 regional centres, and then returned to care of local specialists, and primary care, including support from specialist outreach nurses from regional centre or childrens community nursing team (Children with complex health needs and disabilities 📖). Survival rate for many cancers has increased dramatically in last 30yrs. Estimates of 1 in 1000 young adults are survivors of childhood cancer. The diagnosis has enormous and long lasting impact on the whole family. In the early days:

- Parents need opportunities to discuss diagnosis and feelings as well as written information on the disease, implications and treatments.
- The child and siblings need age appropriate explanations and opportunities to discuss their feelings:
- Family may need help with practical issues such as transport, accommodation, finance, care of siblings while attends tertiary centre.

Once treatment is established and the disease is under control, families are encouraged to return to as normal life as possible:

- Early return to school is encouraged.
- Child and family should be offered ongoing opportunities to discuss feelings and find ways of coping with the unknown of the long-term outcome.
- Parents should be supported in having time out from caring and focusing on themselves and their own needs (Carers assessment and support 📖).

General overview of treatment and management

Treatment: may involve chemotherapy, surgery, and radiotherapy. Bone marrow transplantation may be used to treat patients after administering very high does of chemotherapy and/or radiotherapy that damages normal tissue particularly bone marrow. Side effects of chemotherapy include: immunosuppression, bone marrow suppression, gut mucosal damage, anorexia, nausea and vomiting.

Long-term follow-up: monitors residual problems, risks of second tumours and specific problems as a result of the treatment such as poor growth or sexual dysfunction.

Palliative care: despite treatment, some children progress to the terminal stages of their cancers. Specialist palliative care or hospice teams may be involved. General principles of palliative care at home apply (Palliative care in the home 📖):

- Address pain relief and symptom control.
- Provide emotional support for child and family.
- Ensure continuity with as few professionals as possible.
- Provide on-going support to family members after the child has died.

---

[1] 🖳 Office for National Statistics: www.statistics.org.uk

Main types

Acute leukaemia: peak presentation age 2–4yrs. 80% acute lymphoblastic leukaemia (310 cases/yr), others acute myeloid or acute non-lymphocytic. Usually presents with a short history (wks) of pallor, fatigue, irritability, fever, bone pain, and/or bruising/petechiae.

Lymphomas: malignancies of the cells of the immune system. Peak presentation age 10–14yrs.
- **Hodgkin's disease:** usually presents as painless lymphadenopathy, often in neck. May also have a long history of weight loss, sweating, priutius, fever.
- **Non-Hodgkin's lymphoma:** usually presents with painless lymphadenopathy, often in neck, and/or disease in abdomen. There tends to be a rapid progression of symptoms. Referred for urgent paediatric opinion.

Brain tumours: 280 cases/yr. Almost always primary tumours and present with signs of raised intracranial pressure e.g. headache (worse when lying down), vomiting, squint, nystagmus, personality, or behaviour change. Tumour identified on CT or MRI scan. Outcome influenced by position and size. Survivors may have very complex problems.

Neuroblastoma: derived from neural crest tissue in adrenal medulla and sympathetic nervous system. Tends to affect children <5yrs. Most present with abdominal mass. Children with extra-abdominal tumours, and those who are <1yr at diagnosis have better prognosis.

Wilms' tumour (nephroblastoma) kidney tumour from embryonal renal tissue. 70 cases/yr. Usually affects children <5yrs old. Presents with fever, weight loss, anaemia, abdominal mass and pain.

Retinoblastoma: Rare tumour of the eye. 30 cases/yr Usually affects children <5yrs old. Usually detected by a white pupillary reflex found at routine developmental screening, or with squint or inflammation of the eye.

Rhabdomyosarcoma: presents with a mass at any age. May be at any site.

Osteosarcoma (bone tumour): 10–14yrs. Present with persistent bony pain—most commonly in a limb.

Further information for children, families, and professionals

- 🔲 Association for children with life threatening or terminal conditions and their families (ACT): www.act.org.uk ☎ 0117 922 1556
- 🔲 Association of Children's Hospices (ACH): www.childrenshospice.org.uk
- 🔲 Cancer and Leukemia in Children (CLIC): www.clic.org.uk ☎ 0845 301 0031
- 🔲 CancerBacup: www.cancerbacup.org.uk/Cancertype/Childrenscancers
- 🔲 Help adolescents with cancer (HAWC) ☎ 0161 688 6244 www.hawc-co-uk.com

Cleft lip and palate

Cleft lip: failure of fusion of frontonasal and maxillary processes.

Cleft palate: failure of fusion of palatine processes.

Affects about 0.8 per 1000. Most inherited but may be part of a syndrome.

Usually referred to regional specialist cleft lip and palate multidisciplinary team at diagnosis. As with all families and children with special needs, primary care professionals work in conjunction providing their services and long-term support.

Surgical repair
- Lip: surgical repair may be performed in first wks or first 2–3mths.
- Palate: usually repaired by 1yr.

Feeding
Babies may have difficulty combining reflex actions, creating vacuum, and correctly positioning tongue. Regional team provides specialist advice as does CLAPA (see below). Parents need lots of reassurance as milk and foods may pass into nose and cause sneezing. Babies with cleft lip:
- Can breast feed (Breast feeding 📖), may need to try different positions and holding breast differently.
- If bottle fed may need larger hole in soft teat (CLAPA has catalogue of types of soft bottles, teats and feeding systems).
- May be fed with cup and spoon after repair till heals.

Babies with cleft palate and lip:
- May be given an orthodontic plate to help feeding.
- Many can breast feed if breast held in area that palate complete, well latched-on, with good supply of milk.
- Many can bottle feed with teats with larger holes.
- Some babies may need nasogastric tubes to feed or be fed by cup and spoon.
- After repair depends on age but may be asked to use cup and spoon rather than bottle.

Other issues
The specialist team will monitor speech development and provide therapy if any difficulties, Hearing is also monitored as middle ear infections common. If the gum is affected by the cleft, then teeth may also be missing, twisted, or be misaligned. Orthodontic referral may be required when adult teeth coming in (Dental health in older children 📖).

Related topic
📖 Children with complex health needs and disabilities.

Further information and support
🖥 CLAPA: www.clapa.com/ ☎ 020 7833 4883

Congenital heart defects

Congenital heart defects

Affects about 6–8 babies per 1000 live births.[1] ↑ defects detected at antenatal ultrasound. ↑ diagnosed by non-invasive echocardiography. ↑ number of defects can be treated non-invasively. The 8 most common congenital heart lesions:

- Non-cyanotic:
  - Ventriculoseptal defect (VSD) 32%—a hole connects the 2 ventricles
  - Patent ductus arteriosus (PDA) 12%—ductus arteriosus fails to close after birth
  - Pulmonary valve stenosis 8%
  - Atrial septal defect (ASD) 6%—a hole connects the 2 atria
  - Coarctation of the aorta 6%—localized narrowing of the descending aorta
  - Aortic valve stenoisis 5%.
- Cyanotic:
  - Tetralogy of Fallot 6%—large VSD and pulmonary stenosis
  - Transposition of the great arteries 5%—aorta and pulmonary artery.

Signs and symptoms

- Heart murmur but only 54% of murmurs heard at neonatal examination are due to cardiac defects, most are innocent.
- Heart failure includes:
  - Breathlessness particularly when crying/feeding
  - Cyanosis
  - ↑ respiratory and pulse rates
  - Failure to thrive or weight ↑ due to fluid retention
  - Recurrent chest infection
  - Heart and/or liver enlargement
  - Cool peripheries.

Treatment

Referred for specialist paediatric and/or cardiology opinion. Specialist treatment of valve lesions depends on the size. Most congenital cardiac lesions require medical treatment plus surgery. May have oxygen therapy at home (Oxygen therapy in the community 📖).

Care management issues

Feeding

Slow feeding is a common problem (Breast feeding 📖). Long feeds ↑ tiredness in babies and mothers. Vomiting after feeds often a problem. Encourage ↓ amounts, ↑ frequency. If bottle fed then may need to experiment with teats and bottles to aid feeding but ↓ wind. Night feeds often need longer than other babies. Weight gain may also be a problem. Usually seen by dietitian in specialist team. May need high calorie formula feed (in addition if breast feeding). Introduction of high calorie weaning food at 4mths often aids weight gain. Some babies at home may have NGT or PEG (PEG feeds 📖).

---

[1] 📖 National Congenital Anomaly System. Office of National Statistics www.statistics.org.uk

Immunization
Usual programme (Childhood immunization 📖) plus flu vaccine every year to children with heart conditions (check contra-indications flu vaccination) from the age of 6mths–12yrs. Vaccinations against pneumonia and bronchiolitis may also be recommended by cardiologist.

General
Most children recover quickly after surgery and are back at nursery, playgroup, school within a month. Exercise tolerance varies and each child is encouraged to find own limits. Antibiotic prophylaxis for dental and surgical procedures given as ↑ risk of developing bacterial endocarditis. Many adolescents and adults require revision of surgery performed in early life e.g. replacement of artificial valves.

Related topics
📖 Children with complex health needs and disabilities; 📖 Children with special education needs.

Further information for parents
🖵 Children's Heart Federation: www.childrens-heart-fed.org.uk ☎ 0808 808 5000

Congenital impairments

Congenital impairments are present in approximately 2% of live births, more common in pre-term and small for dates babies.[1] Approximately 30% genetic and chromosomal, 10% teratogenic (viral, bacterial, medications, alcohol, drugs), remainder multiple causes or unknown. Individual child and family needs should be identified and addressed accordingly (A child or young person in need 📖).

Congenital adrenal hyperplasia

Caused by autosomal recessive disorders in 1 per 5000 births. Cortisol deficiencies causes over production of adrenal androgens. Results in:
- Virilization of external genitailia of girls requiring corrective surgery.
- Penis enlargement and precocious puberty (Growth disorders 📖) in some boys.
- Adrenal crisis in some male babies within first 3wks requires emergency treatment.

All require long-term glucocorticoid therapy (BNF 6.3.2) and monitoring of growth by specialists.

Babies with ambiguous genitalia: see below.

Congenital infections

- Cytomegalovirus: affects 4 per 1000 births. 90% of affected develop normally. Remainder have neurological problems e.g. cerebral palsy, epilepsy and developmental delay.
- Rubella, usually intrauterine <18wks gestation from infected mother. Preventable (Antenatal care and screening 📖). May cause deafness, congenital heart defects and cataracts and other problems.
- Toxoplasmosis: 0.1 per 1000 births. About 10% of affected have problems, usually neurological e.g. hydrocephalus and retinopathy.

Uro-genital problems

Babies with ambiguous genitalia

Require full biochemical and sometimes surgical (laparoscopic) investigation prior to assigning sex. Time to correctly assign often causes additional distress to parents but important as has lifelong social, psychological, medical, and legal consequences. Caused by chromosomal (Genetic problems 📖) or adrenal problems. Parents, and later child, need psychological support as well as information at different stages. Surgery may be required at different stages of development as well as long-term glucocorticoid therapy and hormone therapy.

Male genito-urinary problems

- Hypdospadias: urethral opening on the underside of the penis. 1 in 300 boys. Corrected surgically <2yrs.
- Undescended testes occurs in 5% full-term boys. Most descend by 3mths. Those that don't are corrected surgically (orchidopexy) about 2yrs.

---

[1] 📖 National Congenital Anomaly System. Office of National Statistics www.statistics.org.uk

Urological malformations

Increasingly diagnosed by antenatal USS (ultrasound). Horseshoe kidney or double elements in the system common and in themselves are not a problem. However, predispose to reflux and recurrent UTIs (Infections in children ☐) and cause renal damage. Often prophylactic antibiotics started at birth to prevent renal damage. USS again within first 6wks, some malformations may have resolved. Prophylactic antibiotics continue if malformation remains. Obstructions such as posterior urethral valve require surgical intervention.

Related topics

See also other topics of congenital impairments:
☐ Bone and joint problems; ☐ Cerebral palsy;
☐ Cleft lip and palate; ☐ Congenital heart defects;
☐ Cystic fibrosis; ☐ Endocrine problems;
☐ Gastrointestinal problems in children; ☐ Neural tube defects.

Further information and support for parents and children

▣ Great Ormond St Hosptial and Institute of Child Health Family Fact sheets:
   www.ich.ucl.ac.uk/factsheets/family/
▣ The National Kidney Association: www.kidney.org.uk
▣ The UK Intersex Association: www.ukia.co.uk

Constipation and encopresis

Constipation

Painful passage of hard, infrequent stools. Affects about 5% children at some time, more ♂ than ♀ (see also Constipation in adults 📖). NB Babies show considerable variation in bowel habit according to diet (and if breast fed). Babies can change colour when passing a stool and look as if they are straining even when passing a liquid stool. Changing from breast feeding to artificial feeds and/or solids results in change of stool colour and consistency (Bottle feeding and weaning 📖).

Causes

- Babies:
  - Rare causes include: congenital abnormalities e.g. spinal cord lesions, imperforate anus (after surgical repair); Hirschsprung's disease; hypothyroidism; cerebral palsy
  - May occur from hunger, overstrength feeds, and poor hydration.
- Older children:
  - Developmental problems (learning disability, autism)
  - Poor or chaotic diet and inadequate fluid intake
  - Failure to establish toileting routine during toilet training
  - Behavioural or psychological problems
  - Fear of toilets, especially school toilets
  - Vicious cycle created of ignoring sensation, hard stool, anal pain, deferring defecation as long as possible
  - Severe loading i.e. rectum and colon filled with faeces: may also have faecal incontinence or staining.

Management of short-lived or mild consitpation

- Explanation of reasons for problems, engage child and parents in dietary, fluids, and exercise promotion, including increased fibre and fluid intake.
- Ascertain if afraid of the toilet, suggest make toilet appealing.

Advice includes:

- Ensure adequate fibre and fluid intake (not easy with some children).
- Allow sufficient time and privacy for bowel emptying in the morning.
- Eat breakfast and try 20–30min later.
- On the toilet sit comfortably with feet supported (footstool if needed).
  - Avoid holding breath and straining
  - Push using abdominal muscles and relax anus.
- Consider simple rewards (e.g. star chart).
- Avoid punishments/reprimands.
- Always respond to 'urge', do not defer (arrange with teacher).

Mild bulk-forming laxatives used with caution as last resort. Referred for specialist opinion if not resolving or severe.

Management of severely constipated child

Referred for medical review. May have painful anal conditions e.g. anal fissure. May need several months of laxatives to establish a pattern. Senna most commonly used, sometimes up to 1yr in severe cases.

Encopresis

Most children are continent of faeces by $2^1/_2$–3yrs. Faecal soiling during daytime after this age usually occurs when:

- Child has bowel control but passes stool in socially unacceptable places. Cause is often emotional. Consider referral to CAMHS/or via GP as local policies suggest.
- Firm stool passed occasionally in the toilet but usually in the pants. Try a consistent training programme similar to those used for enuresis (📖).
- Soft stool causes child to soil themselves and smell of faeces. Consider possibility of overflow faecal incontinence due to underlying chronic constipation (see above).

Related topic

📖 Toilet training.

Further information for professionals

Clayden, GS, Hollins, G. (2004). Constipation and faecal incontinence in childhood. In: Norton C, Chelvanayagam S, (eds). *Bowel Continence Nursing. Beaconsfield Publishers*, Beaconsfield. pp. 217–228.

🖥 Clinical Knowledge Summaries (Prodigy) guidance on management of constipation in children: www.cks.library.nhs.uk

🖥 Royal College of Paediatricians and Child Health clinical effectiveness guidelines management of diarrhoea and constipation: www.rcpch.ac.uk/

Further information for parents and carers

🖥 Websites for patient information: www.digestivedisorders.org.uk

Cystic fibrosis (CF)

Most common serious pulmonary and genetic disease, affecting 1 in 2500 children (UK). About 1 in 22 of the UK white population are carriers of a copy of CF gene. Rare in children of African or Asian descent. CF affects movement of salt and water across cell membranes and causes thickened secretions; a multi system disease characterized by life-threatening pulmonary and GI problems. There is no cure for CF.

- Inherited as an autosomal recessive trait
- A multi symptom disorder primarily affecting the exocrine glands
- Survival rate has ↑ dramatically, with good management >40yrs
- Majority of CF sufferers in UK are <25yrs (6000)
- Neonatal blood spot screening being introduced (Child Screening tests 🕮).

Presentation

Clinical manifestations vary among children and can change as the disease progresses. Some children display symptoms at birth as gut becomes blocked by extra thick meconium → meconium ileus requiring surgery.

Most affected children display both pulmonary and gastrointestinal symptoms, a few have only pulmonary disease or pancreatic insufficiency. Symptoms include:

- Failure to thrive despite increased appetite
- Abdominal pain
- Oily, foul smelling stools (steatorrhoea)
- Frequent bacterial chest infections and pneumonia
- Persisitent cough, wheezing, dyspnoea
- Excessive production of mucous
- CF sufferers are prone to chronic sinusitis and nasal polyps
- Cyanosis
- Clubbing of fingers and toes
- Some parents notice child tastes 'salty' when they kiss them due to high sodium and chloride concentration in the sweat, a unique characteristic of cystic fibrosis.

Referred for specialist investigations if necessary: sweat chloride test, chest X-ray, pulmonary function tests, stool fat/enzyme analysis.

Care and management

Children with CF should be linked to specialist centre with aims of:

- Promoting independence, improve quality of life and life expectancy
- Preventing infection as long as possible and stabilize respiratory infections
- Maintaining good nutritional state
- Long-term support for child and family
- Good multidisciplinary team working especially with school.

NB Children and families with CF quickly become the experts in their own condition (Expert patients 🕮).

Care for lung associated problems

- 2x daily chest physiotherapy and postural drainage to loosen thick mucous. Parents are taught how to do this by hospital staff and ongoing support from community paediatric nurses. Patients can do this themselves as they become adult.
- Immunizations and flu vaccination (Childhood immunization schedule (UK) 📖 and Targeted immmunisations in adults 📖).
- Rapid treatment with antibiotics with any sign of chest infection. IV antibiotic therapy in the community offered in many areas. Some children are prescribed prophylactic antibiotics.
- Some children will have inhalers for asthma and inhaled medication to reduce stickiness of secretions(pulmozyme) as well as corticosteroids.
- Home oxygen to aid breathing and in severe cases candidates for heart lung transplants (Oxygen therapy in the community 📖).

Care for GI associated problems

- Pancreatic enzymes with each meal to aid digestion (BNF 1.9.4)
- Vitamin supplements especially A and D
- Medicines to reduce/relieve constipation
- High protein high calorie diet.

Complications and associated issues

- Behavioural and psychological problems arising from having life threatening disease
- CF related diabetes
- Fertility problems and genetic counselling (Fertility problems 📖).

Screening for CF

Preconceptual screening available for prospective parents (Buccal smears).

Related topics

📖 Antenatal care and screening; 📖 Child screening tests.

Further information for relatives and health professionals

🖥 Cystic Fibrosis Trust: www.cysticfibrosis.co.uk; www.cftrust.org.uk

Deafness in children

Deafness

The prevalence of confirmed childhood hearing impairment (>40Db HL) in the UK is 1.3 children per 1000 live births at age of 5yrs (UK Screening Committee 2005).

Causes

Prenatal
- 50% genetic
- Infections in pregnancy e.g. cytomegalovirus, measles, toxiplasmosis
- Ototoxic medications in pregnancy.

Post natal
- Prematurity, sequalae of prematurity e.g. jaundice
- Infections e.g. measles, meningitis, mumps
- Otoxic medications for other infections.

Types

Conductive: also known as glue ear (Infections in children 🕮). Sound cannot pass through outer and middle ear to cochlea and auditory nerve.

Sensori-neural: fault in inner ear of auditory nerve.

Mixed: e.g. problem with glue ear and auditory nerve.

Management

Hearing loss problems or deafness are identified through screening (UK screening programmes 🕮) and 🕮 Child health promotion programme. Children are referred to specialists, including audiology, according to local care pathways and protocols. As in all situations where special needs are identified, the parents and child need support, services and information from a multi-disciplinary team (Children with complex health needs and disabilities 🕮).

Management depends on type, severity of loss and impact. It may include; *Hearing aids*: acoustic aids come in a range of shapes and sizes and may be analogue or digital and some children may use radio transmitter systems to reduce background noise e.g. in classrooms. When a child gains no benefit from acoustic aids a cochlear implant may be considered, the electrodes are inserted surgically and directly stimulate the auditory nerve.

Communication: deaf children, like hearing children, needs lots of attention and interaction to learn and develop communication skills. Special needs team advise on learning additional communication methods e.g. oral-auditory systems e.g. lip reading, sign bilingualism e.g. British Sign Language, total communication e.g. multiple methods.

Further information for professionals and parents

⊠ National Deaf Children's Society Factsheets: www.ndcs.org.uk/

Depressive behaviours

This includes depressive feelings, depressive behaviour, depressive cognitions or beliefs as well as depressive disorders. Increase in prevalence as children get older. Girls outnumber boys in diagnosed problems in adolescence, 2:1. Predisposing factors include genetic, temperament, biological factors, chronic life adversity. Factors associated with a high risk of depression include:

- Psychosocial: family discord, bullying, all forms of abuse.
- Other disorders, including drug and alcohol use, and a history of parental depression.
- Social problems, including homelessness, living in institutional settings.
- Single life event losses.

Presentation

Common to suffer >1 internalizing disorder, e.g. anxiety, social withdrawal, loneliness.

- Pre-school:
  - Apathy and food refusal, miserable, irritable, cries, and rocks
  - Growth failure may occur.
- 5–12yrs:
  - Children use language of emotional affect
  - Psychosomatic symptoms
  - Poor concentration, failure to progress at school
  - Irritability, social withdrawal, temper outbursts
  - Usually complain of being bored.
- Adolescence:
  - Alike to adulthood depression
  - Complaints of boredom, sadness, apathy, lacking energy
  - Appetite and sleep disorders more common.

Assessment in primary care (from NICE guidance see below)

- Identify if 1 of following key symptoms present most days, most of the time >2wks:
  - Persistent sadness or low (irritable) mood
  - Loss of interests and/or pleasure
  - Fatigue or low energy.
- If any key symptoms present, ask about associated symptoms:
  - Poor or increased sleep
  - Poor concentration or indecisiveness
  - Low self-confidence
  - Poor or increased appetite
  - Suicidal thoughts or acts
  - Self harm thoughts
  - Agitation or slowing of movements
  - Guilt or self-blame.
- Find out about past history of depression, life events, family history, associated disability, school contexts, quality of family and peer relationships, and availability of social support.

Action on assessment

- If 4 or less above symptoms, no family history, social support present, not actively suicidal then general advice and watchful waiting. Reiterate advice on good nutrition (Nutrition and healthy eating 📖), good sleep patterns and need for exercise. Offer emotional support/active listening (Counselling skills 📖) or referral to self-help groups or other forms of support e.g. Connexions, faith group. Respond to identified adverse events/problems such as action in instances of bullying.
- If 5 or more symptoms, past or family history, low level of social support, associated social disability, child or relative requests, self-neglect then more active primary care intervention and/or referral to CAMHS tiers 2 or 3.
- Urgent referral to CAMHS/tier 3 or 4 psychiatrist if active suicidal ideas, psychotic symptoms, severe agitation, severe self neglect.

Mental health treatments

Depends on severity of depression.

- Ongoing mild depression beyond 4wks: non-directive supportive therapy, group cognitive behavioural therapy CBT (Talking therapies 📖), or guided self-help.
- Moderate to severe depression: specific psychological therapy e.g. individual CBT, interpersonal therapy or shorter-term family therapy.
  - If unresponsive, different and combined therapies considered including the use of medication e.g. fluoxetine.
- Exercise therapy: regular programme of exercise.
- Inpatient care considered when child or young person at significant risk of self harm.

Advice for family members

- Encourage child to talk about worries; listen and offer help.
- If suspect more than passing phase contact GP/get professional help.

Outcomes

- Most children (2 out of 3) improve but full recovery may take years.
- Liability to further episodes.
- Increased risk of depression in adulthood.

Related topics

📖 Emotional development in babies and children; 📖 Working with teenagers; 📖 People with depression.

Further information

- 🖥 NICE (2005). *Depression in children and young people: Clinical Guideline* 28. www.nice.org.uk/
- 🖥 Understanding Childhood: www.understandingchildhood.net. Leaflets on helping parents and children cope with loss events e.g. divorce, death
- 🖥 Young Minds for childrens mental health: www.youngminds.org.uk ☎ Parents Helpline 0800 018 2138

Eczema in childhood

Atopic eczema is an inflammatory skin condition characterized by dry, itchy, red, and inflamed skin. A genetically determined disorder with hypersensitivity to certain antigens such as pollen, feathers, house dust, household pets, dairy, wheat, soy products which can lead to eczema, asthma, and hay fever. It affects approximately 15% of the child population usually starts <6mths and 90% are in remission by 15yrs. <10% eczema result of food allergies. Can range in severity from mild flexural involvement to severe and chronic inflammatory disease.

Symptoms and signs

- Dry, itchy skin
- Erythema, papules, vesicles
- Exudation, crusting, scaling, fissures
- Lichenification (leathery skin)
- Hyper or hypo pigmentation on some areas.

In the acute stages the skin is red and inflamed leading to vesicles exudations and crusting. In the chronic stages the skin is dry and thickened from repeated scratching.

Babies

Itchy exudative eczema onset can be around 3mths of age and usually affects the face, neck, and distal flexures it is symmetrical in appearance. Sleep maybe disturbed because of itch.

Children

>18m often have eczema on flexural areas, wrists, ankles, and feet, excoriation and dry skin common. Adolescents are more prone to have eczema on face, sides of neck, hands, and feet. Often impacts on self-esteem and behaviour problems can be common.

Care and support

Eczema in a family can cause an increase of stress for other family members. Explain condition and overall good prognosis. Advise:

- Avoid the use of soaps and detergents on the skin.
- Cotton clothing next to the skin.
- Nails kept short to reduce damaging the skin if scratching.
- Damp dusting, vacuuming the room and bed, changing the bedding regularly to help reduce house dust mite that can aggravate eczema.
- Favorite soft toys need to be washed frequently.
- Keep pets away.

Food allergies and eczema

Breast feeding should be encouraged in all babies to 6mths (Breast feeding 📖). If bottle feeding extensively hydrolysed cows' milk formula should be recommended in families where parents and/or siblings have atopic conditions. Babies allergic to cows' milk should be referred to specialist allergy services and dietician for specialist testing and advice on dietary manipulation.

Specific treatment

Treatment aims to replace moisture loss on skin and provide a water-proof barrier to prevent further moisture loss and to protect skin. It aims to ↓ inflammation and relieve the intense itch.

Complete emollient therapy (BNF 13.2)

All soaps and detergents should be replaced with emollient soap substitute, emollient bath oil, and emollient ointment. Emollients help to repair the broken skin barrier by acting like an artificial fat filling the cracks and allowing water to be retained by the skin cells. Emollient ointments such as E45®, Diprobase®, Epaderm®, or 50:50 liquid and white soft paraffin (WSP) are applied to the skin as often as needed to prevent skin from getting dry.

A daily soak for at least 15mins. in the bath removes dead skin cells and debris from the skin. A cool bath hydrates the skin and provides a good base for the applications of emollients. The efficacy of topical emollients is ↑ tenfold when applied immediately after a bath; once the skin has been patted dry.

Wet wrapping is a very effective method to achieve rapid control. It has

significantly ↓ the need to admit children into hospital with severe eczema. Wet wraps are warm or cool, wet occlusive dressings that help to:

- Rehydrate and cool the skin
- Treat inflammation and promote skin healing
- ↓ itching
- Protection against scratching
- ↑ comfort and ↑ sleep if applied before bed.

The wet wrap technique involves the following: bath the child with emollients added, pat dry then apply generous amounts of emollient ointment, then apply wet layer of tubifast (BNF A8.2.3) garment and then a dry layer. It should not be used if child's skin is infected. The community children's nurse, dermatology nurses, or HVs can teach the parents how to apply the wet wrap garments.

Other treatment

- Antihistamines (BNF 3.4.1) to stop the itching and scratching. Short-term use in acute phases only. They are used an hour before bed time, daytime use should be avoided.
- Topical steroids (BNF 13.4) can be used in some cases to control the inflammatory component of atopic eczema and offers dramatic relief of symptoms.
- Antibiotic therapy to treat any 2° infection.
- Chinese herbal treatment increasingly used and evening primrose oil *but* still in experimental stages. Referred to dermatology specialists for advice.

Related topic

📖 Eczema/dermatitis.

Further information for professionals and relatives

- National Eczema Society Fact Sheets (including diet and children with eczema): www.eczema.org
- Clinical Knowledge Summaries (Prodigy) Guidance on the management of atopic eczema: www.cks.library.nhs.uk/
- Skincare campaign: www.skincarecampaign.org
- Systematic review of atopic eczema treatments: www.ncchta.org/execsumm/summ437.htm

Emotional problems in children

This includes a range of internalising disorders including fear, anxiety, and phobias. Management and treatment approaches are similar.

Fear and anxiety

Fear focuses on specific object or situation.

Anxiety is diffuse and anticipatory (has developmental variations).

- Both fear and anxiety result in the same physiological manifestations: unhappiness, irritability, tantrums, sleep disruption.
- Age and sex trends: no consistent sex differences during infancy and pre-school years. In school years it is suggested that girls have more specific fears than boys.

Anxiety in infants

- Stranger anxiety—by 4–5mths, peaks 12mths.
- Separation anxiety—related to stranger anxiety, from 8–24mths, peaks 9–13mths, decreases from 30mths.

Anxiety in childhood and adolescence

- Separation and stranger anxiety diminish as capacity to anticipate events develops.
- Stranger fear may manifest itself as shyness.
- At school age most common fears are for harm coming to others.
- May start to exhibit anxiety about personal adequacy and achievement, e.g. test anxiety.
- Adolescents may show anxieties relating to social situations e.g. rejection and may develop phobias or sexual fears.

Generalized anxiety disorder

Characterized as 'worriers'. Approx. 2% of children. Key features:

- Not related to environmental circumstances.
- Four broad features: worries; restlessness, nervousness, inability to relax; physical symptoms; difficulty concentrating; irritability.

Separation anxiety disorder

Anxiety related to separation from people to whom child is attached. Approx 3% of children. Onset occurs before adolescence, may continue into early adulthood. May result in school refusal: peak occurs at time of transition, also in adolescence, 5yrs, 11yrs, 14–15yrs are most common (~1%).

Specific phobias

These are fears that results in avoidance behaviour to the point of interfering with daily functioning. May involve certain objects, situations. May develop anticipatory anxiety for phobic situation. Prevalence unknown.

Aetiology

- Genetic and constitutional—runs in families.
- Temperament.
- Parental behaviour—e.g. overprotection, criticism.
- Specific experiences and life events.

- Cognitive appraisal of stressful events e.g. abuse.
- Social adversity.

Treatment/management

Referred to local CAMHS as per local guidance.
- Generalized anxiety: remove/reduce stresses, enhance coping mechanisms, psychotherapy, medication may help.
- Separation anxiety: brief, focused counselling; improve understanding of anxiety, behavioural treatment e.g. behavioural control skills.
- Other specific phobias: behavioural methods.
- Panic disorder: behavioural methods, medication may help.
- Social phobia: behavioural methods.

Behavioural methods

Modification of acceptable and unacceptable behaviours. Reinforcement of good/wanted behaviour, ignore/distract from unacceptable/bad behaviour. May use training procedures—rewards (reinforcement) and punishments.

Generally children with anxiety disorders have reasonably good prognosis, but may experience some remissions and some exacerbations throughout childhood and into adulthood.

Advice for parents

Follow guidance on basics for emotional support (see Emotional development in babies and children 📖) as well as specifics as provided by 📖 CAMHS.

Further information

- Association for Infant Mental Health: www.aimh.org.uk
- National Mental Health Association: www.nmha.org
- Royal College of Psychiatrists: www.rcpsych.ac.uk/
- Understanding Childhood: www.understandingchildhood.net
- Young Minds: www.youngminds.org.uk

Enuresis

About 30% of children 4yrs and under have no bladder control at night, reduces to about 15% at 5yrs, 10% at 7yrs, 5% at 10yrs. More ♂ than ♀. NB Most urinary incontinence in children fades away naturally.

Causes

- *Not* deep sleep or laziness.
- Idiopathic often represents a delay in maturation: resolves in time.
- Often runs in families.
- In girls may have an underlying cause e.g. UTI.
- Neurological disabilities or congenital deformities.
- Emotional distress especially if was consistently dry at night before.
- Nocturnal polyuria (failure to produce sufficient vasopressin).
- Overactive bladder syndrome.

Assessment

Includes history, current symptoms, developmental problems, neurological or congenital conditions, soiling (double incontinence suggests neurological causes or developmental delay), family dynamics, and child's motivation to be dry. Invasive tests and examination not usually indicated initially.

Management

- Engage child and family.
- Review fluid and diet intake.
- Support for the child and family.
  - May be distressed or unconcerned.
  - May be causing strife (or result of it).
- <6yrs not treated as usually resolves spontaneously.
- >6yrs more actively managed often by school health service run enuresis clinics. Stepwise management as per Table 7.1 opposite starting with motivational counselling.
- Incontinence nappies/pants may be needed for neurogenic incontinence and if laundry is causing an intolerable burden.

Daytime urinary incontinence

See also 🕮 Toilet training. Losing control during the day is more unusual if it persists should consider and manage/refer as indicated:

- UTI may also be other symptoms such as fever.
- Inherited abnormality of the urinary tract.
- Diabetes occasionally urinary incontinence is the first sign.
- Extreme anxiety.
- Consider possible related cause of constipation.

Table 7.1 Management of enuresis

Method	Features
Motivational counselling	• The child avoids drinks for 2–3hrs before bed; urinates before going to bed; records wet and dry nights and changes clothing and bedding when wet. • Rewards (e.g. star chart) are given for dry nights. • The child is reassured throughout that the problem is not their fault and is just a developmental problem likely to resolve in time.
Enuresis alarms	• An alarm is triggered when the child starts to pass urine. • In the first few weeks, the child wakes after complete emptying of the bladder; in the next few weeks partial inhibition usually occurs; eventually the child wakes up in response to bladder contractions before he wets the bed. • The alarm should be used for at least 3wks. after the last bed-wetting episode. • ~70% effective. Relapse occurs in 10–15%.
Desmopressin nasal spray	• Synthetic version of antidiuretic hormone. • Initial dosage—1 puff to each nostril (20µg in total) at bedtime. If effective the dose halved; if ineffective the dose is doubled. • Adverse effects include headache, nausea, nasal congestion, nosebleed, sore throat, cough, flushing, and mild abdominal cramps. • Effective in the short term (for 4–6wks) e.g. to cover holidays.

Adapted with permission from Simon, C., Everitt, H., and Kendrick, T (2005). *Oxford Handbook of General Practice*, 2nd edn. By permission of Oxford University Press, Oxford.

Related topics
📖 Toilet training.

Further information for professionals and families
🖥 Enuresis Resource and Information Centre (ERIC): www.ERIC.org.uk ☎ 0117 960 3060

Endocrine problems

Diabetes

(See also Diabetes: overview 📖, Insulin therapies 📖.)
Incidence increasing now affects 2:1000 children <16yrs. Almost all are insulin dependent (type 1 diabetes) with peak years of presentation at 12–13 with polyuria, polydipsia, and weight loss. Very occasionally type 2 in children but usually older and mostly obesity related. Referred to specialist. Commenced on insulin by subcutaneous injection. Young children usually given insulin twice a day, with about $^2/_3$ of total dose before breakfast and $^1/_3$ before evening meal. Older children and teenagers often have 3 or 4 injections a day relating insulin more closely to food and exercise, diet, and insulin have to be closely matched. Parents and children need intensive education to cover:

- Nature of diabetes.
- Injecting insulin.
- Diet-regular meals and snacks, reduced refined carbohydrates, healthy diet with no more than 30% fat.
- Sick day rules during illness to prevent ketoacidosis.
- Blood glucose monitoring or in young urine testing.
- Recognition and treatment of hypoglycaemia.
- How to get help and advice 24hrs a day.

Children have special needs (Children with special educational needs 📖) and schools need to be included in addressing specific needs through the day e.g. a snacks and what to do if child becomes hypoglycemic.

Hypoglycaemia: most complain of hunger, dizziness, wobbly feeling in legs, irritablitiy. Treated with easily absorbed glucose e.g. glucose tablets, gels. Parents and schools should be provided and taught how to use IM glucagon injection kit for hypoglycaemia not responding.

Neonatal (congenital) hypothyroidism

~1 per 4000 live births. Usually due to congenital absence of the thyroid gland. One of few preventable causes of severe learning difficulties. Normally detected by heel prick testing (Child screening tests 📖). Refer for specialist advice. Treatment is with lifelong thyroxine replacement. In most treated infants development is normal.

Hyperthyroidism

Usually the result of Graves' disease—characterized by anxiety, restlessness, weight loss, thyrotoxicosis, and exopthamlus. Referred to specialist for drug therapy lasting up to 2yrs. and then possible surgery if relapse.

Inborn errors of metabolism

Many hundreds of enzyme defects have been identified mostly with an autosomal recessive inheritance. Individually very rare and consequently managed at specialist centres. Includes:

- Phenylketonuria: deficiency of the enzyme phenylalaninehydroxylase. 1 in 10,000–20,000 live births, detected by heel prick test (Child screening tests 📖). Treated with restriction of dietary phenylaline for at least 10yrs and possibly life (Genetic problems 📖).

- Galactactosaemia: deficiency of galactose-1-phosphate uridyl transferase. Inability to mobilize glucose from galactose resulting in hypoglycaemia. When lactose containing milk feeds (including breast) are introduced results in vomiting, jaundice, hepatic failure. Management is by lactose and galactose free diet. Even if treated early, severe learning difficulties are common.

Related topic
📖 Growth disorders.

Essential reading
📖 National Service Framework for Diabetes. Guidance on standards of care and best practice: www.dh.gov.uk/PolicyAndGuidance/HealthAnd SocialCareTopics/Diabetes/fs/en

Information and resources for parents, children, and professionals
📖 British Thyroid Foundation: www.btf-thyroid.org/
📖 Diabetes UK: www.diabetes.org.uk/home.htm
📖 National Society for Phenylketonuria: www.nspku.org/

Febrile convulsions and epilepsy

A seizure or fit is when there is a sudden disturbance of neurological function associated with an abnormal neuronal discharge. Occurs in 3–5% of children. Referred for paediatric assessment.

A febrile convulsion is a seizure associated with fever in the absence of another cause.

Epilepsy (see Epilepsy, drugs, and side effects 📖) is recurrent seizures other than febrile convulsions and not due to intracranial infection. 60% of adult epilepsy starts in childhood. Affects 5 per 1000 school children.

Febrile convulsions

- 3–5% of children aged 6mths–5yrs.
- Seizures are usually brief (last <5min) and generalized.
- The risk of subsequent epilepsy is low.

Management

- Most children do not need admission.
- Parent reassurance and education important. Give practical advice given on how to prevent attacks by reducing fevers e.g. early use of paracetamol and tepid sponging (The sick baby and child 📖).
- Those with recurrent or complex febrile convulsions referred to paediatrician. Sometimes treated with rectal diazepam (BNF 4.8.3)— parents need to be taught when and how to administer the diazepam.

Epilepsy

See 📖 Epilepsy for diagnosis, treatment, and management. Surgery is increasingly being used for some types of childhood epilepsy. Every child is reviewed at least annually by specialist paediatric services.

Support and education for parents and children

Epilepsy is a diagnosis that can cause great alarm and fear. Education is very important. Parents, children, and young people need clear information on:

- What to expect.
- What to do during an attack and how to brief other people e.g. school staff.
- Avoiding risks e.g. swimming or cycling alone—but not being over-protective.
- Importance of concordance with medication, particularly teenagers.
- When drug withdrawal may be considered if fit-free.
- Adolescent girls in particular may need specific advice around contraception and pregnancy.

School health staff may have a particular role in helping educate school staff and other children about the condition. Some children with recurring and frequent seizures, usually attending special schools, may require rectal diazepam in particular circumstances as prescribed by the paediatrician. See also 📖 Working in schools.

Further information for professionals

▣ Royal College of Paediatricians and Child Health clinical effectiveness guidelines and summary of NICE guidance on the diagnosis and managment of adults and children with epilepsy in primary and secondary care. www.rcpch.ac.uk/

Further information for parents and children

▣ Epilepsy Action www.epilepsy.org.uk ☎ 0808 800 5050

Gastrointestinal problems in children

Most children experience gastrointestinal problems e.g. vomiting. In most instances the symptoms are mild and transient. Parental advice given on nursing a sick child and identifying signs as to when to seek medical advice (The sick baby and child 📖).

Vomiting

Posseting and regurgitation: terms used to describe the non-forceful return of milk. Usually resolved with introduction of solid food and by 1yr.

Vomiting is the forceful ejection of gastric contents. It may be linked to specific events e.g. travel sickness or a symptom of an infection.
- Projectile vomiting is a symptom of pyloric stenosis. Infantile hypertrophic pyloric stenosis usually develops in the first 3–6wks of life (rare after 12wks). Failure of the pyloric sphincter to relax → hypertrophy of the adjacent pyloric muscle. Requires paediatric assessment. Treated with surgery with no long-term effects.

Vomiting and diarrhoea

Parent information important to determine nature and seriousness of problem, including:
- Nature and duration of symptoms
- Presence of blood in the stool
- Other accompanying symptoms e.g. fever
- Contact with anyone else with similar symptoms
- History of recent foreign travel.

Possible causes
- Breast-fed babies have loose, often explosive 'mustard grain' stools.
- Toddlers often have intermittent loose stools related to diet. Usually resolves by 5yrs.
- Gastrointestinal infection: the child may have diarrhoea, vomiting or a combination of the 2. Usually viral (rotavirus, norwalk) in origin—common in winter. Parents encouraged to ensure adequate fluids, may need rehydration fluids, to prevent dehydration. Advised to eat normally, especially in cases of diarrhoea. Advise on nursing sick infant and when to seek medical help.
- Malabsorbtion (see Coeliac disease 📖).
- Acute interabdominal problems includes:
  - Intussusception: the invagination of one part of the bowel into the lumen of the immediately adjoining bowel. 2 per 1000 live births. Usually between 5–18mths. Presents with acute pain, vomiting, passage of reccurrent jelly like stool. Is a medical emergency treated surgically.
  - Appendicitis (📖).

See also 📖 Constipation and encopresis.

Further information for professionals
🖥 Royal College of Paediatricians and Child Health clinical effectiveness guidelines management of diarrhoea and constipation: www.rcpch.ac.uk/

Further information for parents
🖥 NHS Direct (England Wales) www.nhsdirect.nhs.uk
☎ NHS Direct helpline is open 24hrs 0845 4647 for nurse advice and health information
☎ Scotland:. NHS 24 is a free 24hrs helpline offering advice on personal health care 0141 225 0099

Genetic problems

There are 46 chromosomes: 22 are matching pairs with matching genes (autosomes); the remaining pair are sex chromosomes which may match (XX—♀) or differ (XY—♂). Parents of any child affected by a genetic problem are offered genetic counselling and pre-natal diagnosis, if available, for any subsequent pregnancies.

Care, support, and treatment depends on specific problems of each child and family. The primary health-care team, specialist health care services, social services, community paediatric services, education services and voluntary organizations involved as necessary. Should be reviewed regularly (Children with complex health needs and disabilities 📖).

Down's syndrome

Trisomy 21 (an extra chromosome number 21). Commonest chromosomal abnormality affecting 1:600 births. Life expectancy is ↓ but ~¹/₂ live to 60yrs. Incidence ↑ with maternal age at conception but, as most babies are born to mothers <40yrs. old, the majority are born to younger women.

Clinical features
- Facial abnormalities: flat occiput, oval face (mongoloid facies), low set eyes with prominent epicanthic folds
- Single palmar crease
- Hypotonia
- Developmental delay
- Congenital heart disease.

(See also People with learning difficulties 📖.)

Edward's syndrome

Trisomy 18. 1 per 8000 births. Life expectancy is ~10mths (♀ >♂).

Clinical features
- Facial abnormalities: Low-set malformed ears, receding chin, protruding eyes, cleft lip or palate
- A short sternum makes the nipples appear too widely separated.
- Fingers cannot be extended and the index finger overlaps the 3rd digit
- Developmental delay
- Umbilical or inguinal hernias
- Rocker-bottom feet
- Rigid baby with flexion of the limbs.

Patau's syndrome

Trisomy 13. 1 per 7500 births. 50% die in <1mth. Usually fatal in the first year. Multiple abnormalities including:
- Small head and eyes
- Brain malformation
- Heart malformations
- Polycystic kidneys
- Cleft lip/palate
- Skeletal abnormalities e.g. flexion contractures of hands ± polydactyly with narrow fingernails.

Cri du Chat syndrome

Deletion of the short arm of chromosome 5 is the most common deletion syndrome. 1 per 25000–50000 births. Life expectancy unpredictable. Presents with:
- Abnormal cry (cat-like)
- Microcephaly
- Developmental delay
- Marked epicanthic folds
- Moon-shaped face
- Alert expression

Other common infections

See also 📖 Infectious diseases in childhood.

Conjunctivitis: infection (bacterial or viral) of the conjunctiva. Young children very susceptible to repeated episodes and severe forms. Presents with red eye(s), swollen eyelid(s), discharge often sticks lids together. 64% resolve in 5d without treatment.

- Treatment with antibiotics eye drops or ointment (BNF 11.1).
- Up to 25% physical transmission in household so advise to avoid sharing towels etc. No need for exclusion from day care or school (see HPA website below).
- If presenting with these symptoms <1mth, (different from new born sticky eye see minor problems of New babies 📖) swabbed for MS & C. Possibly contracted STI through the birth canal (opthalmia neonaotrum a notifiable disease).

Impetigo See 📖 Bacterial skin infections.

Related topic

📖 Infectious diseases in childhood.

Further information for professionals

📟 BMJ International clinical evidence website: www.clinicalevidence.com/ceweb/conditions/index.jsp
📟 Health Protection Agency: www.hpa.org.uk
📟 Clinical Knowledge Summaries (Prodigy) guidance: www.cks.library.nhs.uk/index

Further information for parents

📟 NHS Direct Encyclopedia: www.nhsdirect.nhs.uk/alphaindex.asp

Infectious diseases in childhood

Primary immunization (Childhood immunization general 📖) has virtually eliminated all traditional childhood diseases with the exception of chickenpox. Key aspects of these diseases are summarized in Table 7.2. Parents should be advised on caring for a sick child and reminded of key indicators when to seek medical advice (see The sick baby and child 📖).

See also 📖 Infectious disease exclusion times.

Further information for professionals
🖥 Health protection agency Topics A–Z: www.hpa.org.uk/
🖥 Clinical Knowledge Summaries (Prodigy) guidance: www.cks.library.nhs.uk/index

Further information for parents
🖥 NHS Direct Encyclopedia: www.nhsdirect.nhs.uk/alphaindex.asp

Table 7.2 Infectious disease in childhood

Disease	Transmission/incubation	Presentation	Treatment	Complications	Infectious
Chickenpox	Physical contact, droplet, airborne. 11–20d	Rash ± fever. Spots progress from macule → papule → vesicle. Crops appear for 5–7d. Vesicles dry out and scab over (usually in <14d.)	Supportive: paracetamol, fluids, topical calamine lotion to lesions	Eczema herpeticum, encephalitis, pneumonia	Until 5d after skin eruption
Diphtheria (very rare in UK)	Droplet 2–5d	Inflammatory exudate which forms a greyish membrane in the respiratory tract	Hospital admission for anti toxin and antibiotics	Respiratory obstruction	
Haemophilus influenzae (very rare in UK)	Respiratory droplet. Nasal secretions	Meningitis: 60%	Antibiotics	Permanent neurological sequelae; mortality—5%	Until antibiotic treatment for 24hrs
Erthema infectiosum (5th disease)	Respiratory droplet. 4–7d	Erthematous maculo-papular rash starting on face, then lacy rash on trunk and limbs. Mild fever	Tepid sponging, paracetamol and fluids		Probably only during prodome. Important for pregnant ♀ to report contact to GP
Measles	Respiratory droplet. 10–14d	Early: fever, conjunctivitis, cough, cold. Later: Koplik's spots (white spots on bright red background inside mouth) red maculopapular rash appears after 4d Last ≈ 10d	Tepid sponging, paracetamol and fluids	Bronchopneumonia, otitis media, gastroenteritis, encephalitis	Highly contagious for up to 18d to non-immune

Table 7.2 (Contd.)

Disease	Transmission/incubation	Presentation	Treatment	Complications	Infectious
Mumps	Respiratory droplet. 16–21d	Fever, malaise, tender enlargement of 1 or both parotids ± submandibular glands	Tepid sponging, paracetamol and fluids	Aseptic meningitis; epididymo-orchitis; pancreatitis	Up to 29d
Pertussis (whooping cough)	Respiratory droplet. 7d	Catarrhal stage as URTI, coughing stage paroxysmal cough with spasms of coughing followed by a 'whoop' lasts 4–6wks	Antibiotics in catarrhal stage	Pneumonia, bronchiectasis, convulsions	Up to 5d after start of antibiotics
Poliomyelitis (rare in UK)	droplet or faeco-oral. 7d	Flu-like prodrome then fever, tachycardia, headache, vomiting, neck stiffness and unilateral tremor, paralysis	Hospital admission	Permanent disability may result. <10% of those developing paralysis die	
Rubella (German measles)	Respiratory droplet. 14–21d	Pink maculopapular rash for 3d, mild fever	Paracetamol and fluids	Birth defects if infected in pregnancy, arthritis (adolescents); thrombocytopoenia (rare)	15–23d
Roseola infantum (<2yrs)	?Oral secretions. 4–7d	High fever, sore throat, macular rash appears after 3–4d as fever drops	Tepid sponging, paracetamol and fluids		5–15d
Scarlet fever	Respiratory droplet. 2–4d	Fever, malaise, headache, tonsillitis, rash, 'scarlet' facial flushing	Penicillin	Rheumatic fever	Not known

Infectious diseases exclusion times

Table 7.3 Infectious diseases exclusion times

Disease	Exclusion period from early years care/schools
Chickenpox (varicella)	5d from start of skin eruption
Conjunctivitis	None
Gastroenteritis	Usually 24hrs after last episode of diarrhoea or vomiting but if cause of diarrhoea is *E.coli*, salmonella, shigella then until negative stools
Haemophilus influenzae infections	24hrs after treatment started
Headlice	None
Hepatitis A	<5yrs of age: 5d (recommendations made on the basis that exclusion is largely ineffective, but recommended in day-care centres and pre-schools because of the risk to adults) >5yrs: none
Herpes simplex	None
Impetigo	Until lesions healed/crusted
Infectious mononucleosis	None
Measles	5d from onset of rash
Meningococcal disease	Duration of illness
Mumps	5d from onset
Pertussis	5d from starting antibiotics otherwise >3wks
Rubella	5d from onset of rash
Scabies	Until treated
Scarlet fever	5d from start of antibiotic treatment
Tinea (ring worm)	None
Threadworms	None
Tuberculosis	Smear positive: 2wks after starting treatment
Typhoid and para-typhoid	24hrs after last episode of diarrhoea
Warts and verrucas	None

Source: ▣ Health Protection Agency Guidelines on the management of communicable diseases in nurseries and schools exclusion www.hpa.org.uk/infections/topics_az/schools/schools.pdf

Insects and infestations

Insect bites and stings

Response depends on the insect involved and the individual's response to the bite. Ranges from blisters through papules to urticarial wheals. Stings should be removed if still embedded.

- Itching resulting from bites from fleas, flies, and mosquitoes can be treated with topical antihistamine (BNF 3.4.1), although greater allergic reactions may need oral anti-histamines.
- Anaphylactic reactions (see Anaphylaxis 📖).

Prevention includes:

- Use of mosquito deterrent (see Travel health care 📖).
- Animal flea infestation in homes needs treatment of animals and carpets. Sprays available OTC, severe infestations may needed wide spread spraying by a commercial company or local environmental heath department (Environmental health services 📖).

Headlice (*Pediculus capitis*)

Wingless insects. Most common in children age 4–16yrs. (♀ > ♂) but can infest anyone. Spread by lice walking from head to head. Eggs known as 'nits' and laid at base of hair shaft, hatch within 7–10d. Empty white shells remain 'glued' to hair. Nymph stage 7–10d to adult and able to reproduce. Lice pierce the scalp to feed on blood.

Prevention: no evidence of effectiveness of prophylactic treatment or use of herbal based lotions. Health promotion schemes with children and parents (e.g. Bug Busters see below), particularly in early years facilities and schools, encourages:

- Hair management strategies.
- Early detection by weekly combing wet, conditioner covered, hair with light coloured fine-tooth comb.
- Early treatment to prevent spread.

Symptoms: itchy scalp and scratching. Detection of a moving louse, not old egg shells, confirms infestation. Difficult to detect moving louse on dry or damp hair unless very severe infestation. Experts continue to debate effectiveness of wet combing and insecticides,

Treatment by mechanical removal

- After washing hair, apply conditioner and systematically comb all hair with fine-tooth detector comb (available from local pharmacies). Rinse comb after each stroke to remove trapped lice and not comb back into hair.
- Repeat every 4d until no more lice are found for a minimum of 2wks to remove nymphs. Bug Busters web site provides detailed instructions, Bug Buster™ kit NHS prescribable (BNF 13.10.4).

Chemical treatments with insecticides

- Available OTC and on NHS prescription.
- Malathion, phenothrin, permethrin, and carbaryl mostly effective against lice. To overcome the development of resistance, a mosaic strategy is used rotating to different insecticide if treatment fails (BNF 13.10.4).
- Application as per instructions for contact time of 12hrs, repeated 7d later. Aqueous formulations preferred for small children and those with severe eczema, or asthma. Shampoos are not effective—use lotions or liquids.
- Some community concerns about using pesticides including organophosphates on children (see Pesticide Action Network, website below).

Other treatments: herbal therapies—e.g. tea tree oil, herbal treatments. No evidence of effectiveness.

All close contacts e.g. family, school friends should check their heads and be treated as necessary.

Scabies (*Sarcoptes scabie*) The scabies mite is ~$^1/_2$ mm long and spread by direct physical contact.

Symptoms: appear 4–6wks. after infection. Red burrows, tracking in irregular lines, commonly between fingers and toes. Intense itching. Scratching results in excoriations.

Treatment: treated with permethrin 5% aqueous preparation over whole body and washed off after 8–12hrs (BNF 13.10.4). All close contacts need treatment. All worn clothing and bedding should be washed. Itching may persist for some time after elimination often alleviated by topical antihistamines.

Threadworm (*Enterobulus vermicularis*)

Common among children. Worm lives about 6wks. Causes anal itch as it leaves the bowel to lay eggs on the perineum. Often seen as silvery thread-like worms in stools or at the anus. Scratching transfers eggs to nails and hands, then ingested. Child >2yrs and household members treated with mebendazole. Piperazine for children <6mths. OTC (BNF 5.5.1). Prevention includes promoting good hand washing before meals and after going to the toilet, ensuring short and clean nails.

Further information

Royal College of Paediatricians and Child Health clinical effectiveness guidelines: www.rcpch.ac.uk/

Clinical Knowledge Summaries, Infections and Infestations. www.cks.library.nhs.uk

Further information for parents

- Bug Busting: www.chc.org/bugbusting/
- NHS Direct (England Wales): www.nhsdirect.nhs.uk ☎ NHS Direct helpline is open 24hrs 0845 4647 for nurse advice and health information; ☎ Scotland NHS 24 is a free 24hrs helpline offering advice on personal health care 0141 225 0099
- Pesticide Action Network: www.pan-uk.org/default.htm

Neural tube defects

The neural tube fuses in first 28d after conception. Incomplete fusion leads to 4 types of malformation (see below). Prevention is through folic acid supplements in ♀ planning pregnancy and in first 12wks (Pre-conceptual care and advice 📖). Most defects detected antenatally (Antenatal care and screening 📖). Incidence now about 0.15/1000 births. Mothers who have had one fetus with a neural tube defect have a very high risk of second and should take high dose folic acid preconceptually and for first 12wks.

Malformations

- Anencephaly: absence of most of cranium and skull. Born stillborn or die shortly after birth. Antenatal termination offered if detected.
- Encephalocele: midline skull defect and brain and meniges herniated through. Corrected by surgery but may be underlying malfomations.
- Spina bifida occulta: failure of fusion of the vertebral arch. May be associated with skin lesion or tuft of hair. Usually asymptomatic.
- Spina bifida. Two types:
  - Meniges only protrude (meningocele) and repaired surgically with a good prognosis.
  - Myelomeningocoele (meniges and spinal cord) protrude. 80% of spina bifida cases. Surgically treated soon after birth. Problems can include hydrocephalus, scoliosis, paralysis of legs, sensory loss, neuropathic bladder and bowel. Hydrocephalus may be treated by endoscopic surgery or introduction of ventricular shunt to drain CSF (cerebro spinal fluid).

Long-term care for the parents and child with spina bifida

These children will be treated and managed by specialist multi-disciplinary paediatric teams with long-term follow-up as needs change with age and they become adults. Primary care professionals provide long term support and primary care services as with all children with special needs (Children with complex health needs and disabilities 📖). Need for emotional support as well as physical care and information important for parents and child. Particular issues primary care professionals may need to be aware of include:

- Prevention of renal problems: many parents are taught intermittent catheterization when child very young to ensure bladder empting. More require support at school.
- Recognition of shunt blockage or infection problems: onset may be gradual including headaches, irritability, vomiting, general malaise. Schools and other child carers need to be informed of signs. Needs assessment and attention at specialist centre not local hospitals.

Further information and support

📖 Association for spina bifida and hydrocephalus (ASBAH): www.asbah.org.uk ☎ 01733 555 988

Sickle cell disorders

Haemoglobinopathies refers to a range of genetically inherited disorders of red blood cell haemoglobin (Hb). Sickle cell disorders refers to a inherited sickle Hb disorders including sickle cell anaemia. Sickle cell anaemia (Hb SS) is an autosomal recessive genetic condition inheriting two Hb S genes from both parents. Hb S refers to haemoglobin that is deformed, rigid and 'sickle' shaped, unable to transport oxygen effectively. Sickle cells have a reduced life span, and block small capillaries, reducing oxygen transportation and resulting in thrombosis and ischaemia. This is made worse by factors such as dehydration and cold or situations of reduced oxygen availability e.g. anaesthesia, high altitudes. About 300 children a year in the UK are born with sickle cell anaemia (NHS Sickle cell screening programme, see below). Mainly affects people of African or Caribbean descent, but also affects people from Asia, the Middle East, and the eastern Mediterranean. The UK has antenatal (Antenatal care and screening 📖) and new born screening programmes (Child screening tests 📖).

Those with one HbA gene and one HbS gene have sickle cell trait and are carriers of sickle cell anaemia. They have enough normal HbA to not experience the problems of those with sickle cell anaemia.

Children identified with HbSS are referred to a named paediatrician. Children (and adults) with sickle cell anaemia will vary in the severity of symptoms and problems. Symptoms include:
• Anaemia.
• Pain as a result of vaso-occlusive crises. Can vary in frequency and severity. Can occur anywhere in the body but often occurs in the limbs, back and abdomen. Also presents as dactylitis—hand/foot syndrome is a painful swelling of the hands, feet, or both and affects children <3yrs old. Often the pain is excruciating. Boys can also experience priapism. Types of vaso occlusive crisis that may require blood transfusions include:
  • *Sequestration crisis*: a sudden ↓ haemoglobin concentration due to pooling of a large volume of blood in the spleen or liver or lungs, painful swelling of the organ with worsening anaemia. Can affect children within the first 5yrs, and in rare instances, can result in death from circulatory collapse, anaemia and hypovolamic shock.
  • *Haemolytic crisis*: when events such as infections cause a serious ↓ in the number of red blood cells.
  • *Aplastic crisis*: occurs at any age as a result of a ↓ of bone marrow activity. May be life threatening.
  • *Megaloblastic changes/crisis*: this is rare due to folic acid deficiency.
• Infections, due to splenic dysfunction causing increased susceptibility.
• Jaundice due to chronic haemolysis.
Long-term problems may include cardiac problems from chronic anaemia, and gall stones due to chronic haemolysis of red blood cells, CVA, ulcerated legs.

Advice and management

There is no cure or specific treatment for sickle cell disease. Prevention of illnesses includes prophylactic antibiotics and full child immunization schedule (📖) plus annual influenza vaccination. Key areas of advice are:

- As normal life style as possible but act early in any illness.
- Ensure a healthy lifestyle and good nutrition (including folic acid).
- Avoid triggers to crisis e.g. dehydration, cold, strenuous exercise in damp or wet conditions.
- Seek medical advice early for any infections.
- Travel advice: ensure adequate malaria prophylaxis: sickle cell disease offers no protection. NB Crisis can be precipitated by anti malarials.
- Recommend wearing a medic alert bracelet.

Sickle Cell Society suggests CBT (Talking therapies 📖) can help young people and adults.

Important to ensure child care and school staff understand the condition and support the active management to avoid triggers e.g. drinking lots of fluids, avoiding cold.

Management of crises

Minor ones are managed at home with support of GP and primary care team. Key management elements are analgesia, ↑ fluid intake, and warmth. Pain can be helped by:

- Careful assessment, child diaries useful insight into patient's pain experience and coping strategies.
- Warmth, massaging and rubbing, and by heat e.g. hot water bottles.
- Bandaging to support the painful region.
- Resting the body. Deep breathing exercises and distraction techniques.

Pain relief prescribed according to severity (see Children's BNF)

- Paracetamol, tds (30–60mg 1–3mths, 60–120mg 3–12mths, 120–250mg 1–5yrs, 250–500mg 6–12yrs, 500mg 12–18yrs).
- Codeine phosphate, qds, at 3mg/kg daily in divided doses.
- Stronger analgesic non-steroidal anti-inflammatory agent, such as diclofenac, which is tds, of 1mg for every kg of body weight.

Children with more severe crisis will be admitted to hospital e.g. severe pain, high fever or other symptoms such as dyspnoea or neurological signs.

Related topic

📖 Children with complex health needs and disabilities.

Further information for professionals and patients

▦ NHS Sickle Cell and Thalassaemia screening programme. Useful leaflets for practitioners: http://kcl.phs.ac.uk/haemscreening/

▦ The Sickle Cell Society: www.sicklecellsociety.org ☎ 0208 961 4006

Thalassaemia

Thalassaemia is a less common haemoglobinopathy than sickle cell in the UK. Estimated to be about 700 people having the most severe form β thalassaemia (UK Thalassaemia screening programme see below). Highest prevalence in Cypriot, Italian, Greek, Indian, Pakistani, Bangladeshi, Chinese, and South Asian populations. Also (less common) Northern European population. The UK has antenatal (Antenatal care and screening 📖) and new born screening programmes (Child screening tests 📖). Any child identified with thalassaemia is referred to a named paediatrican.

B thalassaemia major

Children (and adults) with this condition are unable to produce haemoglobin resulting in life threatening anaemia and jaundice from about 6mths. They require regular blood transfusions for life accompanied by regular chelation therapy to prevent iron deposition. Even with treatment, these children often have complex problems including growth and sexual development problems, enlarged spleen, diabetes and heart problems. Life expectancy is of 2 or 3 decades. A bone marrow transplant can offer a cure.

Thalassaemia intermedia is another less severe form and may require less frequent transfusions.

Management of care
• These children and their families are primarily supported by specialist services.
• Families and children need continual support and recognition of problems being faced over a lifetime.

Related topics
📖 Children with complex health needs and disabilities; 📖 Blood transfusion.

Further information for professionals and patients
▣ NHS Sickle Cell and Thalassaemia screening programme. Includes information leaflets for midwives and community practitioners: www.kcl-phs.org.uk
▣ UK Thalassaemia Society: www.ukts.org ☎ 0800 73 111 09

Sudden unexpected death of an infant (SUDI)

SUDI that cannot be explained, also known as cot death, affects >300 babies in UK each year. Most <1yr, majority <6mths, more ♂ than ♀. Since 1991 the number has decreased in incidence by 75%.

Risk factors are thought to include: prematurity, low birth weight, laying baby face down to sleep (Babies and sleeping 📖), parental smoking smoke, and overheating. FSID (see below) produce parent leaflets on reducing risk.

Protocols

Most areas have joint inter agency protocols for SUDI agreed with coroner. May be part of local child protection procedures (Child protection 📖). All sudden, unexpected deaths are under the jurisdiction of the coroner and post mortems have to be carried out. The police investigate if there is any suspicion it may have been unnatural. Protocols likely to include:

- Ambulance staff attempt resuscitation and always take to ED.
- Immediate notification to coroner's office, GP, police team, and named paediatrician.
- Home visit by paediatrician and police within 24hrs to talk with parents and inspect the scene.
- Paediatrician collates all medical records and asks social services to check child protection register, keeping in close contact with police and coroner.
- Post mortem carried out and findings reported to parents as soon as possible by pathologist, paediatrician and/or GP.
- Case discussion within 6wks involving all professional involved with family to scrutinize all aspects of death and contributory factors, to plan ongoing support for family at that point, and when they plan another pregnancy. Paediatrician and/or GP and/or HV meet with parents to share conclusions and offer ongoing support.

Best practice guidance for HVs and primary care nurses

- If first to visit home when SUDI discovered:
  - Check that an ambulance has been called.
  - If in doubt, resuscitation should always be attempted.
  - Ensure parents and siblings have support from friends and family.
  - Spend time listening to the parents. Mention the baby by name and don't be afraid to express sorrow.
- If learn later that a baby has died, HV team should liaise with GP to avoid duplication and visit as close to the death as possible to offer:
  - Condolences, an opportunity for the parents to talk.
  - Information and support though post mortem, coroner procedures funeral, and Bereavement (📖).
  - If the mother was breast feeding, discuss methods of suppression of lactation.

- Ensure the parents have information from FSID and its befriender scheme (see below).
- Ensure parents have been given and content discussed of DoH's leaflets *A guide to the post mortem examination procedure involving a baby or child* (ref 29768/A) and *Post mortem examination on a baby or child ordered by the coroner* (ref 29773).
- Check the following agencies have been informed of the baby's death:
  - Medical records departments of maternity/children's hospitals to avoid follow-up appointments being sent.
  - Child Health records department to avoid letters being sent about immunizations and development checks.
  - The school, if there are school age children in the family.
- Later revisit following funeral and then follow-up to case discussion to:
  - Offer further time to talk.
  - Information about local bereavement services.
- Remember to talk about the deceased baby by name, at anniversaries and during any subsequent pregnancies and births.
- Offer information about local Care of Next Infant Scheme (CONI).

CONI

This is a programme set up in many areas of the UK where a local coordinator supports parents and professionals through subsequent pregnancies and first year of child's life. Programme includes additional visits from a HV, symptom diary, loan of apnea monitors, room thermometer, and additional advice.

Further information for professionals and parents

Foundation for the Study of Infant Deaths (FSID) provides guidelines and information for professionals as well as information, support, befriending scheme for parents

FSID booklet *When a baby dies suddenly and unexpectedly.* Available at: www.sids.org.uk/fsid/coni.htm; FSID's Helpline ☎ 0870 787 0554

Adult health promotion

Models and approaches to health promotion

There is no universally accepted model of health promotion. There are 3 main types of approaches:
- Individual focused
- Group focused
- Community focused.

Table 8.1 summarizes the main theories and key concepts within these approaches.

Individual focused approaches can involve:
- Medical/nursing input: acting to ensure that the individual is prevented from developing a disease or protected from an agent that might cause a disease, for example immunization against disease and screening for disease.
- Educational input: giving individuals information, or helping them to interpret evidence, so that they can make life choices. Lecturing and multiple leaflets are likely to be ignored.
- Behavioural input: giving people the information and support to help them cope, or move on with making lifestyle changes e.g. stopping smoking. Persuading an unwilling client to make lifestyle changes will only result in failure → resistance to attempting the change at a later date.

Group focused approaches normally a combination of educational and behavioural change approaches, although can also be community development focused. Requires a knowledge of group dynamics.

Community focused approaches to health promotion involves one or a combination of the following:
- Epidemiological focused approaches: based on information on the prevalence and/or incidence of a condition in a geographical area. Use standardized statistical information to initiate health promotion initiatives e.g. TB prevention.
- Social/societal change: initiating or lobbying for change involving policy or legislation change or innovation. Often based on epidemiological evidence, but may be initiated by the expressed need of a community or policy initiative e.g. physical activity promotion.
- Community development: interventions are identified and carried out by the community. This may involve health and other professionals working with communities to empower them to identify their own health promotion and health improvement needs. These may differ radically from the agenda of health and social care professionals.

Table 8.1 Summary of theories: focus and key concepts of health promotion

Theory	Focus	Key concepts
Stages of change model	Individual's readiness to change or attempt to change toward healthy behaviours	• Pre-contemplation • Contemplation • Decision/determination • Action • Maintenance
Health belief model	Person's perception of the threat of a health problem and the appraisal of recommended behaviour(s) for preventing or managing the problem	• Perceived susceptibility • Perceived severity • Perceived benefits of action • Cues to actions • Self-efficacy
Social learning theory	Behaviour explained via a 3-way, reciprocal theory = personal factors, environmental influences, and behaviour continually interact	• Behaviour capability • Reciprocal determinism • Expectations self-efficacy • Observational learning • Reinforcement
Community organization theories	Emphasizes active participation and development of communities that can better evaluate and solve health and social problems	• Empowerment • Community competence • Participation and relevance • Issue selection • Critical consciousness
Organizational change theory	Strategies for ↑ the chances that healthy policies and programmes will be adopted and maintained in formal organizations e.g. NHS	• Problem definition (awareness stage) • Initiation of action (adoption stage) • Implementation of change • Institutionalization of change

Further information

⌸ England NICE Public Health: www.publichealth.nice.org.uk
⌸ Health Promotion Agency for Northern Ireland: www.healthpromotionagency.org.uk
⌸ Health voice network: www.healthvoice-uk.net
⌸ Scotland Health Promoting Health Service site: www.hebs.com/healthservice/

Group health promotion

Group work is an effective method of health promotion. HVs and other public health nurses are often more involved in group health promotion work than other nurses in primary care but all nurses are encouraged to use these techniques. Involvement in group work can mean a range of activities including:

- Teaching health topics as a formal lecture or one off talk e.g. antenatal education classes, to a school class.
- Using principles of participatory adult learning in community group situations e.g. session on contraception in youth group.
- Forming and/or supporting groups for self-help, mutual support, and health information e.g. carers support group.
- Becoming part of a group, made up of local people/professionals to influence policy and/or services e.g. estate action group or campaigning group on housing problems.

Each of these types of group work require different skills and knowledge, some of which may have been part of formal education. Often CPD or local NHS health promotion services (may be part of public health) run short courses e.g. small group work skills or presentation skills for teaching health topics.

Principles of participatory learning in small groups

Beforehand:

- Plan how to use the time together.
- Plan how the environment will help the group work e.g. seats in circles, crèche for small children separately.
- Plan to use materials that are appropriate to the group.

In the session:

- Involve everyone from the beginning of the session by getting them to introduce themselves and saying what they'd like to get out of the session (i.e. icebreaking activities).
- Establish any ground rules the group think necessary e.g. listen to each other.
- Activities that include active participation and sharing by the members. Techniques include:
  - Brainstorming e.g. what are the different types of contraception?
  - Problem solving e.g. 3-year-old John has a full blown temper tantrum at the supermarket checkout, what would you advise his mum to do?
- Break up the time and change activities using additional inputs/health promotion materials.
- Summarize the activity at the end of the session, offer time for participants to summarize/raise any issues and offer written materials e.g. leaflets to back up or provide detailed information e.g. local directory of services aimed at carers.

Principles for helping to establish and run a group

- Identify a need and partners to help, check there is not already a similar local group that you could support, be clear about its purposes e.g. a support/social opportunity for carers with 'sitting' facilities for the person cared for.
- Consider any finance required and possible local sources.
- Find a suitable local venue for the purpose of the group. Consider issues such as access, acoustics, comfort, refreshment opportunities, insurance cover for the purpose intended, separate space if need to split into 2 e.g. for crèche.
- Personal invitations to target members plus wider local publicity.
- Plan the first meeting and tasks for the facilitators such as arranging the space, greeting people, starting and ending the meeting.
- Consider how to involve others in group roles to share the workload and increase commitment.
- Consider how the group could become self-sustaining.
- Recognize that many groups have their own life cycle and ending a group or watching it change into something completely different is often appropriate and healthy.

Further information

Ewles, L. and Simnett, I. (2003). *Promoting Health a Practical Guide.* Chapter 13. Working with Groups. Baillere Tindall, London
Local PCO public health/health promotion services

Community approaches to health

Three inter-linked concepts relate to community approaches to health.

Social capital

Social capital describes the connections and networks among people in a social group or community. The ↑ interaction between people, the ↑ sense of being part of a community. Main aspects include:

• Trust and reciprocity
• Informal and social networks
• Civic engagement.

Higher levels of social capital in a community → better health, ↑ educational achievement, better employment outcomes, and ↓ crime rates. NB Also has the potential to exclude others.

LAs have to have a community strategy through Local Strategic Partnerships. Within this, they may also use community development approaches and employ specific community development workers.

Partnership approaches

All PCOs and health-care professionals are increasingly involved in partnerships with local organizations outside of health care to address health and social issues in the broadest sense e.g. regeneration programmes, Sure Start, crime and disorder partnerships, health, employment, education action zones, Health Living Centres. Primary care nurses are encouraged to participate in these partnerships as well as network with local statutory, voluntary and self-help organizations to improve service response to local need and develop innovative approaches to locally identified need.

Community development approaches

Community development work aims to bring about social change and address inequalities by working with communities (defined geographically and/or by specific interests). The community members themselves:

• Identify their needs and acceptable ways to address them
• Plan and take action
• Evaluate the impact and identifies what else needs to change.

HVs and SNs often take these sort of approaches and in some areas, may not have a caseload of individual families or schools so they can focus on these types of community development approaches to health.

Weight management: overweight, obesity

All opportunities in primary care should be taken for promoting the principles of good nutrition and healthy eating (📖) and exercise (📖). Particularly important to teach children and young people these principles as eating patterns continue into adulthood.

Overweight

People who take in more energy than they require, store the energy as excess fat and become overweight, and if this continues will become obese. The main contributory factors are sedentary lifestyle and increased energy intake. Obesity is directly linked to increased risks of morbidity e.g. DM, CHD, hypertension. Classification of BMI:

- 25–29.9 overweight
- 30–34.9 obese Class I
- 35–39.9 obese Class II
- >40 severely or morbidly obese.

NB People of Asian origin are at greater risk of morbidity at lower BMI levels.[1]

Obesity

Obesity is a major public health issue. Levels of obesity in UK have trebled since 1980. In 2001, 46% of men and 34% of women were overweight, 17% and 21% respectively were obese. Many factors interact to cause weight gain e.g. behavioural, genetic predisposition, lifestyle. Weight gain increases with age, women gain weight more easily, ↑ risk in lower socio-economic groups, higher prevalence in some minority ethnic groups e.g. women of Carribean and Pakistani origin. 80% smokers who cease increase weight, but benefits of cessation outweigh not ceasing.

People who are obese have a shorter life expectancy, are at a greater risk of developing coronary heart disease and type 2 diabetes as well as ↑ risk of other problems e.g. respiratory, musclo-skeletal, stress incontinence.

Raising the issue

Overweight and obesity is an issue that needs to be raised in an open, empathetic manner that acknowledges the complexity of the person's experiences, the causes, and their feelings. Listening to the patient's experience and views establishes their perception of the problem and their willingness to address it. For those not interested in weight reduction at this point it is important to let them know they can come back or give information where else to go if they choose to address the issue later.

Supporting those interested in weight reduction

For those willing to address the issue:

- In general aim to promote good nutrition and healthy eating (📖), ↑ physical activity (Exercise 📖) and ↓ sedentary behaviour, ↑ self-awareness about day-to-day behaviours.
- Make time to clarify patient expectations and ability to engage.

[1] DH (England) (2006). Best Practice Guidance *Care Pathway for the Management of overweight and obesity*. www.dh.gov.uk/publications Reference 274537–40.

- Discuss the options on how to support weight reduction. This may be in or outside of the NHS e.g. Weightwatchers or the community dieticians, GP practice may have a weight management protocol, or weight management clinic, or HVs may have a weight management group.

Supporting weight reduction in primary care

The aim is for a realistic, modest weight loss over no more than 12wks. Some local areas are supported by community dietician programmes and protocols. Supporting protocols and resources on websites (see below). Protocols usually include:
- Agreement between person and professional on goals and means of achieving them.
- Structured assessment, recording and regular follow-up.
- Specific dietary advice and menu sheets for weight loss:
  - ↓ calorific intake by about 600kcal/day to total of 1200–1600kcal will usually achieve target weight loss.
  - ↓ fat intake with accompanying increase in fruit and vegetables.
- Advice supported with weight management leaflets, activity and eating diaries, information on local organizations, increasing exercise.

Obese people with attendant health problems and difficulties in losing weight may be considered by GPs for drug therapies or as a last resort surgical intervention.

Further information for professionals and public

- Food Standards Agency pages on nutrition: www.food.gov.uk/
- Health Scotland Learning Centre Weight Management: www.hebs.scot.nhs.uk/Learningcentre/ obesity/intro/index.cfm
- National Obesity Forum: www.nationalobesityforum.org.uk/

Weight management: malnutrition

(See also Eating disorders ▢.)

Many factors can lead to under nutrition and/or dietary deficiencies. Factors include: socio-economic (e.g. social isolation), disabilities (e.g. osteoarthritis), physical (e.g. swallowing problems, dental problems), pathological (e.g. dementia), psychological (e.g. depression). Some conditions have specific nutritional consequences (e.g. cancer). Poor nutrition leads to muscle wasting, problems with the immune system, apathy, depression, poor wound healing, and altered drug metabolism. Older people are particularly at risk of the effects of undernutrition. Unexplained weight loss may be an early indication of cancer and should be referred for medical assessment.

Assessment

Assessment of nutritional status should include all medical, physical, psychological, and social factors, dietary intake over a few days/week plus BMI repeated over time or evidence of weight loss over time. BMI <18.5 chronic protein–energy undernutrition probable.[1] Nutritional risk factor scoring systems use BMI, plus evidence of unintentional weight loss over time e.g. over last 3mths[1] plus dietary intake in last 5d.[2] If weight and measurement not possible then assessment by checking factors such as clothes and rings becoming too loose. Height can be estimated from length of ulna.[2]

Management

- Address any problems identified in assessment e.g. ill-fitting dentures or the need for help in preparing food e.g. Meals on Wheels or to eat in company e.g. luncheon clubs.
- Advice for people with low BMIs and/or malnourishment:
  - On the components of good nutrition and healthy eating.
  - To fortify diet with more high energy/high protein foods e.g. milk, cheese, butter and eat small high energy/high protein snacks and drinks in between meals e.g. whole milk coffee, whole milk yoghurt, peanut butter sandwiches.[3]
  - On simple measures such as fresh air and exercise increase appetite.
- Monitor and refer to GP or dietician as appropriate.
- Nutritional supplements (e.g. SIP feeds) should only be considered if fortifying diet has had no effect after about 4wks.
  - Likely to benefit people with BMI <20.[1]
  - Should be chosen with consideration of nutritional profile and patient preference.
  - Typically 300–400kcal (1–2 cartons) a day can be of benefit.

---

[1] ▢ British Association for Enteral and Parenteral Nutrition, Malnutrition Advisory Group (2000). *Malnutrition Screening Tool and Advisory Notes for primary care*: www.bapen.org.uk/screening.htm
[2] ▢ British Association for Enteral and Parenteral Nutrition. *Malnutrion Universal Screening Tool*: www.bapen.org.uk/the-must.htm
[3] ▢ National Prescribing Centre (1998). MeReC *Bulletin Oral Nutrition Support* (parts 1 and 2), **9**. Available at: www.npc.co.uk

successfully sustained than exercise on an individual basis and the support from family, peers, community and health care professionals is beneficial.

Community/environmental strategies and partners for PHC team include
- Walking and cycling to work in partnership with employers.
- Preserving and encouraging use of playing fields and open spaces in partnership with LAs.
- Local walking groups including 'Walking the way to health' in partnership with voluntary organizations, local walk leaders, environmental planners, transport professionals.

Individual exercise promotion strategies should include
- Identification of patient/client's current daily/weekly activity levels as opportunities present e.g. consultation for contraception or assessment home visit.
- Routine advice giving in primary care, including written materials, on recommended levels of physical exercise and how to ↑ levels of physical activity in daily routines e.g. use the stairs, cut down on watching TV/screen time, walk faster, do household chores/garden more energetically and most days.
- The use of client-centred, individualized, action plans, based on agreed, targeted behaviour change.
- The use of exercise referral schemes to LA exercise groups (sometimes known as prescription for exercise schemes).

Older people—special considerations
- For frailer older people, strength should be built up before progressing to dynamic exercise e.g. through chair-based exercises, which some community nurses now provide following training (often through local physiotherapists or specific NVQ level courses).
- Moderate physical activity results in physical and emotional health improvements as well as modifies risks/impacts of falls (Falls prevention 🕮).
  - Training specifically in balance, strength, coordination, and reaction time leads to reduction of injurious falls (Falls prevention 🕮).
  - Weight bearing exercise, plus the above, leads to a decrease in fractures (see also Osteoporosis 🕮).

Further information and resources for health professionals and patients
🖳 BBC Keeping Fit at work: www.bbc.co.uk/bigchallenge/makeadifference/keepfitwork.shtml#seated_exercises
🖳 Health Development Agency: www.hda-online.org.uk/html/improving/physical/activity.html
🖳 NICE (2006). *Public Health Intervention Guidance No 2. Four commonly used methods to increase physical activity.* www.nice.org.uk

Smoking cessation

Smoking is the leading cause of preventable disease and death in the UK. Cigarette smoke contains 50 known carcinogens and metabolic poisons as well as nicotine. About 27% ♂ and 24% ♀ smoke but the rates are higher in people in lower social class groups, in younger people, and in vulnerable groups e.g. those with mental health problems. Nicotine is addictive and has psychological and physiological effects. There are about 120,000 smoking related UK deaths each year, most from lung cancer, COPD, coronary heart disease. Smoking reduces life expectancy—half die in middle age. Around £1500 million per year is spent by the NHS treating smoking related illness. Environmental tobacco smoke (ETS) in the home is estimated to cause over 10,000 deaths a year. ETS for children is linked to ↑ hospital admissions, SUDI (🕮), asthma (🕮), and later life COPD. Health promotion for young people is aimed at preventing them starting smoking.

Helping people stop smoking

It is an NHS priority to help smokers quit. Ceasing smoking at any age brings health benefits. About 4 million smokers try each year but only 3–6% succeed. There are smoking status recording standards for general practice in the QOF (🕮). Smokers who are helped to quit by NHS services are 4x more likely to succeed than those trying by other methods.[1] The National No Smoking Day is always the second Wednesday in March in the UK.

Brief smoking-cessation advice in primary care should include:
- Asking about smoking status at each contact, recording it (at least annually in general practice), including intention to quit.
- Giving advice of the benefits of stopping, particularly if a link can be made to the person's ill health or the effects on children, fetus etc., and provide leaflets.
- Assessing motivation to stop e.g. are you ready to give up for good?
  - If the person is not ready to quit then provide information for the future e.g. quit smoking helpline.
  - If the person is ready to quit then refer them to the local smoking cessation service (see below), and/or offer NRT prescription and stop smoking support, as below. NB Most cessation services offer specific stop smoking training for primary care professionals.

Supporting a smoker to quit
Elements include:
- Helping the smoker set a date to quit and advising them to seek support of friends and family.
- Identifying triggers to smoking e.g. alcohol, coffee, and advise the person to plan to reduce these during the first days.
- Encouraging smokers to persist as it can take 3–4 attempts to stop.

[1] 🖵 Clinical Knowledge Summaries (Clinical Knowledge Summaries (Prodigy)) Smoking Cessation: www.cks.library.nhs.uk/Portal/Index.aspx

- Breathe slowly, deeply, effortlessly.
- Working your way from your feet to your head, tense, and then relax each part of the body:
  - Starting with the feet, tense them, counting to 5 in your head, and then release the muscles and count to 5.
  - Repeat with small areas of the body, including the face until every part of the body has been tensed and released.
- Finally, tense all parts of the body, count 5, release and then remain in that position, breathing slowly and deeply for at least 5–20min.

There are many different types of guided relaxation exercises. Self-help tapes and books are available at most book stores.

Related topic
📖 Counselling skills.

Further information
📺 BBC Health self-help information on stress management: www.bbc.co.uk/health/conditions/mental_health/coping_stress.shtml
📺 Health and Safety Executive Information on workplace stress: www.hse.gov.uk/stress/
📺 Royal College of Psychiatrists Fact Sheet on Stress: www.rcpsych.ac.uk/info/index.htm

Alcohol

Sensible drinking limits are defined as:
- <21 units of alcohol a week for ♂, spread over the week and no more than 3–4 a day.
- <14 units of alcohol a week for ♀, spread over the week and no more than 2–3 a day.
- Plus 2 alcohol-free days a week.

1 unit of alcohol:
- $\frac{1}{2}$ pint of ordinary strength beer, lager, or cider
- $\frac{1}{4}$ pint of extra strength beer, lager, or cider
- 1 small glass of white (8 or 9% ABV (alcohol by volume)) wine
- $\frac{2}{3}$ small glass of red (11 or 12% ABV) wine
- 1 single measure of spirits (30 ml).

Alcohol should be avoided in pregnancy (risk of fetal alcohol sysndrome), before driving, operating machinery, swimming, working at heights, or using electrical equipment.

Harmful/hazardous drinking is associated with physical problems e.g. hypertension, cirrhosis of the liver, injuries and accidents e.g. falls/fights, mental health problems e.g. depression, social problems e.g. loss of work, family breakup, homelessness, and offending behaviours e.g. violence to others.

Promoting sensible drinking

Nurses in primary care have a wide range of opportunities to promote sensible drinking for example:
- As part of other clinic/surgery consultations e.g. for travel advice, review consultation for LTC.
- As part of specific health promoting care e.g. preconceptual or antenatal care.
- In group health promotion e.g. PSHE in schools, parenting groups.

Harmful/hazardous drinking

Harmful/hazardous drinking is defined as:
- >28 units of alcohol a week for ♂.
- >21 units of alcohol a week for ♀.

Signs and symptoms of harmful/hazardous drinking include:
- Feeling depressed
- Feeling nervous or on edge
- Having difficulty in sleeping
- Physical symptoms, e.g. gastritis
- History of accidents or injuries due to alcohol
- Poor concentration or memory
- Neglecting themselves, e.g. hygiene.

Interventions and management

Aim to help people reduce drinking at harmful levels. Strategies include:

- Give information on sensible drinking levels and risks of harmful drinking and encourage the person to consider ways of reducing this.[1]
- Encourage patient/client to keep a drinking diary and feed back to patient/client the units of alcohol s/he drinks a week.
- Discuss how and why the patient/client believes s/he benefits from drinking.
- Discuss how much drinking costs the patient/client each week.
- Discuss how to avoid situations where patient/client feels the need to drink, e.g. social situations, stressful events.
- Discuss strategies for ↓ intake, e.g. low-alcohol beer, water to quench thirst, and in between drinks, drink with food, switch to half-pints, avoid buying rounds, avoid friends who drink heavily.
- Discuss benefits of ↓ alcohol intake, e.g. sleep better, ↑ energy, ↓ lose weight, ↑ money.

Dependent drinking is when 3 of the following are present:

- Patient/client has difficulty in controlling drinking.
- There is a very strong urge to drink.
- Patient/client can drink large amounts of alcohol without feeling intoxicated.
- Drinking continues despite the harm it causes.
- Day-to-day activities are neglected due to alcohol use.
- If drinking is stopped, withdrawal symptoms, e.g. tremors, anxiety, and sweating occur.

Patients who are drinking at high levels and who are dependent drinkers need longer and more detailed interventions, determined by whether the patient/client wish to change their drinking behaviour. These patients need to be referred to the GP and/or NHS specialist alcohol services.

Related topic

📖 Substance misuse.

Further information for patients

- 🖳 Al-anon UK is for anyone effected by another persons alcohol misuse: www.al-anonuk.org.uk/index.asp
- 🖳 Alcohol Concern tips for reducing alcohol intake: www.howsyourdrink.org.uk/home.php
- 🖳 www.alcoholics-anonymous.org.uk

Helplines:
- ☎ Alcoholics Anonymous: 0845 769 7555
- ☎ National Alcohol Drinkline: 0800 917 8282

---

[1] Alcohol Concern on-line 6wk programme to help people reduce their drinking to sensible limits www.downyourdrink.org.uk/main.php

Menopause

The cessation of menstruation, usually occurs between 45 and 55yrs. Peri menopause is the time from when the ovaries start to fail, ↓ oestrogen production and symptoms experienced (see below), until 12mths after the last period. Women experience menopause in many different ways. Most experience peri-menopause over 4–5yrs, some experienced abrupt cessation. Contraception advised for 2yrs after last period if <50yrs and 1yr if >50yrs.

Premature menopause is the cessation of menstruation <45yrs. Occurs in some syndromes e.g. Turner's, and as a result of some gynaecological surgery or radiotherapy. Lack of oestrogen associated with ↑ risk osteoporisis, cardiovascular disease. Premature menopause may be treated with HRT (see below).

Signs and symptoms

- Hot flushes and night sweats experienced by about 80% of women.
- Menstruation changes: cycle may shorten or lengthen to many months. Often increases in menstrual loss.
- Thinning of the skin, brittle nails, hair loss, headaches, and generalized aches and pains.
- Urinary symptoms, stress urinary incontinence (📖) and recurrent lower UTI common.
- Vaginal discomfort and dryness, leading to dyspareunia (Sexual problems 📖).

In addition some women may experience a range of emotional changes but mostly related to other life events and not a sequalae of menopause. Some mood changes such as irritability and difficulties in concentration may be a result of disturbed sleep through night sweats. Loss of libido may occur but non-hormonal factors such as conflict between partners, inadequate stimulation, depression, and life stresses are usually main contributors.

Consequences of the menopause

- Many women experience the end of menstruation as very liberating.
- Reduction in oestrogen causes ↑ risk of osteoporosis, urogenital atrophy, cardiovascular disease, and CVA. Increase weight, at or around menopause, to central abdomen area is an additional risk factor for cardiovascular disease.

General advice
- Osteoporosis prevention (Falls prevention 📖).
- ↓ cardio vascular risk through exercise (📖), nutrition and healthy eating (📖), weight management (📖), smoking cessation (📖).
- Pelvic floor exercises (Urinary incontinence in women 📖).
- Stress management through ↑ exercise and relaxation techniques (Managing stress 📖).

Managing symptoms

Many women experience very mild symptoms and manage them easily. About 40% experience symptoms that are distressing at some point.

Hot flushes and night sweats

- May be helped by ↑ exercise, ↓ stress, avoiding triggers such as caffeine, smoking, alcohol.
- Managed through lighter clothing, wearing layers, sleeping in cooler room etc.
- HRT (see below).
- Herbal therapies e.g. red clover, black cohosh, isoflavines, soya products used by many women to some benefit but research evidence is inconclusive (see British Menopause Society Fact Sheets[1]).

Urinary symptoms (Urinary incontinence in women 📖). HRT may also help with recurrent UTI.

Vaginal dryness. Helped with lubricants. Short-term topical oestrogens (BNF 7.2.1) may be required. Use limited to 3–6mth. NB Some damage condoms and diaphragms (Barrier methods 📖).

Hormone replacement therapy (HRT)

HRT provides oestrogen (and progesterone in women with a uterus or premature menopause). HRT ↑ risk of DVT, breast cancer, and endometrial cancer (see British Menopause Society consensus statement[1]). HRT only indicated for short-term use for alleviating symptoms (as above). Long-term HRT use advised only with premature menopause or hysterectomy before menopause. HRT not advised as preventative to cardiovascular disease or osteoporosis. Choice of HRT preparation according to symptoms, medical history, and preferences (BNF 6.4.1.1).

Key principles in use of HRT

Start with lowest dosage, review after 3mths for side effects and improvements. Side effects may be oestrogen related e.g. headaches, fluid retention, or progesterone related e.g. bloating, headache, depression. Side effects may be alleviated by change of preparation. Bleeding may be erratic for first 1–2mths and spotting may occur up to 12mths with combined preparations. Reviewed every 6–12mths including BP, weight, bleeding pattern, and symptoms.

Stopping HRT

- Can be withdrawn once menopause symptoms no longer a problem. Trial withdrawals after 1–2yrs of use. Warn women symptoms may reappear. Some experts advise a staged withdrawal. Clinical Knowledge Summaries (Clinical Knowledge Summaries (Prodigy))[2] provides suggested regimens.
- In premature menopause HRT continued to about 50yrs.

Further information and support for patients

📓 The Menopause Amarant Trust: www.amarantmenopausetrust.org.uk

[1] 📓 British Menopause Society www.the-bms.org for fact sheets
[2] 📓 Clinical Knowledge Summaries (Clinical Knowledge Summaries (Prodigy)) menopause guidance www.cks.library.nhs.uk/Portal/Index.aspx

Healthy ageing

1 in 5 people >65yrs in the UK with estimates that by 2025, 1 in 3 of the population will be >65yrs.[1] However, older people are not homogeneous. Health means different things to different people and may include: ability to lead an active life, ability to get out, independence, financial security. It is important to recognize that:

• Infirmity is *not* inevitable, but disability, dependency, accidents, death, and mental health problems are more common with older people.
• Chronic disease and disability in older people is related to social class. Life expectancy at 65yrs is 2.5yrs greater in social classes I and II than IV and V.[1] Chronological age is therefore less appropriate than class as an indicator of potential illness and disability.

Work and retirement

The traditional view of retirement as 'non-work' is challenged by the concept of the 'third age' as one of productivity, creativity, and contribution to community. Changes in occupational and pension schemes mean people are working in paid employment at older ages. Many employers organize pre-retirement courses including information on: financial management, getting the best from the NHS, skills training/retraining, and how to cope with change.

Health promotion

Many potential problems which can accompany ageing are amenable to a preventive approach (e.g. falls, grief and loss, depression see below). NB Ageism in public services may mean that older people are not offered access to screening or health promotion. Health promotion interventions should be addressed at individual and community/environmental levels (Models and approaches to health promotion 📖).

Community/environmental interventions are important as healthy lifestyles information is insufficient if issues such as access to local healthy food, transport, housing, carer support, tackling crime and improving the environment (e.g. street lighting, pavements) are not addressed.

Specific topics for health promotion include

• *Smoking*: older people and health professionals tend to take a fatalistic approach, but smoking cessation (📖) is effective for all ages.
• *Diet and nutrition*: older people are at risk of poor nutrition due to disease, drugs, social circumstances, income, and cognitive impairment. Healthy eating programmes and lunch clubs also provide social interaction. Alcohol is related to depression and suicide. Safe drinking levels should be emphasized.
• *Activity*: inactivity is strongly associated with falls. Falls prevention programmes (Falls prevention 📖) and exercise referral schemes (Exercise 📖) are beneficial.

---

1 📖 National Statistics Office: www.statistics.org.uk

Life course issues related to age can mean older people are more vulnerable and would benefit from statutory and informal services to support them through times of adjustment. Health professionals should be aware of particular issues including:

- Emotional and mental health:
  - Grief and loss. Older people may experience multiple losses: spouse/partner, family, friends, also loss of independence and autonomy, mobility, social connections, dignity, privacy, confidence and self-esteem (Bereavement, and coping with loss grief 📖).
  - Depressive illness. Depression is the commonest mental health problem of old age, often due to bereavement and changing life events such as retirement (People with depression 📖).
- Physical health:
  - Hearing. About 1 in 3 people >65yrs have a hearing impairment (Deafness 📖).
  - Vision. Presbyopia (blurring of close vision) is a feature of ageing experienced by 90% of >65yrs (Partial sight and blindness 📖).
  - Respiratory function. Physiological deterioration in lungs due to the ageing process (Asthma 📖, COPD 📖).
  - Cardiovascular disease and hypertension problems are more likley (Hypertension 📖).
  - Musculo-skeletal system. Reduced bone density may lead to Osteoporosis (📖) while wear and tear on large weight-bearing joints may lead to Osteoarthritis (📖).

SPICE[2] is a mnemonic for remembering the 5 aspects of older people's health that can be addressed but are often overlooked. It is particularly useful in general practice or clinic consultations:

- **S**enses (hearing and vision)
- **P**hysical activity
- **I**ncontinence
- **C**ognition
- **E**motions.

Related topic

📖 Individual health needs assessment.

Further Information for health professionals and the public

📖 Age Concern (England): www.ace.org.uk Includes Ageing Well UK and ActivAge Unit a health promotion initiative

📖 Department of Work and Pensions (2004) Link-Age: developing networks of services for older people: www.dwp.gov.uk/publications/dwp/2004/linkage/link_agepdf

---

[2] Iliffe, S. et al. (2004). A short instrument to identify common unmet needs in older people in general practice. *British Journal of General Practice* **54** 914–18.

Falls prevention

A fall is an unintentional event that results in a person coming to rest on the ground or another lower level. While accident prevention is a public health issue for all ages, falls and their sequalae are a particular issue for older people. Over 30% people >65yrs have a fall in any one year. Falls are a major cause of disability and the leading cause of mortality due to injury in people 75yrs+ in UK[1]. 75% of falls related deaths occur in the home. Falls are under-reported to health professionals.

Consequences

Falls ↑ the likelihood of osteoporotic hip fracture, thought to be responsible for up to 14,000 deaths year in the UK, accounting for about £1.7 billion NHS spending. Other consequences include: other fractures (e.g. Colles), loss of confidence, restriction of activities. The inability to get up after a fall can result in hypothermia, pneumonia, dehydration, and pressure sores.

Risk factors

Can be divided into physical, environmental, iatrogenic. NB There is often no one clear cause.
- Physical:
    - Age >75y, ♀
    - Orthostatic hypotension
    - Cognitive impairment, depression
    - Parkinson's disease, CVA, balance disorders, acute illness, visual impairment
    - Urinary urgency
    - Inability to rise from chair of knee height without use of arms
    - ↓ mobility, lower limb weakness, foot problems
    - History of fall in previous year/fear of falling
- Environmental factors:
    - In the home e.g. bed or chair too low, poor lighting, loose rugs
    - Outside the home e.g. ice on pavement, uneven pavements.
- Iatrogenic:
    - 4+ medications per day
    - Antihypertensives, sedatives, diuretics.

Key policy interventions

Public health strategies to identify, assess and prevent those at risk of falling exist in each PCO. Strategies also link to activity promotion (Exercise 📖). Most PCOs have developed an integrated falls services (see below). Most PCOs use clinical guidelines on assessment and prevention of falls, case/risk identification, risk assessment and interventions (e.g. NICE guidelines see below). Many have a falls prevention service.

---

[1] NICE (2004) *Clinical Guideline 21: the assessment and prevention of falls in older people.* www.nice.org.uk/CGO2NICEEguideline

Falls prevention services

Usually has a named falls prevention coordinator (e.g. clinical nurse specialist) who coordinates information systems, involvement of older people and carers, education for health professionals, and inter-disciplinary and interagency collaborative programmes. A Falls Prevention Service promotes:

- The identification of people at risk through:
  - The promotion of asking older people whether they have experienced falls at each contact with health and, social services, ambulance services, independent sector or voluntary groups.
  - Promoting the comprehensive assessment of people, who report falling, against the risks reported above (also see NICE guidelines below).
- Multi factorial interventions of:
  - Strength and balance retraining programmes by trained professional (Exercise 📖).
  - Home hazard assessment and modification programmes.
  - Personal, body-worn alarm systems.
  - Optician assessment of vision and correction of visual impairment.
  - Medication review.
  - Education and information provision.

Related topic

📖 Osteoporosis.

Key reading

Gillespie, LD., Gillespie, WJ, Robertson, MC, *et al.* (2003) Interventions for preventing falls in older people. *Cochrane Database of Systematic Reviews, Cochrane Library*, issue 4.

Further information and resources for professionals

📖 Help The Aged: Dedicated section on falls for practitioners: www.helptheaged.org/Health/HealthyAgeing/Falls/_practitioners.htm

📖 *How can we help older people not fall again? Implementing the Older People's NSF falls standard (2003)*: Includes a workbook of ideas for making the case for investing in falls and fracture prevention www.dh.gov.uk/assetRoot/04/07/85/44/04078544.pdf

Weather extremes

Heat waves

Even during relatively mild heat waves death rates are significantly but avoidably raised in the UK. In extreme hot weather there is a risk of developing dehydration leading to **heat exhaustion**:

- Symptoms include headaches, dizziness, nausea and vomiting, muscle weakness or cramps, pallor, high temperature.
- Treatment includes move somewhere cooler, cool down in water or shower or sponge down, rest and drink lots of water.

Untreated heat exhaustion leads to heatstroke

Symptoms include intense headaches, nausea, intense thirst, sleepiness, hot, red and dry skin, sudden rise in temperature, confusion, aggression, convulsions and loss of consciousness. Requires urgent medical attention. Can result in organ failure, brain damage, or death.

Groups at particular risk

- >over 75yrs old and/or living on their own, or in a care home
- People suffering from mental ill health, or with dementia
- People who are bed bound
- People with serious chronic heart or respiratory conditions
- Babies and young children, especially <4yrs.

Each country has a heat watch system for high day and night temperatures in June–September. Each PCO has to plan with social services to identify individuals vulnerable to heatstroke, especially >75yrs, and actions to support them if a heat wave alert is issued by central government.

Prevention advice if a heat wave is forecast

- Keep out of the heat:
  - Especially in the hottest part of the day 11am–1pm.
  - If have to go out stay in the shade, wear a hat, carry water.
- Keep cool:
  - Stay inside in the coolest room as much as possible.
  - Close curtains in rooms that get sun, keep windows closed while the room is cooler than outside, open windows when temperature rises above outside and at night.
  - Take frequent cool baths, showers or splash water over face, neck.
- Drink regular fluids—water or fruit juice best, avoid tea coffee, alcohol, eat cool foods.
- Be alert to signs of heat exhaustion and act as above, seek help if concerned.

Cold weather

Hypothermia occurs when body temperature <35°C (95°F). Caused by exposure to cold environment and an inability to maintain body temperature. When body energy resources drained trying to cope with low temperature then hypothermia becomes life threatening. Those at risk include:

- Babies who cannot regulate their body temperature.
- People exposed to extreme weather conditions or cold water.

- Older people, especially if they are not very active, or have other illnesses.
- People with dementias may not be able to tell when they are cold.
- People with reduced mobility or health conditions that change the body's ability to respond to temperature changes.

Symptoms
- Mild includes shivering (person can still stop shivering), feeling cold, low energy, red skin. Treated by moving to warmer place, additional or dry clothing especially for head and torso, warm drinks and carbohydrates, activity.
- Moderate includes violent, uncontrollable shivering, confusion, memory loss, difficulty moving around or stumbling, drowsiness, slurred speech, listlessness and indifference, slow, shallow breathing and weak pulse. Requires urgent medical attention in hospital.
- Severe includes loss of control of hands, feet, and limbs, shivering stops, unconsciousness, shallow or no breathing, weak, irregular or no pulse, stiff muscles, and dilated pupils. Requires urgent medical attention in hospital.

Action
In mild cases as above. In moderate or severe cases while waiting for assistance preserve body heat and prevent any more being lost e.g. additional layers especially for head and torso (change out of wet clothing), warm drinks if conscious (not alcohol), don't apply heat to limbs (as forces cold blood back to main organs), don't massage or rub (may cause heart attack in severe cases).

Prevention advice
- Maintain body warmth through activity, eating well, including warm food and drinks, dressing in layers to trap heat and covering head.
- Keeping home heated or at least one room and use that for all activities. Use thermometer to check room is between 16°C and 20°C. Government support for heating costs for people on low incomes, disabled and older people (Benefits for disability and illness 💷).
  See also 💷 Homes and housing.

All PCOs and social services have to collaborate on identifying individuals vulnerable to hypothermia in cold weather and plan to ensure support is given, particularly for extreme weather conditions.

Further information

Each central country's central health department web pages for heat wave plans (Useful websites 💷)

💷 National Energy Action: www.nea.org.uk/Campaigns/Keep_Warm_Keep_Well

Skin cancer prevention

Skin cancer, including non-melanoma skin cancer (NMSC) and malignant melanoma, (MM) is the most commonly diagnosed cancer in the UK (Skin cancer prevention 📖). Around 80% of MM are 2° to exposure to sunlight or artificial ultraviolet (UV) light. UV rays from the sun classified into: UVA and UVB. Majority of UV radiation is UVA. UV light is natural in sunlight, or artificial e.g. sunbeds. UV penetrates cloud, water and UVA penetrates glass, sand, snow, concrete.

❶ Most skin cancers are preventable.

Risk factors

- UV radiation is most intense between 11am–3pm British Summer Time (BST) or 10am–2pm Greenwich Mean Time (GMT).
- Burning from over exposure to UV light, doubles the risk of MM, regardless of age.
- Repeated intense exposure to UV light ↑ risk of development of MM.
- UV damage to skin in the first 15yrs linked to risk of MM in later life.
- Those with naturally fair skin are at ↑ risk of DNA damage.
- Those with fair skin which burns and freckles easily and light eye colour, red or fair hair.
- Large number of moles, >50.
- Family history of skin cancer.

Prevention

Most effective preventative measure is to stay out of direct sunlight and protect skin from UV damage. Health promotion advice includes:

- A tan only offers the equivalent protection to a sunscreen with sun protection factor (SPF) 3.
- In the first 18yrs regular sunscreen use can significantly ↓ risk of NMSC.
- Sun **Smart** code (Cancer Research UK):
  - **S**tay in the shade 11am–3pm.
  - **M**ake sure you never burn.
  - **A**lways cover up: ↑ protection increased by dark coloured, close woven, dry (wet fabrics allow more UV through), wide brim wide hats, wrap around sunglasses (British Standard 2427, or marked with CE mark or a UV 400 label protect vulnerable eyes).
  - **R**emember to take extra care of children.
  - **T**hen use factor 15+ sunscreen (see below).
- Also report mole changes or unusual skin growths promptly to the GP.

The Solar UV index indicates the strength of UV. It is shown in weather reports as a number in a triangle. The level of danger depends on skin type i.e. fair burns, fair tans, brown, black (see Table 8.2). UV Index 10 means high levels of UV and advice for people of all skin types is to try to stay in the shade. Daily UV ratings are on UK Government Meterological Office (see below).

Index	Fair, burns	Fair, tans	Brown	Black
1 2	Low	Low	Low	Low
3 4	Medium	Low	Low	Low
5	High	Medium	Low	Low
6	Very high	Medium	Medium	Low
7	Very high	High	Medium	Medium
8	Very high	High	Medium	Medium
9	Very high	High	Medium	Medium
10	Very high	High	High	Medium

Table 8.2 Meterological Office Solar UV Index (reproduced with permission from the UK Meteorological office)

Sunscreens

Sunscreens with a SPF of 15+ filters 93% of UVB. ❶ Sunscreens should not be used to ↑ time in the sun. No sunscreen has 100% protection.
- Choice of sunscreen should include:
  - With an SPF of 15+. Labelled 'broad spectrum'—to protect against UVA and UVB.
  - Water resistant, to prevent being washed or sweated off.
  - With a valid 'use by' date. Most sunscreens have a shelf life of 2–3yrs. Expensive sunscreens are not more effective than cheaper ones.
- Advice on application of sunscreen:
  - Apply 15–30min before going out in the sun and reapply every 2hrs or more frequently if washed/rubbed off.

Signs of skin cancer

Advise people to know what their skin normally looks like by looking regularly in a full-length mirror. ❶ The following abnormalities and changes should be referred to the GP for further investigation.
- *Changes of non melanoma skin cancer:* occurs mainly in older people, often on head, neck, and/or hands:

- A new growth or sore that does not heal within 4wks.
- A spot or sore that continues to itch, hurt, crust, scab, or bleed.
- Persistent skin ulcers that are not explained by other causes.
- *Signs of abnormality of malignant melanoma:*
  - Moles which are asymmetrical or have blurred or jagged edges.
  - Moles that have changed colour, or with multiple colours in them.
  - Moles which are new, growing, or bigger than other moles.
  - Moles which are raised and/or have an uneven surface.
  - Moles which are bleeding, oozing, crusting, itchy, or painful.

Related topic

📖 Skin cancer prevention.

Further information

🖥 Cancer Research UK SunSmart: www.cancerresearchuk.org/sunsmart/
🖥 UK Meteorological Office UV information: www.metoffice.com
🖥 WHO (2002). *A global solar UV Index: a practical guide*. WHO, Geneva. www.who.int/uv/ publications

Early signs of cancer

Key advice for prevention against cancer is summarized in the Europe against cancer code:[1]

- Do not smoke/smoke in the presence of non-smokers (Smoking cessation 📖).
- Avoid obesity (Weight management: overweight, obesity 📖).
- Undertake brisk physical activity each day (Exercise 📖).
- ↑ daily intake and variety of fruit and vegetables to at least 5 portions daily and ↓ foods containing animal fats (Nutrition and healthy eating 📖).
- Moderate alcohol consumption (Alcohol 📖).
- Avoid excessive exposure to sunlight especially children, adolescents, and those with tendency to burn (Skin cancer prevention 📖).
- Adhere to safety regulations about exposure to known carcinogens.

Early signs of cancer

Many cancers are easier to treat and cure if found early, with ↑ likelihood of longer life expectancy and better quality of life both during and post treatment. Cancer is not just 1 disease, there are at least 200 different types, therefore there is a wide range of possible symptoms which may or may not be early symptoms of cancer.

Health promotion on early signs of cancer

Signs and symptoms to consult a medical professional about:

- *Ongoing chest or throat problems:* coughing or hoarseness that lasts >3wks, haemoptysis.
- *Changes in bowel function:* unexplained changes in bowel movements, such as chronic constipation, diarrhoea, or a change in the size of the stool, which last for >6wks. Blood in the stool, melaena, occult blood, frank blood.
- *Changes in bladder function:* dysuria, heamaturia, or unexplained changes in micturition.
- *Unexplained intermenstrual bleeding or discharge.*
- *Skin changes:* skin changes can occur in internal cancers as well skin cancers. These can include: hyperpigmentation, erythema, pruritus, hirsutism, and ulceration.
- *Changes in skin moles:* changes in colour, shape or sensation i.e. pain or itching; bleeding or crusting; moles which have multiple colours in them, moles with irregular edges; moles which are new or growing; moles which are raised and/or have an uneven surface (Skin cancer 📖).
- *Lumps, or thickening that does not go away.*
- *Ongoing indigestion or swallowing problems.*
- *Unexplained fatigue.*
- *Unexplained pain.*
- *Unexplained weight loss.*

Related topic

📖 UK screening programmes.

---

1 📖 The European Code Against Cancer (third version 2003). www.cancercode.org/code.htm

Further information for professionals

- Macmillan Cancer Relief: www.macmillan.org.uk/cancerinformation/disppage.asp?id=127
- NHS Cancer Screening Programmes website for more information on national cancer screening programmes: www.cancerscreening.nhs.uk

Breast awareness and cancer prevention

Breast awareness in UK, focus on ↑ self-awareness of breast changes, rather than just routine self-examination for lumps. 2° prevention is by breast screening by mammography (see below) and clinical breast examination. The rationale for the promotion of breast awareness:

- Approximately 90% of breast cancers are detected by women themselves or their partners.
- Early detection of cancer equates to increased chances of survival.

Teaching breast awareness

Primary care workers are a key information source for women. The most effective methods of promoting breast awareness are: provision of verbal and written information; demonstration and return demonstration on the woman's own breast; and feedback to the woman regarding her own ability.

Women should practice breast awareness from the age of 18yrs onwards as part of overall bodily awareness. The Breast Awareness Five Point Plan:

1. *Know what is normal for you:*
   - During activities e.g. bathing, showering, and dressing become aware of the normal state of the breasts.
   - Understand the anatomy and physiology of the breast and what to expect at different life stages. Breasts are glandular sensitive to the presence of oestrogen and progesterone. In pre-menopausal ♀, and ♀ taking HRT, normal breasts feel different at different times of the month. Post-menopausal women breasts may become softer, and less lumpy.

2. *Look and feel:*
   - Look: stand in front of the mirror, undressed to the waist, and raise the arms above the head and drop them to the sides. Then place the hands on the hips and clench the chest muscles.
   - Look at the outline and rise and fall of each breast.
   - Feel: the breast is pear shaped and extends into the armpit, richly supplied by lymph nodes so ensure whole breast and surrounding area is felt, including into the armpit, the nipple, the clavicle, and the sternum.
   - Feel: use the pads of the fingers which are more sensitive and accurate at detecting change than the finger tips.
   - Feel for: lumps, thickening or bumpy areas in one breast or armpit which seem to be different from the same part of the other breast and armpit.
   - Feel for: discomfort or pain in one breast that is different from normal, particularly if new and persistent.

3. *Know what changes to look for:*
   - Change in the outline or shape of the breast.
   - Skin puckering or dimpling anywhere on the breast including underneath the breast.

- Changes in the nipple: position, shape, discharge.
- Nipple rash (on or around the nipple), or bleeding or moist reddish areas that don't heal easily.
- Veins that are more prominent than normal.

4. Report any changes without delay.
5. Attend for breast screening if aged 50yrs or over.

Mammography screening

Mammography is part of the UK screening programme (□) offered every 3yrs for ♀ aged 50–70yrs. It detects 85% of breast cancers in women aged >50yrs (60% of which are impalpable). Women have a good prognosis in 70–80% of cancers detected by screening. Screening more regularly does not improve outcomes.

Related topics

□ Menopause; □ Breast problems; □ Breast cancer.

Further information for women

- BBC Health: www.bbc.co.uk/health/womens_health/body_breast1.shtml
- NHS direct have an online self assessment and advice page that women can complete: www.nhsdirect.nhs.uk/SelfHelp/symptoms/breastchanges/start.asp

Further information for health care professionals

- Breast Screening Resource Pack for Training Primary Care Nurses (NHSBSP 2003): www.cancerscreening.nhs.uk/breastscreen/publications/nhsbsp39.pdf ☎ DH publication order-line: 08701 555 455, Fax: 01623 724 524, Email orders: doh@prolog.uk.com
- Guidelines for Referral of Patients with Breast Problems (National Health Service Breast Screening Programme (2003)): www.cancerscreening.nhs.uk/breastscreen/publications/pc-rgfw-01.pdf

Testicular self-examination (TSE)

Aim of TSE is the early detection of any changes from normal that may indicate testicular cancer. There is no effective method of primary prevention for testicular cancer. TSE is method of 2° prevention. TSE is part of overall body awareness, to familiarize a man with the normal size, shape, and weight of his testicles and the area around the scrotum. The majority of testicular cancers are first detected by men themselves. Testicular cancer responds extremely well to treatment with a cure rate of 95% for testicular cancer which is detected early. Most of the testicular cancer deaths in UK occur in males aged 30–50yrs of age.[1]

Risk factors for testicular cancer
- More common in white Caucasian men
- Relationship to social class: ↑ with higher social class
- Risk ↑ in men with cryptorchidism (undescended testis). Risk is ↓ if the testicle is repositioned by the age of 10yrs[1]
- Previous testicular cancer
- Klinefelter's syndrome
- HIV +ve status.

Teaching TSE

Primary health care professionals are a key sources of information for men. Barriers to performing TSE are embarrassment, ignorance, and lack of confidence in the ability to perform TSE. TSE instruction is usually necessary. Testicular models are available which help in demonstrating the technique, although men can also be provided with written illustrated literature (see below).

TSE guidelines

The easiest time for men to self examine is after a bath or a shower, when the scrotal skin is relaxed.

1. Know what is normal:
- Hold the scrotum in the palm of the hand and feel testicles' size and weight. It is usual for one testicle to be larger than the other, or one that hangs lower.
- Feel each testicle and roll it between a thumb and finger. It should feel smooth. The soft, tender tube toward the back of each testicle is normal (i.e. the epididymis).

2. Know what changes to look for:
- A lump or swelling in part of the testicle, NB most are not cancer. The lump may be small and hard (pea sized) although it may be much larger.
- A dull ache in the testicle and/or lower abdomen. NB there may be no pain.
- A heavy feeling in the scrotum.

3. Report any changes without delay.

---

1 ▣ Cancer Research UK 2005. www.cancerresearchuk.org

Related topics
📖 Health promotion in schools; 📖 Sexual health: general issues.

Further information for men
📓 Cancer Research UK leaflets: www.cancerresearchuk.org/images/11632/leaflet_testicular.pdf
http://info.cancerresearchuk.org/images/publicationspdfs/leaflet_testicular.pdf
📓 Royal Marsden Hospital Patient Information: www.royalmarsden.nhs.uk/patientinfo/booklets/
testicular_cancer/testicular4.asp
📓 Young people website: www.soyouwanna.com/site/syws/testexam/testexamFULL.html

UK screening programmes

There are internationally agreed criteria for appraising the viability, effectiveness, and appropriateness of screening before a condition screening programme is initiated[1]. These include:

- The condition is an important health problem
- Its natural history is well understood
- It is recognizable at an early stage
- Treatment is better at an early stage
- A suitable test exists
- An acceptable test exists
- Adequate facilities exist to cope with abnormalities detected
- Screening is done at repeated intervals when the onset is insidious
- The chance of harm is less than the chance of benefit
- The cost is balanced against benefit.

Each country has a committee which appraises the evidence and advises the central health department on implementation of screening programmes. It also lists conditions which are not recommended for screening because insufficient evidence exists or evidence that screening does more harm than good (and provides links to reasons for decisions). Examples of conditions not recommended for routine screening are diabetes, depression, prostate cancer, domestic violence, speech and language delay in children.

Current national screening programmes

- Cancer:
  - Breast (Breast awareness and cancer prevention 📖).
  - Cervical (Cervical cancer screening 📖).
  - Bowel cancer screening is to be phased in in England from late 2006 for men and women aged 60–69, every 2yrs, using faecal occult blood tests sent direct by the individual to laboratory for analysis.
- Cardiovascular screening. Currently pilots being undertaken in high-risk communities to determine the benefits of screening.
- Antenatal (Antenatal care and screening 📖) and newborn (Child screening tests 📖).
- Sexually transmitted diseases.
  - See 📖 Antenatal care and screening.
  - Chlamydia (Sexually transmitted infections 📖).
- Child health (Child screening tests 📖).

Further information

- 🖳 Conditions which should not be screened for in whole populations: www.screening.nhs.uk/noscreen/index.htm
- 🖳 UK NHS cancer screening programmes: www.cancerscreening.nhs.uk/index.html
- 🖳 NHS electronic specialist library on screening: www.library.nhs.uk/screening/

---

[1] 🖳 UK National Screening Committee www.screening.nhs.uk/home.htm

Cervical cancer screening

Cervical cancer accounts for 2% of all female cancers. Diagnosed in 9.3 per 100,000 women. ↑ Risk with some types of HPV, multiple partners, smoking. Very low risk if never had penetrative vaginal sex. Screening by smear test reduces a woman's chance of developing cervical cancer by 80–90%. There is a national call and recall system for women registered with a GP.

Screening
Frequency: first invitation at 25yrs; 3-yearly between 25–49yrs; 5-yearly 50–64yrs,. At 65+ only those are screened who have not been screened since age 50 or have had recent abnormal tests; ♀ 65+ who have had 3 consecutive negative smears are taken out of the call–recall system.

Cervical cell sampling
Currently done by a smear test (Cervical smear taking 🕮) but liquid-based cytology (LBC) is being introduced to ↓ inadequate smear rate. LBC uses a special device to collect the cells, which is broken off or rinsed into a small vial with preservative fluid.

Quality assurance
Each PCT, general practice, and community clinic has a named co-ordinator responsible for ensuring the service meets the national quality Cervical Cancer Screening Programme (see website below) standards, including:
- Providing information to allow eligible women to make an informed decision about the screening.
- Adequately train and equip all staff performing the test.
- Ensure results are appropriately followed up (see Table 8.3) and recorded.
- Ensure regular auditing of smear taking and all aspects of the programme.

Cervical screening is an additional service in the nGMS contract (General practice 🕮) and specified in the QOF (🕮).

Smear results
Smear results are sent to the woman either by her GP or the clinic where the smear was taken. Table 8.3 describes the action taken on different results.

Table 8.3 Cervical cancer screening results and action

Smear result	Action
Inadequate (10%)	Repeat smear in 3mths. If 3 inadequate in a row then refered for colposcopy
Negative (93%)	Routine recall as per national programme
Normal plus candida, trichomonas, or herpes	Routine recall plus treatment as indicated (see Sexually transmitted infections 📖)
Actinomyces-like organisms (ALO)	Common in presence of IUCD. Clinical examination then possible treatment and change of IUCD. Repeat smear 3mths later (see Interuterine devices and systems 📖)
Atrophic cells	Common in peri/post menopausal women. No action (see Menopause 📖)
Borderline changes <4%	Repeat in 3–6mths. If recurs, referred for colposcopy according to local care pathways
Mild dyskaryosis (outer third epithelium abnormal = CIN1)	Repeat in 3–6mths. If recurs refer for colposcopy according to local care pathways
Moderate dyskaryosis (half to two-thirds epithelium abnormal = CIN2)	Referred for colposcopy according to local care pathways
Severe dyskaryosis (full-thickness epithelium abnormal/ carcinoma *in situ*)	Referred for urgent colposcopy/gynaecological opinion (see Gynaecological cancers 📖)

Related topics

📖 Sexual health: general issues; 📖 Sexually transmitted infections; 📖 Gynaecological cancers.

Patient information

Leaflets are available from the NHS screening programme (below), including those for women with learning disabilities and other languages.

Further information

📖 National Cervical Cancer Screening Programme: www.cancerscreening.nhs.uk/cervical

Cervical smear taking

See also 📖 Cervical cancer screening.

This procedure will be replaced by LBC over the next few years.

Timing

Optimum time is mid-cyle between days 10 and 16. Avoid days immediately before and after menstruation.

Patient comfort

Aim to minimize embarrassment, anxiety, and discomfort. A sensitive approach is required to ensure women continue in the programme for subsequent smears.
- Explain the procedure before and during
- Offer the opportunity to empty bladder before
- Offer a chaperone (Chaperones 📖)
- Ensure privacy in the examination room
- Use modesty paper sheet while on the couch
- Offer tissues after procedure
- Offer an opportunity to ask questions after.

Protection against infection

Ensure PPE is used to minimize exposure to blood borne viruses. If centrally supplied sterilized equipment is not available, ensure all equipment is sterilized after use (Cleaning, disinfection, and sterilization of equipment 📖).

Request form

The national request form HMR101 is used although there may be some local variations. Ensure that patient contact details and GP address are correct. Results are sent to the GP (and community clinic if the sample was taken there), who is responsible for ensuring that the woman receives the results.

Smear taking

- Cells must be taken from the area where columnar cells change to squamous cells (known as the transformation zone TZ), which is usually in the cervical canal.
- Use a warm speculum to keep the vaginal walls apart and visualize the cervical os.
- Do not use oil-based lubricants, as they may affect the smear reading.
- Coughing or bearing down by the woman helps move the cervix into view.
- A Winterton speculum may be helpful when the cervix is very posterior, as may the woman pressing on her lower abdomen.
- Insert the extended tip of the spatula (Aylesbury) into the canal, turning 360° × 2. A cyto-brush can be used in addition.
- Sometimes the lining of the cervical canal turns outwards, so the TZ is over the lip of the cervix, known as ectopy. This is common if the COC pill is used, or the woman is multiparous or pregnant.

- If ectopy is seen, use the rounded end of the spatula in addition to sample peripherally.
- If an IUCD is *in situ*, the 360° sweep starts and ends at the thread position, gently moving it aside.
- Record clinical observations of the cervix, such as contact bleeding, on the request form.
- Take additional bacterial and viral swabs if indicated clinically.

The glass slide

- Use a pencil to label the slide
- Smear cells along the length of the slide as soon as the sample is taken
- Cover gently with about 1ml of fixative immediately
- Leave to dry flat for 10min
- Do not flood the slide, tilt, or shake off excess fluid.

The slide should be placed in a plastic slide container. This should be sealed in a bag with the request form and sent to the laboratory.

Related topics

📖 Sexual health: general issues; 📖 Sexually transmitted infections.

Information for women

📖 Women's Health: www.womenshealthlondon.org.uk/leaflets/cervical/cervical.html

Further information

📖 UK National Cervical Cancer Screening Programme: www.cancerscreening.nhs.uk/cervical

New patient health check

GP practices offer new patient (i.e. new registration to the practice) checks, and each practice decides its own protocols. Good practice suggests a new patient check should be offered within 6mths of registration with the practice. The aim is to reduce the incidence of preventable conditions, to encourage good health in the practice population and record any relevant QOF (📖) indicators.

NB Ideally practices should offer a routine health check to all patients aged 16–75yrs who have not been seen by a health professional in the last 3yrs and to all patients >75yrs who have not been seen in the last year.

Suggested elements of the new patient health check

- Review current and past illnesses and operations.
- Identify FH of illnesses with particular reference to diabetes, CHD, stroke, hypertension, cancers, and other significant problems.
- Check and record current medications, OTC medications, and allergies. Refer to GP regarding medication requirements.
- Check any screening tests are up-to-date e.g. cervical smear, mammography, and advise or offer an appointment as appropriate.
- Check immunization status and offer as appropriate (Targeted immunization in adults 📖).
- Check and record smoking status and offer smoking cessation (📖) advice.
- Measure weight, height for BMI calculation, and waist circumference. Offer as appropriate weight management (📖), exercise advice (📖).
- Review alcohol units/wk and possible advice or intervention required (Alcohol 📖).
- Undertake urinalysis.
- Measure BP. All adults should have their BP measured at least every 5yrs (QOF 📖). Optimal BP in adults is <120/80, normal BP is <130/85, high normal is 130–139/85–89.[1]
- Measuring BP:
  - In both arms, arm with the highest value should be used for BP monitoring.
  - Use appropriate size cuff i.e. bladder encircles at least 80% upper arm and arm must be supported at heart level.
  - Korotkoff phase I and phase V sounds used for systolic BP and diastolic BP respectively.
  - At least 2 measurements 1–2min apart taken on each BP check.

NB Hypertension is sustained BP>140/90 on 3 or more occasions (Hypertension 📖). Lifestyle advice for high normal BP and reassess yearly.

- Offer other healthy life style advice e.g. nutrition and healthy eating (📖) exercise as appropropriate.
- Arrange appointments with appropriate health-care professional if additional intervention necessary.

Related topics

📖 Healthy ageing; 📖 General practice nursing.

1 British Hypertension Guidelines 2004. 🖳 www.bhsoc.org

Targeted immunizations in adults

Flu immunization programme

Flu immunization provides 70–80% protection against influenza and lasts ~1yr. Antibody levels reach protective level 10–14d post vaccination September–early November is ideal time for vaccination. Most general practices identify target recommended groups, invite them to flu vaccination sessions or ensure home visits (often by district nursing service) for housebound patients. Flu immunization is an enhanced service under nGMS contract (see General practice 🕮). Recommended groups:

- All patients 65yrs and over
- Patients aged 6mths and over in a clinical risk group(s):
  - Chronic respiratory disease including asthma
  - Chronic heart, renal, or liver disease
  - Diabetes
  - Immunosuppression.
- Health and social care workers with direct patient care involvement
- Residents of long-stay care facilities
- Main carer for an older or disabled person
- Consider household contacts of immunocompromised individuals

Children and adults >13yrs: single injection 0.5mL
<13yrs see Children's BNF.

Meningitis C

Recommended for adults at ↑ risk meningococcal disease:

- Adults 18–25yrs if no prior immunization. Single vaccination
- Those with asplenia or splenic dysfunction. Single vaccination followed by booster dose >2mths

See 🕮 Childhood immunization.

Pneumococcal

Recommended for adults where infection is more common or serious:

- All patients 65yrs and over and clinical risk groups:
  - Asplenia or splenic dysfunction
  - Chronic respiratory disease
  - Chronic heart, renal, or liver disease
  - Diabetes
  - Immunosuppression
  - Individuals with cochlear implants
  - Individuals with potential for CSF leaks.

Single dose of 23-valent polysaccharide vaccine recommended for at risk adults.
Reimmunization 5-yrly for patients who are asplenic, splenic dysfunction or chronic renal failure.

Hepatitis A

Recommended for:

- Patients with severe liver disease of whatever cause
- Haemophiliacs receiving plasma derived clotting factors. ❶ Need SC immunization

Anti-malarial medication

Anti-malarial medications (BNF 5.4.1) are <100% effective against malaria. Choice of anti-malarials depends on:

- Presence of chloroquine-resistant malaria in the travel area.
- Patient's medical history.

Commonly recommended anti-malarials include: chloroquine, proguanil, mefloquine, doxycycline, proguanil, and atovaquone. Specific advice on dosages for children are available at the BNF website (Useful websites 📖). Specialist advice is usually sought for long-term prophylaxis. Tablets must be taken in accordance with instructions. All are started pre-travel (most 1wk; except mefloquine, started $2^1/_2$ wks before travel) and continued for 4wks on return to UK (except Malarone® 1–2d before travel, 1wk on return). Anti-malarials are best taken after meals to ↓ side effects. Malaria prophylaxis is not prescribed from the NHS so requires a private prescription or some are available OTC.

Anti-malarial precautions to avoid being bitten

- Cover arms and legs from dusk to dawn.
- Use effective anti-mosquito repellent: most effective ones contain DEET. Reapply regularly.
- Sleep with windows closed, use a permethrin-impregnated mosquito net, spray room with knockdown spray, burn a mosquito coil overnight, air conditioning is an effective deterrent. NB Electronic buzzers are not effective.

Post-travel care

Health professionals have to consider the presence of imported diseases, as well as usual UK health problems, in travellers consulting for up to a year (particularly in first 3mths) on return. Assessment should include details of dates, place, animal contact, swimming in inland waters, sexual contact with people, previous vaccinations, and health of others in travel party.

- *Fever in travellers*: suspect imported disease, including malaria, typhoid, and paratyphoid. Investigations include full blood screen, including thick and thin films for malaria.
- *Diarrhoea in travellers*: suspect imported disease such as giardisis, amoebic dysentery, and cholera. Investigations include M, C & S of fresh stool sample.

Further information for professionals and public

📖 Department of Health England: www.dh.gov.uk/PolicyAndGuidance/HealthAdviceForTravellers

📖 Fit for travel, provided by NHS (Scotland): 24-hr hotline, journey-specific advice: www. fitfortravel.nhs.uk/ ☎ 09068 44 45 46

📖 Chiodini *et al* (2007) Guidelines for malaria prevention in travellers from the UK. Health Protection Agency www.hpa.org.uk

📖 MASTA (recommended by DoH England as an authorative source): www.masta.org

📖 Travax, an NHS UK-wide resource: http://travax.scot.nhs.uk

Travel health promotion

This may form part of a pre-travel assessment or be offered opportunistically during other consultations. The emphasis is on prevention for a wide range of issues tailored according to travel plans, age, type of activity planned on travel, length of stay. Key areas include the following:

On the journey

- DVT prevention advice for any travel involving sitting for long periods: avoid alcohol, drink ↑ water, foot and leg exercises.
- Remind women using COC and travelling across time zones to keep track of the hours, not day of the week, for the next pill.

Out and about

- Accidents and injuries: main cause of death in travellers aged <40yrs, often alcohol related.
  - Advise on using same level of preventive measures as in UK, e.g. crash helmets with mopeds.
  - Need for first aid kit.
  - Need for adequate travel health insurance cover.
- Safe sex, supply condoms if appropriate (Sexual health: general issues 🕮).
- Sun protection (Skin cancer prevention 🕮).
- Remote areas, advise:
  - Purchasing a sealed sterile medical kit (obtainable from MASTA).
  - Perhaps taking antibiotics, discuss with GP.
  - Avoiding blood transfusion.
- Danger of altitude sickness if travel to altitudes >2500m.
- No-go areas because of risk of violence (contact Foreign Office help line, see below).
- Avoid insect bites, advise:
  - The use of insect repellents, cover up, especially between dusk and dawn (see anti-malarial precautions, Travel health care 🕮).
  - Travellers to areas at risk of tick-borne encephalitis to wear long trousers tucked into socks and to spray clothes with insect repellant.
- Avoid animal bites:
  - Rabies occurs in animals in Europe and North America as well as less-developed countries. Advise not to touch any wild or seemingly tame animals.

Food and drink

- Traveller's diarrhoea is common, ~50% travellers (Food poisoning 🕮).
  - Remind people of basic hygiene, e.g. hand cleaning after toilet.
  - Avoid foods kept warm or likely to be touched by flies.
  - Advise on oral rehydration, e.g. 1tsp sugar, pinch salt to 250mL boiled or bottled water.
  - Anti-motility medicines available OTC in UK for adults and some older children (patient to be advised by pharmacist).

• In areas with ↑ risk of cholera, typhoid, hepatitis A, advise people to avoid tap water, salads, seafood, and ice cubes, drink bottled or boiled water, peel fruit.

Travel health insurance

Required for foreign travel in case of needing access to health services. In Europe a European Health Insurance Card provides evidence of eligibility for health services under reciprocal EAA agreements.

Further information for patients

DH leaflet *Health Advice for Travellers*: www.dh.gov.uk

Fit for travel provided by NHS (Scotland): 24-hour hotline, journey-specific advice: www.fitfortravel.nhs.uk/ ☎ 09068 44 45 46

☎ Foreign and Commonwealth Office Advice to travellers: 0870 606 0290

▣ MASTA (recommended by DoH England as an authorative source): www.masta.org

Travel vaccinations

All travellers should have had primary childhood immunization programme (Childhood immunization 🕮), and up-to-date tetanus and polio.

Children
Routine child immunization may be given earlier if:
- Travelling to high-risk areas for prolonged stay.
- Travel is likely to delay the routine programme.

Live vaccines
Special considerations for pregnant women, people with a suppressed immune response, people treated with chemotherapy or radiotherapy (see BNF 14.1). If 2 live vaccines are required (and no combination available), they should be given simultaneously at different sites or 3wks apart.

Immunization advice by country
- Authoritative up-to-date information on requirements for area and countries of travel should be consulted (see below).
- No special immunization required for travel to USA, Europe, Australia, New Zealand, although all should have up-to-date tetanus and polio.
- Table 8.4 lists vaccine information against each disease.

Prescribing and administration of vaccines
Prescribing and administration of vaccine should follow legal and good practice guidelines as well as relevant protective procedures against blood born viruses and sharps injuries.

Payment and availability of vaccines
Travel vaccination can be supplied at commercial travel clinics and in general practice. Some immunizations are charged for and individual practices can set administration fees. Yellow fever vaccination and international certificates (required for entry to some countries) are available only at DH designated centres.

Further information for professionals and public
- 📖 DH *Immunization against infectious disease,* known as the 'Green book', and its supplement, *Health information for overseas travel,* known as the 'yellow book'. Available at: www.nathnac.org/yellow_book/01.htm
- 📖 NaTHNaC National Travel Health Network and Centre: www.nathnac.org/index.htm; Advice line for professionals ☎ 020 7380 9234
- 📖 Travax is a NHS UK-wide resource: 📖 www.travax.scot.nhs.uk

Table 8.4 Travel vaccination: always seek current advice on recommendations e.g. Travax (www.travax.scot.nhs.uk)

Disease	Vaccination schedule	Comments
Cholera	Oral; 2 doses separated by a week; complete 1wk before travel	Not official requirement for entry to any country. May be advised for prolonged stay or close contact with local people in endemic areas
Typhoid	IM; single dose	70% protection for 3yrs, 3yr booster required if at continued risk. The oral vaccine is live (strain Ty2la available through MASTA): ❶ as per all live vaccines
Hepatitis A	IM; 2 doses; interval 6–12mths	Can be given in combination with typhoid vaccine
Hepatitis B	IM; 3 doses; interval 0, 1, 6mths	Accelerated monthly regimen can be used if time is short. Booster 5yrs if continued risk
Tetanus, diphtheria, polio	5-dose course usually given in childhood	Boosters at 10yrs if travelling ↑ risk area
Meningitis A&C	IM; single dose	Required for those making haj to Saudi Arabia
Rabies	SC or IM; 2 or 3 doses if risk; 2 doses 0 and 1mth; 3 doses 0, 7, and 28d	Boosters every 2–3yrs if at continued risk, especially if in remote areas
Japanese B encephalitis	IM; 2 or 3 doses; intervals according to age and vaccine	Protection lasts 2–3yrs but only commences 1mth after vaccination. Unlicensed vaccine available on named patient basis only
Yellow fever	IM, single dose	Protection lasts 10yrs. ❶ As per all live vaccines
Tick-borne encephalitis	IM, 3 doses, intervals 0, 4–12wks, 9–12mths	Unlicensed vaccine available named patient basis only. Booster at 3yrs

Contraception: general

Fertility control is important for the health of ♀, families, and societies. Contraceptive services are available in NHS clinics, some sexual health clinics, young people's clinics, general practice, and not-for-profit organizations e.g. Marie Stopes and Brook Advisory Service (under 25yrs). Contraception free if provided in NHS clinics, prescribed in general practices, or commissioned by the PCT. Barrier methods, oral EC, fertility monitoring can be bought OTC.

Choice of method

Informed by:
- Patient preference and accurate knowledge of methods, effectiveness (see Table 8.5), benefits, and risks.
- Patient age, medical history, immediate family medical history, gynaecological history.
- Past contraceptive history and experience.

All consultations are an opportunity for health promotion

Includes:
- Smoking cessation (Ⅲ)
- Weight management (Ⅲ)
- Exercise (Ⅲ)
- Breast awareness (Ⅲ), self examination, and mammography programme for >50yrs
- Cervical cancer screening (Ⅲ)
- Safer sex practices, STIs particularly chlamydia in under 25s
- Pre-conceptual (Ⅲ) care
- Menopausal symptom management and osteoporosis (Ⅲ) prevention
- Emergency contraception (Ⅲ) provision.

Under 16s and contraception

Sexual and reproductive health advice and treatment

Fraser Guidelines (a House of Lords ruling) applies. A health professional is able to provide contraception, sexual and reproductive health advice and treatment, without parental knowledge or consent provided that:
- The young person understands the health professional's advice.
- The health professional cannot persuade the young person to inform his or her parents or allow the health professional doctor to inform the parents that s/he is seeking contraceptive advice.
- The young person is very likely to begin or continue having intercourse with or without contraceptive treatment.
- Unless he or she receives contraceptive advice or treatment, the young person's physical or mental health or both are likely to suffer.
- The young person's best interests require the health professional to give contraceptive advice, treatment or both without parental consent.

See also Ⅲ Consent, Ⅲ Confidentiality.

Menopausal women and contraception

- ♀ <50yrs contraception required 2yrs after last period.
- ♀ >50yrs contraception required 1yr after last period.

Table 8.5 Effectiveness of all contraceptive methods

Method	Effectiveness
Male condom	98%*
Female condom	95%*
Diaphragm, cervical cap, and spermicide	92–96%*
Fertility awareness methods	98%*
Combined hormone contraception: oral and patch	>99%*
Progesterone only pill (POP)	99%*
Progesterone sub dermal implant	>99%
Progesterone injection	>99%
Intrauterine system (IUS)	99%
Intrauterine device (IUD)	>99%
Sterilization: male and female	>99%

* If used according to instructions

Further information for professionals
Key reference text
▣ Faculty of Family Planning and Reproductive Health. Clinical Effectiveness Guidance Publications available at www.ffprhc.org.uk/

Guillebaud, J. (2004). *Contraception: Your Questions Answered.* 4th edn. Churchill Livingstone.

Further information for the public
Family planning association (FPA)
FPA UK Helpline ☎ 0845 310 1334; FPA Scotland ☎ 0141 576 5088; FPA Northern Ireland ☎ 028 90 325 1334 ▣ www.fpa.org.uk

Young people advice and information
Brook Advisory Centres for under 25yrs: www.brook.org.uk/content/Brook ☎ 0800 0185 023
▣ RU Thinking About It www.ruthinking.co.uk/ (both national Teenage Pregnancy Unit initiatives)
☎ Sexwise Helpline for under 18s: 0800 282 930

Combined hormonal methods

Combined oral contraceptive pill (COC)

Oral drug containing synthetic oestrogen and progestogen. Prevents pregnancy by suppressing ovulation, thickens cervical mucus, thins endometrium. 1 pill 21d at same time each day then 7d pill free (unless everyday preparation). 24hrs window to take the next pill before efficacy ↓.

Advantages: ↓ bleeding, ↓ dysmenorrhoea, ↓ pre-menstrual symptoms. Protects against uterine and ovarian cancer. ↓ ovarian cysts, ↓ PID.

Risks in taking COC: venous and arterial thrombosis (resulting in MI, CVA, PE), breast cancer—risk returns to normal within 10yrs.

Absolute contraindications for taking COC

- Smokers >35yrs
- BMI >39kg/m^2
- Unexplained vaginal bleeding
- Focal migraines
- Pregnancy, breast feeding

- First degree relative with arterial or venous disease diagnosed <45yrs
- 4wks before and 2wks after major or leg surgery
- Oestrogen dependent neoplasm
- Active liver disease, heart disease, lipid disorders, conditions affected by sex steroids
- Past VTE, arterial thrombosis, CVA, TIA

Conditions that are relative contraindications

Sickle cell disease, severe depression, IBD, splenectomy, diseases with HDL, DM diseases with drug treatments that interact e.g. epilepsy, TB, BMI >30kg/m^2.

Choice of COC

First choice COC = low in progestogen and low in oestrogen. COC with gestodene and desogestrel (e.g. Femodene®, Femodene ED®, Femodette®, Marvelon®, Mercilon®, Minulet®, Triadene®, and Tri-Minulet®), known as '3rd generation' pills associated with a slight ↑ VTE risk.

Starting COC

Starting routines for immediate efficacy (otherwise additional contraception required for 7d);
- Day 1 menstruation
- Day 21 postpartum and not lactating
- Same day as miscarriage/TOP
- Instant switch to higher dose COC
- Switch to lower dose COC after 7d break
- Day 1 of menstruation switch to POP.

Advice on starting COC

- To seek medical attention if: chest pain, pain and swelling in calf, shortness of breath, ↑ headaches or with speech or visual disturbances, jaundice, severe stomach pain, blood pressure >160mmHg systolic, 100mmHg diastolic.

- Situations of ↓ effectiveness. Additional contraception e.g. condoms required if.
  - Severe vomiting and/or diarrhoea >24hrs.
  - Taking interacting drugs e.g. enzyme inducing drugs e.g. anticonvulsants, antitubercule. Broad spectrum antibiotics (penicillin, ampicillin, tetracyclines, cephalosporins). Long-term antibiotics need extra contraception for first 3wks only.
  - Taking St Johns Wort herbal preparation.
- Missed pill rules (see Contraception: missed COC rules 📖).
- How to obtain EC if required.
- Follow-up 3mths after starting or changing COC (earlier if problems) and then 6mths, (or 1yr according to local protocols).

At each consultation review/check the following
- Age, BP, weight, smoking habits, change in health or family health status
- Any minor side effects (see below)
- Date and any problems with last menstrual period
- Problems with missed pills or missed pill rules
- Any questions or concerns.

Minor short-term side effects
- *Break through bleeding*: not unusual in first months but check pill routine/missed pills/diarrhoea and vomiting/drug interactions/disease of cervix. If persistent may need higher dose pill.
- *Nausea, bloating, weight gain, breast tenderness, loss of libido, depression*: may need change of pill.

Contraceptive patch

A transdermal patch, releasing oestrogen and progestogen, stuck on skin for 7d x 3 then patch-free 7d. As COC for advantages, risks, contraindications, starting regimens, follow-up and minor short-term effects. If patch falls off:
- <24hrs apply new patch immediately, no additional contraception needed
- >24hrs apply new patch immediately, then additional method for next 7d
- >48hrs after usual start day apply new patch immediately, then condoms for next 7d

Evra helpline for patients ☎ 0845 850 1601.

Related topics

📖 Prescribing; 📖 Sexual health: general issues.

Further information

BNF 7.3.1.

Key reference text

Guillebaud, J. (2004). Contraception: Your Questions Answered. Churchill Livingstone.

Patient advice and information

📖 Family Planning Association (FPA) www.fpa.org.uk; FPA UK Help-line ☎ 0845 310 1334; FPA Scotland ☎ 0141 576 5088; FPA Northern Ireland ☎ 028 90 325 1334

Contraception: missed COC rules

The basic principles (see Fig. 8.2) are:
- Whenever a woman realizes that she has missed COC pills she should take a pill ASAP and then resume her usual pill-taking schedule.
- **Also,** if missed COC pills are in **week 3**, she should omit the pill-free interval.
- **Also**, a back-up method (usually condoms) or abstinence should be used for 7d if the following numbers of pills are missed:
  - 'Two for twenty' (i.e. if 2 or more 20mcg ethinylestradiol pills are missed).
  - 'Three for thirty' (i.e. if 3 or more 30–35mcg ethinylestradiol pills are missed).

Further information for professionals
📖 Faculty of Family Planning and Reproductive Health at the Royal College of Obstetrics and Gynecology (2005) *Missed Pills*. www.ffprhc.org.uk

Further information for patients
📖 Family Planning Association (FPA): www.fpa.org.uk; FPA UK Help line ☎ 0845 310 1334; FPA Scotland ☎ 0141 576 5088; FPA Northern Ireland ☎ 028 90 325 1334

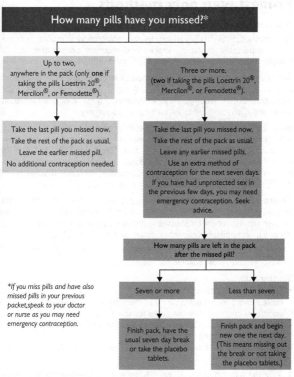

How many pills have you missed?*

Up to two,
anywhere in the pack (only **one** if
taking the pills Loestrin 20®,
Mercilon®, or Femodette®).

Three or more,
(**two** if taking the pills Loestrin 20®,
Mercilon®, or Femodette®).

Take the last pill you missed now.
Take the rest of the pack as usual.
Leave the earlier missed pill.
No additional contraception needed.

Take the last pill you missed now.
Take the rest of the pack as usual.
Leave any earlier missed pills.
Use an extra method of
contraception for the next seven days.
If you have had unprotected sex in
the previous few days, you may need
emergency contraception. Seek
advice.

How many pills are left in the pack
after the missed pill?

**If you miss pills and have also
missed pills in your previous
packet, speak to your doctor
or nurse as you may need
emergency contraception.*

Seven or more

Less than seven

Finish pack, have the
usual seven day break
or take the placebo
tablets.

Finish pack and begin
new one the next day.
(This means missing out
the break or not taking
the placebo tablets.)

Fig. 8.2 Missed pill rules diagram (reproduced with permission from the Family
Planning Association www.fpa.org.uk/guide/contracep/compillchart05.pdf © **fpa** All
Rights Reserved)

Progestogen only methods

Progestogen only pill (POP, also known as mini-pill)

Oral method. Prevents pregnancy by thickening cervical mucus, in some cycles suppresses ovulation, makes endometrium unreceptive and ↓ fallopian tube function. Efficacy: see ▢ Contraception: general.

Advantages: alternative to COC when oestrogens are contraindicated (Contraception: missed rules COC ▢) e.g. ♀ >35yrs and smokes, focal migraines, breast feeding. May ↓ dysmenorrhoea and pre-menstrual symptoms. Can continue to be taken prior to surgery.

Initial consultation: opportunity for health promotion topics (Contraception: general ▢), discussion of POP method, benefits and side effects — particularly alteration of menstrual pattern (see below). Risks: ↑ ovarian cysts, if became pregnant ↑ risk of ectopic, small ↑ risk breast cancer but returns to normal within 10yrs, NB Cerazette® contains desogestrel = ↑ VTE risk (see Contraception: missed rules COC ▢).

Contra-indications to POP: pregnancy, previous ectopic pregnancy, past or present severe arterial disease, severe lipid abnormalities, liver disease or liver cancer, recent trophoblastic disease, concurrent enzyme-inducing drugs e.g. anti-epileptics (Epilepsy, drugs, and side effects ▢).

Choice of POP: one that gives least side effects to individual ♀. Microval® and Norgeston® most suitable for breast feeding.

Starting POP
- Day 1–5 (i.e. 1st day of the period–day 5) offers immediate protection (unless short menstrual cycle <23d then day 1–2). Otherwise— additional contraceptive measures for the 1st 2d.
- Changing from a COC. Immediate protection if POP from day 21 of COC pill i.e. omitting the 7d break.
- Postpartum to start on day 21 otherwise additional contraceptive measures for the 1st 2d.

Taking the pill: daily pill with no pill-free breaks, taken at the same time each day within 3hrs of usual time (12hrs for Cerazette®). ♀ >70kg are often prescribed 2 pills/d (unlicensed use see Prescribing ▢) but not if prescribed Cerazette®.

Missed pills: if a pill is later than 3hrs from usual time of taking (12hrs Cerazette®) continue taking POP at usual time and use additional precautions for 2d. Ensure ♀ knows about EC (Emergency contraception ▢).
- *Severe diarrhoea or vomiting within 2hrs of taking pill*: continue taking POP but assume pills 'missed' and additional precautions for 2d.
- *Antibiotics*: do not affect the POP (except enzyme-inducing rifampicin and griseofulvin when additional precautions or different method required).

Review: 3mths after starting POP, earlier if problems, then 6mthly (or yrly according to local protocols). Check age, BP, weight, change in health or family health status, minor side effects (see below), any problems with menstruation or missed pills, any questions.

Side effects
- *Menstrual irregularities*: duration, volume, and flow may alter, may experience inter-menstrual episodes, may experience amenorrhoea. This is the commonest reason for stopping method. Pathology needs to be excluded, and pregnancy test if amenorrhoea. Consider changing type of progestogen i.e. to a different POP.
- *Others*: breast discomfort, bloatedness, depression, weight changes, nausea, skin problems (e.g. acne or chloasma), changes in libido. Consider changing progestogen i.e. to a different POP.

Progestagen injectables
Main preventative action through suppression of ovulation. Efficacy see ▢ Contraception: general.

Advantages: as POP above, lasts 8–12wks.

Disadvantages: irregular bleeding, amenorrhoea, fertility may take up to 1yr to return, may ↑ weight, may ↓ mood, cannot be withdrawn. Long-term use has a possible link ↓ oestrogen levels and requires medical review after 5yrs use.

Contraindications: as POP

Initial consultation: as POP

Preparations
- Depo-Provera (DMPA): 150mg IM injection lasts 12wks. Licensed for long-term use.
- Noristerat (NET EN): 200mg IM lasts 8wks. For short-term use only.

Contraceptive effect immediate if 1st injection is given:
- Within 5d of onset of menstruation
- <5d post partum if not breast feeding
- 6wks post partum if breast feeding
- 1–5d after miscarriage or TOP.

Otherwise advise ♀ to use additional contraception for 7d after the 1st injection.

Repeat injections: effective immediately if given <12wks + 5d after previous injection (<8wks for Noristerat) If not, exclude pregnancy before repeat injection and use additional contraception for 7d. Consider EC >94d (DMPA), >66d (NET EN) (Emergency contraception ▢).

Progestogen subdermal implants (e.g. Implanon®)
Small (40mm), thin rod inserted (and removed by specially trained doctor or nurse) into upper arm. Lasts for 3yrs with no checkups required. Action: as injectables above. Contraindications and side effects as POP above. Effect rapidly reversible.

Further information
BNF 7.3.2. Also details on ▢ Contraception: general
▣ NICE (2005). Long Acting Reversible Contraception Clinical Guidelines. www.nice.nhs.uk

Interuterine devices and systems

Interuterine devices (IUDs)

IUDs are inserted via the cervical canal into the uterus. It is a small plastic device often incorporating copper, with threads hanging into vagina and tucked around the cervix. Prevents pregnancy by impeding sperm transport, altering gametes, and blocking fertilization.

Disadvantages: heavier and more painful periods, ↑ risk of ectopic if pregnant, ↑ risk of pelvic inflammatory disease, rare risk of perforation of the uterus during insertion, risk of explusion.

Advantages: effective immediately (Contraception: general 🕮), not reliant on user for efficacy, safe. Easily removable.

Contraindications: previous ectopic pregnancy, abnormalities of uterus, allergy to copper, at risk of STI e.g. multiple partners or short-term partners. History of fibroids and endometriosis, dysmenorrhoea, menorrhagia need careful individual assessment.

Pre-insertion
- Health promotion (Contraception: general 🕮).
- Counselling on advantages and disadvantages particularly menstrual impact.
- Chlamydia screening (Sexually transmitted infections 🕮).
- Ensure very effective method of contraception until insertion or abstinence from day 1 of period in that cycle. If changing IUD no sex for 7d before in case new IUD cannot be inserted and sperm survive.
- Information about insertion procedure, and likelihood of cramping pains that day.

Insertion
- Performed by specially trained doctors and nurses.
- Optimum time for insertion.
  - End of main menstrual flow to day 14–28 of cycle.
  - 4–6wks post-partum (6–8wks post Caesarean section).
- Mefenamic acid 500mg orally pre-insertion ↓ pain post insertion.
- Emergency equipment should be available in case of vasovagal attack or anaphylaxis. Insertions usually performed with 2 professionals for reassurance and in case of emergency.

Post insertion
- ♀ encouraged to rest, then get up slowly.
- Use sanitary towels not tampons until next period.
- Advised on feeling threads monthly and to return if cannot.
- Abstain from sex for 3d or use condoms as insertion interferes with protective mechanism of cervix.
- Advised to seek medical attention if pelvic pain ± vaginal discharge.
- Give patient a record of date of insertion and type of IUD.

Review and follow-up
- Reviewed 4–6wks post insertion.
- Ask about periods, pelvic pain, vaginal discharge, discomfort to partner, frequency of thread checks. Threads should be checked visually (through speculum) also felt as well as cervix moved gently side-to-side to detect partial expulsion of device.
- Subsequent reviews according to local protocols. Many now state only required if woman has a problem or cannot feel threads.

Life span of IUDs
- Check BNF 7.3.4 by brand. Modern copper devices e.g. T-safe® Cu 380 A effective for 10yrs. Older types 3–5yrs.
- ♀≥40yrs: most IUDs effective until the menopause.

Removal
- Any time if considering pregnancy.
- 7d after alternative method of contraception established.
- 1yr after menopause (Contraception: general 📖).

ALOs
See 📖 Cervical cancer screening.

Inter uterine systems (IUSs)
IUSs have slow release progestogen (levonorgestorol) reservoir around the vertical stem. Mirena® is the only IUS in UK and licensed for 5yrs use.

Advantages: as IUDs plus:
- ↓ heavy periods
- ↓ dysmenorrhoea
- Protects against ectopic pregnancy
- Suitable for women with history of PID.

Disadvantages
- Associated with irregular bleeding, may be constant spotting over first few months although this settles down
- Amenorrhoea after first few months
- More expensive than IUDs so it is important ♀ fully understands disadvantages
- Expulsion and possible increased risk of ectopic pregnancy.

Pre-insertion, insertion, post insertion, and removal: as IUDs.

Further information
📓 Faculty of Family Planning and Reproductive Health (2004) *Copper IUD and IUS systems.* www.ffprhc.org.uk
📓 NICE (2005). *Long Acting Reversible Contraception Clinical Guidelines.* www.nice.nhs.uk

Further information for patients
📓 Family Planning Association (FPA): www.fpa.org.uk
📓 FPA UK Helpline ☎ 0845 310 1334; FPA Scotland ☎ 0141 576 5088; FPA Northern Ireland ☎ 028 90 325 1334

Barrier contraceptive methods

Male condoms

Single use latex sheath. Applied to erect penis before contact with vulva. Closed end squeezed to expel air before unrolling down length of penis. After ejaculation penis removed holding condom firmly in place. Efficacy see 📖 Contraception: general.

Advantages: protection against STIs, no systemic effects, easily available OTC. Disadvantages: perceived as an interruption to sex, loss of sensitivity. Plain ended and thin condoms ↑ sensitivity. Contraindications: erectile problems.

Allergy problems: Hypoallergenic brands available if allergic to latex. Local irritation can be caused by spermicidal lubricant on some brands—change brand.

❶ Should only be used with water based lubricants e.g. KY jelly®. Oil based products e.g. baby oil, Vaseline® damage latex and ↓ effectiveness.

Female condoms

Lubricated polyurethane tube with inner and outer ring, inserted into vagina. Inner ring aids insertion (see Fig. 8.3). Outer ring at open end, sits flat against vulva. Only Femidom® licensed in UK. Advantages: as male condom above. Can be used with oil based products. Disadvantages: can be perceived as noisy during sex.

Vaginal diaphragms and caps

A diaphragm is a latex rubber dome used with spermicide and inserted into vagina to cover the cervix (see Fig. 8.4). Advantages: non-systemic, can be used in menstruation. Disadvantages: requires motivation, may be perceived as messy.

Contraindications: poor vaginal tone or prolapse, allergy to rubber or spermicide, recurrent UTI, past history of toxic shock syndrome.

Type of diaphragm: flat spring type is suitable for ♀ with anterior or mid plane cervix. Coiled spring type is suitable for those who find flat spring uncomfortable. Arcing spring type is suitable for ♀ with posterior cervix.

Fitting: must be performed by a doctor or nurse trained to fit diaphragms. The woman then practises in the clinic room:
- Insertion.
- Checking the diaphragm covers cervix.
- Removal.

Then ♀ has a trial period for >1wk in which she uses the diaphragm while using another form of contraception. Any problems of insertion, fit, removal, comfort are addressed at a follow-up appointment and the size and fit checked before prescribing the diaphragm for contraceptive use.

Advice on correct use
- Diaphragm used with 2cm strips of spermicide on both sides. Spermicide effective for 3hrs. If intercourse takes place ≥3hrs later, more spermicide is needed (either as cream or pessary).
- Insert diaphragm before intercourse and leave in place ≥6hrs afterwards but no longer than 24–48hrs, depending on the brand.

- Some oil based products, e.g. Vaseline®, baby oil, and vaginal medications e.g. Nystan® cream damage caps (full list in leaflet in box).
- After use, wash diaphragm in warm soapy water, dry, and store in its box.

Follow-up: fit and comfort checked after ~1wk. Advice on use and care discussed. Advised to return for check of fit if problems, or weight changes by 5kg or more, or after pregnancy. New diaphragm prescribed: annually, or if develops hole, or after a vaginal infection treated.

Cervical/vault caps: attach by suction. Otherwise used in the same way as a diaphragm. Useful for women with poor muscle tone, absent retropubic ledge, or recurrent cystitis when using a diaphragm.

Spermicides

Are used in combination with barrier methods and are not protective on their own (see BNF 7.3.3).
Different forms:
- Cream—Ortho-Crème®
- Pessaries—Orthoforms®.

Some contain perfumes and may be irritant, consider different type in this instance.

Further information for professionals

Key reference text

Guillebaud, J. (2004): *Contraception: Your Questions Answered*, (4th edn). Churchill Livingstone.

Further information for the public

⊞ Family Planning Association (FPA): www.fpa.org.uk; FPA UK Help line ☎ 0845 310 1334; FPA Scotland ☎ 0141 576 5088; FPA Northern Ireland ☎ 028 90 325 1334

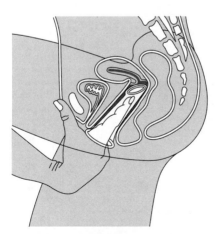

Fig. 8.3 Inserting the female condom (reproduced with kind permission of The Female Health Company (UK) Plc).

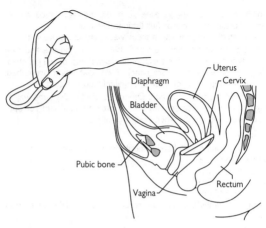

Fig. 8.4 Inserting a diaphragm. Reproduced with permission from Szarewski A. and Guillebaud J. (2000) *Contraception*. By permission of Oxford University Press.

Natural family planning and sterilization

Natural family planning involves fertility awareness through observation of changes that indicates ovulation (usually between 12–16d before menstruation). From this the couple decide to either abstain, use additional contraception (or have sex for a pregnancy). Methods of estimating ovulation are:

- A hand-held computerized system for testing early morning urine for hormone changes. Commercial system (Persona®) available to buy plus additional urine dip sticks. Not suitable if: menstrual cycle <23d or >35d, or menopausal, or breast feeding, or has kidney or liver disease, or using hormonal treatment.
- Temperature. Taken orally in the morning prior to drinking or getting up (ovulation thermometer available on FP10). Charted from 1st day of period. An ↑ 0.2–0.4°C indicates progesterone release from the corpus luteum. Once temperature has ↑ and been maintained for 3d then intercourse can be unprotected until the next period.
- Mucus texture (Billing's method). The texture of vaginal secretions is felt between finger and thumb daily (more frequently at first). Prior to ovulation the mucus becomes profuse, clear, stretchy (looks like raw egg white). 4d after peak mucus changes to thick, sticky, and opaque. Advised no unprotected intercourse from the day the mucus becomes more profuse until 3d after it becomes sticky.
- Termperature and mucus texture often used in combination as a double check method.

Further information for professionals and patients

🖳 Fertility UK: www.fertilityuk.org/

Sterilization

Sterilization is a surgical, permanent procedure preventing egg and sperm meeting. It is used by people who are certain they do not want children or more children. In the UK about 45% couples >40yrs rely on sterilization of one partner. Referred to specialist services (NHS or private) after initial counselling.

Counselling and information process

Very important particularly with those <25yrs, without children, pregnant women, those in reaction to a loss of relationship, or those who may be at risk of coercion by their partner or others. Prior sanction by a high court judge sought in all cases where there is doubt over an individual's mental capacity to consent (Mental capacity 🕮). Key information should include:

- Alternative long-term contraceptive methods.
- Sterilization should be thought of as permanent, reversal is <50% successful.
- Post-procedure pregnancy rate: 1:200 ♀ (plus ↑ increased ectopic risk); 1:2000 ♂.

- Procedures:
  - ♀: laparoscopic tubal occlusion with clips or rings. Usually done under general anaesthetic as a day case.
  - Men: vasectomy. Usually done under local anaesthetic as a day case.
- Risk of operative complications.
- Need for contraception before and after operation:
  - ♀ other contraception until 1st post-procedure menstruation.
  - ♂ other contraception until 2 consecutive but 2–4wks apart semen analyses (>8wks post vasectomy) shows sperm free.

Further information
Key reference text
Guillebaud, J. (2004). *Contraception: Your Questions Answered.* 4th edn. Churchill Livingstone.

Further information for the public
🖳 Family Planning Association (FPA): www.fpa.org.uk; FPA UK Helpline ☎ 0845 310 1334; FPA Scotland ☎ 0141 576 5088; FPA Northern Ireland ☎ 028 90 325 1334.

Emergency contraception (EC)

Two time-limited forms of EC are available to prevent pregnancy post unprotected sexual intercourse (UPSI):
- Levonorgestrol tablets.
- Insertion of copper IUD.

Choice depends on; time from earliest UPSI in that cycle, and medical, contraceptive, and menstrual history.

Levonorgestrel (Levonelle®)

May be used <72hrs after UPSI. Given as a single dose of 1.5mg. Most effective closest to UPSI in time. Acts to prevent ovulation or blocking implantation of egg. If pregnant ↑ risk of ectopic. Unlicensed use on named patient basis by doctor only between 72–120hrs after UPSI. (BNF 7.3.1.)

Contraindications: porphyria.

Cautions: liver disease, enzyme inducing drugs (may need ↑ dose), severe malabsorption syndromes, breast feeding.

Side effects: nausea and vomiting, menstrual irregularities, breast tenderness.

Advice to ♀
- Take tablet(s) immediately.
- Not 100% effective and if pregnant may ↑ risk of ectopic.
- If vomit within 2hrs of taking tablet to return for replacement dose.
- Levonorgestrol deals with past UPSI not future: so use a barrier method until next period.
- The next period may be late.
- To seek medical attention if lower abdominal pain.
- To re-consult if period unusual or >5d late.
- Discuss future contraceptive needs (Contraception general 🕮). If starting oral hormonal contraception should start on day 2 of bleeding to ensure it is a period.

Insertion of copper IUD

Acts as a post-coital method by preventing implantation and may also block fertilization (100% effective). May be inserted up to 5d after single UPSI or if several UPSI in that cycle up to 5d after the most probable calculated date of ovulation (usually 12–16d before next menstrual period).

Pre-insertion counselling, insertion, post insertion care, and removal: as IUD (🕮). As the pre-insertion chlamydia results will not be available prophylactic antibiotics are given.

Rape and sexual assault

See 🕮 Crime and victims of crime.

Further information for professionals

🖳 Faculty of Family Planning and Reproductive Health (2006) Emergency contraception: www.ffprhc.org.uk

Further information for patients

🖳 Family Planning Association (FPA): www.fpa.org.uk; FPA UK Helpline ☎ 0845 310 1334; FPA Scotland ☎ 0141 576 5088; FPA Northern Ireland ☎ 028 90 325 1334

Young people advice and information

🖳 Brook Advisory Centres for under 25yrs: www.brook.org.uk/content/Brook ☎ 0800 0185 023
☎ Sexwise Helpline for under 18s: 0800 282 930 and 🖳 RU Thinking about it www.ruthinking.co.uk/ (both national Teenage Pregnancy Unit initiatives)

Pre-conceptual care and advice

Pre-conceptual care and advice can be offered as part of other consultations as well as those for contraception, cervical screening checks etc. It may be given opportunistically or as part of a planned consultation. The aims are to:
- ↓ problems in pregnancy.
- ↑ chances of conceiving in an optimum state of health.

Key areas to discuss

Rubella

Rubella infection in early pregnancy results in a high risk of fetal abnormalities including deafness and blindness. Rubella status should be checked. If not immune, should be immunized with MMR (exclude pregnancy beforehand) and advised to avoid pregnancy for 1mth.

Screening

♀ should be encouraged to ensure any screening is up to date e.g. cervical cancer screening (📖) or undertaken if at risk e.g. STI, HIV.

Genetic screening and counselling

Aimed at detecting carriers, identifying levels of risk, and then couples having informed choices about pregnancy. Sometimes direct access to services e.g. some haemoglobinopathy centres or offered through referral from GP to couples who:
- Have personal or family history of genetic abnormality.
- Have had a previous pregnancy, baby with genetic abnormality.
- Have an ethnic background in which high risk of carrier status e.g.
  - South East Asia and Southern China: thalassaemias.
  - Mediterranean, parts of N. and W. Africa, Middle East and Indian subcontinent: thalassaemias and sickling disorders (Sickle cell disorders 📖).
  - Black African and Caribbean: sickling disorders (Sickle cell disorders 📖).
  - Ashkenazi Jewish: Tays–Sachs, Gaucher's disease, and cystic fibrosis.

Diet

- Encourage health diet and BMI in normal range (Nutrition and health eating 📖) plus:
  - Folate rich foods (e.g. breakfast cereals, leafy green foods) prior to pregnancy and in the first 12wks.
  - Avoid high levels of vitamin A e.g. in liver.
  - Avoid unpasteurised dairy products (e.g. brie and camembert cheeses), uncooked eggs, undercooked meat, pâtés, pre-prepared salads to prevent infection (e.g. Listeriosis, salmonella) during pregnancy as associated with ↑ risk of stillbirth and miscarriage.
- Start folic acid supplementation (OTC or prescribed) which ↓ risk of neural tube defect by 72%.
  - All ♀ should take 0.4mg daily when pregnancy is being planned and for 12wks after conception.

- ♀ at higher risk of pregnancy with neural tube defect take 5mg daily until 12wks after conception. This group includes: women who have had a previous affected pregnancy, one of the couple has a neural tube defect, ♀ has coeliac disease, or takes anti-epilepsy medication, or has sickle cell disease.

Smoking

Encourage cessation (Smoking cessation 📖) in both partners because:
- In ♀ it affects ovulation.
- In ♂ it ↓ the sperm count and sperm motility.
- In pregnancy, smoking increases the miscarriage rate (x2), increases the risk of pre-term delivery, and is associated with a low birth weight.

Alcohol

Opportunity for brief intervention on reduction of alcohol consumption. Current advice: avoid alcohol in pregnancy but if alcohol is taken it should be a maximum of 1 unit a day. Heavy drinking associated with increased risk of miscarriage. Fetal alcohol syndrome (brain damage, growth retardation, facial malformations) occurs to approx 1/3 of ♀ drinking >18 units a day (see also Alcohol 📖).

OTC medicines

Few have been established as safe in pregnancy so avoid use while trying to conceive.

Toxoplasmosis

Parasitic infection causing fetal brain damage and blindness. Avoid raw meat, cat faeces, sheep and goat milk.

Fertility awareness

Review knowledge of fertile period and optimum days in menstrual cycle to have sex for conception. Ovulation usually 12–16d before period.

♀ with pre-existing medical conditions

Should consult their GP for review and advice particularly on suitability of medication in pregnancy.

♀ with previous problems in pregnancies

Should consult their GP for review, advice and possible early referral to specialist.

Related topic

📖 Antenatal care and screening.

Further information for professionals

▣ Clinical Knowledge Summaries (Clinical Knowledge Summaries (Prodigy)) guidance on preconceptual counselling: www.cks.library.nhs.uk/

Further information for patients

▣ Family Planning Association: *Planning for pregnancy* (also a leaflet). www.fpa.org.uk

Pregnancy

Pregnancy is a continuous process of growth and development from the time of conception to the birth of the baby. The early signs and symptoms include:

- Missed period (or very light spotting)
- Sickness and/or nausea
- Breast tenderness and enlargement
- Tiredness
- Frequency of urine, constipation.

Urine dipstick pregnancy tests can detect hormone human chorionic gonadotrophin at about 14d (see instructions on different brands) after conception. OTC pregnancy testing kits are available.

The length of a normal pregnancy is 280d from the date of conception, or 38wks. The date of the last menstrual period (LMP) is used as a marker for calculating the length of a pregnancy and expected date of delivery (EDD). It is usual to confirm length of gestation (and thus EDD) with USS which is accurate to within 3–5d.

The first trimester

- During the first 12–14wks of pregnancy the baby develops from an early embryo into a fetus with all its organs and systems in place. The placental circulation also becomes established.
- If a woman is going to experience a miscarriage it is more likely to happen in the first trimester. This is most likely due to developmental problems with either the fetus or the placenta, or genetic defects.
- Antenatal screening for fetal abnormality takes place towards the end of the first trimester.

The second trimester

- From 14–30wks, the mother experiences a growing sense of well-being as early symptoms like nausea diminish.
- The baby continues to grow and develop with the nervous system progressively maturing so that fetal movements become more pronounced.
- He/she is also able to experience sensations like warmth and can taste the amniotic fluid swallowed. Some even develop hiccups from time to time. A baby born late in this trimester would be unable to sustain independent life and would require both respiratory and nutritional support.

The third trimester

- From 30wks to birth is a time of continued growth and maturation.
- The baby doubles its weight between 34–40wks. Every week spent in the mother's uterus is significant in respect of maturity of the respiratory and digestive system.
- The baby also develops a layer of subcutaneous fat which helps to protect it from hypothermia and hypoglycaemia in the neonatal period, so it is essential that the mother maintains an adequate healthy diet throughout pregnancy.

Further information for professionals and the public

- Midirs Informed Choice Information Leaflets for professionals and expectant parents www.infochoice.org/
- NCT www.nctpregnancyandbabycare.com/ ☎ 0870 444 8707

Maternity rights and benefits

Pregnant women and new mothers who are in employment are protected by a number of regulations specific to their welfare and well-being while at work and protect against discrimination on the basis of their pregnancy.

Employers of pregnant women must

- Carry out a risk assessment.
- If aspects of the job pose a risk to the health of the woman, adjust working conditions, working hours or offer another job.
- Provide a rest area, preferably smoke free.
- After returning to work provide a private room for breast-feeding mothers to express and store their milk.

Pregnant women in employment have

- Paid time off to attend antenatal care.
- Normal sick pay rights for pregnancy related illness.
- Accrual of contracted holiday entitlement while on maternity leave.
- A right to return to the same job.

Maternity leave

All employed women are entitled to 26wks ordinary maternity leave and 26wks additional maternity leave (if EDD on or after 1 April 2007) irrespective of whether they are entitled to maternity benefits (see below). For those with EDD before 1 April 2007 a further 26wks additional maternity leave can be taken by women who have been in employment for 26wks by the beginning of the 14th wk before the week of the birth. Key regulations for all are:

- They must inform the employer, preferably in writing with a medical certificate (MATB1), by the end of the 15th wk before the baby is due, when they wish to commence maternity leave. MATB1 is signed by midwife or GP to verify pregnancy and EDD at 20wks before EDD.
- The leave can start anytime after 11wks before EDD.
- Maternity leave starts automatically if a woman is sick with a pregnancy related illness during the 4wks before the EDD.
- A woman may not return to work within 2wks of the birth (4wks if they work in a factory).
- Maternity leave rights remain if baby is still born after 24wks or born earlier than EDD.

Maternity benefits

Statutory maternity pay (SMP) is

- A weekly payment made by employers to employees or former employees if they meet the qualifying conditions:
  - Employed for 26wks continuously by the 15th wk.
  - Earning at least an average of £82/wk before tax.
- An entitlement whether or not they intend to return to work for that employer.
- Paid for a maximum of 39wks, can start 11wks before EDD.
- The first 6wks of SMP are 90% of weekly earnings (with no upper limit). Then 33wks of £108.85 or 90% of earnings if less than £108.85.

Maternity allowance is
- Available to some employed and self-employed women who don't qualify for SMP but meet criteria on wks of continuous employment and earning on average £30/wk.
- Paid by DWP and claimed on form MA1 from Jobcentre Plus.
- Paid for 39wks at rate of £108.85 or 90% of weekly earnings.
- Reduces amount received from other state benefits e.g. (income support 📖).

Paternity leave and pay
Fathers are entitled to statutory paternity leave of 1 or 2wks at time of birth if they have been employed continuously for 26wks at the 15th wk before EDD. They have to inform employer in writing. A self-certification form is available at DWP website (see below). This leave is paid if they are earning enough to pay National Insurance otherwise the father may be able to claim income support (Benefits for people with a low income 📖).

Sure Start maternity grants
These are:
- Available to parents on low incomes receiving Jobseeker's Allowance, Income Support, Pension Credit, Child Tax Credit at a rate higher than the family element, or Working Tax Credit where a disabled worker is included in the assessment.
- A social fund payment of £500 which does not have to be paid back (see also Benefits for people with a low income 📖).
- Claimed on SF100 Sure Start form from local Jobcentre Plus office, Social Security office.

Other benefits
Pregnant women and up to 12mths after birth are entitled to:
- Free prescriptions on production of exemption card (MATEX) from prescription pricing authority on completion of form FW8 (obtainable from GP or midwife).
- Free NHS dentistry.
- Tokens for milk—if receiving low income benefits, from 10wks of pregnancy by claiming on form 'Free Milk for Pregnant Women', countersigned by GP or midwife. ☎ Helpline 0845 1032.

Related topic
📖 Benefits for mothers, parents, and children.

Further information for parents-to-be
🖳 Department of Trade and Industry Tailored Interactive Guidance on Employment Rights (TIGER): www.tiger.gov.uk/index.htm
🖳 DWP *Leaflet NI17A: A guide to Maternity Benefits*. Available from Directgov, a government information web site, parent pages: www.direct.gov.uk/Parents/fs/en
🖳 Local Citizens Advice Bureau and online guide: www.adviceguide.org.uk/

Antenatal care and screening

Pregnancy is a time of tremendous physical, psychological, social, and emotional change. For the majority of women, pregnancy is a time of well-being and good health and should not be regarded as an illness.

The need for early antenatal care

- Professional care and advice at an early stage of pregnancy allows identification and management of any initial problems.
- Most women seek advice from their GP as a first point of contact. The GP makes early referral to either a midwife or an obstetrician according to need. Women who are at risk of experiencing problems in their pregnancies may also be referred to an early pregnancy assessment unit or a high risk day care unit.

Midwives

The midwife is responsible for antenatal, intranatal, and postnatal care, and is the expert in normal pregnancy. Midwives are employed by a NHS Trust, working in community teams (3–6), or in hospital, or both. Some midwives provide all the care needed by the woman throughout. Other midwives are responsible for all the pregnant women in their locality but can only provide antenatal and postnatal care.

The pattern of antenatal care

It is best delivered at a venue easy to reach for the mother and provided by same midwife or team for continuity of care. The aim of antenatal appointments is to check on the mother's and baby's progress, and provide information, explanations about care and health promotion advice. The pattern varies according to need and is regularly reviewed.

Antenatal care appointments

The schedule for low-risk women varies according to whether they are nuliparous or having a subsequent baby (parous). All women should have appointments as follows:

- Their first appointment before 12wks when a full assessment is undertaken. This may be a lengthy appointment.
- Around 14wks to perform ultrasound dating and serum Down's risk screening.
- 16wks to review the results of the scan and screening tests.
- 18–20wks if the mother requests a fetal anomaly scan.
- 28wks to offer prophylactic anti-D to women who are Rhesus negative (2nd dose at 34wks) and to obtain a FBC to monitor the mother's haemoglobin level.
- 34, 36 (presentation of baby checked), and 38wks to monitor mother and baby.
- All women not delivered by 41wks have a further visit to arrange an induction of labour.

Nuliparous women: have another 3 appointments interspersed to a total of 12 visits.

Parous women: usually require 7–8 appointments.

Monitoring

BP and urinalysis for proteinuria is undertaken at each visit. Also the measurement of symphysis fundal height at each visit from 25wks. Pregnant ♀ are also offered the opportunity to disclose domestic violence (🕮). If at any time a complication were to arise the woman would be referred to an obstetrician for advice.

Women whose pregnancies are assessed as medium or high risk

Because of the presence of long-term condition e.g. diabetes, previous problems in pregnancies, age >40yrs or <18yrs, BMI >35 or <18, mental health problems or problematic social circumstances these women will have extra visits according to their needs and the progress of the pregnancy.

Screening tests

The midwife will advise on, offer, or arrange the following screening tests:

- Blood tests: will be obtained by the midwife during the first or second visits.
  - Routine: FBC, blood group and Rhesus factor, VDRL, rubella antibodies.
  - Recommended but optional: Down's risk, HIV, hepatitis B.
- Ultrasound scans: dating/fetal anomaly/nuchal fold measurement.

The majority of tests are performed before the 14th wk of pregnancy for early detection of problems. This can be a time of anxiety for the woman especially if she has chosen to have fetal screening tests. Diagnostic tests are offered and if a congenital abnormality is detected the woman and her family will need to choose whether or not to carry on with the pregnancy. Genetic counselling is available for all women in this situation.

Pregnancy records

Mothers hold their own pregnancy record so that continuity is maintained.

Essential information for professionals

🖳 National Institute of Clinical Excellence/National Collaborating Centre for Womens's and Child Health (2003). *Antenatal Care: Routine care for the Healthy Pregnant Woman.* www.nice.org.uk

National Service Frameworks for maternity services in all countries available on central health departments' websites (Useful websites 🕮).

Further information for parents

🖳 Public Information version of *Antenatal Care: Routine care for the healthy pregnant woman* at www.nice.org.uk

The Pregnancy Book (published by Health Departments in England and Wales). *Ready Steady Baby* (Scotland).

VICTORIA INFIRMARY
MEDICAL STAFF LIBR

Antenatal education and preparation for parenthood

Antenatal education can take place during any encounter a pregnant woman may have with a health professional, for instance during antenatal visits to a midwife.

Parent education classes

Women are also invited to locally-held, free NHS parent education classes. Some localities offer a range of different preparation to suit local needs for instance, Aquanatal classes that take place in a swimming pool under the direction of a midwife or other specially trained instructor. In many areas HVs work with midwives to provide community antenatal classes. Other organizations e.g. The National Childbirth Trust (NCT) also offer parent education but will charge a fee for attendance at their classes.

Aims of classes

The aim of antenatal education is to build confidence to enable parents to take control over their labour and the birth of their child. Antenatal classes provide a place to discuss fears and worries, and exchange views with other parents-to-be. Parents attending classes find meeting new friends who will be going through the same experiences beneficial, particularly if first time parents. The needs of parents attending antenatal classes are broadly:

- To obtain balanced realistic information so they know what to expect.
- To learn skills that will help them to cope during labour.
- To learn about the emotional and social aspects of birth and being a parent.
- To learn about life after birth and caring for their new baby.

The content of a series of classes might include:

- Development and growth of the baby and what the mother might expect during pregnancy.
- Common screening tests/blood tests.
- Healthy eating for pregnancy.
- Going into hospital to give birth/what to take.
- Recognizing that labour has started and when to seek advice. Coping skills for labour. What happens if help is needed to give birth (assisted birth, Caesarean birth).
- Common types of pain relief available during labour.
- Breast feeding and caring for the new baby.
- Life at home with the new baby/how partners can help.
- Common problems in the postnatal period.

Most sessions would probably include practising labour coping skills such as relaxation and breathing techniques.

Further information for professionals and the public

- Midirs Informed Choice Information Leaflets for professionals and expectant parents: www.infochoice.org/
- NCT: www.nctpregnancyandbabycare.com/ ☎ 0870 444 8707.

Common problems in pregnancy

During pregnancy a woman may experience a range of problems for which she can be given timely advice, making these easier to manage and improving her well-being. Problems include nausea, constipation, indigestion, varicosities, backache, and frequency of micturition. These so-called minor disorders of pregnancy are a series of commonly experienced symptoms related to the effects of pregnancy hormones and the consequences of enlargement of the uterus as the fetus grows during pregnancy.

Nausea

- Nausea and vomiting are common, with about 50% of pregnant women suffering anything from mild nausea on awakening, to nausea throughout the day with some vomiting, during the first half of pregnancy.
- For many women the symptoms subside after the 12th–14th wk of pregnancy coinciding with the ability of the placenta to take over support of the growing embryo.
- Advice includes maintaining a good fluid intake, eating little and often throughout the day, and avoiding alcohol, caffeine, spicy, and fatty foods.
- A doctor should be consulted if the woman is vomiting more than 4 times a day, if she is losing weight, or fluids are not being kept down.

Indigestion

- This is caused when progesterone relaxes the smooth muscle in the cardiac sphincter, leading to a reflux of acid into the oesophagus.
- Taking fluids at separate times to mealtimes, and sleeping with more than 2 pillows so the chest is raised slightly higher than the abdomen can ease the symptoms.
- The woman can be prescribed a suitable antacid if the above advice doesn't work and she needs additional help to manage the symptoms.

Constipation

- Caused by progesterone relaxing the smooth muscle in the bowels.
- The woman can be advised to take extra fluids, increase the amount of fruit and vegetables consumed, and that exercise such as walking may help (Nutrition and healthy eating 📖).
- If constipation is very difficult to manage a gentle laxative may be prescribed by the midwife or doctor dependent on the stage of pregnancy.

Varicosities

- They are caused when the weight of the growing uterus creates back pressure in the veins of the lower body overcoming the normal flow of blood.
- This is accompanied by smooth muscle relaxation in the vessel walls due to the influence of progesterone.
- These can occur in the legs, vulva, or anal canal (haemmorhoids).

- Support tights, and close fitting supportive underwear will minimize the leg and vulval varicose veins. If the legs are aching, resting with them elevated will ease the symptoms.
- Haemorrhoids can be treated by avoiding constipation (see above). A soothing haemorrhoidal preparation (BNF 1.7.1) may be prescribed in a cream or suppository form.

Backache

- This complaint is common both during and after pregnancy.
- The ligaments supporting the lower spine and pelvis become softer and stretch more readily during pregnancy, and poor posture exacerbates this leading to backache.
- Advice includes not standing or sitting for long periods, attention to posture particularly if the woman uses a keyboard or computer at work. Using a chair with good lumbar support at work and at home, and regular gentle exercise such as walking can all be beneficial.

Frequency of micturition

- This is usually apparent during early pregnancy when the uterus is still a pelvic organ, and later in pregnancy when the fetal head enters the maternal pelvis.
- Both these situations create pressure on the bladder reducing the amount of space available, hence the need to pass urine more often.
- This does not normally inconvenience the woman but she should be asked about other symptoms such as burning, stinging, or discomfort during micturition to rule out urinary tract infection.

Further information for professionals and parents-to-be

National Childbirth Trust: www.nctpregnancyandbabycare.com/ ☎ 0870 444 8707

National Institute of Clinical Excellence/National Collaborating Centre for Womens's and Child Health (2003). *Antenatal care: Routine care for the healthy pregnant woman*: www.nice. org.uk and full guideline at www.rcog.org.uk/resources/Public

The Pregnancy Book (published by Health Departments in England and Wales). *Ready, Steady, Baby* (Scotland).

Birth options and labour

For most mothers-to-be, planning the birth of the baby is an exciting prospect. Previous experience can however make this a daunting prospect. The midwife usually discusses options with the mother and her family once a risk assessment (includes medical history, pregnancy, and previous complications) is completed as it may limit the woman's choices.

Place

A mother may give birth at home, in a birth centre, or midwife-led unit, or in a hospital consultant led unit. Healthy, low-risk mothers whose pregnancies are progressing normally can deliver with their midwife at home or in a midwife-led setting. Arrangements may change if complications occur in pregnancy and mother is referred to a consultant obstetrician. A mother may have a preference for a particular type of care e.g. epidural pain relief, which requires she is cared for in hospital.

Care in labour

During labour the mother will be cared for on a one-to-one basis by either her named midwife, if she is low risk, or another midwife from the same team. Mothers with high-risk pregnancies are cared for by a midwife from a high-risk team working alongside the consultant obstetrician. In a hospital setting also available if required are an obstetrician, anaesthetist, paediatrician, and operating department staff. It is very rare that mothers being cared for at home will require any assistance other than that of the midwife, however the midwife can call to her aid any of the above named individuals should the situation warrant this. A decision to transfer into hospital is made if there is any deviation from normal during the labour or birth.

Pain relief

Usually a discussion about such choices will have taken place during pregnancy and any preferences included in the birth plan. During labour in any setting a mother also has choices about how she will be cared for. She may wish to be upright and mobile and give birth in a standing, kneeling, squatting, all fours, or seated position. A range of pain relief is available including epidural analgesia (not in home deliveries), opiates, nitrous oxide, and oxygen. A range of complementary therapies may be available if the mother wishes to use these.

During pregnancy the uterus contracts painlessly and passively to assist circulation of blood to the uterine muscles and placenta. These are called Braxton Hicks contractions. At the end of pregnancy, hormone changes result in the uterus becoming more sensitive to oxytocin and so these formerly passive contractions become more active.

The process of labour

Initiation of labour

The cervix has to become softer and stretchier to allow it to dilate during labour. In a first time mother these changes start to occur from 36wks gestation. Prostaglandins are responsible for these changes and some mothers might experience a blood-stained mucous discharge as the cervix alters. This is because the protective plug sealing the cervix is disturbed as the cervix alters its shape and size.

First stage

- Effacement of the cervix i.e. the cervix gradually becomes shorter (3cm long to almost flat) as early labour contractions pull the cervical tissues up into the lower part of the uterus. These contractions can stop and start again several times before labour establishes.
- The cervix then gradually dilates until it is completely open in response to contractions and pressure from the baby's head.
- Meanwhile the membranes containing amniotic fluid in front of the baby's head start to bulge through the opening cervix. This 'bag' of water does not normally break until the cervix is fully open.
- The first stage of labour can last anything upto 12–18hrs.

Second stage

- This is characterized by the contractions becoming more expulsive in nature creating an almost uncontrollable urge to push as the descending baby's head is pressed against the rectum.
- The mother will push during contractions and gradually this stretches the perineum allowing the baby's head to be born. The next contraction delivers the baby's body.
- The second stage of labour can last from 30min to 1hr or more depending on the type of analgesia used. Use of epidural analgesia lengthens this stage as the mother does not experience bearing down sensations.

Third stage

The uterus continues to contract until the placenta and membranes deliver. Most women are offered an injection of syntocinon to prevent excessive bleeding during this stage which lasts 5–15min.

Further information for professionals and the public

- Midirs Informed Choice Information Leaflets for professionals and expectant parents: www.infochoice.org/
- NCT: www.nctpregnancyandbabycare.com/ ☎ 0870 444 8707

Complicated labour

Induction of labour

Labour may be induced with the mothers consent if the mother is 10d overdue, or if there are any concerns about maternal or fetal well-being at any other point during late pregnancy.
Key points:

- Induction methods aim to mimic normal labour so synthetic prostaglandin gel or pessaries are used to soften the cervix, followed by IV oxytocin which causes regular contractions to become established.
- The process of labour then continues as normal. Because the contractions are artificially induced they may be more painful, especially if rupture of the membranes is also performed.

Caesarean section

This operation is performed with the mother's consent if it is anticipated that a vaginal birth poses unacceptable risks to the mother and/or the baby. This can be planned in advance if a problem is identified before labour or be carried out in an emergency should a problem develop unexpectedly either during pregnancy or during labour.
Key points:

- It is common for this operation to be performed under epidural anaesthetic as this leads to reduced post-operative complications.
- Caesarean section on demand is discouraged as it is statistically more likely for a woman to die as a result of a caesarean birth than a vaginal birth.
- Postnatal recovery can be delayed due to giving birth by Caesarean section.
- Complications such as infection, urinary problems, haemorrhage, and thrombo-embolic disorders are managed by administering prophylactic antibiotics and low molecular weight heparin.
- Before surgery an indwelling urinary catheter is inserted to prevent urinary complications.
- Analgesia is usually required for a number of days/weeks after the birth. The mother stays in hospital 3–4d afterwards.
- Caesarean section can sometimes lead to delay in lactation so extra support is required by breast-feeding mothers (Breast feeding 📖).
- There are also some risks to the baby of being delivered by this method. These include difficulties establishing respiration, transient tachyapnoea of the newborn which requires admission to a special care baby unit (if delivered before 39wks gestation) scalpel cuts to the head, face, or neck area.

Forceps/ventouse

These instruments are used in 12% of births when either the mother or baby become tired or distressed or the second stage of labour is considered too slow. Having an epidural increases the risk of needing an instrumental delivery. After use of ventouse, oedema on baby's head can take up to 2wks to resolve (New babies 📖).

Episiotomy

This is a cut made by the midwife or doctor into the perineum under local or epidural anaesthetic. Its purpose is to enlarge the vaginal opening and assist birth. It can be performed if the baby is in distress and needs to be born quickly, or during an instrumental delivery to protect the vaginal wall, or to assist a slow birth. 12% of births are aided by episiotomy. Repaired with dissolvable stitches (as are tears). Heals in about 2wks. Advised by midwife on perineal hygiene, pain relief, and other remedies e.g. ice packs, warm baths that may ease discomfort.

Further information for professionals and the public

Midirs Informed Choice Information Leaflets for professionals and expectant parents www.infochoice.org/

NCT: www.nctpregnancyandbabycare.com/ ☎ 0870 444 8707

NICE Clinical guideline (2004). *Caesarean Section*: www.rcog.org.uk/

Postnatal care

The postnatal period is the time when the mother recovers from the birth, her reproductive and other organs regain their normal function, and lactation is established if she is breast feeding. She adjusts to motherhood and becomes confident in the care of her baby receiving advice and support initially from the midwife and subsequently from the HV. The midwife visits according to the needs of the mother and baby up to 28d (although may be involved up to 6wks. NB There is variation according to national and local frameworks), visiting frequently in the first 10d. The midwife liaises with the HV and in most instances the HV makes contact from day 10 (New birth visits 📖).

Most of the physical changes take place in the first 6wks after the birth. Social, psychological, and emotional adjustment can take considerably longer even up to a year after the birth. The rate at which a woman recovers will depend on several factors:
• Her health during pregnancy.
• The length of her labour.
• Whether the birth was complicated or uncomplicated.
• Whether the baby is healthy and makes normal progress.
• Whether there were any problems for mother or baby in the immediate postnatal period.
• The level of support she receives as she recovers.

Maternal health

At the first postnatal contact the mother will be offered information on the physiological process of recovery after birth and that some health problems are common. The midwife will advise the mother about the signs and symptoms of potentially life-threatening conditions and to contact a health-care professional immediately if any of the following occur:
• Sudden and profuse loss of blood or persistent increased blood loss.
• Signs and symptoms of infection.
• Headache in the first 72hrs accompanied by visual disturbances, vomiting, or feeling faint.
• Signs and symptoms of thrombo-embolism.
• If the mother has not passed urine within 6hrs of birth.

During the 1st wk after birth the mother is given guidance and advice on the following:
• Tiredness, a normal consequence of new parenthood.
• Perineal hygiene or care of a Caesarian wound.
• Involuntary leakage of small amounts of urine, commonly experienced after birth.
• Haemorrhoids, common in the postnatal period.
• The importance of an appropriate diet and fluid intake.
• Contact details for expert contraceptive advice.
• Intercourse: may be uncomfortable at first and that contraception (Contraception: general 📖) should be used by 21d post birth.
• Normal patterns of emotional changes.

The mother is advised to contact a midwife, GP, or HV if:
• Any changes in mood outside of the normal pattern
• Itching or bleeding around the anus
• Faecal urgency or frank faecal incontinence.

Between 2–6wks the mother advised to contact a midwife, GP, or HV if:
• Still bleeding after 6wks
• If sex still painful
• If severe, long-lasting backache stopping normal daily activities.

Midwife and HV remain alert to signs of domestic violence during this period (Domestic violence ▢).

Infant feeding

Infant feeding information and advice is given during the 1st wk. The midwife will support each mother in her feeding method of choice (Breast feeding ▢ and Bottle feeding and weaning ▢) and knows to contact midwife or GP urgently if signs of mastitis (flu-like symptoms, red and painful breasts).

Infant health

At each postnatal contact the parents are offered information and advice to help them to assess their baby's general condition, identify warning signs to look for if their baby is unwell, and how to contact a health-care professional or emergency service if required.

The midwife will assess the physical well-being of the baby during each postnatal contact as well as advising the parents on:
• Parenting and attachment, the social capabilities of the baby.
• Neonatal screening: obtaining the neonatal blood spot screen.
• Health promotion and well baby care including skin, thrush infection, nappy rash, constipation, diarrhoea, colic, fever, jaundice, vitamin K, and care of the umbilicus before and after cord separation.
• Each visit is an opportunity to evaluate relevant safety issues, safety equipment, and reinforce the recommendations about sudden infant death and co-sleeping.
• The midwife will be alert to risk factors and signs of child abuse and children in need.

Either the midwife or the HV will give the parents PHCHR and a NHS produced child health promotion book e.g. the *Birth to Five* book according to local protocols.

Further information for professionals and parents

NICE (July 2006). *Postnatal Care: routine postnatal care of women and their babies.* Professional and public versions www.nice.org.uk

Postnatal depression

Definition

A depressive illness, occurs following childbirth during the first 12mths and lasts for several wks/mths. It appears more long-lasting and debilitating than depression at other times. It occurs in 10–15% of women. It is distinguishable from postnatal 'blues' (i.e. brief low mood felt at some point by many women in first 2wks postnatally) by greater severity and longer duration. It is also distinguishable from more severe postpartum psychosis (symptoms include loss of contact with reality, hallucinations, severe thought disturbance) which only occurs in 2:2000 births and requires immediate medical assessment and treatment.

Causes

- Unknown, probably no single reason.
- In some cases, it is the result of hormonal changes.
- Stress of looking after a young baby, having sleep disrupted may also help to bring on illness in susceptible people.

Risk factors

- Main risk factor is a previous history of depression.
- Others include:
  - Stressful life events especially during pregnancy (negative life events, previous miscarriage/stillbirth).
  - Family and marital difficulties (poor marital relationship, conflict between woman and parents).
  - Inadequate levels of social support.
  - Personality factors, attitudes (perfectionism, low self-esteem, negative maternal attitudes towards child rearing).
  - Mood during pregnancy.
  - FH of depression.
  - Infant temperament and mother–infant difficulties.
  - Early experiences (poor relationship with own mother, history of sexual abuse).
  - Unrealistic expectations of motherhood.

Symptoms

- Variable but persist most of the time.
- Low mood, tearfulness/crying, anxiety/panic attacks, self-blame/guilt, undue health worries, lethargy/tiredness, irritability, ↓ appetite, inadequacy, emotionally labile, loss of interest in activities.

Onset

- Usually develops within the first 3mths following childbirth.
- Second peak at 6–8mths postpartum.

Assessment and management

Assessment

- Should be a through, simple, brief self-report on symptoms of depression as above (People with depression 📖).

- Edinburgh Postnatal Depression Scale (EPDS) is *not* a screening tool but it is however incorporated within many HVs' routine postpartum care. Many treat the EPDS as a screening tool but it has not been ratified by Screening Committee (see UK screening programmes ⏚). SIGN guidance (see below) suggests EPDS should only be administered by trained professionals at about 6wks and 3mths, and a score of 10 or above should be used in whole population use. Local protocols apply in the management and referral to GP and mental health services of women identified at different levels of risk.
- Primary prevention focuses on raising awareness antenatally, and provision of extra support and the prevention of social isolation e.g. through schemes such as Homestart and Newpin (see Working with parents ⏚ and Parenting programmes ⏚). Additional 'listening visits' may be offered by HVs to women identified as at 'at risk' of depression.
- Management of women diagnosed with postnatal depression is as for any depression (see People with depression ⏚). It may include 'listening visits' by HVs, non-directive counselling, dynamic psychotherapy, CBT (see Talking therapies ⏚), and antidepressants. Occasionally hospital admission to a mother and baby unit is necessary. Additional support may be required to aid the mother and child relationship (see Working with parents ⏚ and Parenting programmes ⏚), and prevent social isolation.
- Women diagnosed with puerperal psychosis are managed in the same way as any psychotic illness (see People with schizophrenia ⏚) and may be admitted to a mother and baby unit.

Potential long-term effects
- Woman's mental health, may predispose for future postnatal depression.
- Mother–infant relationship. It may have a negative influence on this relationship and future child development.
- It may have a negative effect on partner/marital relationship.

Further information for professionals
📖 NICE (2006). *Postnatal Care: routine postnatal care of women and their babies*. Professional and public versions: www.nice.org.uk
📖 Royal College of Psychiatrists: www.rcpsych.ac.uk
📖 SIGN Guideline 60 (2002). *Postnatal Depression and Puerperal Psychosis*. www.sign.ac.uk/guidelines/fulltext/60/index.html

Further information for parents
📖 Association for Postnatal Depression: www.apni.org
📖 Net Mums: www.netmums.com

Vulnerable groups with extra needs

Asylum seekers and refugees

The UK is signatory to the 1951 UN Convention relating to the Status of Refugees. Most refugees and asylum seekers in the UK are from areas of conflict and are single men <40yrs. In 2004 it was estimated 250,000 asylum seekers and refugees were living in London (see essential reading below).

In the UK:
- A person is recognised as a **refugee** only when their application for asylum has been accepted by the Home Office.
- An **asylum seeker** is a person that has lodged an asylum claim with the Immigration and Nationality Directorate at the Home Office and is waiting for a decision on their claim.

Refugees

Refugees have full entitlement to family reunion, welfare benefits, housing and health care, and have the right to work. Since August 2005 refugees have been granted limited (rather than indefinite) leave to remain, initially for 5yrs. At which point their case will be reviewed again and they may have to return to their own country or be given indefinite leave to remain. Those not recognized as refugees, within the terms of the Refugee Convention, but can demonstrate a need for international protection, may be granted Humanitarian Protection or Discretionary Leave.

Asylum seekers

The National Asylum Support Service (NASS) is the government body that normally looks after people who are seeking asylum in the UK. Policy is to disperse asylum seekers from London and the South East to across the UK. Asylum seekers are not dispersed from London if receiving care from the Medical Foundation for the Care of Victims of Torture. NASS provides support, furnished accommodation, and a weekly allowance (70% income support for adults 100% for children (Benefits for people with a low income)). Asylum seekers are not allowed to work after they make their asylum application. They have a right to primary health care (NHS entitlements). After a decision on their application:
- If asylum claim unsuccessful, NASS support stops 21d after the decision (unless appealed against).
- If the decision is to give leave to remain, indefinite leave to remain, humanitarian protection, or discretionary leave to remain, NASS support stops 28d after the decision, including leaving the NASS accommodation (Homes and housing).

Unaccompanied children

See Children in special circumstances.

Health issues

The health problems of asylum seekers and refugees are dependent on:
- The communicable diseases, disease patterns, and availability of health services to them in their home country.
- The events that led them to flee their country e.g. civil war, persecution, imprisonment, and torture.

- The events that have happened to them while travelling to the country of asylum and their treatment in the UK.

Refugees and asylum seekers are not homogeneous. Health-care needs have to be assessed individually. While all refugees and asylum seekers have experienced loss, they also demonstrate great resilience and courage in facing enormous challenges and losses. Key issues for health-care professionals:

- Ensuring good communication (Communication with people who have English as an additional language 📖) using interpreters and advocates.
- A recognition of different cultural attitudes to norms in health and expectations of health-care services.
- Recognizing that asylum status may make accessing health-care services problematic. e.g. temporary accommodation, may be moved on at short notice, if in hostel accommodation may have to be present at meal times or may not eat.

Essential reading

📖 Burnett, A. and Fassil, Y. (2002). *Meeting the health needs of refugees and asylum seekers in the UK*. A NHS UK wide Information and Resource Pack. Available at: www.dh.gov.uk/publicationsandstatistics

Further information for professionals

📖 HARPWEB information, practical tools in health issues relating to refugees in UK: www.harpweb.org.uk/

Further information for patients and clients

📖 National Asylum Support Service: www.ind.homeoffice.gov.uk
📖 Refugee Council: www.refugeecouncil.org.uk/

Homeless people

The UK has legal definitions of homelessness (Homes and housing 📖).
LAs have a legal duty to provide advice to all those who meet the criteria
and duty to provide accommodation to groups legally eligible for assistance (see Homes and housing 📖).

Homeless people who do not meet these criteria are referred to as
single homeless people and include:

- Hostel residents
- Rough sleepers
- Homeless asylum seekers who are no longer receiving support from the
  National Asylum Support System (Asylum seekers and refugees 📖).

Single homeless

Numbers are difficult to estimate but thought to be 310,000 and 380,000
single homeless people in the UK. One-quarter of these live in hostels or
bed and breakfast accommodation, or are facing imminent threat of evic-
tion through debt. Three-quarters like in what are known as concealed
households, with friends or family, often in unsatisfactory accommodation.
Rough sleepers account for approx. 1000 of this population. The average
life expectancy of a rough sleeper is 42yrs.

> Rough sleepers will access primary care health services provided that
> they are provided in an appropriate and sensitive way.

Causes of homelessness

Complex interrelated and different for different age groups (see Related
topics below).

- Mental health needs
- Family breakdown
- Abuse or violence in the home
- Alcohol, drug, and substance misuse
- Debt and unemployment
- Leaving armed forces, prison, or residential care (e.g. looked-after children).

Policy in all countries of UK is to address complex problems of single
homeless and ensure minimal numbers of rough sleepers.

Health needs

In addition to health needs that have contributed to homelessness people are vulnerable to a wide range of health problems:

> However homeless people 40 times more likely not to register with a
> GP than members of the general population.

- 30–50% of homeless people have mental health problems including
  depression
- 70% misuse drugs (Substance misuse 📖)
- TB (📖) and respiratory problems
- Hepatitis (📖)
- Skin problems (Bacterial skin conditions 📖; Eczema/dermatitis 📖;
  Fungal infections 📖)

- Malnutrition
- Antenatal and postnatal complications.

Needs of homeless children: see 📖 Children in special circumstances.

Access to health care

Government priority is to improve homeless peoples' access to health care. Expectations that:
- Primary care organizations and LA have local plans for improving access to health care of families in temporary accommodation and homeless people particularly in areas of known health need.
- Close liaison between mental health service providers, charitable providers, and primary health care.
- In urban areas where there are higher numbers of homelessness more likely to be specialist providers/teams and GPs offering enhanced services (General practice 📖).

Access to help with housing

Local CABs and Housing Advice Centres are key resources for advice and help on housing issues.

Emergency accommodation found through Shelter national helpline ☎ 0808 800 4444 and local council: provision variable.
- Night shelters: free, often found in redundant public buildings e.g. old churches and halls. One night's accommodation.
- Hostels: provide a few nights to a few mths, require payment and often need to book ahead (payment through housing benefits, jobseekers allowance etc.). Some have entry criteria e.g. age, no substance abuse, religious and cultural background.
- Nightstop for young 16–25-year-olds single homeless for 1 night only provided by people with spare rooms (see below).
- Foyers for young people provide accommodation up to 9mths and provide support to acquire new skills and long-term housing.
- Support and advice for other forms of accommodation such as bed and breakfast (subject to eligibility), housing association, council housing and private rental can be accessed through local council, homeless outreach teams (charitable or council based) and main homeless charities e.g. Shelter, Crisis.

Related topics

📖 Asylum seekers and refugees; 📖 Alcohol; 📖 People with depression; 📖 Substance misuse; 📖 Homes and housing.

Further information for health professionals

📓 Crisis Homeless Charity: www.crisis.org
📓 Nightstop services for young homless people: www.nightstop-uk.org
📓 Policy briefing on homelessness Office of the Deputy Prime Minister: www.odpm.gov.uk
📓 Shelter advice for homeless people: www.shelter.org.uk

Travellers and gypsies

Definition of terms

- *Traveller*: overarching term covering various groups of *gypsies and travellers* in the UK.
- *Romany Gypsies, Irish Travellers* (recognized minority ethnic groups).
- *New Travellers* (not a recognized ethnic group).
- Also covers *Scottish Travellers, European Roma, Show people* (fairground and circus people), and *Bargees* (occupational boat dwellers).

Gypsies and travellers in the UK

- Estimated numbers of Romany Gypsies and Irish Travellers: 300,000.[1]
- Legally covered under the terms of the Race Relations (Amendment) Act (2000).
- One of most marginalized ethnic minorities in the UK; subject to widespread prejudice.

Accommodation

Trailers (caravans) on privately owned or rented sites, or on unauthorized encampments (due to limited site availability). Cultural importance of close proximity to extended family for support and well-being. Possibly half the population lives in houses. House dwelling is associated with long-term illness, poorer health state, and anxiety.

Health profile

Gypsies and travellers have significantly worse health than the general population. ↑ respiratory problems, anxiety and depression, excess prevalence of stillbirths, neonatal deaths, and premature death of older offspring. Possibly the highest maternal death rate among all minority ethnic groups. Research in Leeds and Ireland shows ↓ life expectancy and ↑ mortality rates for all causes, than the general population.[1]

Access to services

There is an inverse relationship between their health needs and use of health and related services. Contributory factors:

- Reluctance of GPs to register travellers or visit sites.
- Practical problems of access.
- Mismatch of expectations between travellers and health staff, accompanied by travellers' defensive expectation of racist attitudes from health staff.
- Attitudinal barriers and cultural inappropriateness of service delivery.
- Lack of readily available health records for continuity of care.
- Low literacy levels and poor knowledge of services amongst travellers.

Good practice guidance

- Never make assumptions about cultural practices—ask!
- Use client-held and PHCHR health records (Client- and patient-held records 📖).
- Seek advice and support from specialist health workers for gypsies and travellers.

[1] Parry, G. et al. (2004). *Health status of gypsies and travellers in England*. Department of Health Research Report 121/7500, University of Sheffield.

- Maximize opportunistic health promotion and protection, e.g. 📖 Child immunization.
- Consider provision of services to sites if no specialist health workers are already doing so.

At an organizational level:

- Involve gypsies and travellers in cultural competence training of health service staff.
- Use specialist health workers in partnership with gypsy and traveller communities and agencies to address wider determinants of health through community development and capacity development (Community approaches to health 📖).
- Include in NHS ethnic monitoring to address 'invisibility' in public health terms.

Related topics

📖 Anti-discriminatory health care; 📖 Professional conduct.

Further information for professionals

A better road: An information booklet for health care and other professionals. Derbyshire Gypsy Liaison Group, c/o Ernest Bailey Community Centre, Office 3, New Street, Matlock DE4 3FE

📓 CPHVA special interest group: www.msfcphva.org/sigs/sigtravellers.html
📓 Friends, Families and Travellers: www.Gypsy-Traveller.org
📓 Gypsy & Traveller Law Reform Coalition: www.travellerslaw.org.uk
📓 Irish Traveller Movement: www.itmtrav.com
📓 Irish Travellers organization in Dublin: www.paveepoint.ie
📓 The Gypsy Council: www.thegypsycouncil.org

Domestic violence

'Any incident of threatening behaviour, violence, or abuse (psychological, physical, sexual, financial, or emotional) between adults who are or have been intimate partners or family members, regardless of gender or sexuality'.[1] Describes a continuum of behaviour ranging from verbal, physical, emotional, and sexual abuse, to rape and murder.

In the UK:
- Majority of victims (>90%) are women
- Affects about 1 in 4 ♀, 1 in 6 ♀ in life time
- 2 ♀ murdered every week by partners, 40% after separation
- Estimated that ♀ suffer at least 35 assaults before contacting police
- Violence starts in 30% cases during pregnancy
- >52% of reported ♀ rapes committed by current or former partner
- Estimated over 30,000 children affected each year
- In 50% cases where mother abused, children also abused
- >50% child protection cases involve domestic violence.

Impact not just on ♀ health but also on children—both ♀ and children likely to have long-term emotional and mental consequences. ♀ stay in abusive relationships for many reasons including self-blame, shame, loss of confidence, fear of losing children, financial dependency, fear that no one will believe them.

Potential indicators of domestic violence
Include:
- Multiple injuries at various stages of healing to areas such as breast, genitals, and abdomen.
- Explanations vague or inconsistent with injuries.
- Partner insists on being present at all appointments, speaks for ♀.
- ♀ appears depressed, or overly anxious.
- ♀ fails to attend for medical appointments, comply with treatment.
Women are particularly at risk during pregnancy and following separation from a violent partner.

Key principles in the role of health professionals
- Create a supportive environment that allows ♀ to talk.
- Ask ♀ (only if alone) direct questions about domestic violence (see selective and routine enquiry below).
- Have information on local agencies that can help, readily available and in a format that ♀ can easily conceal.
- Keep the ♀'s safety in mind and that of any children (see risk assessment below).
- Know how to refer the ♀ to local support agencies if that is what the ♀ chooses, respecting their decisions.
- Document all discussions and assessments accurately.
- Never try to mediate between partners, ensure own and colleagues' safety.

[1] 🔲 Home Office (2005). *Domestic Violence a National Report Plan*: www.crimereduction.gov.uk/domesticviolence51.htm

Selective enquiry is asking the ♀ directly if she is experiencing violence or fear of violence from another adult in the home when there are indicators suggesting it might be a possibility.

Routine enquiry is undertaken when HVs, midwives, and GPs routinely ask women about domestic violence as part of their overall health assessment. All PCOs are developing inter-agency policies/training on the introduction of routine enquiry as part of UK wide government initiatives to reduce domestic violence. Routine enquiry includes being clear on the limits of confidentiality (Confidentiality 📖).

On disclosure of domestic violence

- Reassure, support, give national helpline (see below) and local specialist domestic violence services contact details e.g. women's refuge, police domestic violence unit.
- Undertake a risk assessment with ♀ to determine extent of danger.
- High risk includes children present, pregnant, previous violence, alcohol and/or drug misuse, weapons present, stalking, separation, suicide threat.

❶ If immediate risk e.g. partner acting aggressively in the same building, call police.

❶ If children in household follow local child protection procedures (Child protection processes 📖).

❶ If high risk seek senior clinician/manager support to follow multi-agency guidelines.

- If low risk of danger then help ♀ think through need for a safety plan if still living with perpetrator (e.g. think about escape routes, calling 999 if violence starts, keep money and keys easy to grab) and if now living separately (e.g. changing locks, think about escape routes).
- Document fully in records all observations, actions, and events.

Related topics

📖 Abuse of vulnerable adults.

Further information for professionals

DoH (England) (2005). *Responding to domestic abuse: A handbook for health professionals* DoH, London. NB All county's updating guidance.

Further information and sources of help for victims of domestic violence

🖳 Refuge www.refuge.org.uk (includes links to UK wide domestic violence services and information)

🖳 The hideout web based support for children and young people experiencing domestic violence www.thehideout.org.uk

☎ UK National Domestic Violence 24hrs Helpline Freephone 0808 2000 247

🖳 Womens' Aid www.womensaid.org.uk/

Abuse of vulnerable adults

A vulnerable adult is one who is unable to take care of themselves and/or unable to protect him or herself against significant harm or exploitation through mental or other disability, illness, and/or age.

Abuse is a violation of human and/or civil rights and may be one off or repeated acts of physical, psychological, sexual, financial (includes theft as well as intimidation about wills), discriminatory (includes hate crime) abuses, or acts of omission or neglect. Most abuse is a criminal offence and the police lead the investigations (see below).

Patterns of abuse may take different dynamics e.g. may be opportunistic or involve repeated acts by person in position of power over another or long-term slow increase in violations (e.g. grooming). Perpetrators may be household members, carers, neighbours, professionals, or multiple staff members in institutions where neglect, acts of omission, use of punishment e.g. withholding medication, have become a cultural norm.

Predisposing factors may include: carer stress, vulnerable adults living with financially dependent family members, vulnerable person isolated, personal or family history of violence, abuse, alcohol, or drug misuse.

Acting on concerns

Often when anxieties or concerns are raised about possible abuse of a vulnerable adult, it is not clear the extent or nature of the harm.

All primary care staff receiving allegations or having concerns about harm or possible harm to vulnerable adults (either by informal carers/family/neighbours or professional/carer) should discuss this with their line manager or named senior clinician and follow local agreed multi-agency procedures for protection of vulnerable adults (POVA).

All areas should have agreed multi-agency procedures, often follows the model of those for child protection. Social services has the key coordinating role. Every PCO should ensure that each surgery and nursing team has copies or internet access to the policies.

Concerns for vulnerable adults at home should be referred to social services as per local guidance. Many areas have a facility for a pre-referral consultation with the designated social service officers (DSO). The procedures usually involving in-depth assessment of the level and impact of the abuse, the individual's safety, rights, and views. This may lead to police involvements and decision to offer an immediate place of safety or the DSO may convene a multi-agency case conference to establish the facts, and plan to prevent further abuse.

Key principles include:
• Active interagency collaboration
• Active empowerment of the individual through the services provided

- Supports the rights of the individual to lead an independent life
- Recognizes the right to self determination involves risk
- Ensures the individual receives the full protection of the law.

Concerns about a care service

Everyone has a duty to report any allegations or suspicions of abuse or potential abuse of a vulnerable adult either to their immediate line manager or to discuss their initial concerns with the social services agency, the regulatory authorities, or the police. Local agreed procedures should be followed. Suspected abuse by staff of a regulated service e.g. care agency, care home, is also reported to the relevant regulatory bodies.

Whistle blowing

Individual staff members should also be aware of policies supporting 'whistle blowing' (Whistle blowing 📖).

Situations of immediate danger or need for emergency treatment

Primary care staff should call for police or ambulance without referring to a senior staff member.

Disclosure of abuse

- Listen carefully and allow them to tell as much as they want to at that point, don't press for details.
- Be sympathetic, non-judgmental, reassure them it is not their fault.
- Explain this has to be shared to get them the help they require.
- Discuss with senior staff member and refer to social services/police as per local guidelines.
- Document in detail the disclosure conversation as soon as possible.

Related topics

📖 Domestic violence; 📖 Crime and victims of crime; 📖 People with learning difficulties; 📖 Child Protection; 📖 Key facts on carers and caring.

Further information for professionals and public

- Action on Elder Abuse: www.elderabuse.org.uk ☎ Response line: 020 8679 7074
- DoH (England) (2000). *No secrets: guidance on policies and procedures to protect vulnerable adults*: www.dh.gov.uk
- Practitioners Alliance Against Abuse of Vulnerable Adults: www. pavauk.org.uk//home/home
- Witness. A UK charity supporting victims of abuse by health and care staff: www.popan.org.uk ☎ Helpline: 08454 500 300

Crime and victims of crime

UK public perceive levels of crime and anti-social behaviour as higher than surveys and reporting suggest:

- <80% of all crimes are reported to the police. Common assault and sexual assault least likely to be reported.
- Young men aged 16–24yrs most at risk of being a victim of violent crime.
- Eight metropolitan areas account for >40% of all recorded crimes in England and Wales, 40% of all UK reported robberies occur in London. No geographical variation in reported domestic violence (Domestic violence 📖).
- Distraction burglaries (i.e. bogus callers) target older people.
- About 15% of victims of violent crime require medical attention.
- No injuries in >70% mugging, >50% assaults by acquaintances or strangers, <30% domestic violence (Domestic violence 📖).
- Sexual offences account for 5% of recorded crime. 93% of victims of reported rapes ♀.

Source: 🖥 *Home Office Crime Reduction resource:* www.crimereduction. gov.uk

Crime reduction

- Crime & Disorder Reduction Partnerships (CDRPs) involve the police, local authorities, PCOs, other organizations and businesses in developing local strategies for tackling crime and disorder. This may include schemes such as Neighbourhood Watch.
- All police forces have crime prevention officers to give public and victims of crime advice on personal and property security.
- LAs usually have a lead contact for addressing anti-social behaviour (includes problem neighbours, vandalism, fly-tipping, graffitti).
- Anti-Social Behavior Orders (ASBO) are court orders to protect public from behaviour that is likely to cause distress, alarm, or harassment.

Reporting crimes

Important in order to catch criminals and prevent further crime. For some types of crime also require a police crime number to claim compensation through insurance or to claim criminal injuries compensation (see below).

- *Emergencies*: dial 999.
- *Non-emergency crimes* reported at local police station, some crimes like thefts, criminal damage, vehicle damage, hate crimes and hate incidents (defined as any incident on persons or property because of a particular persons ethnicity, sexual orientation, religion, political opinion, or disability), can also be reported to the police online (🖥 www.online.police.uk).
- *Anonymously* via Crimestoppers, an independent charity for reporting information about crime and criminals and passes on to police. 🖥 www.crimestoppers-uk.org ☎ 0800 555 111.

Post-assault consultations with health professionals

Victims may need physical and psychological care, as well as considering the need to collect forensic evidence.

Assault: any professional consulted should document carefully extent of injuries as may be required for legal purposes. Measurements and photos if possible of injuries should be taken. Encourage victim to report to police.

Rape or sexual assault: if victim is willing to report assault then should not be examined except by specialist trained in collecting forensic evidence. Most areas now have sexual assault referral centres i.e. one stop shop offering medical care, counselling, collection of forensic evidence, and police investigation into the alleged offences.

Victims unwilling to access such services should be offered medical examination, assessed for need for EC, STI screening, offered prophylactic antibiotics, assessed for need for HIV prophylaxis. Also offered counselling and information on support organizations.

Victims of crime

Many people experience a range of emotions including anger, fear, anxiety, sorrow after a crime, depending on the type and consequences. Counselling and opportunities to talk through the experience may help many victims (see victim support below). Some assault victims and many sexual assault victims develop post traumatic stress disorder (PTSD), with symptoms such as flashbacks, leading to insomnia, depression etc. Referral to either counselling services or psychology services as appropriate.

Victim Support: national charity that works with police, in some areas receives referrals and provides free and confidential support for victims of crime and witness support (see below).

Criminal Injuries Compensation Scheme: aims to provide blameless victims with material recognition of their pain and suffering and to allow society to express its regret to them. Level of compensation set in a tariff determined by Parliament. Individual applies directly. England, Wales, and Scotland: 🖥 www.cica.gov.uk Northern Ireland: 🖥 www.compensationni.gov.uk/

Further information for professionals and public

🖥 Rape Crisis Centres for advice, support, and counselling www.rapecrisis.org.uk/
🖥 Sexual Assault Referral Centres locations in England and Wales:
  www.homeoffice.gov.uk/crime-victims/reducing-crime/sexual-offences/
🖥 UK Police Services: www.police.uk
🖥 Victim Support UK: www.victimsupport.org ☎ 0845 30 30 900

Standards of care for people with mental health problems

Each country of the UK is working to improve and develop a long-term strategy, for mental health services. The NSF for Mental Health (DH1999) across England for adults up to 65yrs clarifies what the National Standards are for service provision and what they aim to achieve (see equivalent guidance on websites for Wales, Scotland, and Northern Ireland, NHS in Northern Ireland, Scotland, and Wales 📖). The following summarizes the key principles:

Aims

- To ensure that health and social services promote mental health and reduce discrimination and social exclusion.
- To deliver better primary mental health care, and to ensure consistent advice and help for people with mental health needs, including primary care services for individuals with severe mental illness.
- To ensure that each person with severe mental illness receives the range of mental health services they need and that crises are anticipated and prevented where possible.
- To ensure that people in crisis receive prompt and effective help, and timely access to an appropriate and safe mental health place or hospital bed, including a secure bed, as close to home as possible.
- To ensure health and social services assess the needs of carers for those with severe mental illness, and provide care to meet their needs.
- To ensure that health and social services play their full part in achieving the target of reducing the suicide rate.

Mental health promotion

- Promote mental health for all, working with individuals and communities.
- Combat discrimination against individuals and groups, and promote their social inclusion.

Primary care and access to services

Service users who contact their primary health team with a common mental health problem should:

- Have their mental health needs identified and assessed.
- Be offered effective treatments, including referral to specialist services for further assessment, treatment, and care if they need it.
- Be able to make contact with local mental health services 24hrs a day and receive adequate care.
- Be able to use NHS Direct for first level advice and referral to specialist helplines or to local services.

Effective services for people with serious mental illness

- Receive care that optimizes engagement and anticipates or prevents a crisis thereby reducing risk.
- Have a copy of their written care plan which:
  - States the action to be taken in a crisis by the service user, their carer, and their care coordinator.

- Advises the GP how they should respond if the service user needs additional help.
- Is regularly reviewed by the care coordinator.
- Enables them to access services 24hrs a day, 365d per year.

Service users who are assessed as needing a period of care away from their home should have:

- Timely access to an appropriate hospital bed or place which is:
  - In the least restrictive environment, and consistent with the need to protect them and the public.
  - As close to home as possible.
- A copy of a written care plan, agreed on discharge, which sets out their care and rehabilitation, identifies their care coordinator, and specifies the action to be taken in a crisis.

Caring about carers

All carers or people who provide regular and substantial care for a person on CPA (Care Programme Approach) should:

- Have an assessment of their caring, physical, and mental health needs repeated on at least an annual basis.
- Have their own written care plan given to them, and implemented with them.

Preventing suicide

Local health and social care services should aim to prevent suicides by:

- Combining all the above standards into a local delivery plan based on local need.
- Support local prison staff in preventing suicides among prisoners.
- Ensure that staff are competent to assess the risk of suicide among individuals.
- Develop a local system for suicide audit, to learn lessons and take any necessary action.

🖳 The full document is available at www.dh.gov.uk

Related topics

📖 Key facts on carers and caring; 📖 Mental capacity.

Further information for professional

🖳 DH (1998). A First Class Service: Quality in the new NHS: www.dh.gov.uk
🖳 DH (1999). Saving Lives: Our Healthier Nation: www.dh.gov.uk
🖳 DH (2002). Modernising mental health services: www.dh.gov.uk

Adapted from Callaghan P., Waldock, H. *Oxford Handbook of Mental Health Nursing*. By permission of Oxford University Press.

Patients receiving antipsychotic medication

Antipsychotic medication is a common form of treatment for psychotic illnesses such as schizophrenia. It can be administered either orally or by depot injection. Choice of administration depends on past history of drug effectiveness, preference, tolerability and adherence. It is often prescribed alongside psychosocial interventions. (Talking therapies 📖.)

Monitoring

Antipsychotic medication can cause distressing and disabling side effects. These include extra pyramidal symptoms i.e.:
- Parkinsonism
- Dystonia
- Akathisia.

Need to be monitored to help the patient cope with them, help to ↓ effects and ↑ adherence.

If a patient is taking antipsychotic medication, any consultation is a good opportunity to assess the patient's general health, monitor for side effects, and liaise with GP or Community Mental Health Team (CMHT) key worker if there are problems.

Assessment tools

- Liverpool University Neuroleptic Side Effect Rating Scale (LUNSERS).
- A simple 14 item checklist to use is the Side Effects Scale/Checklist for Antipsychotic Medication (SESCAM).[1]

Face/mouth/neck

- Unchanged facial expression (e.g. rigid looking face with little spontaneous movement)
- Increased salivation
- Involuntary movements of mouth, lips, or tongue
- Looking sleepy.

Extremities

- Tremor/involuntary movements of fingers, hands, arms ie pill rolling
- Restlessness of feet/legs.

Trunk/posture/gait

- Pelvic gyrations
- Rigid shuffling gait
- Reduced arm swinging
- Slowness and reduced spontaneity.

General

- Dizziness
- Drowsiness
- Sexual problems (ejaculatory/erectile/libido/menstrual)

---

[1] Walker, H. and MacAulay, K. (2005). Assessment of the side effects of antipsychotic medication *Nursing Standard* **12**, 40, 41–46.

- Constipation
- Urinary problems
- Skin problems
- Excessive weight gain
- Blurred vision
- Lack of energy.

Management of side effects and support

Side effects need to be managed in discussion with GP or whoever is prescribing medical treatment; patient's case worker and/or CMHT Commonly achieved by dose titration and/or addition of other pharmacological treatments.

Some general advice on side effects and strategies

- Appetite increase: eat a low fat, high fibre diet; avoid sugary or fatty foods; drink low-calorie soft drinks.
- Constipation: increase exercise, dietary fibre and fluid intake (Constipation in adults 📖).
- Dizziness: get up slowly from lying or sitting; avoid excessively hot showers or baths; avoid alcohol, sedatives or other sedating drugs e.g. marijuana.
- If possible take medication before bedtime (discuss with GP first).
- Dry mouth: ensure regular fluid intake; limit alcohol and caffeine; use sugarless gums, fruit pastilles and lollies; suck on ice cubes.
- Sensitivity to sunburn: avoid midday sun; regularly use sunscreen and wear a hat, sunglasses and shirt (Skin cancer protection 📖).

Related topics

📖 People with bipolar affective disorder; 📖 People with schizophrenia.

Further information for health professionals, patients and families

Callaghan, P. and Waldock, H. (2006). *Oxford Handbook of Mental Health Nursing.* Oxford University Press, Oxford.

📖 Rethink www.rethink.org ☎ General Enquires 0845 456 0455; National Advice Service 0208 974 6814

People with eating disorders

Anorexia nervosa

A condition where there is a marked distortion of body image, low weight, and weight loss behaviours. 0.5% of adolescent and young women develop anorexia nervosa. 1:10 ratio of ♂:♀ with an equal distribution across social classes with mostly upper and middle class people seeking treatment. Mortality rate of 10–15% ($^2/_3$ due to physical complications and $^1/_3$ due to suicide).[1]

Presentation

- Low body weight: 15% below expected BMI (BMI charts 📖).
- Self induced weight loss; vomiting, purging, excessive exercise, use of appetite suppressants.
- Body image distortion: dread of fatness, imposed low weight threshold.
- Patients with symptoms of starvation: sensitivity to cold, bradycardia, low BP, hypothermia, constipation.
- Children with poor growth.
- Amenorrhoea, reduced sexual interest or impotence, small body frame, altered thyroid function.
- Delayed puberty: if the onset is prior to puberty.
- Endocrine disorders: involving the hypothalamus, pituitary, or adrenal glands.

Causes

- Genetic: 6–10% of female siblings develop the condition.
- Life events: physical or sexual abuse can be a risk factors.
- Psychodynamic:
  - Family relationships may be rigid, over protective, weak parental boundaries, lack of conflict resolution.
  - Individual: disturbed body image due to dietary problems in early life, parents' preoccupation with food, lack of sense of identity.
  - Analytical: regression to childhood, fixation on the oral stage, avoidance of problems in adolescence.

Related problems and complications

Patients who are pregnant or have diabetes are at particular risk, everyone involved in their care should be aware of the eating disorder.

- Mental health problems: poor memory, irritability, depression, low self-esteem, loss of libido, reduced decision making.
- Physical problems: fatigue, cold, fainting and dizziness, reduced immunity, amenorrhea, hair loss, dry skin.
- Loss of muscle mass, brittle nails.
- Anaemia.
- Calluses on finger joints, eroded teeth enamel.
- Hypotension, bradycardia.
- Atrophy of the breasts.
- Swollen tender abdomen.
- Loss of sensation in extremities.

[1] 📖 Eating Disorder Association www.edauk.com

Screening questions

- Do you worry excessively about your weight?
- Do you think you have an eating problem?

Treatment

Referral to specialist eating disorder clinic where available. If treated, $^1/_3$ of patients make a full recovery, $^1/_3$ make a partial recovery, and $^1/_3$ have chronic problems.

- Often treated as an outpatient, with a combined approach including:
  - Pharmacological: antidepressants, medication to stimulate appetite.
  - Psychological: family therapy (may be effective if early onset). Individual therapy such as CBT (Talking therapies 🕮) may improve long-term outcomes.
  - Education: nutritional, self-help manuals.
- Hospital admission if there are serious medical problems. Compulsory admission when feeding is regarded as treatment. Ethical issues around a person's right to die, and their right to treatment.
- Offer ongoing support and information to patient and families if no ongoing 2° care patients should receive annual physical and mental check up.
- Poor prognostic factors include: chronic illness, late age onset, bulimic features, and anxiety when eating with others, excessive weight loss, poor childhood social adjustment, poor parental relationships, males.

Bulimia nervosa

Characterized by:

- Recurrent episodes of binge eating well in excess of normally accepted amounts of food.
- Inappropriate behaviors to prevent increase in weight e.g. vomiting, use of laxatives and diuretics, appetite suppressants.
- People with bulimia can be divided into those who purge and those that just use fasting and exercise to control their weight.

Management

- Evidence based self-help programmes (see below).
- Refer to GP for assessment for antidepressants. If unsuccessful referral to eating disorders clinic or CBT.
- Advise patients to avoid brushing teeth after vomiting and rinse with a non-acid mouthwash.
- Where laxative abuse advise to gradually reduce intake. NB laxatives do not significantly reduce calories intake.

Related topics

🕮 Overview of the child health promotion programme; 🕮 The assessment of children, young people, and families; 🕮 Growth and nutrition 12–18yrs; 🕮 Child and adolescent mental health services.

Further information for professionals and patients

Callaghan, P. and Waldock, H. (2006). *Oxford Handbook of Mental Health Nursing*. Oxford University Press. Oxford.

🖳 Eating Disorders Association (EDA): www.edauk.com

🖳 NICE (2004). Core interventions in the treatments and management of anorexia nervosa bulimia nervosa and related eating disorders www.nice.org.uk

🖳 *Overcoming Bulimia*. CD Rom from Calipso: www.calipso.co.uk

Substance misuse

Substance misuse refers to the harmful use of any substance, such as alcohol (Alcohol 📖), a street drug or the misuse of a prescribed drug. 1 in 10 adults report using illicit drugs in the last year, most frequently abused drugs: cannabis, amphetamine, ecstasy, and cocaine but opiod drugs are main drugs of abuse (e.g. heroin and methadone). Solvent abuse common among teenagers. Likelihood of substance abuse influenced by:

● Availability of drugs
● Peer and social pressure
● Vulnerable personality.

Individuals may present with inappropriate behaviour, lack of self care, constricted or dilated pupils, evidence of injecting, hepatitis or HIV (HIV 📖).

Features of substance misuse disorder

● **Acute intoxication**: pattern of reversible physical and mental abnormalities caused by direct effect of the substance such as disinhibition, ataxia, euphoria, visual, and sensory distortion.
● **At risk use**: where the person is at increased risk of harming their physical or mental health. Not dependent on how much taken, but on the situations and associated behaviours e.g. cannabis use while driving.
● **Harmful use**: the continuation of substance misuse despite damage to the mental health, social, occupational, or familial well-being. Damage is denied or minimized.
● **Dependence**: includes both physical and psychological dependence.
● **Withdrawal**: where abstinence leads to features of withdrawal. Different substances have different symptoms; often the opposite of acute effects of the substance. Clinically significant withdrawals are recognized in alcohol, opiates, benzodiazepines, amphetamines, and cocaine.
● **Complicated withdrawal**: development of seizures, delirium, or psychotic features.
● **Substance induced psychotic disorder**: hallucinations and/or delusions occurring as a direct result of substance neuro-toxicity. Differentiated from primary psychotic illness by non-typical symptoms e.g. late first presentation, prominence of non-auditory hallucinations.
● **Cognitive impairment syndromes**: reversible cognitive deficits occur during intoxication, persist in chronic misuse → dementia. Occurs in alcohol, volatile chemicals, benzodiazepines, and possibly cannabis.
● **Residual disorders**: continuing symptoms exist despite discontinuing the substance.
● **Exacerbation of pre-existing disorder**: all other psychiatric illnesses, e.g. anxiety, mood disorders, and psychotic disorders may be associated with co-morbid substance misuse → an exacerbation of the patient's symptoms and a decline in the effectiveness of treatment.

The Dependence Syndrome describes the features of substance dependence:
● Primacy of drug seeking behaviour—it is the most important thing in the person's life, taking priority over all activities and interests.
● Narrowing the drug taking repertoire—the person takes a single substance in preference to all others.

- Increased tolerance to the effects of the drug—increased amounts are needed for same effect, the person explores other routes such as IV.
- Loss of control of consumption—inability to restrict consumption.
- Signs of withdrawal on attempted abstinence, and drug taking to avoid withdrawal symptoms.
- Continued drug use despite negative consequences, such as marital break up, prison sentence, loss of job.
- Rapid reinstatement of previous pattern of drug use after abstinence.

Aims of care

- Reduce or modify drug abusing behaviour.
- Reduce risk of other health problems e.g. infections, depression, psychoses, threats to personal safety.
- Reduce social consequences of substance abuse e.g. family crisis, criminality, financial crisis, and homelessness.

Care and management

Achieved as part of MDT and should involve community substance misuse teams when available.

- Education, safer routes of administration, risks of overdose, hepatitis immunization for injecting drug users and close contacts, needles exchange.
- Treatment of dependence: provided as part of PHCT, involving community pharmacist and specialist services: work to set realistic goals, reduce dosages, and review regularly.
- Family and carer support liaison with voluntary agencies and support groups.
- Talking therapies, counselling (□), and possible alternative therapies such as acupuncture.

Related topics

□ Homeless people; □ Alcohol.

Further information and support for professionals, patients and carers

▣ Adfam charity supporting families of drug abusers: www.adfam.org.uk
▣ ANSA association of nurses in substance abuse: www.ansa.uk.net
Callaghan, P. and Waldock, H. (2006). *Oxford Handbook of Mental Health Nursing*. Oxford University Press, Oxford.
▣ Drugscope: www.drugscope.org.uk
▣ Drugs-Info: Information about substance abuse for addicts and families: www.drugs-info.co.uk
▣ Talk to FRANK: government run information and referral services: www.talktofrank.com
☎ 0800 77 66 00

People with depression

Most common mental disorder in primary care. Depression and mixed depression/anxiety = 17 per 1000 in ♂, 25 per 1000 in ♀. Often undetected and often linked to long-term conditions. Characterized by:

- Feelings of unhappiness that interfere with everyday life
- Everything is a struggle
- Feelings of hopelessness about the future
- Unable to see any positives in life
- Feel apathetic and unable to participate in activities once enjoyed.

Severity of depressive symptoms varies. At its worst, depression → feelings of helplessness and lack of worth that people begin to consider suicide.

Causes/risk factors

Multidimensional including:

- Biological, genetic
- Stress, vulnerability
- Social and physical reasons e.g. health inequalities.

Patients should be screened who have:

- A past history of depression
- Significant physical illnesses/events causing disability and other mental health problems (People with dementias 📖; Postnatal depression 📖; Alcohol 📖; Parkinson's 📖; Principles of rehabilitation following stroke or sudden deterioration in health 📖).

Signs and symptoms

If experiencing 4 or more, for most of the day nearly every day, for >2 weeks: consider referral to GP or other mental health specialist.

- Tiredness and loss of energy
- Persistent sadness
- Loss of self-confidence and self-esteem
- Difficulty concentrating
- Not being able to enjoy things
- Undue feelings of guilt or worthlessness
- Feelings of helplessness and hopelessness
- Sleeping problems
- Avoiding other people, sometimes even your close friends
- Finding it hard to function at work/college/school
- Loss of appetite
- Loss of sex drive and/or sexual problems
- Physical aches and pains
- Thinking about suicide and death
- Self-harm.

Screening and assessment

See the NICE guidelines for management of depression in primary and 2° care (see 'Further information for professionals').

Two initial screening questions recommended with patients:

- 'During the last month, have you often been bothered by feeling down, depressed or hopeless?'

and

- 'During the last month, have you often been bothered by having little interest or pleasure in doing things?'

If patients answer yes to these, further symptoms to assess for are:

- Low energy
- Changes in appetite, weight, or sleep pattern
- Poor concentration
- Feelings of guilt or worthlessness
- Suicidal ideas.

Assessment tools: see below.

❶ Risk. Always ask depressed patients about suicidal ideas and intent; a common misconception is to believe asking will introduce suicidal ideas.

- Advise patients and carers to watch out for changes in mood, negativity and hopelessness, and suicidal intent.
- If a patient expresses suicidal ideas refer to GP.
- If a patient is of considerable immediate risk to self or others, refer urgently to specialist mental health service.
- Contact depressed patients not attending follow-up appointments.

❶ Some cultures do not have a term for depression and may present with physical symptoms or use culturally specific phrases like 'sadness in my heart'.

Treatment

The stepped care model of the NICE guidelines should be followed.

Step 1: recognition and assessment of depression by the GP or nurse.

Step 2: treatment of mild depression by primary care team and primary care mental health worker; watchful waiting—if patient does not want treatment or may recover with no intervention ask patient to return within 2wks for further assessment.

Sleep and anxiety management

- Encourage sleep pattern
- Avoid caffeine and excess alcohol before bed
- Advise relaxation methods, encourage structured problem-solving
- Advise patients to exercise (Exercise 📖)
- Consider guided self-help programmes i.e. booklets or leaflets
- If access to it—consider computerized cognitive behavioural therapy; and, refer on for psychological therapy such as brief cognitive behavioural therapy and counselling (Talking therapies 📖).

Step 3: Treatment of moderate or severe depression by primary care team and primary care mental health worker. Antidepressant medication is usually routinely offered to patients. Key advice for patients:

- They do not cause addiction or craving
- Patients should not suddenly stop taking their medication
- Medication takes time to start working—as much as 4wks
- Patients should take medication exactly as prescribed
- Antidepressants should be continued for at least 6mths after remission.

Monitor for side effects (BNF4.3) Selective serotonin reuptake inhibitors (SSRIs) may cause nausea, vomiting, abdominal cramps, diarrhoea, anorexia, weight loss, headaches, anxiety, tremor, dizziness, drowsiness, sexual dysfunction.

Tricyclic Antidepressants (TCAs) may cause arrhythmias, drowsiness, dry mouth, constipation, blurred vision, urinary retention, dizziness, syncope, hyponatraemia. If symptoms persist refer to GP.

❶ Monitor risk of suicide frequently; Review patients regularly if an acute risk refer to 2° care (see below).

Steps 4 and 5: treatment for patients with treatment-resistant, recurrent, atypical, and psychotic depression or at significant risk. Refered to mental health specialists, crisis teams, and inpatient care.

Related topics
📖 Risk of suicide and deliberate self harm; 📖 People with dementias; 📖 Alcohol; 📖 Stress.

Further information for patients
📺 Depression Alliance: www.depressionalliance.org ☎ 0207 768 0123
📺 Samaritans: www.samaritans.org.uk ☎ 08457 909090
📺 Geriatric Depression Scale public domain: www.jr2.ox.ac.uk/geratol/GDSdoc.htm

Further information for professionals
DoH (1999) National Service Framework for Mental Health. DoH, London.
📺 NICE Guidelines for management of depression in primary and secondary care: www.nice.org.uk/pdf/CG023quickrefguide.pdf

Talking therapies

Talking therapies provide an opportunity to talk in a way that assists the person to understand themselves better and then work out ways of living in a more positive, constructive way. May be used as part of a staged approach to mental health problems e.g. depression (People with depression 📖).

There are a wide variety of talking therapies including:
- Self-help and support groups
- Individual counselling or therapy
- Couple or family therapy
- Group therapy
- Therapeutic communities.

The most common types in the NHS are counselling, cognitive behaviour therapy (CBT), and psychoanalytic or psychodynamic psychotherapy, usually provided by counsellors, psychologists, psychiatrists, or psycho-therapists but also by nurses and social workers in some services. There may be variation in local NHS availability. Anyone seeking a private therapist should ensure they belong to a recognized professional body such as the UK Council for Psychotherapy.

Counselling

Counselling can help with ordinary problems of living and life crises e.g. bereavement (📖), relationship problems, minor depression, disability, or loss. Can help prevent mental health problems. A key element is active and reflective listening to encourage people to think about their own difficulties and feelings and try to find ways to address them. It does not involve giving advice. Usually short term e.g. 6 sessions of 45–50min. Counsellors may be available in general practice, local mental health services, or sometimes primary care nurses may be involved in offering brief intervention counselling or active listening sessions to particular groups e.g. women with postnatal depression. Often also available through local voluntary sector e.g. Cruse (bereavement counselling), Relate (relationship counselling).

Cognitive behaviour therapy

Cognitive behaviour therapy (CBT) aims to help people change patterns of thinking or behaviour that are causing problems. The focus is on the thoughts, images, beliefs, and attitudes and how this relates to the way the person behaves. This also changes how they feel. Shown to be effec-tive for a variety of mental health problems including depression, anxiety, panic attacks, phobias, obsessive compulsive disorder, and some eating disorders, especially bulimia. Also thought to be helpful for people with psychoses. It is a structured approach, with goals for treatment and activities to try out between sessions. Usually up to 15 sessions weekly for about 1hr.

Psychoanalytical and psychodynamic therapies

Psychoanalytic/psychodynamic therapy can help people get to know themselves better, improve their relationships and get more out of life. The therapist listens to the person's experiences, explores connections between present feelings, actions, and past events. Therapists have different approaches and different styles of working. Psychoanalytic and psychodynamic therapy often continues for a year of more. It can help people with long-term or recurring problems get to the root of their difficulties. Some evidence that it can help depression and some eating disorders (People with eating disorders 📖), however, some people, e.g. those who feel vulnerable or who are experiencing psychosis, can find psychotherapy unhelpful.

Benefits and risks

- Talking therapies work for some but not all people.
- Some people find that just knowing a therapist is there and focused on their concerns makes them feel valued.
- Some people can find it disappointing, or feel they did not relate to the therapist or the therapist did not seem to understand them.
- A bad experience with a therapist can leave some people feeling worse.
- One of the most important ingredients in effective talking therapies is whether the person feels they can make a good relationship with the therapist.

Further information and support

📖 British Association for Counselling and Psychotherapy provides information on counselling, choosing a counsellor, and lists of private counsellors: www.bacp.co.uk

DH (England) (2001). *Public Information Leaflet. Choosing Talking Therapies?* (Product code 20797). DH, London.

📖 MIND produces public information leaflets on all talking treatments: www.mind.org.uk

People with dementias

Dementia: a descriptive term for symptoms affecting the brain = generalized impairment of memory, intellect, and personality. >100 different kinds of dementia. Average lifespan of dementia sufferers 7yrs but can live for 15yrs.

- Alzheimer's disease most common in people aged 65+ and can occur as early as 30yrs.
- ↑ with advancing age. >750,000 people in the UK with dementia. 1:5 people >80yrs. By 2050 it has been estimated that there will be 1.5 million dementia sufferers in the UK.
- Prevalence ↑ in people with learning disabilities.

Types

- Alzheimer's disease is characterized by amyloid plaques and neuro-fibrillary tangles in the brain.
- Vascular dementia = 20% of all dementias. Is caused by brain damage from cerebrovascular or cardiovascular problems—usually CVA. Can also result from genetic diseases, endocarditis, or amyloid angiopathy.
- Lewy body dementia: fluctuating but persistent dementia, cognitive impairment hallucinations, and Parkinsonianism.

Signs and symptoms

Patients (carers may also seek help) may describe the following features and may have compensated for these deficiencies for some time before seeking help (also see Table 9.1).

- Steady ↓ in memory for recent events and forgetfulness
- ↓ mental functioning e.g. getting muddled
- Difficulty finding words
- Feeling depressed
- Steady ↓ in thinking, judgement, orientation, and language
- Patient appears indifferent or subdued but can appear alert
- ↓ in daily activities such as washing and dressing
- Changes in personality or emotional control
- In some cases, persecutory delusions.

Assessment tools

(See 🖳 www.alzheimers.org.uk)

- Clifton Assessment Procedures for the Elderly (CAPE). CAPE assesses both functional ability and cognitive function.
- Mini Mental State Examination (MMSE). The MMSE effective instrument for assessing cognitive function. NB Influenced by educational level.
- Abbreviated Mental Test Score (AMTS). A quick ten-item cognitive function test. **Note: none of these tests are diagnostic.**
- Carer Strain Index. Use scale to profile the carer, particularly when considering a request for a needs assessment under the Carer's Act (Carers assessment and support 📖).

NB Depression and delusional states can be confused with or coexist with dementia.

Table 9.1 Features of dementia at different points in its path

	Early changes	Later changes
Emotional changes	• Shallowness of mood, frustration • Lack of emotional responsiveness and consideration of others • Depression and/or anxiety	• Irritability and hostility • Aggression
Cognitive changes	• Short-term memory deficit with particular difficulty in registration and recall of new information • Thinking becomes concrete with a reduced range of concerns • Perseveration of thoughts and actions, accompanied by repetitive speech	• Language disorder: both receptive and expressive dysphasia can occur • Thought process becomes fragmented, so that speech becomes disordered and fragmented • Psychotic features in 30–40% • Persecutory ideas and delusions • Auditory and visual hallucinations—not mood congruent
Behavioural changes	• Social withdrawal • Emotional and physical disinhibition • Difficulty in carrying out purposeful tasks; domestic tasks, dressing, etc. • Socially inappropriate behaviour, self-neglect • Disorientation progressively for time, place, and eventually for person	• Wandering and restlessness • Evening and nocturnal restlessness prominent • Turning night into day • Aggression and violence

Adapted from Iliffe, S. and Drennan, V. (2001). *Primary Care and Dementia* JKP, with permission from Professor Steve Iliffe, Department of Primary Care and Population Sciences, UCL.

Functional capacity

Is more important than a test score.

Assessments of functional impairment can ↑ quality of life and ensure networks of support from social services, voluntary organizations, and specialist medical services are established.

Points to consider:

• Continence
• Dressing
• Self-care
• Cooking ability and nutrition
• Shopping/housework
• Degree of orientation in the home
• Social contacts
• Safety in the home
• Financial capacity.

Physical problems

Toxic confusional states and other physical disorders can coexist with and/or complicate dementia. Consider referral to the appropriate specialist:

- State of nutrition
- Drug regimen, if any
- Hearing
- Eyesight
- Mobility
- Continence.

Related topics

📖 Principles of working with someone with dementia; 📖 People with depression.

Further information

🖥 Alzheimer's Society: www.alzheimers.org.uk ☎ 0845 300 0336
🖥 For Dementia: www.fordementia.org.uk

People with bipolar affective disorder

People with bipolar affective disorder can experience recurrent attacks of depression and mania or hypomania. It is commonly called manic depression, and is more common in women, with the average age of onset at around 21 years. Children of a parent with bipolar disorder have a 50% chance of developing a mental illness. There is no significant racial difference. Morbidity and mortality rates are high in terms of lost work, productivity, effects on marriage and the family. 25–50% of people with bipolar affective disorder attempt suicide and 10% with the disorder kill themselves.

Poor prognosis is associated with poor employment history, alcohol abuse, psychotic features, depression in between episodes of mania, being male, and not complying with medication.

Good prognosis is associated with manic episodes of short duration, later age at onset, few thoughts of suicide or symptoms of psychosis, good treatment response and compliance.

The course of the illness is extremely variable. The onset can be hypomanic, manic, mixed, or depressive; and this may be followed by 5 or more years without a further episode. The length of time between episodes may then begin to diminish. People with hypomania share the same symptoms as mania, but to a lesser degree, and the condition may not significantly disrupt work or lead to social rejection.

Table 9.2 Core features of mania

Elevated mood, usually out of keeping with circumstances	
Increased energy, which may manifest as:	• Over activity • Pressured speech (flight of ideas) • Racing thoughts • Reduced need for sleep
Increased self-esteem, evident as:	• Over optimistic ideation • Grandiosity • Reduced social inhibitions • Over familiarity (may be over amorous) • Facetiousness
Reduced attention span or increased distractibility	
Tendency to engage in risk behaviour that could have serious consequences	• Preoccupation with extravagant impractical schemes • Spending recklessly • Inappropriate sexual encounters
Other behavioural manifestations:	• Excitement • Irritability • Aggressiveness or suspiciousness • Disruption of work, usual social activities, and family life

Reproduced from the Oxford Handbook of Mental Health Nursing, Callaghan, P. and Waldock, H (2006). By permission of Oxford University Press.

Psychotic symptoms

In severe mania, psychotic symptoms may develop:

- Grandiose ideas may become delusional with special powers or religious content.
- Suspiciousness may develop into well-formed persecutory delusions.
- Pressured speech may become so great that clear associations are lost and speech becomes incomprehensible.
- Irritability and aggression may lead to violent behaviour.
- Preoccupation with thoughts and schemes may lead to self-neglect, not eating or drinking, and living in dishevelled circumstances.
- Catatonic behaviour, also termed manic stupor.
- Total loss of insight and connection to the outside world.

Supporting a patient and their family or carers

Important to have good multidisciplinary working with GP, the CMHT, and, where appropriate, the care co-coordinator for the patient (England and Wales have implemented a care programme approach (CPA)) which draws on case management to deliver care to people with mental health problems.

- Acute episodes may require hospitalization and if patient is unwilling to be hospitalized may need to be reviewed under the Mental Health Act for compulsory admission.
- Treatment: lithium drug of choice. To avoid nephrotoxicity it is important that levels are checked weekly until the dose is constant for 4wks, then every 3mths as long as the dose is constant.
- Plasma creatinine and TFTs checked every 6mths.
- Patients may need encouragement to continue with drug therapy.
- Over time patients can come to recognize situations and events that can trigger episodes of mania or depression. Encourage them to seek help and review of treatment when they think they are at risk.
- Talking therapies (☐) may be helpful and ensure both patient and family have adequate social support and access to disability benefits (Benefits for disability and illness ☐).
- Living with someone with bipolar disorder can be very stressful and particular attention should be given to individual needs of family, children, and carers of sufferers (Carers assessment and support ☐).
- Patients must inform DVLA.

Related topics

☐ People with depression; ☐ Talking therapies; ☐ Alcohol.

Further information for professionals, patients and carers

Callaghan, P. and Waldock, H. (2006). *Oxford Handbook of Mental Health.* Oxford University Press.

Fink, C. Kraynak, J. (2005). *Bipolar Disorder for Dummies.* John Wiley & Sons Ltd.

▣ MDF—The bipolar organization: www.mdf.org.uk

▣ MIND: www.mind.org.uk

Adapted from Callaghan, P., Waldock, H. (2006) *Oxford handbook of Mental Health Nursing.* By permission of Oxford University Press.

People with schizophrenia

Schizophrenia is a highly variable disorder characterized by disordered perception, disordered thoughts (hallucinations and delusions), and withdrawal of the individual's interest from other people and the world.

Schizophrenia is a form of psychosis, it typically develops in the late teens or early twenties, although males tend to have an earlier onset than females, and may develop a more serious illness.

- Prevalence: lifetime risk is between 7–13 per 1000 of the population.
- Mortality: suicide is the most common cause of premature death; accounting for 10–38% of all deaths.
- Genetic factors.
- Environmental factors: complications of pregnancy, delivery, and the neonatal period; delayed walking and neurodevelopmental difficulties; early social services contact, and disturbed childhood behaviour.

The symptoms of schizophrenia are divided into positive (new symptoms) and negative (loss of a previous function) symptoms.

Positive symptoms	Negative symptoms	Other symptoms
• Delusions	• Loss of motivation	• Thought disorder
• Hallucinations	• Loss of social awareness	• Agitation
	• Flattened mood	• Depression
	• Poor abstract thinking	• Poor sleep
		• Cognitive impairment

The following symptoms have a special significance as they occur often in schizophrenia and more rarely in other disorders (sometimes referred to as first rank symptoms):
- Auditory hallucinations:
  - Voices heard arguing
  - Thought echo
  - Running commentary on what the person is doing.
- Delusions or thought interference:
  - Thought insertion
  - Thought withdrawal
  - Thought broadcasting.
- Delusions of control:
  - Passivity of affect
  - Passivity of impulse
  - Passivity of volitions
  - Somatic passivity.
- Delusional perceptions:
  - A primary delusion of any context reported by the person as having arisen from a normal perception.

Prognosis

- Approximately 15–20% of first episodes will not occur again
- Few people will remain in employment

- 52% will be without psychotic symptoms in the last 2yrs
- 52% are without negative symptoms
- 55% show good/fair social functioning.

Supporting patients, families, and carers

Patients will be under the care of a psychiatrist and all care should be in liaison with CMHT and where appropriate the care co-coordinator for the patient (England and Wales have implemented a care programme approach which draws on case management to deliver care to people with mental health problems).

- Antipsychotics treatment of choice for sufferers (BNF 4.2.1). Many have side effects. Long acting depot injections often used in maintenance therapy. Administered with Z track technique. There is a reduced risk of relapse if medication is maintained.
- Encourage healthy lifestyle and discourage use of illicit drugs.
- Patients may benefit from CBT and related talking therapies.
- Patients must inform DVLA.
- CMHT regularly review patients and include review social support available for patients and their carers addressing the individual needs of family, children, and carers who are living with and supporting patients.
- Many areas now have crisis intervention teams to provide a rapid community-based response to out-of-hours crisis and prevent hospital admission.

Related topics

📖 Risk of suicide and deliberate self-harm; 📖 Social support; 📖 Carers; 📖 Benefits for disability and illness; 📖 Talking therapies.

Further information for professionals, patients, families and carers

Callaghan, P. and Waldock, H. (2006). *Oxford Handbook of Mental Health.* Oxford University Press.

📟 Rethink (formerly National Schizophrenia Fellowship): www.rethink.org

Adapted from Callaghan, P., Waldock, H. (2006) *Oxford handbook of Mental Health Nursing.* By permission of Oxford University Press.

Mental capacity

Approximately 2 million people in Britain are thought to lack mental capacity including those that suffer from dementia. Mental capacity is highly complex and care must be taken to consider the person's rights and responsibilities. As a basis for assessment the following should always be considered:

- **Everyone** has capacity unless it is established otherwise.
- A person is not to be treated as being unable to make a decision unless all attempts to help them have been tried and been unsuccessful.
- Any assessment should consider who the person was and is (especially where the sense of self alters or diminishes, as in dementia).
- How to achieve a balance between an older person's last-known wishes and current wishes (as expressed through words and behaviour).
- Previously communicated directives or instructions.
- The person's unique responses to their physical and mental health, and how the person sees their future.
- How capacity is being supported or hindered by others on a day-to-day basis.
- Full and open discussion of multiple perspectives and not simply clinical interests of one or other professional group or a family member.
- How capacity has been formally assessed and in what situations it does and does not exist.

Lack of capacity is defined in regards to:
- Inability to make a decision because of impairment of the brain or mind at the material time whether temporary or permanent.
- Inability to make a decision is based on the central tenets of informed consent (); i.e. understanding, weighing up, using and communicating information.

The Mental Capacity Act

(See below.) This governs decision-making on behalf of adults, where they lose mental capacity at some point in their lives or where the incapacitating condition has been present since birth. The Act covers all decisions made, or actions taken on behalf of people lacking capacity on:
- Personal welfare including day-to-day and major life-related health care.
- Financial matters and also provides substitute decision-making by attorneys, court-appointed 'deputies', and clarifies the position where no such formal process has been adopted.

Key principles underpinning the Act are:
- A person must be assumed to have capacity unless it is established that (s)he lacks capacity.
- A person is not to be treated as unable to make a decision unless all practicable steps to help him/her to do so have been unsuccessful.
- A person is not to be treated as unable to make a decision merely because they make an unwise decision.

- An act or decision made, under this Act, or done on behalf of the person who lacks capacity must be in the best interests of the person.
- Before the act, or the decision, consider if it can be effectively achieved in ways less restrictive of the person's rights and freedom.
- *There is a two stage test of incapacity:*
  - Stage one considers the presence of impairment and its likely consequences.
  - Stage two considers if the person has been unable to make a decision. Attention is given to minimizing disability. Situational capacity is recognized as is fluctuating capacity.
- Assessing capacity should be done when the person is at their highest level of functioning. Assessment is to be carried out by the relevant professional. Within health care this is the doctor or the professional proposing treatment. Multi-disciplinary consultation is recommended. Refusal to consent to capacity assessment must be respected.

NB Decision making regarding capacity is contextual and varies between persons and within a person over time.

Professionals have a duty to ensure they take reasonable steps to establish consent *first*. So professionals must have assessed a person's lack of capacity prospectively i.e. before care is given. Where professionals are satisfied advance directives are valid *and* applicable to the proposed treatment they should be followed.

Act also provides guidance on:
- Paying for goods and services
- Lasting power of attorney and financial issues
- Court of protection and court appointed deputies
- Advance decisions to refuse treatment
- Protection and supervision of those responsible for making decisions or taking actions on behalf of those who lack capacity and links with mental capacity and finally data protection.

Related topics

📖 Professional conduct; 📖 Consent; 📖 People with dementias; 📖 End-of-life issues.

Further information

📖 Department for Constitutional Affairs (2004). *A Guide to the Mental Capacity Bill: what does it mean for me?* DCA, London. Available at: www. dca.gov.uk/family/mi/
📖 Making Decisions Alliance: alliance of national disability and older peoples' organizations: www.makingdecisions.org.uk
📖 Mental Capacity Act: www.dca.gov.uk

Risk of suicide and deliberate self-harm

UK suicide rate is 1:6000 and in ♂ <35yrs is the most common cause of death.

Aims of risk assessment

To establish:

- *If there is ongoing suicidal intent* such as a continuing wish to die, sense of hopelessness, or ambivalence about survival.
- *If there is evidence of mental illness* e.g. depressive illnesses or alcohol dependence.
- *If there are any non-mental health issues to address* e.g. emotional problems, family and/or relationship difficulties, school, employment, debt, or legal problems.

Assessing suicide risk

Should consider (see useful questions below):

- History
- Information from relatives and carers
- Ideation/mental state
- Intent
- Planning
- Person's awareness of risk
- Benefits and harm from risk
- Formulation.

Predictors of suicide risk

- History of self-harm
- Depression
- Dual diagnosis
- Inpatient care
- Loss of contact with mental health services
- Within one week of discharge from psychiatric in patient care
- Member of an ethnic minority
- Homelessness.

People at higher risk of suicide

- ♂ >65yrs, ♂ 15–30yrs
- Separated, widowed, divorced
- Live alone, socially isolated, or loss of supports
- Poor physical health
- Poor mental health
- Substance misuse
- Previous episodes of self-harm
- Suicide by relative
- Hopelessness, despair, loss of interest
- Mild learning difficulty.

Deliberate self harm[1]

Deliberate non-fatal act committed in the knowledge that it was harmful e.g. drug overdose, poisoning. Self-harm is often aimed at changing a

---

[1] Adapted from Simon, C., Everitt, H., Kendrick, T. (2005). *Oxford Hanbook of General Pratice.* Oxford University Press, Oxford.

situation (e.g. where there has been a relationship breakdown), a communication of distress/cry for help or a genuine failed suicide attempt.

Common misconception that asking about suicidal intention can plant the idea into the patient's mind and make it more likely.

Useful questions if you consider someone to be at risk

- Do you feel you have a future?
- Do you feel that life is no longer worth living?
- Do you ever feel completely hopeless?
- Do you ever feel you would be better off dead?
- Have you ever made any plans to take your life?
- Have you ever attempted to take your life?
- What prevents you doing it?
- Have you made any arrangements for your affairs after your death?

Hopelessness is a good predictor for subsequent and immediate risk of suicide. Any concerns about a patient should be shared with their GP and relevant primary health care team members.

Suicide risk is high when:

- Direct statement of intent, severe mood change, hopelessness, alcohol or drug dependence, abnormal personality. Refer to GP for admission to ED as a psychiatric emergency, may involve using the Mental Health Act for compulsory admission if voluntary admission declined.
- If risk of suicide believed to be lower (decision should be made as part of multidisciplinary team) then arrange for someone to stay with the patients until follow-up and remove all potentially harmful drugs. Community Mental Health Team should be involved.

People who have attempted suicide/self-harmed should be treated with the same care, respect, and privacy as any other patient.

Support of those bereaved through suicide

Those bereaved following a suicide need extra support to help deal with the death and possible stigma. Self-help groups or counselling may help.

Related topics

📖 People with depression; 📖 Social support; 📖 Bereavement, grief, and coping with loss.

Further information for professionals

🖳 National suicide prevention strategy for England: www.dh.gov.uk
🖳 NICE. *Self harm: the short term physical and psychological management and secondary prevention of self harm in primary and secondary care:* www.nice.org.uk

Further information for patients and relatives

Callaghan, P. and Waldock, H. (2006). *Oxford Handbook of Mental Health.* Oxford University Press.
☎ Samaritans 24h emotional support: 08457 909 090
🖳 Self injury and related issues: www.siari.co.uk
🖳 Survivors of bereavement by suicide: www.uk.sobs.org.uk ☎ 0870 241 3337

Key facts on carers and caring

A carer is someone who provides care on an unpaid basis and provides that care either in association with paid carers (e.g. care workers, nurses, and social workers) or instead of paid carers.

NB Confidentiality is an issue when involving carers in discussions about a patient's care. Consider a 'carer contract' where the patient gives written consent for their medical information to be shared with their carer. GPs both through QoF and DES (Scotland) should record care, status, and provision of services for carer.

Estimated to be >6 million carers in the UK who are key to the support of dependent family members and friends in the community of carers, believed to save the NHS £57 billion pa.

Contribution

Many carers derive high levels of personal satisfaction in their role but this does not mean they do not need support and regular review.

1.9 million carers provide 20hrs or more care a week. Caring is often provided in conjunction with other work/family responsibilities. Majority of carers look after older people.

Carers may provide:
- Personal care
- Physical help with daily activities
- Practical support e.g. help with medication and shopping.

Women more likely to be carers (58% of carers). Peak age for caring 50–59yrs. 1 in 4 of ♀ in this age group provide care (see young carers, below).

Impact of caring

- Significant financial consequences from being a carer—70% of carers worry about finances.
- Caring often detrimental to health, carers providing high levels of care 2½x more likely to experience mental health problems than non-caring counterparts.
- Spouse carers and mothers of disabled children increased likelihood of psychological distress.
- Carers may benefit from respite from their caring responsibilities. For those who are already depressed respite care alone is unlikely to be sufficient.

NB Carers are not a homogenous group. The quality of the relationship between the carer and the dependent person prior to a person taking on a caring role directly affects emotional health and reciprocity in caring relationships.

Carers need their role and knowledge acknowledged and respected by health and social care professionals. Primary Care nurses are well placed to offer ongoing support, advice, and help with direct care.

Health professionals that are in contact with carers should ensure that the carer's needs are considered *independently* of the dependent person.

Important that:
- Individual has made an informed choice about being a carer and does not feel coerced into the role through guilt or expectations of others.
- Carers have access to proper assessment of their needs and are aware that they are entitled to a carer's assessment from social services.
- Carers are fully consulted on decisions that affect them.
- Receive information about benefits services (Sources of information on benefits and support 📖) and sources of peer and voluntary/charity-based support.
- That services are coordinated between health, social care, housing, and, when relevant, education.
- Services are *not* withheld because a carer is present.
- Risks of being socially excluded are addressed: carers often cannot take up paid employment because of need for flexible working or give up holidays and ↓ leisure activities because of low incomes and costs.
- That black and ethnic minority carers are not overlooked by mainstream services.
- That practice complies with the Carers (Equal Opportunities) Act 2004 and carers and those considering becoming a carer have access to a full assessment.
- NB confidentiality is an issue when involving carers in discussion about patient care. Consider 'carer contract': patient gives written consent for information to be shared with carer. GPs through QoF and Direct Enhanced Services (Scotland) should record carer status and services received.

Young carers (see also Children in special circumstances 📖). Anyone <18yrs whose life is in some way restricted because of the need to take responsibility for someone who is:
- Ill.
- Has a disability, is experiencing mental distress, or is affected by substance misuse.

Caring responsibilities can have adverse affects on:
- Schooling: learning and attendance.
- Relationships with peers.
- Relationships within the family.

Health professionals should consider:
- The need to be proactive in identifying children who may be carers.
- Term 'young carer' is important and differentiates from a child of someone who has a disability or needs extra help.
- Carers Act 1995 and the Framework for the Assessment of Children in Need should be a starting point in assessment a young carer's needs.

Related topics

📖 Carers assessment and support; 📖 Children with complex health needs and disabilities; 📖 Social support; 📖 Aids to daily living and equipment for home nursing.

Further information for professionals and patients and carers

- 📄 Age Concern: www.ageconcern.org.uk
- 📄 Carers UK: www.carers.uk.org.uk
- 📄 Caring about Carers; Carers Strategy: www.carers.gov.uk
- 📄 Childrens Society Young Carers Initiative: www.youngcarer.com
- 📄 Help the Aged: www.helptheaged.org.uk
- 📄 Princess Royal Trust for Carers: www.carers.org

Carers assessment and support

Carers (Equal Opportunities) Act 2004 gives carers rights to information and places a duty on LAs to inform carers of their right to a carers assessment (see below). Gives LA powers to enlist the help of housing, health, education, and other LAs in providing carer support.

Carers assessment

Anyone who is a carer or who is contemplating becoming a carer has the right to an assessment by social services. They can request an assessment directly or ask the GP or nurse to do so on their behalf. The assessment does not assume that the individual wants to take on or should take on the caring role. The purpose is to:
- Discuss with social services the help needed to support the caring role.
- Explore how an individual feels about being a carer.
- Provide information about benefits.
- Discuss how to balance caring responsibilities with other responsibilities and interests.
- Plan and consider how caring responsibilities might change.
- If caring is likely to continue for the foreseeable future then a review date should be set.

Assessment should include review of:
- Housing: possible needs for aids and adaptations.
- Health and likely health needs of the carer.
- Work: if there is a need to ↓ working hours because of caring role, desire to return to work, challenges of balancing demands.
- Other interests e.g. leisure access to lifelong learning.
- Time spent on caring, where support is needed and opportunities for respite/care breaks.
- Relationships, feelings, and emotional consequences of caring.
- What contingency plans are in place for emergencies or situations where it is not possible to carry on caring.

Types of help and support that should be available to carers and their dependents

(NB There is considerable local variation.)
- Help at home: means tested support from social services is available to carers in need of support. Voluntary organizations e.g. Crossroads can offer sitting services.
- Involvement of district nursing service to provide support and relevant specialist nursing support e.g Admiral nurses, MS CNS.
- Day care: social services will have a list of centres providing day care for older people and children.
- Respite care: care homes and specialist residential settings can provide short-term care to provide carer with planned breaks. Social services may provide support with costs.
- Involvement of district nursing services.
- Aids and equipment (Aids and equipment: general ▢).

- Adapting the home environment: the person being looked after may be eligible for a home improvement grant.
- Carer specific support services: local carer support groups, carer services offered by social services e.g. help with taxi fares for hospital visits.
- Access to financial support e.g Carers allowance, Direct payments, vouchers to purchase care Independent Living Fund.
- Pharmacy support: e.g. delivery of repeat prescriptions.

LAs are required to set out how they make decisions arising from the needs identified according to their eligibility criteria. If carers are dissatisfied with the support they have been offered then carers' organizations provide support and advice about how to appeal and what it is reasonable to expect.

Related topics

📖 Key facts on carers and caring; 📖 Sources of information on benefits and support; 📖 Children with complex health needs and disabilities; 📖 Social support; 📖 Aids to daily living and equipment for home nursing.

Further information for professionals and patients and carers

📱 Carers UK: www.carers.uk.org.uk
📱 Caring about Carers; Carers Strategy: www.carers.gov.uk
📱 Children's Society Young Carer's Initiative: www.youngcarer.com
📱 Princess Royal Trust for Carers: www.carers.org

Principles of rehabilitation following stroke

Definition

Stroke: a focal neurological deficit due to local disturbance in the blood supply to the brain; may have abrupt onset but which lasts for longer than 24hrs.

Prevalence

Stroke is the third commonest cause of death in developed countries; 200 per 100,000 will have a stroke each year. Incidence ↑ with age; 80% are >65yrs and ♂:♀ equal. 20% die within the first month, 5–10% within the year, 40% achieve full recovery. Recovery can take years.

Risk factors

↑ blood pressure, smoking, DM, heart disease, PVD, past TIA, raised lipid levels, excessive alcohol intake.

Effects of stroke

- Motor deficits: speech difficulties (e.g. dysarthria, dysphasia), hemiplegia and hemiparesis, facial paralysis → difficulties in swallowing.
- Sensory deficits: visual deficits, poor response to heat and cold, perceptual deficits (e.g. environment), lack of awareness of disabled part of body.
- Altered consciousness: memory loss, short attention span.
- Emotional deficits: personality change, loss of self-control, confusion, depression.
- Bladder and bowel dysfunction: incontinence, frequency, urgency.
- Altered sexual function.

Secondary prevention

Control risk factors, asprin or warfarin may be prescribed by GP/hospital consultant if an embolic stroke.

Rehabilitation

Is an active process in which people with a disability work together with multidisciplinary team, relatives, and members of the wider community to achieve optimum well-being. Should have a systematic approach to assessment (Integrated assessment process 📖) that considers the physical deficits arising from stroke, emotional consequences, immediate physical needs e.g. adjustments to clothing, equipment aids, and housing, ability to be independent in and outside the home and range of social support networks.

Principles

- Patients and carers should have active involvement in the rehabilitation process, agree care plans that have realistic goals, and be offered information e.g. voluntary stroke services, benefits such as disability living allowance and attendance allowance (Sources of information on benefits and support 📖).

- Early mobilization exercises (passive, assisted or active) and weight-bearing and mobilization should be encouraged (see below).
- Based on the pattern of recovery. Recovery of leg function occurs before arm function, and arm function prior to hand function.
- Prevention of deformity and damage based on maintaining the correct position which opposes the direction of flexion. Avoid overusing the unaffected side.
- Monitor progress through use of valid tools eg Barthel Index. (Standardized assessment tools for adults ☐.)
- Psychological rehabilitation e.g. engaging the patient in conversation, encouraging participation in social activities.
- Multidisciplinary teamwork: rehabilitation team includes patient, family/carers, nurses, GP, physiotherapy, OT, speech and language therapy, and social services. Specialist referral where necessary.
- Carer support: stroke often called the family illness.
- Provision of stroke family care workers/nurses where they exist.
- Driving after a stroke: patients with a stroke who make a satisfactory recovery should not drive for at least one month after their stroke. Patients with residual disability at one month must inform the DVLA and can only resume driving after formal assessment by the GP or other professional.

Related topics

☐ Aids to daily living and equipment for home nursing; ☐ Carers assessment and support; ☐ People with depression; ☐ CHD.

Further information for professionals

☐ Chest, Heart and Stroke Association: www.chss.org.uk
☐ Effective Stroke Care. Database of summaries of best interventions for people with stroke: www.effectivestrokecare.org
☐ National Clinical Guidelines for Stroke. Series of pdf publications on stroke: www.rcplondon.ac.uk/pubs/books/stroke/index.
☐ SIGN (Scottish Intercollegiate Guidelines Network) (2002). *Management of patients with stroke*: www.sign.ac.uk/fulltext/64
☐ Stroke Association: www.stroke.org.uk

Further information for patients and carers

☐ Connect. National charity providing services to people with communication difficulties after stroke: www.ukconnect.org
☐ Different strokes. Charity for young people who have suffered a stroke: www.differentstrokes.co.uk
☐ Speakeasy. Charity and support group for people with Aphasia: www. buryspeakeasy.org.uk

Principles of working with someone with dementia

For definitions, prevalence, risk factors and signs, symptoms and assessment see 📖 People with dementias.

People living through the early stages of dementia often adopt strategies to hide symptoms. Important to recognize that presentation of dementia involves an interplay of factors that all influence an individual's experience.
- Neurological impairment
- Personality (temperament, psychological defences, coping style)
- Biography and recent life events
- Physical health and sensory awareness
- Individual's existing relationships with individuals and groups.

❶ Health professionals and carers can rob people with dementia of their self-esteem, confidence, and sense of personhood by their actions e.g. being patronizing and infantalizing them, using deception to gain compliance, not acknowledging feelings and subjective reality, ignoring their presence, denying them choices, blaming them.

Very unhelpful to characterize dementia as a condition of relentless decline where patients and carers have no control, process of normalization as individuals family and carers adjust to living with the disease.

Needs of people with dementia
- Comfort: feeling of security, people with dementia experience sense of loss and bereavement
- Inclusion and feeling of connectedness
- Occupation
- Identity: continuity with individual's past.

Management information and advice
- Encourage patient to live as full life as possible and make full use of remaining abilities; promoting choice.
- Monitor the patient's safety in daily activities e.g. cooking.
- It is important to work with carers and family, sharing information and providing ongoing support.
- Restore self-esteem in patient by encouraging recall of early memories of childhood, school, family, work etc.
- Referral to specialist services as indicated e.g. consultant, old age psychiatrist, geriatrician, neurologist, memory clinics, community mental health team, social services.
- Encourage full use of remaining abilities, interests and hobbies by e.g. writing things down, making lists.
- Encourage maintenance of physical health and fitness through good diet, exercise, and swift treatment of physical illness.
- Suggest membership of a support group or organization which may help the caring, though some find these distressing in the short term.
- Financial and legal matters need to be discussed, including benefits and power of attorney (Mental capacity 📖).

- 'Challenging behavours' e.g. screaming, wandering, shouting, may be attempts to communicate: can benefit from careful listening and affirmation of what is being expressed.
- Medication and medicines management includes observation for effects and side effects:
  - Antipsychotics for some behavioural problems should be reviewed regularly to see if still indicated, since problems often change over course of the disease.
  - Avoid sedative or hypnotic medications if possible.
  - In Alzheimer's disease patients may be referred to primary care for assessment and initiation of anticholinergic drugs, to postpone onset of more severe symptoms (NICE recommendation).
- Arrange for carers to receive advice on help with caring, accommodation, financial advice, benefits, and support groups e.g. Alzheimer's Society.
- As dementia and its effects ↑, more intensive care will be required utilising statutory and voluntary services (Care homes ; Mental capacity ; Palliative care in the home).

Needs of family care givers
- To know someone will provide care when they no longer can
- Access to telephone support
- Strategies for dealing with stress
- Respite
- Strategies for dealing with feelings of being trapped.

Admiral nurses
(Not available across whole of UK check For Dementia website.) Specialist nurses that:
- Work with family carers as their prime focus
- Provide practical advice, emotional support, information, and skills
- Deliver education and training in dementia care
- Provide consultancy to professionals
- Promote best practice in person-centred dementia care.
Also available in some areas: Dementia care centres and Memory clinics.

Palliative care teams will also provide support to people with end stage dementia.

Further information for health-care professionals
- Age Concern England: www.ace.org.uk
- Alzheimer's Society: www.alzheimers.org.uk Advice for all types of dementia not just Alzheimer's disease.
- For Dementia: www.fordementia.org.uk
- Forthcoming guidelines from NICE. Dementia: management of dementia, including use of antipsychotic medication in older people. www.nice.org.uk
- Help The Aged: www.helptheaged.org
- National Library for Health Mental Health Specialist Library (2005) Dementia: www.nelh.nhs.uk Click on mental health

Principles of working with someone with compromised immunity

Healthy people fight infections through the immune system, mainly the lymphatic system. This can be compromised by age, infection, burns, neoplasms, metabolic disorders, irradiation, foreign bodies, cytotoxic drugs, steroids. Causes include:

- Immunodeficiency:
  - Primary causes.
  - Secondary e.g. lymphoma, myeloma, malnutrition, chemotherapy, HIV, post transplant.
- Hypersensitivity i.e. excessive immune response e.g. asthma, hay fever, eczema, anaphylactic shock.
- Autoimmune diseases e.g. pernicious anaemia, rheumatoid arthritis, systemic lupus erythematosus, myasthenia gravis.
- Graft rejection and transplantation.

Principles of care

Most people with compromised immunity live independently. Care is related to the severity and type of symptoms. Many of the associated disorders have support groups and organizations providing information.

Principles of care for people with immunodeficiency disorders

- Lack of awareness about antibody defects → considerable under-diagnosis. Be alert to patients with multiple infections per year (ear, sinus, chest, skin), failure of an infant to gain weight, or when family history of immune deficiency.
- Aim to prevent infections and complications and to enable a normal working capability and life expectancy.
- Involve patient in self-care and disease management.
- Involve: MDT, medical, and other specialists.
- Smoking should be discouraged.

Prevention of infection: NB adhere to principles of infection prevention and control

- Patients exposed to specific infections (e.g. rheumatic fever, TB, meningitis (should receive prophylactic antibiotics)).
- Treat prohylactically patients with HIV and pneumocystis and granulo-cytopaenifor prevention of bacterial infections.
- Immunization against influenza, meningococcal, and pneumococcal infections.
- Hepatitis B immunization given to people who regularly receive blood products.

Related topic

Principles of working with someone with an infectious disease.

Further information for professionals

Primary Immunodeficiency Association: www.pia.org.uk

Principles of working with someone with an infectious disease

Infectious or communicable diseases are illnesses caused by micro-organisms which would not normally be present in the body. These contrast with those acquired as a result of poor asepsis, antibiotic therapy, immunosuppressive drugs, or inadequate hand washing (see also 📖 Principles of working with someone with compromised immunity).

Causes

- Bacteria e.g. *streptococcus, salmonellosis, meningococcal* meningitis
- Viruses e.g. influenza, hepatitis, chickenpox
- Protozoa e.g. malaria, toxoplasmosis
- Infestation e.g. head lice.

Knowledge of the organism causing the disease is important in planning care.

Transmission

May be by ingestion, inhalation, innoculation (through a cut, skin abrasion or needle stick injury) and direct contact.

Care principles

- For common infectious diseases (e.g. herpes simplex, chickenpox) only general care is needed with precautions to prevent spread (e.g. hand hygiene (📖), contact avoidance, washing cutlery, not sharing toiletries).
- Isolation precautions for being nursed at home include wearing gloves and apron when in contact with body fluids or contaminated surfaces is likely, hand washing after removing gloves and before leaving the house.
- It is useful to carry some paper towels and a small container of alcohol handrub, if available, when visiting premises with inadequate hygiene facilities.
- Advice to patients and relatives should be given on washing clothes and dishes. Hot, soapy water is adequate for dishes and a hot wash (60°C) for clothes.
- Clinical waste should be disposed of in appropriately coloured bags designated for clinical waste in the community. (See also Managing health-care waste 📖.)
- Other isolation precautions are rarely necessary in the home.
- There should be referral to specialist advice if available and indicated (e.g. nurse or HV TB specialists).

Related topics

📖 Infectious disease notifications; 📖 Sterile cleaning, disinfection, and sterilization of equipment; 📖 Managing health-care waste; 📖 Sharps injuries; 📖 Bacterial skin infections; 📖 Fungal infections; 📖 Viral skin infections; 📖 Viral infections; 📖 MRSA; 📖 Viral hepatitis; 📖 Pandemic influenza; 📖 Tuberculosis.

Further information and resources for professionals

▣ CLINICAL KNOWLEDGE SUMMARIES (PRODIGY) (2004) has also produced guidelines on particular infectious diseases:
   www.cks.library.nhs.uk/guidance

▣ RCN (2005). Good practice in infection prevention and control:
   www.rcn.org.uk/resources/mrsa

Stewart, M.C. (2000). The immune system and infectious diseases. In Alexander, M.F. *et al* (eds). *Nursing practice: hospital and home*. 2nd edn. Churchill Livingstone, Edinburgh.

▣ The Health Protection Agency (2003). Guidelines on the management of communicable diseases in the community: www.hpa.org.uk/infections

Care provision

Urinary incontinence in women

Involuntary loss or urine is a common problem with 38% ♀ admitting to having had symptoms of incontinence over a 12mth period. Prevalence of daily incontinence ↑ with age:

- 12.2% in women 60–64yrs
- 20.9% in women 85yrs+.

Some evidence that it is hereditary. ♀ with incontinence often have lower self-esteem and physical and emotional health compared to those who do not have continence problems.

Types of urinary incontinence experienced by ♀ include:

- Overactive bladder (see below)
- Stress urinary incontinence (🕮)
- Mixed urinary incontinence i.e. leakage associated with urgency and also with exertion, effort, sneezing, or coughing.

Assessment of problem

- Ask ♀ about severity of incontinence, extent to which it affects every-day life, history, specific symptoms, and her desire for treatment.
- Mobility and access to toilets.
- Consider menopausal status, atrophic vaginal changes.
- General health issues obesity, fitness, smoking.
- Level of fluid intake.
- Consider possibility of constipation.
- Review medication some drugs exacerbate symptoms e.g. diuretics, antihistamines.
- Pelvic floor assessment (Stress urinary incontinence 🕮).

Investigations

- Test urine for UTI (🕮).
- Ask ♀ to complete a frequency and volume chart for 3d (see 🖥 www.continence-foundation.org.uk for example of chart).
- Refer to continence specialist service for bladder ultrasound to ensure voiding to completion and ♀ is not in retention.
- Consider referral to urodynamics service for possibly invasive tests if there is a complex history of previous vaginal surgery, neurological problems and/or the type of incontinence is uncertain.

Overactive bladder/urge incontinence

Occurs when bladder contracts unintentionally cause often unknown though can occur with MS, dementia, Parkinson's, and local irritation e.g. infection. Characterized by frequency and an overwhelming desire to void. Also may experience nocturia (voiding more than once overnight).

Symptoms can be antagonized if women smoke or are obese. Evidence is unclear about the negative effects of caffeine and fizzy drinks (see also Stress urinary incontinence 🕮).

Care and management

- Treat UTI (🕮).
- Advise and address any constipation (🕮).
- Advise on healthy diet and smoking cessation (🕮).

- Discuss the possible benefits of ↓ caffeine and fizzy drinks.
- Advise on bladder re-training (see below).
- Suggest/prescribe topical HRT (BNF 7.2.1) for atrophic changes in vagina (Menopause 📖).
- Pelvic floor exercises (Stress urinary incontinence 📖).
- Consider provision of incontinence pads for those with intractable problems according to local guidance (Continence products 📖).
- If symptoms do not respond to the above refer for specialist assessment and treatment e.g. drug therapy or electrical stimulation.
- Possibility of relapse so review and reassess every 3–4mths.

Bladder training programme: advice for patients

Aim to establish a normal pattern of bladder emptying of between 6–8 times a day by increasing the length of time of holding urine so bladder is trained to fill and stay relaxed

Drink 3–4 pints (2L) of liquid daily—avoiding coffee, tea, cola, hot chocolate, and alcohol.

Based on the recorded frequency of passing urine set a target that lengthens the time before going to the toilet to pass urine and increases the volume passed e.g.:

- Week 1: each time you feel the urge, hold urine and wait before going to the toilet for 5min longer.
- Week 2: hold for 10min.
- Week 3: hold for 15min.
- Week 4: hold for 20min.
- Week 5: hold for 25min.
- Week 6: hold for 30min.

The urge feeling is the first sign that your bladder is filling up but it will subside. When going to the toilet, do not rush. Sit down on the seat, do not hover over it, and do not push or strain to empty. Strategies that can help control the initial urge to pass urine include:

- Sitting on a hard seat or tightly rolled towel to put pressure on pelvic floor muscles.
- 5 quick squeezes of the pelvic floor muscles can help to manage the feeling of urgency.

Related topics

📖 Stress incontinence; 📖 Continence products; 📖 Menopause; 📖 Constipation in adults.

Further information for health-care professionals and patients

📖 Continence Foundation *Urgency, frequency and Treatments.* www.continence-foundation.org.uk
📖 Incontact for people affected by urinary and bowel problems and their carers: www.incontact.org

Stress urinary incontinence

See also ☐ Urinary incontinence in women. Loss of urine (often small amounts) upon physical exertion (cough, exercise). Occurs in 30% ♀ and for up to 10% ♀ it is a significant problem limiting activities; rare in ♂ except post-prostatectomy. Caused by incompetent urethral sphincter mechanism (e.g. following childbirth, surgery, pelvic floor weakness, hormone deficiency, ageing).

Assessment

- Symptoms, history, and patient's desire for treatment
- Childbirth (number, mode of delivery, birth weight)
- Menopausal status, atrophic vaginal changes
- Obesity, fitness, smoking
- Pelvic floor strength, voluntary contraction.

Investigations

- Test urine for UTI
- Fluid-volume chart for 3d.

Invasive tests not indicated unless complex history of previous vaginal surgery.

Care and management

- Advise on ↓ weight, smoking cessation (☐), and management of constipation (☐).
- Pelvic muscle exercises. See box. Exercises should achieve optimum results in 3–6mths.
- If simple exercises do not work, consider referral to continence advisor or physiotherapists, for biofeedback or electrical stimulation.
- Vaginal cones: small graduated weights placed in vagina, intention to use pelvic floor muscles to keep cone in place. Little evidence to support effectiveness but may help ♀ when doing pelvic floor exercises.
- Local HRT for atrophic changes in vagina.
- If symptoms severe, life-limiting, and do not respond to exercises discuss with patients if they want surgical referral. Surgery may be minimally invasive (e.g. tension free vaginal tape (TVT) or via abdominal incision or laparoscopic (e.g. colposuspension)). Good success rates, but some morbidity (e.g. voiding difficulties).

Prevention

Management of labour; lifelong pelvic muscle exercises; ↓ obesity and smoking.

Specialist support

Every primary care organization should have a continence advisor/ continence nurse specialist, practitioners and patients can access for specialist assessment and advice.

Pelvic floor exercises

Exercise 1
- Tighten the muscles around the anus, vagina, and urethra and lift up as if trying to stop passing urine and wind at the same time.
- Hold for as long as possible. Build up to a maximum of 10sec—rest for 4sec repeat to a maximum of 10 contractions.

Advise ♀ to try and isolate their pelvic floor as much as possible by
- Pulling in the abdominal muscles.
- Not squeezing legs together.
- Not holding breath or tightening buttocks.

Practice maximum number of contractions up to 6x a day.

Exercise 2
- Practice quick steady contractions, drawing in the pelvic floor muscles and holding for 1sec before releasing muscles.
- Aim for strong muscle tightening with each contraction up to maximum of 10x.

Advise to do 1 set of slow contractions (exercise 1) followed by 1 set of quick contractions (exercise 2), 6x each day.
Adapted from Continence Foundation advice.[1]

Related topics
📕 Urinary incontinence in women; 📕 Menopause; 📕 Women's health; 📕 Continence products; 📕 Constipation in adults.

1 🗗 Continence Foundation: www.continence-foundation.org.uk ☎ Helpline: 0845 345 0165

Urinary incontinence in men

Involuntary loss of urine that is a social or hygienic problem. 1:3 seek help at first sign of problem, 1:3 later and 1:3 suffer in silence. Opportunistic questioning can reveal problems.

Causes

- Outflow obstruction (enlarged prostate, tumour, neurogenic).
- Under-active detrusor muscle.
- Sphincter damage (e.g. post-prostatectomy).
- Functional incontinence arising from other problems: e.g. toileting difficulties (physical immobility or cognitive impairment/confusion).
- Neurological problems (e.g. stroke, MS, PD, spinal cord injury).
- Constipation/faecal impaction.
- NB Some drugs can exacerbate incontinence e.g. anticholinergics, diuretics, anti histamines, sedatives and hypnotics.

Assessment (see also Urinary incontinence in women 📖)

- Obtain history of symptoms (urgency, urge or stress leakage, nocturia, voiding difficulties, constant dribbling).
- Check urine for infection (MSU).
- Discuss with patient their own goals for treatment.
- Ability to self toilet whether any co-existing problems/morbidities.
- Fluid volume chart for 3d.

Care and management

- Treat reversible causes e.g. altering pattern of medication, UTI.
- Accessible toileting advise on aids.
- For post micturition dribble refer to continence specialist (see Stress urinary incontinence 📖).
- Patients with retention refer to GP for specialist review and possibly intermittent catheterization.
- Patients post prostatectomy may need specialist review.
- Patients with an overactive bladder/urge incontinence referral for bladder retraining to continence specialist (described in Urinary incontinence in women 📖). Antimuscarinics may also be used.
- Psychological support for distress and embarrassment. NB Carer may not be appropriate person to offer support.
- Provide male appliances or absorbent products according to needs and patient's wishes (Continence products 📖).

Related topics

📖 Constipation in adults.

Further information for patients

📟 Continence Foundation: www. continence-foundation.org.uk ☎ 0845 345 0165
📟 InContact: www.incontact.org

Further information for professionals

📟 Clinical Knowledge Summaries (Prodigy) advice on urology: www.cks.library.nhs.uk
Getliffe, K., and Dolman, M. (2003). *Promoting continence a clinical resource.* Balliere Tindall, London.

Urinary catheter care

Indwelling catheters

Used as a last resort due to complications including trauma, urinary tract infection, stricture formation, encrustation, urethral perforation, and carcinoma of the bladder.

Indications for using catheter

- Urethral obstruction with urinary retention
- Where it will enhance QoL or independence
- Occasionally if important to protect healing wounds e.g. pressure sores
- Patient is terminally ill and it increases their comfort
- Intermittent catheterization is an alternative for some, especially patients with neurogenic retention e.g. MS.

Choice of types

	Lengths	Gauges	Balloon sizes
♂	standard 40–45cm	10–22Ch	10–30mL
♀	20–26cm	10–22Ch	10–30mL
Paediatric	30–31cm	size 6–10Ch	3–5mL

- ❶ Only standard length catheters should be used for male catheterizations.
- Obese or chair bound females may require standard length catheters.
- ❶ Use smallest size which provides adequate drainage: sizes 12–16Ch usually adequate for adult, seek guidance if considering larger sizes.
- ❶ 30mL balloons only used post urological surgery or when bladder neck damage present (not routinely).

Catheter materials and coatings

The material and coating determines time it can remain *in situ*.

- Latex or plastic up to 14d
- Teflon-coated latex up to 28d

- Hydrogel coated up to 12wks
- All silicone up to 12wks
- Silicone elastomer-coated up to 12wks

- ❶ Consideration should be given to patients sensitive to latex products.
- Also consider supra-pubic rather than urethral (↑comfort, non-interference with sexual activity ↓ infection rates).

All catheters and bags available on prescription.

Inserting an adult indwelling catheter

- Check local policy regarding catheterization of females by male nurses.
- Check local policy regarding circumstances nurses can undertake male catheterizations e.g. often prohibited if patient is in acute retention, or history of pelvic trauma, and when haematuria present.
- Offer chaperone (🔖) and use aseptic technique.

As many female nurses have little experience of male catheterization, procedure outlined below:

- Retract foreskin if present, cleanse urethral meatus with soap and water and dry thoroughly.

- Instil lubricating/local anaesthetic gel from single use container into urethra and massage gel along male urethra. ❶ Caution with local anaesthetic products in patients taking anti arrhythmic medication, patients with cardiac conditions, hepatic insufficiency, and epilepsy.
- Allow 5min to elapse.
- Hold penis vertically and gently introduce catheter into urethra for 15–25cm until urine flows (if resistance is felt at the external sphincter, increase traction on penis slightly and apply steady, gentle pressure on catheter whilst asking patient to gently strain as if passing urine).
- When urine begins to flow, advance catheter almost to its bifurcation.
- Inflate balloon with sterile water or integral air bulb. ❶ Never inflate balloon until catheter is fully inserted into bladder.
- Observe for pain, discomfort, and bleeding.
- Gently withdraw catheter until slight resistance felt and connect catheter to closed drainage system, then secure drainage system.
- Return foreskin to original position.
- Document type of catheter (size, length, material, balloon size, batch, and manufacturer), lubricant instilled, problems negotiated, colour and consistency of urine, and patient's condition following procedure.

Drainage and support systems

The type of drainage and support system depends on individual assessment.
- *Intermittent drainage* by catheter valves give greater independence but are inappropriate with detrusor over activity, poor bladder capacity, ureteric reflux, or renal impairment.
- *Continuous drainage systems* either body worn systems or suspensory systems and larger capacity, night drainage bags.
  - Care should be taken to prevent infection entering the closed system.
  - Non-ambulant or confined to bed patients can have a sterile, drainable, 2L night bag and emptied as required.
  - Body worn systems should use a non-drainable night bag, discarded in the morning.
  - Drainage bags incorporating a sample port removes the need to break the closed system when obtaining a urine sample.
  - Bags should be changed weekly.

Blockages

Encrustation caused by formation of calcium phosphate and magnesium ammonium phosphate salts when the urine becomes alkaline due to urease-forming bacteria.
- Regular pH monitoring used to predict future blockages and plan individual maintenance programme.
- Prevention may involve acidification of urine by use of catheter maintenance solutions (citric acid solutions) or systemic agents such as ascorbic acid (vitamin C).
- Caution should be exercised as there is evidence that all bladder maintenance solutions increase shedding of epithelia cells within the bladder.

No encrustation: occlusion by bladder mucosa.
- If the catheter blocks and encrustation has not been a problem in the past, gently instil 20–30mL of sterile water into the catheter to flush.

Management

Advice to patients and carers:
- Advise a fluid intake 1.5–2L a day
- Avoid constipation (Constipation in adults 🕮)
- Avoid kinking of tubing and keep catheter bag below bladder
- Meatal care: gentle soap and water bd
- Emptying bag: high risk of contamination and subsequent infection: encourage careful hand hygiene (see NICE ref below).

If no problems with blockage catheter can be *in situ* 3m.

Problems

- People who frequently block their catheters: ↓ risk of blockage: acidify urine by encouraging vit. C and cranberry juice, regular saline washouts, and planned catheter changes.
- Infection: all long-term catheters become infected. Treat symptoms only e.g. fever.
- Leaking catheters: try smaller catheter and/or smaller balloon size.
- Bag can be changed every 5–7d or more often if discoloured, damaged, odourous, or build up of sediment. Also change following catheter change or instilling of maintenance solution.

Valves

Catheter valve can be used in place of drainage bag:
- Bladder drained intermittently.
- Good for patients who can recognize when bladder is full, can operate a valve and with a minimum bladder capacity of 200mL.
- Catheter valves should be changed every 5–7d.

> A spigot must never be used in place of a catheter valve.

Related topics

🕮 Urinary incontinence in women; 🕮 Urinary incontinence in men.

Further information for patients

🖳 InContact: www.incontact.org

Further information for professionals

The Royal Marsden Hospital Manual of Clinical Nursing Procedures. Dougherty, L. and Lister, S. (eds) (2004) (6th edn.), Blackwell Publishing, Oxford.

Getliffe, K., and Dolman, M. (2003). *Promoting continence a clinical resource.* Balliere Tindall, London.

NHS Quality Improvement Scotland (2004). *Best practice statement, urinary catheterization and catheter care*: www.nhshealthquality.org

NICE (2003). *Infection Control: prevention of health care associated infection in primary and community care Clinical Guidelines 2.* NICE, London: 🖳 Available at: www.nice.org.uk

Constipation in adults

3 million GP consultations pa; 10% DNs time spent remedying problems; NHS spends £45m pa on laxatives. Myths abound. (See also Faecal incontinence 🕮.)

Definition: constipation < than 3 stools per week and/or straining, hard stools or sense of incomplete evacuation at least 25% of the time. Associated symptoms:

- Abdominal discomfort, pain and bloating
- Lethargy and malaise
- 'Spurious diarrhoea'/overflow incontinence in frail impacted patients.

Prevalence: 5–10% population. 50%+ in care homes and neurological patients. >People believe that they are constipated than fit the definition.

Causes (may co-exist): 1. Slow colonic transit; 2. Evacuation difficulty. Underlying causes include:

- Poor diet (amount, frequency, fibre), low fluid intake, immobility
- Local anal pathology (e.g. haemorrhoids)
- Neurological disorders affecting sensory or motor function (e.g. spinal cord injury, multiple sclerosis, spina bifida, any neuropathy)
- Pregnancy
- Endocrine disorders (e.g. hypothyroidism, DM, hypercalcaemia)
- Difficulty with toilet access
- Drug side effects (e.g. analgesics, especially opioids)
- Idiopathic (may be associated with laxative abuse, anorexia).

Nursing assessment: need adequate privacy and time for patient to relax. Bowel diary and symptom questionnaire useful aid. Should include:

- History of the problem and former bowel habit
- Current symptoms, severity, and frequency
- Diet (especially fibre) and fluid intake
- Medication (include laxative history) and other medical conditions
- Effects of symptoms and limitations to lifestyle
- Co-existence of faecal incontinence
- Ability to use the toilet independently
- Availability and involvement of carers
- General observation: patient's mobility and ability to self-toilet
- Digital rectal examination for presence and consistency of stool when faecal impaction is suspected.

❶ Consider possibility of serious bowel pathology (rectal bleeding, unexplained change in bowel habit, anaemia, or weight loss) → referral to GP for further investigations.

Management: always try non-drug options first.

- Reassurance and patient education
- Ensure toilet is accessible (supporting feet on footstool may help evacuation)
- Address diet, fluids, mobility as possible
- Eat regularly and do not skip meals

- ↑ fibre slowly and mix types
- Unrefined bran can = bloating, mineral malabsorption, and impaction
- 1.5L fluids per day (but excessive will not help)
- Immobile: passive exercise or abdominal massage may help
- Regular toileting pattern after breakfast or evening meal (capitalize on the gastro-colic response)
- Change constipating medications if feasible
- Consider short-term laxatives or evacuants (see below) to establish a pattern
- Refer for specialist investigations if initial management fails.

Laxatives

Greatly over-used. Most become ↓ effective with continuous use. Abdominal discomfort and bloating may be 2° to laxatives. Re-evaluate regularly. See Fig. 10.1.
- Start with low dose of cheap preparation, discontinue ASAP
- Evacuation difficulty/hard stool: use softener or rectal preparation
- Slow transit: use a stimulant
- If long-term use is likely, find several and rotate.

Rectal preparations (see Constipation in adults 🕮: enemas and suppositories, and manual evacuation).

Related topics

🕮 Constipation and encopresis; 🕮 Faecal incontinence; 🕮 Palliative care in the home.

Further information

🕮 Müller-Lissner, S.A., Kamm, M.A., Scarpignato, C., and Wald, A. (2005). Myths and misconceptions about chronic constipation. *American Journal of Gastroenterology*, 100(1): 232–42.
🖳 www.bowelcontrol.org.uk
🖳 www.digestivedisorders.org.uk

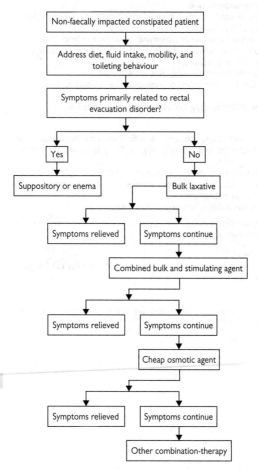

Fig. 10.1 Decision-making flow chart for use of laxatives. (Copyright © 2002 Royal College of Physicians. Reproduced by permission. The use and abuse of laxatives. In: Potter J, Norton C, Cottenden A, (eds). *Bowel care for older people*. Royal College of Physicians, London)

Constipation in adults: enemas, suppositories, and manual evacuation

Used when oral laxatives have been ineffective or when rapid relief of rectal loading is needed. Generally recommended for occasional use, frequent use may cause electrolyte imbalance and disturbance.

May be more predictable in effect and timing than oral laxatives. Especially useful for evacuation difficulties and in neurogenic constipation. May need carer or community nurse to administer.

NB Not all patients have the dexterity or find acceptable, and/or can find procedures distressing. Careful attention should be given to obtaining patient consent before undertaking any procedure.

Aim: to stimulate a complete rectal evacuation. Try to achieve desired result with the least intervention, in the following hierarchy, moving down the list until effect achieved:
- 1, then 2 glycerin suppositories
- 1, then 2 stimulant suppositories (e.g. bisacodyl)
- Micro (5mL) enema
- Water enema
- Phosphate enema. Use with care if tissue fragile (e.g. after pelvic irradiation) or electrolyte disturbance likely.

Suppositories (BNF 1.6.2)
Moisten or lubricate prior to insertion. Position against the rectal mucosa as high as can reach (will not work if embedded in stool). Controversy whether blunt or pointed end first, evidence unclear:
- Glycerin: 1 prn. If no effect, use 2. Paediatric size available. Lubricates stool plus slight stimulant effect on rectal mucosa.
- Bisacodyl: 1–2 daily. Rectal stimulant effect.
- Phosphate (Carbalax®).

Enemas (BNF 1.6.4)
It is customary to administer rectal preparations with the patient in the left lateral position, but sitting on the toilet may be more practical for some. Consider if self-administration is feasible.
- Micro enemas (5mL): sodium citrate.
- Tap water enemas: use 50–200mL warm tap water.
- Arachis oil (peanut oil) enema: as softener for hard stool. Do not use in nut allergic patients.
- Phosphate enemas: 120mL. Acts osmotically. Also as preparation prior to flexible sigmoidoscopy. Use with care if tissue fragile (e.g. after pelvic irradiation) or electrolyte disturbance likely (hyper-phosphataemia and perforation are RARE, but have been reported).

Manual evacuation
Some constipated patients find this helpful, especially those with neurological disorders and associated faecal incontinence (e.g. spinal cord injury, spina bifida). Also indicated with faecal impaction and when other bowel emptying techniques have failed.

Can be a very distressing procedure for patients.

- Check for abnormalities that might contraindicate procedure e.g. prolapse, anal lesions, haemorrhoids.
- Lubricate the finger with gel, if not a regular procedure consider using lignocaine gel on finger and anus.
- If stool is a solid mass push finger into the centre, split it and remove small sections until none remains.
- Encourage patient to assist with valsalva manoeuvre.
- Before and during procedure check pulse: stop if it changes or drops.
- In spinal patients consider risk of autonomic dysreflexia (where BP rises very rapidly) observe for headache, flushing, sweating, hypertension and stop procedure immediately.

Digital stimulation

Possible to stimulate a defecation reflex voluntarily by stimulation of the anus or anal sphincter in spinal injury patients if lesion above the cauda equine.

Related topics

📖 Constipation in adults; 📖 Urinary incontinence in women; 📖 Urinary incontinence in men; 📖 Spinal injury; 📖 Hand hygience; 📖 Managing health-care waste.

Further information

📖 Clinical Knowledge Summaries (Prodigy) guidelines use of laxatives,enemas and suppositories: www.cks.library.nhs.uk

RCN (2000, revised 2006). *Digital rectal examination and manual removal of faeces: guidance for nurses.* RCN, London.

Faecal incontinence (FI) in adults

Definition

'Involuntary loss of stool which is a social or hygienic problem'. Anal incontinence is used to denote involuntary loss of stool or flatus.

Prevalence

5% of community-dwelling adults, 1% having a regular and life-limiting problem. >25% in nursing home care. Very embarrassing, many reluctant to report symptoms. ❶ Active case-finding very important.

Causes

FI is a symptom not a diagnosis. Results from any combination of:
- Anal sphincter disruption or weakness, e.g. obstetric trauma
- Iatrogenic injury during anal surgery
- Impalement injuries
- Idiopathic anal sphincter degeneration
- Neurological disorders affecting sensory or motor function (e.g. spinal cord injury, multiple sclerosis, spina bifida, any neuropathy)
- Severe constipation with faecal impaction and 'overflow spurious diarrhoea' (frail and dependent people)
- Local anal pathology (haemorrhoids, prolapse, skin tags)
- Difficulty with toilet access, drug side effects.

Typical symptoms

- Urgency and urge FI (usually external sphincter disruption)
- Passive faecal soiling (usually internal sphincter disruption)
- Diarrhoea, loose stool or intestinal hurry (inflammation, diet, anxiety, irritable bowel syndrome) (Irritable bowel syndrome 🕮).

Nursing assessment

See checklist opposite.
Takes time, need adequate privacy for patient to relax. Bowel diary and symptom questionnaires give added information. Include:
- History of the problem and former bowel habit
- Current symptoms, severity, and frequency (see checklist)
- Diet (especially fibre) and fluid (especially caffeine) intake
- Medication and other medical conditions
- Effects of symptoms and limitations to lifestyle
- Co-existence of urinary incontinence (about 50%)
- Mobility and ability to use the toilet independently
- Availability and involvement of carers.

❶ Important to consider possibility of serious bowel pathology (rectal bleeding, unexplained change in bowel habit, anaemia or weight loss) referral → GP for further investigation.

Management

- Aim = firm loose stool (eg diet, antidiarrhoeals, loperamide 2–16mg daily)
- ↓ caffeine intake
- Make sure toilet is accessible

- Pelvic muscle exercises (Stress urinary incontinence 📖)
- Bowel retraining for urgency (urge resistance, practice deferment)
- Address constipation if present
- If initial management fails. Refer to GP for referral for specialist investigations.

Checklist for faecal incontinence symptom assessment

- Onset of symptoms
- Usual bowel habit
- Changes in bowel habit
- Stool consistency (Bristol stool form scale)
- Amount and frequency of faecal incontinence
- Urgency or urge faecal incontinence
- Passive soiling
- Difficulty wiping clean after toilet
- Nocturnal bowel symptoms
- Abdominal pain and bloating
- Evacuation difficulty:
  - Straining
  - Incomplete evacuation
  - Pain
  - Digitation
- Control of flatus
- Rectal bleeding or mucus
- Products used to manage faecal incontinence.

Related topics

📖 Constipation in adults; 📖 Urinary incontinence in men; 📖 Urinary incontinence in women; 📖 Continence products.

Further information

Norton, C., and Chelvanayagam, S. (2004). *Bowel Continence Nursing*. Beaconsfield Publishers, Beaconsfield UK.

🖥 Website for patient information: www.bowelcontrol.org.uk

Stoma care

Approx 100,000 people with stomas in UK. Majority in people >50yrs. Many will need an adjustment period after stoma formation. Support for patient and family crucial.

Three main types of stoma (temporary stomas formed to allow intestinal healing post surgery):

- Colostomy (most common). Colonic: 1–2 formed bowel actions per day usual.
- Ileostomy: 15000 in UK. Small bowel content, continuous semi-liquid and corrosive.
- Urostomy (ileal conduit): continuous urine.

Reasons for needing a stoma

- Inflammatory bowel disease (📖).
- Bowel cancer.
- Diverticular disease (Appendicitis, diverticulitis, hernias, and intestinal obstruction 📖).
- Accidental damage to the bowel wall.
- Urostomies rare, → cancer, or pelvic or abdominal surgery, incontinence.

Nursing assessment and management[1]

NB Output from stoma will change in the first 7wks post surgery:

- Discuss with patient, and ask about preferences, concerns and their understanding of how their stoma works.
- Recognize there is a substantial adjustment required to living with a stoma and reassure them that they can lead a normal and active life.
- Note size, colour, and position of stoma and surrounding skin check for any signs of retraction, prolapse, infection, stenosis excoriation etc.
- If possible observe how patient manages stoma, check they can see stoma and their dexterity with equipment.
- Encourage normal balanced diet, emphasize importance of ↑ fluids (2L for patients with ileostomies) some people find sensitivities or flatus from some foods. Occasional blocking of small diameter stoma with nuts/seeds, mushrooms, sweetcorn.
- Leaking appliances usually caused by poor fit. Stoma may change shape, especially postoperatively and if body weight changes. May also be poor siting or skin deformities (can build up by using paste/wafers).
- Sore skin: true allergy is rare. Often a leaking appliance or inappropriate management (changing too often or without due care; use of skin products on sensitive skin). Cleanse with water avoid deodorants and creams. Check bag fit around stoma. Watch bag, change routine. Observe pattern of soreness.
- Flatus: chew food carefully and note foods and drinks that cause flatus.
- Constipation: ↑ fluid and dietary fibre intake.
- Pain: patients with pain associated with the stoma should be referred to the GP.
- Patients do not need to wear an appliance when swimming or bathing.
- Travel: take adequate supplies and avoid heat when storing pouches.

[1] Myers, C. (1996). *Stoma care nursing*. Arnold, London.

Products

Very individual. Trial and error to find the best product for each patient. Many companies will send samples. Two piece: to avoid frequent flange changes. Drainable bag for urostomy and ileostomy (with night extension if needed). In UK all products are on prescription and patients are exempt from prescription charges. Some bags are flushable.

Stoma care nurses

Available for home visits or clinic consultations in most areas.

Related topics

📖 Faecal incontinence; 📖 Constipation in adults.

Further information for patients

🖥 British Colostomy Association: www.bcass.org.uk and links to products and clothing suppliers
🖥 Ileostomy and Internal Pouch Support: www.the-ia.org.uk

Continence products

Most people with continence problems can achieve a successful resolution without continence products. However for others the appropriate product gives confidence and an unrestricted quality of life.

Many continence products provided through NHS (local policies apply) and the range of products available may be determined by local policy. Laundry costs are usually the responsibility of individual and carers.

Points to consider when assessing and choosing a product
- Lifestyle of the patient: e.g. level of activity, cosmetic effect
- Pattern of incontinence e.g. more protection needed at night
- Visual acuity, cognitive ability, and dexterity for using products
- If patient is alone or has help with personal care
- Costs especially if product not provided by NHS.

Reason for choosing a continence product
- Maintenance of skin integrity
- Protection of furniture and equipment e.g. covers and pads
- Protection of individual and their clothes e.g. pads and pants
- Specialist products e.g. sheaths, alarms, catheters
- Need an alternative to the toilet because of access problems or urgency e.g. commode, male or female urinals.

See Continence Foundation Directory and Promocon websites for detailed list of products and prices (below). Local continence specialist staff will also produce information.

Points about bedding protection
- Mattress covers: breathable fabrics preferable (PVC covers often hot and uncomfortable only suitable for short-term use).
- 'No launder duvets' can be wiped down, dried, and reused.
- Covers with terry toweling surface preferable for occasional episodes of incontinence at night.
- Reusable bed pads often used in conjunction with personal body protection. Can be difficult to launder at home.

Points about personal protection from urine and faeces
Wide range of choice to reflect patient preference and type of continence problem. The absorbency of a product depends on the materials used and not its cost, size, or thickness. Barrier creams should not be used with pads as they affect product's ability to absorb urine.
❶ Sanitary towels are inappropriate for urinary incontinence:
- All in one (Pad and pant combined): disposable or reusable: Suitable for heavy urinary or faecal incontinence especially if confined to wheelchair/bed bound. Hip measurements important to ensure good fit. NB Any form of toileting difficult with this product.
- Insert pads (disposable and reusable): cater for slight/moderate and heavy urinary incontinence. Held in place by close fitting underpants (net or stretch pants). If pads do not have waterproof padding then

use with waterproof pants or pants with waterproof pouch. For men with light/dribbling incontinence possible to have pouch pad held in place with adhesive strip in tight fitting underpants.

- Absorbent pants: disposable and reusable. Suitable for slight urinary leaks or faecal staining. Use hip measurements for women and waist measurements for men and children. Useful when travelling or where laundry difficult. Most like ordinary underwear, does not require manual dexterity (i.e. to fit pad etc.). Can be used over insert pad for extra absorbency. Disadvantage: every pad change = change of underwear.
- Penile sheaths: condom urinal, incontinence sheath. Soft rubber sleeve available on prescription, available in one or multiple sizes (some manufacturers provide sizing chart/measuring device). Good for men with physical disabilities, but may not be suitable for:
  - Men with a small or retracted penis
  - If patient is confused or demented and may pull sheath off
  - If patient has limited dexterity and needs help to fix it on
  - Skin sensitivity e.g. latex intolerance.
- Self adhesive sheaths: a strip of double side special adhesive wrapped round the penis and the sheath is rolled up over it. Men with sensitive skin or those who make frequent changes may prefer external fixing around the outside of the sheath: a foam strip with adhesive on one side or a rubber adjustable strap fixed with a button or Velcro. To apply:
  - Make sure foreskin is not pulled back
  - Keep a gap between tip of penis and outlet of sheath to allow for sudden gushing of urine but not enough to allow twisting
  - Avoid pressure on penis and check for soreness/tissue damage.

Aids for the toilet and toileting

- Range of aids designed to promote continence and independence e.g. bottom wipers and customized commodes for use in cars etc. Information from Promoncon (below) see also aids to independent living (Aids to daily living and equipment for home nursing 📖).
- Male and female hand held urinals. Allows people with limited mobility to be continent and independent especially in situations where access to toilets difficult. Useful for carers if moving and handling is difficult. Can be used in bed, seated or standing depending on the users' capabilities.
- Radar Keys for people who need quick access to public toilets when out ☎ 0207 250 3222.

Related topics

📖 Urinary incontinence in women; 📖 Urinary incontinence in men.

Further information for health-care professionals patients and carers

📖 Continence Foundation: www.continence-foundation.org.uk
📖 Promoncon Promoting continence and product awareness: www.promocon.co.uk

Spinal cord injury

Approx 700 new spinal injuries pa in the UK, most common in 16–30yrs and >80% ♂. Most common causes falls (41%) and RTA (37%).

Extent of paralysis depends on level of injury.

- C4 injury = complete paralysis below the neck
- C6 injury = partial paralysis of hands and arms as well as lower body
- T4 injury = paralysis from chest down
- L1 injury = paralysis below the waist.

Where there is incomplete injury there is more variation between patients in the amount of movement they have. Patients with acute spinal injury will be managed in neurosurgery and/or spinal unit, majority will go home to adapted living accommodation often with carer support.

Common longer-term problems patients may encounter include:

- Psychological problems including depression
- Financial hardship
- Family and relationship stress and breakdown
- Bladder and bowel dysfunction
- Autonomic dysreflexia
- Pressure sores
- Temperature regulation
- Cardiovascular and respiratory disorders
- Risk of DVT and PE.

Care and management

- Common responses to spinal injury are disbelief, low self-esteem, anger, guilt, and depression and both patients and their families can take a long time to adjust. Important they receive emotional support from the MDT and voluntary/charitable groups with specialist knowledge of living with a spinal injury (see below).
- People with spinal injury will be eligible for range of disability benefits e.g. higher rate disability living allowance for mobility: schemes like Motobility can provide a car or motorized wheel chair.
- Citizens advice bureau and specialist legal centres can provide advice on employment and welfare rights (see below) and access to education and sport and leisure.
- Patients with complete spinal cord injury do not sweat below the level of their injury therefore in environments of high humidity and heat the body temperature rises. The use of wet towels around the neck and water spray to mimic the effect of sweat can help manage this. In cold environments patients may become hypothermic. Important they have access to warmth and warm drinks and clothes.
- Prevention of UTI and bladder management: retention or urine with overflow incontinence can put patient at risk of long-term renal damage. Ensure bladder drained by self-catheterization or patient may need a urinary diversion formed.
- Bowel care: prevention of constipation and establishing a predictable bowel regime. May require manual evacuation of faeces.
- Autonomic dysreflexia (see also Urinary catheter care 📖) in manual removal of faeces in patients with injury above T6, caused by noxious

stimulus (e.g. full bladder/bowel, pain) occurring below injury. Monitor symptoms of: dramatic ↑ BP, patient appears flushed above level of injury and pale below (due to vasoconstriction), bradycardia, pounding headache, blurred vision, nausea, and profuse sweating. Can lead to cerebral haemorrhage and seizures. ❶ Medical emergency: remove stimulus immediately, give GTN spray 1–2 puffs sublingually or nifedipine 5–10mg capsule sublingual (BNF 2.6).

Related topics

📖 Expert patient; 📖 Carers assessment and support.

Further information for patients carers and health professionals

🖥 Disability law service: www.dls.org.uk
🖥 Spinal injuries association: www.spinal.co.uk
🖥 Spinal injuries Scotland: www.sisonline.org

Pressure ulcer prevention

Pressure ulcers are areas of localized damage to the skin and underlying tissue caused by combination of pressure, shear, and friction. Prevalence is 5–9% and 70% occur in >70yrs. Potential to develop pressure ulcers may be exacerbated by moisture to the skin and certain medications. Pressure ulcers are generally avoidable. Risk factors in individuals include:

- Immobility
- Sensory impairment (especially with spinal injury)
- Acute illness
- Impaired consciousness
- Incontinence
- >70yrs
- Vascular disease
- Chronic or terminal illness
- History of pressure damage
- Malnutrition and dehydration.

Formal risk assessment

Initial assessment should be included within 6hrs of any first contact with patients likely to be at risk. Subsequent assessments as indicated by the patient's condition. Risk assessment tools (e.g. Walsall Community Pressure sore risk calculator) that give scores are an aide memoir and do not replace clinical judgement.[1] Assessment includes:

- Consideration of individual risk factors (as above) and patient and carer's understanding of their at risk status.
- Document skin inspection (frequency determined individually):
  - Inspect heels, sacrum, ischial tuberosities, shoulders, back of head, toes, parts of the body affected by anti-embolic stockings, equipment and clothing, and parts of the body where pressure, friction and shear is exerted.
  - Observe for persistent erythema and non-blanching erythema on light skinned patients, purplish/bluish localized patches on dark skinned patients, blisters, localized heat, localised oedema, and localized induration (see grading system below).
  - Encourage patients to inspect own skin (teach mirror use for wheel chair users).
  - Document skin changes.

Wheelchair users should have specific seating assessments, usually by physiotherapists or OTs. Some areas have wheel chair clinics.

Care plan should include

Essentials of care

- Involve patient and carer in decision making
- Monitor BMI and advise on nutritional status
- Effective management of incontinence and skin cleaning
- Apply moisturisers to dry skin
- Avoid skin rubbing and massage over bony prominences
- Ensure correct moving and handling to avoid shearing.

---

1 RCN (2005). *The prevention and management of pressure ulcers: quick reference guide Clinical Guideline 29.* www.rcn.org.uk developed with the National Institute for Health and Clincial Excellence.

Pressure redistribution devices

- Choice based on patient comfort, lifestyle and abilities, critical care needs, and acceptability of proposed equipment to patient and carer.
- Availability, maintenance, cleaning etc of devices for home use subject to local policies.
- Patients at 'risk' require low-pressure or overlay mattresses.
- Patients at 'high risk' require alternating pressure mattresses.
- ❶ Do not use doughnut type devices, synthetic sheepskins, genuine sheepskins, or water filled gloves as ineffective and potentially harmful.

Positioning and seating

- Frequency of repositioning should be determined an individual basis and aim to minimize prolonged pressure on bony prominences.
- Repositioning to continue even when pressure redistribution devices in use.
- Patients at very high risk should restrict chair sitting to <2hrs.
- Keep bony prominences from direct contact with one another.
- Teach patients and carers to redistribute weight.
- Remove slings and other parts of manual handling equipment from underneath patient after manoeuvring.
- Consider distribution of weight, postural alignment, and support of feet when seating patients.

Pressure sore grading systems

Many classification systems exist and can be useful. 4 grades are the simplest to use as below:

- Grade 1: non-blanchable erythema of intact skin. Discolouration of the skin, warmth, oedema, induration, or hardness.
- Grade 2: partial thickness skin loss involving epidermis, dermis, or both.
- Grade 3: full thickness skin loss involving damage to or necrosis of subcutaneous tissue.
- Grade 4: extensive destruction, tissue necrosis, or damage to muscle, bone, or supporting structures with or without full thickness skin loss. (adapted from 🕮 European Pressure Ulcer Advisory Panel www.epuap.org).

Essential reading

🕮 NICE (2003). Pressure ulcer prevention, pressure ulcer risk assessment and prevention, including the use of pressure-relieving devices (beds, mattresses and overlays) for the prevention of pressure ulcers in primary and secondary care. www.nice.org.uk

Further information

🕮 The Tissue Viability Society: www.tvs.org.uk

Wound assessment

Accurate assessment is vital to provide correct treatment and evaluate its effectiveness. It must always be part of a wider, holistic approach.

> ### Aims of wound assessment
> - Determine cause/aetiology
> - Monitor treatment effect
> - Support clinical decision making
> - Identify healing and non-healing wounds
> - Early detection of complications
> - Resource allocation
> - Improve patient concordance

Practical indications that a wound is responding to treatment include:
- Reduction in exudate production.
- Improvement in condition of the wound bed.

These parameters are subjective and difficult to measure, particularly in chronic wounds, which do not always follow the expected sequence of healing. Wounds can be objectively assessed in a variety of other ways: acidity (pH), temperature, and wound dimension.

> In clinical practice the most commonly assessed objective parameter is wound size.

Wound dimensions
- Simple length and width measurements overestimate size of larger, irregular wounds.
- More accurate results obtained by tracing the wound circumference using acetate sheets and a pen *but* is subjective.
- Use of portable digital planimeters ↑ accuracy of wound circumference measurement.
- NICE (2005)[1] guidelines recommend photographing and/or tracing pressure ulcers at initial assessment.

Wound healing curves[2]
Monitoring wound healing curves particularly within the first 4wks of treatment can determine efficacy of treatment.

Wound healing curves plot the reduction in % area of the wound surface against time on a graph to determine progression towards healing.
This requires 3 key elements:
- Measurement: a recording of wound surface area.
- Time: a recording made at consistent intervals.
- A consistent approach.

A ↓ of wound area between 20–40% from initial assessment, between 2–4wks of treatment = a reliable indicator of healing. A ↓ in surface area <10% per month is indicative of a non-responding chronic wound. Every 7 to 10d measure the % reduction of wound surface area.

1 NICE (2005). *The prevention and treatment of pressure ulcers.* www.nice.org.uk
2 Fette, A. (2006). *A clinimetric analysis of wound assessment tools.* www.worldwidewounds.com

Characteristics of wound bed

Identification of tissue type will indicate the depth of the wound, potential complications (e.g. infection) and length of time to healing. Knowledge of anatomy is important as a relatively shallow wound or a finger may involve tendons, and bone. Need to ask what the tissue involvement is e.g. bone, fascia, muscle, tendon, subcutaneous fat, dermis, epidermis etc.

Colour of wound bed The predominant colour of a wound can be used as a method of classifying wounds to inform treatment.
- Pink: epithelial cells—protection
- Red: granulation tissue—protection
- Yellow: loose = slough; adherent= fibrinous tissue—debridement
- Black: necrotic tissue (wet or dry)—debridement.

Exudate No standard definitions/methods of assessing exist. What is 'normal' varies depending on wound type, size and stage of healing. Exudate is described subjectively:
- Volume: low, medium, high
- Viscosity: low, medium, high
- Colour: straw coloured (serous), red (blood), creamy off-white (purulent) (Infected wounds 🕮).

Wound edges and surrounding skin

Wound margin condition provides information for wound status and dressing suitability:
- Flat migrating sides: healthy, moist, dividing epithelial cells
- Steep non-migrating sides: unhealthy, dry, epithelial cells
- Escar: dry wound secretions, dead cells
- Induration: firm swelling with or without redness
- Inflammation: pink/red, warm indicative of inflammatory process
- Maceration: white, soft, wet tissue. Indicates poor exudate control.

Documentation

The following should be included in wound assessment documentation. (see also related topics below):
- Patient details
- Pressure ulcer risk assessment
- General skin condition
- Wound type, duration, location, dimensions
- Exudate type/amount, wound odour
- Characteristics of wound bed—colour, tissue type
- Condition of wound margin/surrounding skin
- Wound pain/discomfort
- Previous treatment.

Related topics

🕮 Management of chronic wounds; 🕮 Pressure ulcers prevention; 🕮 Infected wounds; 🕮 Principles of leg ulcer assessment and management; 🕮 Fungating wounds; 🕮 Wound dressings.

Further information for professionals

🖵 Website for specialist information on wound care: www.worldwidewounds.com

Postoperative wound care

The aims of postoperative wound care are to reduce discomfort, aid healing, and produce the best cosmetic result possible. Surgical wounds can be closed by primary or secondary intention. Potential wound complications include haematoma, infection, dehiscence, sinus, and fistula formation.

Wounds healing by primary intention

Wound edges opposed and secured using sutures (absorbable and non-absorbable), staples, tissue adhesives, and adhesive skin tapes. The 3 most common suture lines seen in primary care are continuous sutures (a series of stitches taken with one strand of material, proximal and distal ends knotted), interrupted sutures (a number of strands closing the wound, each knotted and cut after insertion), and subcuticular sutures (continuous sutures placed in the dermis, beneath the epithelial layer, proximal and distal ends knotted or secured with an anchoring device). See Fig. 10.2.

A light dry dressing is required until haemostasis is achieved and the wound is sealed by a fibrin scab. Dressings can usually be removed after 24–48hrs. Alternatively a vapour permeable dressing may be applied and left in place until the wound closure material is removed. Any build up of exudate under the film should be removed according to the manufacturer's instructions. Occlusive dressings should not be used with tissue adhesives. Surgical incision wounds should *only* require cleaning when excessive leakage has occurred. Adhesive skin tapes are left in place until they peel off by themselves and tissue adhesives slough off in 7–10d.

Removal of sutures or staples

- Establish number of sutures/staples and when to remove e.g. from discharge letter or referral. Most removed 7–10d (less if on face and more for high tension areas e.g. back).
- Encourage patient to wash area prior to procedure.
- Perform procedure using aseptic technique and PPE (📖).
- Examine wound to assess whether suture/staple removal appropriate.
- Clean wound with normal saline 0.9%.
- For continuous sutures, lift knot of suture with forceps, snip stitch close to the skin, and gently remove entire suture.
- For interrupted sutures, lift knot of suture with forceps, snip stitch close to the skin, and gently remove individual suture. Repeat on alternating sutures. If wound remains intact remove remaining sutures.
- For subcuticular sutures, lift knot or anchoring device e.g. bead, snip stitch close to the skin, and gently remove entire suture.
- For staples, hold staple remover device at 90 degree angle, slip lower jaw under bridge of staple, gently close handles and the staple is automatically released. Repeat on alternating staples. If wound remains intact remove remaining staples. Dispose of staples in sharps box.
- Ensure no sutures/staples have been left in skin unintentionally.
- If wound gapes use adhesive tape to oppose wound edges.
- Record condition of wound closure line and surrounding skin.

(a) Interrupted suture

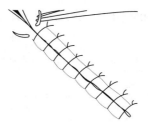

(b) Continuous suture

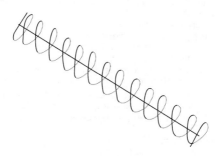

Fig. 10.2 Sutures

Wounds healing by secondary intention

Wound edges come together naturally by means of granulation and contraction (for example, abscess cavities such as peri-anal abscesses). These wounds require a moist healing environment. Dressing materials include alginates, hydogels, foams, hydrocolloids. Cavity wounds should be lightly filled with an absorbent dressing material. Tight packing can lead to tissue ischemia and tissue death. Surgical wounds healing by secondary intention often require cleaning. This can be achieved by the patient having a shower and so irrigating the wound with warm water. Infected wounds should be irrigated with normal saline 0.9%. Hydrocolloids should be avoided on infected wounds.

Essential reading

Dougherty, L. and Lister, S. (eds) (2004) *The Royal Marsden Hospital Manual of Clinical Nursing Procedures*, 6th edition, Blackwell Publishing.

Further information

Website for information on wounds: www.worldwidewounds.com

Management of chronic wounds

In chronic wounds the normal repair process becomes disrupted at one or more of the different stages of wound healing. Chronic wounds are classified according to their underlying pathology e.g. pressure ulcers, venous leg ulcers etc.

Although some chronic wounds heal and respond to conventional therapy, many become unresponsive and need advanced technologies to stimulate healing. It is important to differentiate between a responding chronic wound and a non-responsive wound.

The aetiology of acute and chronic wounds are different (Table 10.1) and require different management approaches. General wound management principles:

- Correct underlying cause of wound
- Improve factors that may delay healing
- Create optimum local environment at the wound site
- Identify realistic treatment objectives
- Prevent further wound deterioration or complications
- Evaluate effectiveness of wound management interventions.

During the continuous process of assessment about the status of the chronic wound the following questions should be asked:

- Prolonged inflammatory response?
- Infection?
- Necrotic tissue?
- Unhealthy granulation tissue?
- Tissue ischemia?
- Delayed epithelialization?
- Skin maceration?
- Skin sensitivities and allergies?

Specific chronic wound management principles

Wound management decisions rely on assessment, complex decision making skills, and experience (Wound assessment 🕮) including wound type, size and location as well as the patient's psychological response.

Wound bed preparation

An approach that can remove barriers associated with chronic non healing and aims at ↓ oedema, ↓ exudate, ↓ bacterial burden and, correcting abnormalities contributing to impaired healing. There are 4 components:

- Tissue management
- Inflammation and infection
- Moisture balance
- Epithelial (edge) advancement.

Tissue management

Chronic wounds have a 'necrotic burden' that accumulates and consists of necrotic tissue, dead cells and exudate that delay healing. Initial debridement: a temporary improvement in healing can be observed followed by gradual deterioration. Recommend steady continuous removal of necrotic burden (Wound debridement 🕮).

Inflammation and infection

↑ bacterial load within chronic wounds can lead to delayed healing. Regardless of the type of organism, substantial impairment of healing occurs, when there is between 10^5 and 10^6 organisms per gram in a wound bed. However, the number of organisms in a wound may not necessarily be as critical as the type and pathogenicity of the organism present (Infected wounds 📖). Removal of bacterial burden at the wound surface ↓ the possibility of infection but also may ↓ the prolonged inflammation response characteristic of chronic wounds. ↓ the bacterial count, by debridement or slow-release antimicrobials can help.

Moisture balance

Moisture balance at the wound/dressing interface is agreed to be a key factor responsible for optimizing wound healing. Control of excess wound exudate is important as it increases the risk of:

- Delayed inflammation
- Cellular inhibition
- Wound infection
- Odour
- Skin maceration
- Excoriation.

Table 10.1 Differences between chronic and acute wounds

	Acute wounds	Chronic wounds
Healing Process	Regulated	Haphazard
Pathology	None	Underlying
Time to healing	Rapid	Slow
Inflammatory response	Short	Prolonged
Exudate	Reduced after 48hrs	Prolonged
	Promotes cellular proliferation	Inhibits cellular proliferation
Bacterial Load	Low	High
Fibroblast proliferation	Active	Inactive
Excoriation/maceration	Infrequent	Frequent
Extracellular matrix	Normal remodelling	Defective remodelling
Vascular network	Good	Poor
Complications	Infrequent	Frequent
Progress	Heal	Fail to heal/recur

Reproduced from Flanagan, M and Fletcher, J (2006) Wound pathologies; causes of acute and chronic wounds in Bale, S and Gray, D (eds). A pocket guide to Clinical Decision Making in wound management. Wounds UK Publishing, Aberdeen. By kind permission of Wounds UK Ltd.

Exudate can be managed using direct means such as:
- Wound cleansing
- Absorbent dressings
- Compression therapy
- Topical negative pressure
- Skin protection.

Or indirectly by alleviating underlying cause e.g. heart failure, diabetes, venous insufficiency, and managing symptoms e.g. infection, excoriation.

Epithelial (edge) advancement

Epithelialization = final stage of wound healing needs well-prepared wound bed and a source of healthy epidermal cells, promoted by:
- Well vascularized granulation tissue
- Absence of infection
- Optimal moisture levels
- Hydration of wound margins
- Minimal dressing trauma.

Healing can be monitored using a series of wound measurements plotted as a graph (Wound assessment 🛄). This allows early detection of complications and prompt intervention.

Related topics

🛄 Wound assessment; 🛄 Infected wounds; 🛄 Principles of leg ulcer assessment and management; 🛄 Fungating wounds; 🛄 Principles of wound management following amputation.

Further information for professionals

🖥 European Wound Management Association: www.ewma.org
🖥 World wide wounds online journal for wound management information: www.worldwidewounds.com

Infected wounds

Wound infection

Defined as the presence of bacteria within a wound with multiplication and an associated host reaction. If a wound contains 10^6 bacteria per gram of tissue = usually defined as being infected. Wound infection initiates the body's immune response locally then systemically if untreated will delay healing.

Bacterial colonization is of no clinical significance and should not be confused with wound infection.

Critical colonization

Is the term used to describe a wound where the bacterial burden is rising due to multiplication of organisms which are beginning to cause a delay in healing. Critical colonization initiates the body's immune response locally but not systemically.

Risk factors
- Number of organisms present
- Bacterial pathogenicity
- Host resistance—immunocompetence
- Local anoxia
- Devitalised tissue
- Haematoma
- Foreign bodies

Surgical wounds
- Presence of an existing chronic infection
- Nature of invasive procedure—especially bowel
- Extent of tissue loss and/or trauma to tissues during surgery
- Adequacy of wound drainage.

Signs and symptoms
- Raised temperature—shivering, fever
- Tachycardia
- Generally feeling unwell
- Confusion (older people)
- Lymphangitis
- Neutrophilia.

Local signs
- Erythema—spreading cellulitis
- Localized oedema, heat
- Loss of function—pain/tenderness
- Increased exudate levels
- Increased odour
- Increased slough/necrosis
- Pus formation
- Bridging/pocketing at the wound base
- Fragile granulation (bleeds easily)
- Dark red (cherry) granulation tissue
- Wound breakdown
- Non-healing wound.

Investigations

- Bloods: FBC, ESR
- Swab for M, C & S if signs above
- Diabetic foot ulcers: if signs above, X-ray foot to exclude osteomyelitis.

Care and management

Objectives of treating infected wounds are:

- Identify the infective organism
- Remove devitalized tissue and excess exudate
- Eliminate wound infection using appropriate antimicrobial agents
- Protect the surrounding skin from the effects of maceration.

Select wound dressings for exudating wounds. Assess wounds daily change dressings frequently. Some evidence that topical antimicrobials could be used selectively for:

- Stimulation of previously unresponsive chronic wounds
- Treatment of infected wounds
- Eradication of MRSA from contaminated wounds (MRSA 📖).

Evidence indicates that some iodine and silver preparations have bacteriocidal effects even against multi-resistant organisms such as MRSA. This suggests that bacterial resistance to such a topical agent is less likely to develop. Critically colonized wound use local formulary for topical, sustained, antimicrobial dressings.

Reserve systemic antibiotics for diagnosed wound infection.

Adjunctive measures

- Wound debridement may be necessary (Wound debridement 📖)
- Exudate management
- Skin protection may be necessary.

Spreading infection i.e. visibly spreading from wound site, requires systemic antibiotics (possibly IV), dressing selection will have little impact on the spreading infection. Seek appropriate medical help immediately.

Complications

- Delayed/non-healing wounds
- Wound dehiscence
- Cross infection
- Oesteomylitis (especially diabetic foot ulcers, sacral pressure ulcers)
- Septicemia
- Death.

Related topics

📖 Wound assessment; 📖 Management of chronic wounds; 📖 Principles of leg ulcer assessment and management; 📖 Fungating wounds; 📖 Wound dressings.

Further information for professionals

European Wound Management Association (EWMA) (2005). *Position Document: Identifying criteria for wound infection.* MEP Ltd; London.

📖 World wide wounds on-line journal for wound management information:
www.worldwidewounds.com

Wound debridement

Removal of non-viable tissue is essential (provided there is an adequate blood supply) to promote wound healing and ↓ the risk of local infection. When necrotic tissue collects at the wound surface it may:
- Delay wound apposition and closure
- Prolong inflammation
- ↑ wound odour
- ↑ risk of infection
- Limits effectiveness of antibiotic therapy
- Inhibits epithelial cell migration
- Prevents accurate wound assessment
- ↑ scarring.

Methods

The most common methods of debridement include:
- Sharp (surgical or conservative)
- Autolytic
- Chemical
- Enzymatic
- Mechanical
- Biological.

Sharp conservative debridement: the removal of dead tissue, with a scalpel or scissors, above the level of viable tissue is quickest and most cost effective method. The decision to use a particular method depends upon a number of factors e.g. wound type, location, extent of tissue damage, amount of exudates. For chronic wounds debridement may take several weeks and require more than one method.

Sharp (surgical or conservative)
Surgical debridement: an extensive procedure performed by surgeons. Sharp debridement is conservative and can be performed in the home or clinic environment. Debridement using a scalpel must be performed by an experienced, competent clinician. Issues to be considered: training, adequate supervised practice, informed patient consent, need for local anaesthesia, and patient reassurance.

Contraindications
- Ischaemic wounds
- Blood clotting disorders/long-term anticoagulant therapy
- Necrotic tissue close to or involving blood vessels/nerves/tendons
- Fungating/malignant wounds
- Patients with reduced sensation
- Debridement of the feet/hands (excluding the heel)
- Debridement of the face.

Autolytic debridement

Autolysis: commonest method of debridement using moist or occlusive dressings e.g. hydrogels, hydrocolloids. These dressings have a high water content that help to soften devitalized tissue. The speed of debridement will vary between products. Speed of autolysis depends on the wound size and the patient's general physical condition. Rapid debridement may occur within 2–3d making it safe and effective in the home care setting. (BNF Appendix 8.1.3).

Chemical debridement

Strong chemical agents e.g. hypochlorites are rarely used due to adverse side effects and increased availability of less toxic and more effective products. Iodine, (either povidone or cadexomer) has a broad spectrum antibacterial activity and a secondary effect of drying out wet slough to facilitate sharp debridement.

Enzymatic debridement

They have limited use for wounds with hard, dry eschar. Enzymatic preparations collaginase may be used on chronic wounds as the active ingredient proteases penetrate soft, devitalised tissue. Enzymatic preparations are applied either in solution or in combination with a hydrogel which makes it difficult to separate the enzymatic activity from the autolytic effect. They may also be inactivated by antimicrobial dressings and detergents.

Mechanical debridement

Is a non-discriminatory method that physically removes debris from the wound and may cause additional tissue damage and patient discomfort. Examples of non-selective mechanical debridement include: wet-to-dry dressings, high pressure wound irrigation, and whirlpool therapy.

Biological debridement

Larvae only digest necrotic tissue, slough and bacteria, leaving the wound bed clean. Larval therapy can quickly eradicate infection and wound odour, may be effective against MRSA. They can be left in place for up to 3d but may require changing sooner in ischaemic wounds. Increased exudate production may occur during early stages of treatment which may be associated with increased odour. Disadvantages of maggot therapy: aesthetic reasons, local discomfort, itching, and application problems. Available on FP10.

Maintaining debridement

In chronic wounds, difficult to fully remove the necrotic burden as non-viable tissue and exudate continues to accumulate. After initial debridement in chronic wounds, a temporary improvement in healing is often observed followed by gradual deterioration. Initial debridement followed by repeated debridement important whilst the wound is open to maintain steady, continuous removal of necrotic burden.

Related topics

📖 Wound assessment; 📖 Management of chronic wounds; 📖 Infected wounds; 📖 Fungating wounds; 📖 Wound dressings.

Further information

📄 NICE (2001 reviewed 2004). *Guidance on the use of debriding agents and specialist wound care clinics for difficult to heal surgical wounds:* www.nice.org.uk

📄 www.worldwidewounds.com

Fungating wounds

Fungating wounds develop from 1° skin tumours, an underlying tumour, or metastatic disease. Occasionally chronic, non-healing wounds e.g. leg ulcers may become malignant. Often develop in older patients (>70yrs) with metastatic cancer. Lesions may develop into a 'cauliflower' shaped nodular growth, or ulcerate into a wound with a crater-like appearance or both. The commonest site of fungating wounds is in the breast, although 25% develop in the head and neck area. Fungating wounds have significant psychological impact, and can be a constant reminder of a condition's progression.

Assessment

Assessment of fungating wounds should consider the patient's views, psychological state, pain and local wound factors (Wound assessment 📖).

Factors delaying healing

- Advanced malignancy
- Immunosuppression—chemotherapy, radiotherapy
- Malnutrition/dehydration
- Psychological stress.

The aim of care is symptom control and to promote patient comfort and sense of well-being.

Exudate

Fungating wounds often produce moderate to high levels of exudate. Use dressings that absorb excess exudate but maintain a moist wound environment to avoid dressing adhesion, trauma, and bleeding. For smaller, ↑ exudating wounds, a wound manager/wound drainage pouch. Skin barriers around the wound can be an effective method of ↓ damage associated with exudates leakage. Alcohol polymer barrier film helps prevent excoriation and gives a surface dressings can adhere to.

Odour

- Debridement: most effective treatment for malodorous wounds. Surgical/sharp debridement, not recommended due to ↑ tendency of wounds to bleed. Autolytic or enzymatic debridement better (Wound debridement 📖), monitor to check no ↑ exudate production.
- Antibiotic therapy may be effective if it destroys the bacteria responsible for malodour. ↓ local blood supply can reduce the effectiveness of systemic treatment. Metronidazole (BNF 5.1.11) can be given systemically, but side effects e.g. nausea, neuropathy can be problematic. Topical preparations of metronidazole gel applied daily for between 5–7d may help, odour may reoccur once treatment stops.
- Charcoal based dressings can help in the management of odour.
- Occlusive dressings contain wound malodour but may not be available in an appropriate size or conform to the wound surface. Meticulous wound hygiene, gentle irrigation with normal saline/water, daily dressing changes and the correct disposal of soiled dressings, can help ↓ odour.

Pain

Assess to determine pain type. Specialist advice should be sought regarding management of cancer pain, persistent, and dressing-related wound pain. Anti-cancer therapies e.g. chemotherapy, radiotherapy, hormone therapy may help to ↓ the wound mass.

Bleeding

Use low-adherent dressings that maintain a moist environment. Cleanse by irrigation rather than swabbing, → ↓ risk of bleeding.

Sucralfate paste or alginate dressings may be applied to the surface of wounds with a small amount of bleeding. NB Alginates should be used with care in fragile tumours: may cause bleeding. Loosen alginates by irrigating with normal saline to ensure complete removal.

Alternative: haemostatic surgical sponges can be left in place and covered with an appropriate dressing.

Topical adrenaline (epinephrine) can also be applied under medical supervision.
- Wounds should be inspected daily and dressings changed regularly.
- Care is required when removing dressings to avoid further trauma and bleeding.
- Skin barriers may minimize skin excoriation/maceration.
- These patients will be at high risk of pressure damage.

Related topics

📖 Wound assessment; 📖 Infected wounds; 📖 Principles of leg ulcer assessment and management; 📖 Wound debridement; 📖 Wound dressings.

Further information for professionals

Grocott, P. (2004). Malignant Wounds. In *Management of Advanced Disease.* (eds) Sykes, N., Edmonds, P., and Wiles, J. (4th edn.) Arnold, London. pp. 295–305.
📖 Naylor, W. (2002). Part 2: Symptom self assessment in the management of fungating wounds. Available at www.worldwidewounds.com
📖 NHS Clinical Knowledge Summaries (Prodigy) guidelines on care of malignant ulcers: www.cks.library.nhs.uk

Principles of wound management following amputation

Amputation has significant social, medical, and economic consequences. Lower limb amputations are the most common. Two-thirds of amputees are ♂. Lower limb amputations are more common in diabetics; 50% of all amputations occur in people with diabetes.

Patients who go on to need an amputation may have had one or more of the following problems/symptoms:
- Cold pale limb
- Absent or ↓ foot pulses
- Altered sensation/paresthesia
- Paralysis
- Pain on limb elevation—note that intermittent claudication is not always present in diabetic people with ischaemia.

Factors delaying stump healing
- Poor health status
- Level of amputation
- Need for revision
- Vascularity of skin flap
- Position of stump wound
- Ability to mobilize with prosthesis.

Complications
Wound complications:
- Oedema (misshapen stump)
- Haematoma
- Ischemia
- Infection
- Wound dehiscence.
General:
- Delayed prosthetic fitting
- Delayed independent ambulation
- Flexion contractures.

Management of post amputation wounds
Assessment should include pain management, specialist advice should be sought regarding postoperative phantom pain e.g. referral/consultation to pain clinic.

Use of appropriate dressings allows earlier mobilization of patients with unhealed trans-tibial stumps with promising results. No strong evidence of clinical or cost effectiveness: wound dressings that best match clinical experience, patient preference, and the wound site. Useful dressing types (e.g. BNF A8.1.1, 8.1.2, 8.1.6).
- Alginates
- Foams
- Hydrofibres
- Low-adherent contact layers.

Care of patient with amputation wound
- Wounds should be inspected daily and dressings changed regularly.
- Stump wounds produce ↑ levels of exudate—use absorbent, non-bulky dressings that do not cause skin tension on transfer.
- Skin barriers may minimize stump excoriation/maceration.
- Tight/elasticated bandages should be avoided in vascular amputees.
- Once healing begins the stump can be shaped with a graduated pressure stump sock.
- Care must be taken to protect the contralateral leg from trauma.
- The patients sacrum and heel will be susceptible to pressure damage.

Related topics

📖 Wound assessment; 📖 Wound debridement; 📖 Infected wounds; 📖 Principles of leg ulcer assessment and management; 📖 Wound dressings.

Further information

🖥 www.worldwidewounds.com

Wound dressings

Range of dressings available, often very little difference between competing brands. No dressings address all the requirements of an ideal dressing and no one dressing is suitable for all wound types. Choose dressings based upon wound characteristics (see Table 10.2 and refer to local formularies).

Passive dressings: products which have no direct effect on the wound. They protect the wound by covering it e.g. low adherent dressings.

Interactive dressings: interact with the wound bed to provide an optimum local environment at the wound/dressing interface.

> **Ideal dressing characteristics** dressings should be:
> - Highly absorbent
> - Resistant to external contaminants
> - Moisture vapour permeable
> - Hypoallergenic
> - Comfortable to wear
> - Low adherent
> - Cost effective

Dressing types

This list excludes those not recommended.

Activated charcoal (Contraindications: dry, black necrotic wounds.) Anaerobic bacteria causes wound malodour. Can be controlled by using active or antimicrobial dressings. Charcoal deodorizes but once in contact with exudate, its odour adsorbing properties are ↓ and will require changing. Dressings containing activated charcoal: charcoal sandwiched between 2 fabric layer (BNF A8.1.8).

Alginates (Contraindications: dry wounds, or those covered with dry necrotic tissue.) Suitable for use with medium to heavily exuding wounds. Available as a loose 'rope' or packing for cavities, a ribbon for narrow wounds or sinuses, and a flat non-woven pad for larger open wounds. Alginates can be soaked off with saline or water (BNF A8.1.1).

Anti-microbials (Dressings containing iodine and silver.)

Dressings containing iodine. A single course of treatment should not exceed 3mths. Contraindications:
- Known or suspected iodine sensitivity
- Impaired renal function, thyroid disorders
- Children, pregnant, lactating mothers
- Iodosorb should not be used on dry wounds.

Suitable for suspected or infected, exuding wounds. Available as: polysaccharide paste between 2 fabric layers, polysaccharide paste/ointment. knitted viscose dressing impregnated with povidone iodine (BNF A8.1.3).

Dressings containing silver. (Contraindications: dry wounds.)
Suitable for suspected or infected, exuding wounds. Powerful antimicrobial capable of killing antibiotic resistant strains of micro-organisms. Ability to kill micro-organisms influenced by:
- Distribution of silver in the dressing
- The chemical/physical form of the silver
- Dressing's affinity to moisture.

Dressings with silver concentrated on the surface have ↑ antimicrobial effect. Dressings with sustained silver-ion release effective against MRSA and VRE. Dressings containing silver: activated charcoal. Plus foams, hydrocolloid, hydrocolloid fibrous, non-woven fabric dressing (BNF A8.1.4).

Films. (Contraindications: highly exudating, deep, cavity or infected wounds.) Suitable for lightly exudating, superficial wounds. Permeable to water vapour and oxygen and impermeable to micro-organisms, moist environment promotes epidermal regeneration in superficial wounds. Variety of uses in securing primary dressings and other medical devices, e.g. OpSite® Flexigrid, Tegaderm®. Adhesive films with absorbent pad e.g. Mepore® Ultra, OpSite® Plus.

Table 10.2 Selection of wound dressings by wound type (BNF Appendix 8)

Wound bed	Necrotic/sloughy	Clinical signs of infection	Clean granulation	Epithelialization
Exudate level				
Heavy	• Alginate • Foam • Honey dressings • Hydrocolloid Fibrous	• Iodine dressings/pastes • Honey dressings • Silver alginate • Silver foam • Silver hydrocolloid fibrous • Silver non-woven fabric	• Alginate • Foam • Honey dressings • Hydrocolloid Fibrous	• N/A
Moderate	• Activated charcoal • Alginate • Foam • Honey dressings • Hydrocolloid Fibrous • Hydrogel + Foam	• Iodine dressings/pastes • Honey dressings • Silver alginate • Silver activated charcoal • Silver foam • Silver hydrocolloid fibrous • Silver non-woven fabric	• Alginate • Foam • Honey dressings • Hydrocolloid Fibrous • Hydrogel + Foam	• N/A
Minimal	• Honey dressings • Hydrocolloid • Hydrogel + foam/film	• Honey dressings • Silver hydrocolloid	• Foam • Honey dressings • Hydrocolloid-film • Low-adherent dressings	• Thin hydrocolloid film • Low-adherent dressings

For further information see BNF A8.1

Hydrocolloids. (Contraindications: highly exudating, or infected wounds.) Suitable for light to medium exuding wounds. Need margin of good skin around wound edges to ensure adhesion. frequent changes with heavily exuding wounds, Thin hydrocolloid without border and fibrous hydrocolloid (BNF A8.1.4).

Hydrogels. (Contraindications: highly exudating wounds.) As they contain 80% water hydrogels hydrate dry wounds and facilitate autolytic debridement of moist, sloughy, or dry necrotic wounds. Although gels look similar, fluid donating properties vary considerably. Some are able to absorb a limited amount of fluid from exuding wounds. Secondary dressing (film or foam) is required to retain amorphous hydrogels at the wound surface (BNF A8.1.3).

Low-adherence dressings. (Contraindications: highly exudating wounds especially if fluid is viscous.) Suitable for light to medium exuding wounds. e.g. perforated plastic film faced dressing, cellulose dressings, knitted viscose primary dressing, adhesive bordered dressings, knitted fabric impregnated with silicone (BNF A8.1.6).

Medical grade honey. (Contraindications: if localized wound pain occurs discontinue.) Suitable for suspected or infected, exuding wounds. Honey has powerful antimicrobial effects capable of killing antibiotic resistant strains of micro-organisms. Medical grade honey. Products containing honey: antibacterial medical wound gel, Mesitran range of products e.g. hydrogel honey dressing, hydrocolloid honey dressing, polyester net honey dressing and ointments.

Polyurethane foams. (Contraindications: dry, necrotic wounds, narrow necked sinus.) Suitable for light to medium exudating wounds, are hydrophilic, highly absorbent, and have low adherence. Absorb excess fluid but maintain a moist wound surface: foam non-bordered, foam bordered, non-adhesive, foam bordered, adhesive. Foams suitable for cavities. Cavity wound dressing is formed from 2 reagents which react together to make a pliable, slightly absorbent foam, which is poured into cavities to promote granulation (BNF A8.1.2).

Related topics

📖 Wound assessment; 📖 Management of chronic wounds; 📖 Wound debridenment.

Further information

🗔 www.worldwidewounds.com

Principles of leg ulcer assessment and management

Prevalence of leg ulcers between 1–2% of adult population ↑ with age. Healing rates range from 45–80% at 24wks for all ulcer types. Ulceration is characterized by alternating phases of ulceration, healing, and recurrence. Estimated that approx 25% of patients have open ulcers at any time. 75% of all leg ulcers are venous in origin, 25% are arterial, mixed aetiology, or neuropathic.

Many leg ulcer patients have never had the aetiology of their ulcer correctly diagnosed. Ulcer aetiology determines the management strategy.

Specific assessment criteria

- How the patient understands what has caused their ulcer and what would be a good outcome for them
- Medical history (damage to arterial/venous system)
- History of previous ulceration, healing, and recurrence
- Presence of foot pulses
- Doppler ultrasound (ankle brachial pressure index (ABPI))
- Wound related pain (persistent/temporary)
- Condition of surrounding skin
- How the ulcer affects ability to sleep
- How the ulcer affects patient's mood and social interaction
- Level of social support available to patient with a leg ulcer.

Management principles

General management principles for patients with leg ulcers are:
- Identification and treatment of the underlying cause of the ulcer
- Provision of optimum local conditions at wound site
- Prevention of avoidable complications and recurrence
- Involvement of the patient in their care and achieving concordance with treatment and after care.

Investigations

- Urinanalysis
- Bloods FBC, ESR
- Ankle brachial pressure
- Duplex scan
- Wound swabs M, C & S
- Patch testing.

Factors delaying healing

- Increasing age
- Ulcer duration
- Ulcer size
- Poor general mobility
- Fixed ankle mobility
- Co-morbidities.

Correct treatment depends upon accurate differentiation between venous insufficiency and arterial disease. The clinical signs summarized in Clinical signs and symptoms of venous and arterial leg ulceration (📖).

Older people with ulcers of venous origin are likely to have co-existing arterial disease. a differential diagnosis should be based on physical examination and Doppler assessment.

Vascular assessment

Hand-held Doppler compares blood flow in the arm with blood flow in the lower limb to calculate the ABPI. Doppler ultrasound ↑ accuracy of ulcer assessment by excluding concomitant arterial disease and defining a safe level of compression bandaging. All patients should have their ABPI calculated prior to treatment (see Table 10.3). For arterial ulcers the ABPI reading provides an indication of severity of the arterial disease. ABPI readings should be re-assessed every 3mths to detect early vascular changes.

Table 10.3 Significance of ABPI readings

ABPI 1 or >1	Normal arterial blood flow
ABPI <0.9	Mild degree of arterial involvement
ABPI 0.8	80% arterial blood flow reaching the foot
	Standard compression contraindicated
ABPI <0.7	Arterial insufficiency. Vascular referral required
ABPI <0.5	Severe arterial disease. Urgent vascular referral

Standard compression therapy should not be applied if ABPI <0.8 due to risk of necrosis. UK national guidelines recommend that all patients with ABPI <0.8 should receive specialist assessment (see below).

NB Specialist advice important for those with arterial disease including diabetes and rheumatoid arthritis. The following should be included in leg ulcer assessment documentation (see also Wound assessment 🕮):

- Family history
- DVT, phlebitis
- Varicose veins, hypertension
- Allergies/hypersensitivities.

Ulcer history (see also Table 10.4.)

- Duration of current ulcer
- Onset of first ulcer
- Number of episodes recurrence
- Location e.g. gaiter area, foot, toes
- Type of ulcer e.g. venous, arterial, neuropathic
- Skin sensitivities/allergies
- Ankle mobility
- Ankle measurement
- Skin condition
- Eczema/dry skin
- Signs of chronic venous insufficiency e.g. ankle flare, lipodermatosclerosis.

Regular re-assessment is important.

Referral criteria

Patients should be referred to medical staff if:

- Younger, mobile individuals
- Unresponsive ulcers within 3mths
- Failure to heal within a year
- ABPI below 0.6 (severe ischaemic disease)
- Individuals with contact dermatitis
- Uncertain aetiology of ulceration.

Related topic

🕮 Compression therapy for venous ulcers.

Further information for professionals

▣ SIGN guidelines Care of patient with chronic leg ulcer: www.sign.ac.uk
▣ World wide wounds online journal for wound management information: www.worldwidewounds.com

Clinical signs and symptoms of venous and arterial leg ulceration

Table 10.4 Comparison of clinical signs and symptoms of venous and arterial leg ulceration (leg ulcer assessment)

	Venous ulceration	Arterial ulceration
Previous medical history	Previous leg fracture, (DVT), skin staining, eczema, FH of leg ulcers, varicose veins.	History of (CVA), heart disease, PVD, hypertension, diabetes.
Site/position	Often near the ankle or between the ankle and knee (gaiter area).	Usually on the foot, between the toes, or close to the medial malleolus.
Appearance	Large, shallow wounds producing copious exudate.	Often small, deep wounds producing less exudate.
Surrounding skin condition	Characteristic pigmentation—lipodermatosclerosis, atrophy blanche. Contact dermatitis and eczema common.	Hairless, shiny skin. Skin colour ranges from white to dusky pink and purple. Dusky pink feet turn pale when raised above heart.
Pain/discomfort	Aching/heaviness of legs, localized ulcer pain.	Severe rest pain, constant ulcer pain, often worse at night.

Venous leg ulcers

Venous ulcers are one of the common types of chronic wound. Patients frequently experience wound leakage, offensive odour, wound pain, and lack of sleep. This can ↑ dependence on carers, ↓ quality of life and affect self-esteem. (See Principles of leg ulcer assessment and management 📖.):

- Venous leg ulcer: a non-healing break in the skin of the lower leg caused by disease in the venous system.
- Lipodermatosclerosis: characteristic skin changes in lower extremities including fat necrosis, skin staining, fibrosis of skin, and subcutaneous tissues that become hard and 'woody'.
- Atrophe blanche: refers to the presence of white satellite scars in the ankle area commonly seen in venous stasis due to occlusion of dermal vessels causing tissue death.

Assessment

Signs of venous hypertension are initially mild and become more pronounced (Principles of leg ulcer assessment and management 📖).

> **Risk factors**
> - DVT
> - Vein trauma/surgery
> - Phlebitis
> - Congenital valve defect
> - Increasing age
> - Gender—female
> - Sedentary lifestyle

Clinical signs of venous hypertension

- Ankle oedema (dependent)
- Ankle flare (distented venous medial aspect of ankle)
- Varicose veins
- Abnormal leg shape 'inverted champagne bottle'
- Brown skin pigmentation
- Lipodermatosclerosis
- Atrophe blanche
- Varicose eczema.

Complications

- Recurrent infection
- Lymphodema (📖): refer to specialist services
- Malignant changes (rare): refer for biopsy
- Contact dermatitis refer for patch testing.

Management

Aim of venous leg ulcer management: reversal of venous hypertension. Compression therapy is the cornerstone of treatment (Compression therapy for venous ulcers 📖).

Exudate can produce high levels of exudate which ↓ with healing. Select dressings that will absorb excess exudate, but still maintain a moist wound environment to avoid dressing adhesion and trauma. Skin barriers can be an effective method of reducing damage and excoriation.

Debridement (Wound debridement 📖). Infection or uncontrolled oedema are the commonest causes of slough accumulation on the ulcer surface and require removal. Uncomplicated venous ulcers generally do not require debridement. Surgical debridement seldom used as ulcers are shallow and risk of damage great.

Pain. Pain is common and often underestimated can contribute to sleep disturbance, anxiety, depression and poor compliance with treatment. Important to assess and manage (Pain assessment and management 📖).

Skin care. Varicose eczema and contact dermatitis are common. Patients often are sensitive to allergens e.g. latex, preservatives, and perfumes. Corticosteroid creams may be helpful. Contact dermatitis should be suspected when eczema does not respond to treatment. All topical products should be discontinued and patch tests performed. Development of irritant dermatitis and maceration often leads to new areas of ulceration.

Prevention of recurrence. Once healed follow-up care is essential as recurrence rates are high. Appropriate skin care, exercise, leg elevation and avoidance of prolonged standing should be emphasized together with the permanent use of fitted compression stockings (BNF Appendix 8) to minimise recurrence.

Useful dressing types (BNF Appendix 8). Refer also to local prescribing formularies for product choice and guidance.

- Alginate
- Antimicrobial dressings
- Foam
- Hydrocolloid fibrous
- Low adherent contact layers
- Secondary absorbent pads
- Clean ulcers with clean water or normal saline solution
- Fluid absorption of dressings may be affected beneath compression bandages as lateral flow of fluid may be affected
- Avoid bulky dressings that under compression can cause local pressure damage and tissue necrosis
- Simple non-adherent dressings are recommended to minimize skin maceration
- To contain leakage distal to ulcer: position dressings slightly off centre
- Topical antimicrobials can used for short duration, if no improvement is seen by 2wks, stop treatment and consider systemic antibiotics
- Skin barriers may minimize skin excoriation/maceration.

Related topics

📖 Wound assessment; 📖 Management of chronic wounds; 📖 Compression therapy for venous ulcers; 📖 Wound dressings.

Further information for professionals

SIGN guidelines. The Care of Patients with Chronic Leg Ulcer. Publication Number 26. (1998). SIGN, Edinburgh: www.sign.ac.uk

📓 World wide wounds online journal for wound management information www.worldwidewounds.com

Compression therapy for venous ulcers

The most effective treatment of venous leg ulcers is high compression therapy; can heal 50–80% of venous ulcers in a 12wks period. It is vital to involve the patient in all stages of care, especially decision making around treatment decisions. (Principles of leg ulcer assessment and management 🕮; Venous leg ulcers 🕮.)

- Multi-layer systems are more effective than single-layered systems.
- High compression is more effective than low compression.

The aims of compression therapy are to:
- Reduce pressure in superficial venous system
- Encourage venous return and tissue perfusion
- Minimise oedema
- Improve lymphatic drainage.

Contraindications

- Arterial disease (ABPI >0.5)
- Co-existing vascular conditions
- Patients with narrow ankles/calves
- Patients with reduced sensation
- Uncontrolled heart failure.

❶ Extreme caution should be exercised for patients with venous leg ulcer and diabetes (🕮) or rheumatoid arthritis (🕮).

Various methods of achieving graduated compression include:
- Compression bandages
- Compression hosiery
- Intermittent compression systems.

Choice depends on resources, size and shape of the patient's leg, patient mobility, and patient preference and local policy.

Bandage types

(See BNF Appendix 8)

Highly extensible (elastic) bandage: contain elastic materials and apply sustained compression over time by applying pressure inwards to the tissues at rest.

Minimally extensible (inelastic) bandage: contain inelastic materials providing a rigid structure: the pressure rises when the calf muscle expands against the rigid cuff during activity causing pressure to be forced into the tissues. Does not sustain pressure over long periods of time.

Bandage application

❶ Should only be done by practitioners trained in compression therapy.

A venous ulcer with a reading of <0.8, standard compression should be applied which exerts a sub-bandage pressure of between 30–40mmHg at the ankle. The highest pressure should be exerted at the ankle, gradually falling to 50% at the knee. Reduced levels of compression may also be safely used in patients with mild arterial disease (ABPI 0.5–0.8). Table 10.5 outlines RCN/SIGN recommendations and a range of regimens that may be used.

Table 10.5 Recommendations for use of compression in relation to arterial status

ABPI (ankle to brachial pressure index)	Compression regimen	Comments
>0.8	High compression	Bandage pressure approx. 40mmHg e.g. Setopress®, Tensopress® Multi-layer, e.g.: Profore®. Caution in patients with concurrent conditions e.g. diabetes and heart failure.
0.5–0.8	Reduced compression	Bandage pressure approx. 20–25mmHg eg: Litepress®, Elset® paste bandage + elastocrepe Rosidal K®, Comprilan®, Reduced multi-layer, e.g.: Profore® Lite. Careful monitoring of vascular signs.
<0.5	No compression	Patients should be referred for urgent vascular opinion.

Three factors affect the amount of pressure exerted onto a limb.

1. Bandage tension
The more the bandage is stretched on application the higher the sub bandage pressure. Generally elasticated bandages (highly extensible) are applied with 50% extension. The aim is to apply the bandage with constant extension.

2. Limb circumference
For effective graduation, ankle circumference should measure approximately 50% of the calf circumference. A bandage applied with constant tension and 50% overlap will exert a higher pressure at the ankle than calf. Bony prominences are prone to high pressure. Apply orthopaedic wool to protect the skin and to increase the size of small ankles. To determine the bandage regimen, remeasure ankle circumference wkly and refer to manufacturer's guidance on bandage application according to ankle circumference.

3. Bandage layers
The more layers applied the higher the sub-bandage pressure gained. When applying a spiral application using 50% overlap 2 layers are being applied, conversely a figure of 8 application applies 4 layers.

Practical application
• Measure ankle circumference.
• Cover ulcer with primary dressing.
• Avoid padding small areas e.g. bony prominences.

- Apply bandage from base of toes to knee (refer to manufacturer's instructions).
- Avoid double turns of the bandage which doubles the pressure exerted in a single turn.
- Do not apply additional layers of bandage under knee in an attempt to use up bandage surplus.
- Ask patient to inform staff if bandage feels uncomfortable and remove if necessary.

Prevention of recurrence after healing

It is important that patients wear below knee support hosiery. Compression hosiery maintains a compression force of between 30–40mmHg at the ankle and maintains venous return. Hosiery should be measured and fitted. Hosiery is tight and patients may initially have difficulty in getting it on, should be applied with care to prevent skin damage. A minimum of one-year follow-up post healing to ↓ risk of recurrence.

Related topics

📖 Wound assessment; 📖 Management of chronic wounds; 📖 Venous leg ulcers.

Further information for professionals

RCN guidelines RCN Institute, Centre for Evidence-Based Nursing, University of York, School of Nursing, Midwifery and Health Visiting, University of Manchester (1998). *Clinical practice guidelines: the management of patients with venous leg ulcers.* RCN Institute, London.

SIGN guidelines. Scottish Intercollegiate Guidelines Network (1998). *The Care of Patients with Chronic Leg Ulcer: a national clinical guideline.* No. 26. SIGN Publications, Edinburgh.

🖥 www.worldwidewounds.com

Lymphoedema

A long-term problem caused by obstruction of lymphatic drainage, causing oedema, affects one or more limbs and adjacent trunk. If not treated lymphoedema becomes resistant to treatment arising from chronic inflammation and subcutaneous fibrosis. Cellulitis causes a rapid ↑ in swelling. NB Swelling can usually be reduced but can take wks or mths before discernible improvement and it may recur.

Secondary lymphoedema caused by:
- Tumour in axilla, groin, or intrapelvic area
- Extensive axillary or groin surgery (including mastectomy involving axillary clearance)
- Post operative infection/radiotherapy
- Trauma.

NB More likely to occur if surgery and radiotherapy on the same area.

Aims of care
- Relieve discomfort by reducing swelling
- Prevent build up of fluid
- Prevent complications e.g. cellulitis.

Care and management
- Important to have good skin care and prevention of infection: moisturize skin everyday with non-perfumed cream/oil, clean and treat small cuts, wear gloves for housework and gardening to reduce risk of cuts, insect repellant to avoid bites, sun protection.
- Treat fungal infections e.g. athletes foot (Fungal infections 📖).
- Avoid BP measurement, vaccination, and taking bloods on affected limb.
- Compression garments e.g. sleeves, stockings, special bras need to be fitted (see below for further information). Use with extreme caution or not at all if skin fragile, limb is very swollen, or skin is pitted. Multi layer bandaging can provide support and immobility to affected limb.
- Support swollen arms when sitting with a pillow and slightly elevate when lying down (do not rest arm above shoulder height). Support affected legs when sitting and avoid standing for long periods.
- Gentle exercises following advice from lymphoedema specialist (see below for directory information). Should always wear compression garment when doing exercise. Stop exercise if skin becomes red.
- Refer for manual lymphatic drainage (MLD) by trained specialist, patient can be taught by specialist to do simple lymphatic drainage (SLD). Gentle fingertip massage to promote drainage.
- Excess heat can exacerbate swelling. Advise to avoid saunas, direct heat very hot showers and baths etc.

Related topic
📖 Breast cancer.

Further information for health professionals

- British Lymphology Society: www.lymphoedema.org/bls
- Lymphodoema Support Network provides directory of services available for sufferers: www.lymphoedema.org/lsn
- In Worldwide wounds www.worldwidewounds.com: Williams, A. (2003). *An overview of non cancer related chronic oedema*: www.worldwidewounds.com/2003/april/Williams/Chronic-Oedema.html

Pain assessment and management

Pain is an unpleasant sensory and/or emotional experiences linked to actual or potential tissue damage. It is a subjective experience and ∴ it is always the patient who defines it and its severity.

NB Health professionals often underestimate patient's pain and overemphasize the risk of addiction or overmedication. Pain can go unrecognized especially in older people or those with cognitive impairment.

Acute pain: the cause often obvious although amount of pain reported often unrelated to injury.

Chronic pain For >3–6 million a significant source of suffering. >7% of adults in the UK and 70% of sufferers experience pain despite analgesia. Causes are multifactoral. Living with pain can:
- Induce depression and exacerbate anxiety
- Affect ability to perform everyday tasks and work
- Damage relationships.

Assessment

Questions should be open ended and allow the patient to define the pain experience. Follow-up with specific questions that will help locate and monitor the pain e.g.
- Where the pain is and how long the patient has had it.
- Whether there were any triggers and if it has changed over time.
- Is it worse at different times of day?
- Pain intensity and what relieves the pain: e.g. analgesia, relaxation, distraction techniques etc.

Pain assessment tools

(See Further information below, Bristol Pain Society.)
Particularly useful when charting effectiveness of different pain reduction strategies and interventions.
- Brief Pain Inventory and McGill Pain Questionnaire.
- Visual analogue scales: a line with 'no pain' and 'worst pain' at each extreme. Patient marks point online that reflects their pain severity.
- Variations on the analogue scales include: verbal rating scales and numerical rating scales.
- Pain diary: can help identify patterns of pain and effectiveness of different treatments.

Pain management

- Fear always increases the pain perception. Important that the patient is reassured supported and involved in decisions on pain control through education and discussion of possible options (See Table 10.6).
- Ensure causes of pain addressed e.g. infection, nerve compression etc.
- Use WHO analgesia ladder: staged approach to pain control (See Fig. 10.3) for cancer pain.
- To maintain freedom from pain in palliative care, pain relief should be given 'by the clock' and not on demand.

Step 1: *Mild pain* non-opioids e.g. NSAID and/or paracetamol	Step 2: *Moderate pain* Weak opioids e.g. tramadol, dihydrocodeine ± non-opioid (paracetamol and/or NSAID)	Step 3: *Severe pain* Strong opioids e.g. morphine, hydromorphone, diamorphine, Fentanyl TTS patch ± non-opioid (paracetamol and/or NSAID)
Co-analgesics: drugs, nerve blocks, TENS, relaxation, acupuncture		
Specific therapies: radiotherapy, chemotherapy, surgery		
Address psychosocial problems		

Fig. 10.3 WHO Pain Relief ladder (reproduced with permission from the Oxford Handbook of Palliative Care by Watson, M (2005), Oxford University Press.)

Management of pain in palliative care (see also symptom control)
Pain is multi-factoral and can arise from:
- Cancer specific causes e.g. bone metastases, nerve compression/infiltration, muscle spasm, lymphoedema, raised intracranial pressure.
- Associated factors: e.g. constipation.
- Arising from treatment e.g. surgery, radiotherapy.
- Co-morbidity e.g. arthritis.

Related topics

📖 Syringe drivers; 📖 Symptom control in palliative care.

Further information for health-care professionals and patients

Bristol Pain Society (2004). *A Practical Guide to the provision of Chronic Pain Service for Adults in Primary Care*: www.bristolpainsociety.org/pub-professional.htm
Doyle et al. (2005). Brief Pain Inventory. In, D., Hanks, G., Cherny, N.I. et al. *Oxford Textbook of Palliative Medicine*. Oxford University Press, Oxford.
Watson, M.S. (2005). *Oxford Handbook of Palliative Care*. Oxford University Press, Oxford.
🖥 The Oxford Pain Internet site: www.jr2.ox.ac.uk/bandolier/booth/painpag

Table 10.6 Management of specific types of pain

Type of pain	Management
Bone pain	• Try NSAIDs. • Consider referral for palliative radiotherapy, strontium treatment (prostate cancer), or IV bisphosphonates (↓ pain in myeloma, breast and prostate cancer). • Refer to orthopaedics if any lytic metastases at risk of fracture, for consideration of pinning.
Abdominal pain	• Constipation is the most common cause. • Colic—try loperamide 2–4mg qds or hyoscine hydrobromide 300mcg tds s/ling. Hyoscine can also be given via syringe driver. • Liver capsule pain—use dexamethasone 4–8mg/d, titrating dose down to the minimum that controls pain. • Gastric distention—may be helped by an antacid ± an anti-foaming agent (e.g. Asilone). Alternatively, a prokinetic may help e.g. domperidone 10mg tds before meals. • Upper GI tumour—coeliac plexus block may help. Refer to palliative care team. • Consider drug causes—NSAIDs are a common iatrogenic cause. • Acute/subacute obstruction
Neuropathic pain	• Often burning/shooting and may not respond to simple analgesia. • Titrate to the maximum tolerated dose of opioid. • If inadequate, add a nerve pain killer e.g. amitriptyline 10–25mg nocte increasing as needed every 2wks to 75–150mg. Alternatives include carbamazepine, gabapentin, phenytoin, sodium valproate, and clonazepam. • If pain is due to nerve compression caused by tumour, dexamethasone 8mg od may help. • *Other options:* TENS; acupuncture; nerve block
Rectal pain	• Topical drugs e.g. rectal steroids. • TCAs e.g. amitriptyline 10–100mg nocte. • Anal spasms—glyceryl trinitrate ointment 0.1–0.2% bd. • Referral for local radiotherapy.
Muscle pain	• Paracetamol and/or NSAIDs. • Muscle relaxants e.g. diazepam 5–10mg od, baclofen 5–10mg tds, dantrolene. • Physiotherapy, aromatherapy, or relaxation. • Heat pads.
Bladder spasm	• Try oxybutinin 5mg tds or tolterodine 2mg bd. • Amitriptyline 10–75mg nocte is often effective. • If catheterized, try instilling 20mls of intravesical bupivacaine 0.25% for 15min. tds.
Acute pain of short duration e.g. dressing changes	• Try a short-acting opiate e.g. meptazinol 200mg po given 20min. prior to procedure.

Reproduced with permission from Simon, C., Everitt, H., and Kendrick, T. (2005). *Oxford Handbook of General Practice*, 2nd edn, Oxford University Press, Oxford.

Syringe drivers

Syringe drivers are a portable battery operated infusion device used to aid SC drug delivery when the oral route is no longer feasible. Indications for use:

- Intractable vomiting
- Severe dysphagia
- Patient too weak to swallow oral drugs
- Decreased conscious level
- Poor alimentary absorption (rare)
- Poor patient compliance.

Advantages of using a syringe driver:

- Avoids repeated injections
- Drug mixtures can be administered
- Infusion timing is accurate
- Allows patient mobility and independence and enables them to stay at home.

> It is best to use one type of syringe driver with standardized procedures across PCO to reduce risk of dose error. Always check manufacturer's instructions before use. Training is essential before setting up and using a syringe driver.

Sims (Graseby) Medical Syringe Drivers are widely used. The most commonly used model in community settings is:

- MS26 administers drugs on a **daily** rate (MS16A administers drugs on an hourly rate but rarely suitable for community use).

The MS26 is calibrated in mm per day. The stroke length in mm is the *length* of fluid to be delivered (i.e. the distance the plunger has to travel irrespective of the number of mL) The rate of delivery is based on a length of fluid in mm per unit time.

- Rate = measured 'length of volume' in mm divided by delivery time in days.
- For example stroke length = 48mm. Delivery time = one day. Rate on dial setting is 48.

NB Alarm system of some syringe drivers only operate if the plunger is obstructed so does not alert patient or nurse if flow is too rapid or if there are problems at the skin site.

Medication

Diamorphine often the preparation of first choice and can be administered SC in a smaller volume than morphine.

Oral morphine: SC diamorphine ratio 3:1 (See 🕮 BNF Section on prescribing in palliative care and syringe drivers for detail on prescribing and dosages over time: www.bnf.org.uk).

The following drugs may be mixed with diamorphine:

- Hyoscine hydrobromide
- Dexamethasone
- Cyclizine
- Levomepromazine
- Haloperidol
- Metoclopramide
- Hyoscine butylbromide
- Midazolam.

Contraindicated are chlorpromazine, prochlorperazine, and diazepam: these can cause skin reactions at the injection site; cyclizine and levomepromazine (methotrimeprazine) may also cause local irritation.

General issues

(Training should be given according to local policies and protocols.)

- Accurate documentation of site, rate, flow, start time, and drugs used is imperative to avoid confusions and errors.
- Ensure patients and carers have explanations and supporting literature on problem solving and guidelines for use.
- Care should be taken when mixing more than 2 drugs in a syringe: ensure the diluent used is compatible with the drugs.
- The diluent of choice is water for injection except in the following where sodium chloride 0.9% for injection should be used: diclofenac, granisetron, ketamine, ketorolac, octreotide, and ondansetron.
- With combinations of 2 or 3 drugs in one syringe, a larger volume of diluent may be needed, e.g. 20mL or 30mL syringe.

Problems

- Infusion running too fast: check rate setting and recalculate.
- Infusion running too slow: check start button, battery, syringe driver, cannula, and make sure injection site is not inflamed.
- Site reaction: firmness or swelling not always a problem. Change needle site if pain or obvious inflammation. A plastic/teflon needle may reduce local irritation if a nickel allergy.
- Check solution regularly for precipitation and discolouration and discard if it occurs. Check compatibility of drugs.
- Light flashing: this is normal. The light flashes: blue—once per sec; green—once per 25sec. Flashing will stop when the battery needs changing. The syringe driver will continue to operate for 24hrs after the light has stopped flashing.
- Alarm: this always sounds when the battery is inserted. Silence by pressing Start/Test button. Check for: empty syringe/kinked tube/blocked needle/tubing/jammed plunger.

Related topics

📖 Chemotherapy in the home; 📖 Controlled drugs.

Further information

Dickman, A. et al. (2005). *The syringe driver: continuous subcutaneous infusions in palliative care* (2nd edn). Oxford University Press, Oxford.

Dougherty, L. and Lister, S. (eds) (2006). *The Royal Marsden Hospital Book of Clinical Nursing Procedures*, (6th edn). Blackwell Publishing, Oxford.

Chemotherapy in the home

Chemotherapy can be used for cure or palliation. The aim is to reduce the number of actively dividing cells in a tumour. Most cytotoxic drugs disrupt cell reproduction either by damaging DNA or affecting mitosis. There is a narrow margin between a therapeutic and a lethal dose. Nurses caring for patients at home should know:

- The name, action, and side effects of drugs the patient is receiving.
- Local policies and procedures for all aspects of cytotoxic drug administration including management of side effects and emergency situations including anaphylaxis and extravasation (see below).
- Transport drugs in labelled, robust, tamper and leak proof container.
- Store drugs in the correct conditions and out of reach of children.
- Disposal methods for cytotoxic drugs and waste as set out in Hazardous Waste Regulations England and Wales (2005).[1]
- Equipment available and access to spillage and extravasation kits.
- Links with 2° care and contact details for advice and support.
- Administration of drugs must comply with Control of Substances Hazardous to Health (COSHH) and HSE Protection legislation.
- Pregnant workers can choose not to be involved in activities involving exposure to cytotoxic drugs.

Cytotoxic drugs are teratogenic, mutagenic, and carcinogenic, and potentially hazardous to patients, staff, families, and the environment. Exposure occurs through ingestion, inhalation, and absorption through skin. Highest risk = reconstituting drugs, connecting and disconnecting IV tubing, and disposing of used equipment and patient excreta.

Measures to reduce exposure to cytotoxic drugs

- Drugs should be supplied ready for administration.
- Personal protective equipment. Gloves should be worn at all times when handling drugs and excreta and be changed regularly.
- Dispose of contaminated needles, syringes, should be intact. All drug containers, unused drugs and equipment such as gloves and aprons must be disposed on in leak proof container clearly marked *cytotoxic*. It is classed as hazardous waste and must be disposed of separately from other types of waste. Consignment note needed so that disposal can be tracked (Environment Agency 2005[1]). Description should include waste codes for cytotoxic drugs, estimate of the weight of the waste in kg, chemical components of the waste and physical form of waste i.e. liquid, solid mixed, and the hazard codes.
- Community pharmacists can receive hazardous waste from patients for disposal in the same way they receive other unwanted medication.
- Patient excreta may contain traces of drugs for up to 72hrs.
- If there is a risk of splashing or generating an aerosol: use eye and respiratory protection. Undertake a COSHH risk assessment for each handling activity to assess if a gown or plastic apron best protection.
- Avoid eating and drinking in areas where drugs are administered.
- Do not handle oral preparations never crush tablets or open capsules.

[1] Environment Agency (2005) www.environment–agency.gov.uk

Spillage

Kits should always be available. Use copious amounts of soap and water for skin contact. Eyes should be flooded with water or isotonic eye wash solution for 5min minimum and seek medical advice. Spillage of a large amount of cytotoxic drug incurring exposure should be reported to RIDDOR (Reporting Injuries, Diseases and Dangerous Occurrences Regulations 1995).

Care and management

- Patients and their carers need education and information about safe handling, side effects of treatment, dose and duration of drug treatment, the importance of strict adherence to the drug regimen, who to contact, and what to do if they experience side effects.
- Absorption of oral drugs may be affected by food, gastrointestinal problems e.g. nausea and vomiting or diarrhoea and concurrent medications.

Venous access devices

For those having lengthy courses of treatment a central venous access device (CVAD) (e.g. Hickman line) is usual. Patients may be sent home with a small battery operated pump connected to a central line for administration of chemotherapy.

- Prevention of infection is vital and strict asepsis.
- Monitor for signs of tissue infiltration/extravasation i.e. infiltration of a drug into the subcutaneous tissues and subsequent tissue damage are major potential problems. Symptoms include: erythema, discoloration, swelling, leakage, change in skin temperature, burning stinging and pain resistance to syringe or slowing of infusion rate, lack of blood return.
- Any prescribed pre-hydration fluids or anti-emetics should be given before chemotherapy is commenced.
- Before giving drug, withdraw blood and flush with NaCl 0.9% to ensure patency NB: *sodium chloride not compatible with all drugs*.
- Nurses looking after patients on chemotherapy should know drug properties, extravasation symptoms, and how to manage an emergency.

Managing extravasation

Management of extravasation is controversial. Local protocols and procedures should be known *before* any drug administration. Administration of chemotherapy should always be done as part of the MDT, following training and with the support of the specialist oncology centre. General principles:

- Stop administration immediately
- Leave cannula in place
- Seek specialist medical help
- Mark affected area with pen.

Related topics

📖 Palliative care in the home; 📖 Syringe drivers.

Further information

🖳 BACUP Cancer Back up services: www.cancerbackup.org.uk ☎ Freephone: 0808 800 1234

🖳 NICE (2003). Infection control: prevention of health care associated infection in primary and secondary care (section on care of central venous catheters): www.nice.org.uk

Tadman, M. and Roberts, D. (2007). *Oxford Handbook of Cancer Nursing*. Oxford Unniversity Press, Oxford

Palliative care in the home

Although the majority of dying people would like to die at home only 19% of all deaths occur at home. However, 90% of the final year of life for most patients is spent at home.

- People live longer at home with serious illnesses.
- GPs and primary care nurses are the main providers of palliative care in primary care.

General palliative care: focus on person centred care, quality of life with good symptom control.

Terminal care: refers to the management of patients from the time it is clear that the patient is in a progressive state of decline i.e. their last few days, weeks of life.

Patients who are dying and their carers value:

- Continuity of care
- Effective symptom control
- Choice, information, and control over care and decisions made
- Being listened to and the time to discuss feelings and worries
- Access to services.

Services available for the dying patient and their carers

- Primary Health Care Team provide generalist palliative care: GP and DNs establish ongoing relationships with patients, assess need, liaise with specialists, social care, secondary services and provide direct care.

NB Provision for the following is locally determined. Often less support available for patients and carers with non-malignant end stage illness than for people with equivalent symptoms and problems who have cancer.

- Out-of-hours care where there is 24hrs DN availability: greater likelihood of maintaining a patient at home.
- Social care: night sitters: through social service or Marie Curie night sitter service. Some social services also provide respite care, carers support groups, and financial advice.
- Specialist palliative care: Macmillan CNS, Marie Curie nurses, hospice home care teams, symptom control teams.
- Hospice care for symptom control, day centre care and short stay, outreach/hospice at home teams.
- Care homes and community hospitals: can provide respite and short stay support particularly for people who live alone.
- Charities can help with respite care, extra nursing care at home and special treats for people who are dying and bereavement support.

(NB See also Prescribing 📖 and Controlled drugs 📖.)

Standards and guidelines for providing palliative care at home

Gold standard framework (GSF): proactive model of care involving whole PHCT that aims to optimize organization of care for patients in their last 6–12mths of life.

Three key processes:

- Identification of key group of patients using a register
- Assessment of their needs
- Plan ahead for problems e.g. out-of-hours care.

Achieved by emphasizing 7 'gold' standards of community care: optimizing communication, coordination of care, control of symptoms, and continuity of care, continued learning, carer support and care in the dying phase. Evidence suggests GSF is helping more people to die in their preferred setting and improves QoL.

Liverpool Care Pathway for the dying patient: integrated care pathway (ICP): a template of care integrating local and national guidelines for best practice for care of patients in dying phase (e.g. last few days/hours of life). Useful educational tool and basis for multidisciplinary working.

Three sections that each identify key goals:

- Initial assessment and care of dying patient
- Ongoing care of dying patient
- Care of family and carers after death of the patient.

Related topics

📖 Syringe drivers; 📖 End-of-life issues; 📖 Carers assessment and support; 📖 Bereavement, grief, and coping with loss; 📖 Controlled drugs; 📖 Palliation of symptoms.

Further information for professionals

🖺 A programme for community palliative care: the Gold standard framework: www.macmillan.org.uk

🖺 Supportive and palliative care for people with cancer: Part A and Part B. www.nice.org.uk

Ellershaw, J.E., Wilkinson, S. (2003). *Care of the Dying: a pathway to excellence*. Oxford University Press, Oxford.

Watson et al (2004). *Oxford Handbook of Palliative Care*. Oxford University Press, Oxford.

Symptom control in palliative care: nausea and vomiting

20–30% of patients with cancer will experience nausea and 70% in last week of life. Vomiting occurs in 20% of patients with cancer. 30% of patients receiving opioids will feel nauseated and/or retch and vomit in first week of treatment. Treatment decisions should be in consultation with patient, other members of the MDT and where available specialist palliative care services. Causes often multifactoral including:

- Metabolic e.g. hypercalcaemia, renal failure (do blood biochemistry screen to check)
- Drugs e.g. opioids. antibiotics, NSAIDs, iron, digoxin
- Toxic e.g. infection, chemotherapy, radiotherapy
- Brain metastases
- Dehydration
- Dysphagia (NB regurgitation can be mistaken for vomiting)
- Psychosomatic factors e.g. anxiety, fear
- Pain
- Strong smells e.g. from fungating wound.

When assessing impact of nausea and vomiting consider:

- Level of hydration
- Functional impact on patient's and family/carer's everyday activities
- Impact on patient's level of anxiety and depression
- Whether patient's overall level of well-being means that they may benefit from chemotherapy to palliate symptoms e.g. ovarian and colonic cancers can respond well.

Care and management

- Identify the cause (NB if multifactoral = separate interventions).
- Correct reversible causes e.g. constipation, dehydration.
- Refer to local formularies and protocols for care.
- Depending on symptoms use first line anti emetic (Table 10.7). If fails to respond consider alternative medication and/or seek specialist opinion.
- Regular small amounts of fluid and food more likely to be tolerated.
- Support and reassurance to patient and family/carers.

> ❶ For prophylaxis of nausea and vomiting use oral medications. Always give antiemetics regularly not prn. For established nausea and vomiting consider a parenteral route e.g. syringe driver as persistent nausea may reduce gastric emptying and drug absorption.

Non-drug measures to palliate nausea and vomiting

- Avoidance of food smells and strong odours
- Diversion and relaxation techniques
- Acupressure/acupuncture.

Table 10.7 Anti-emetic therapy (refer to Clinical Knowledge Summaries (Prodigy) guidelines and BNF for dosage advice, administration routes and possible interactions)

Cause	First choice treatment	Second choice treatment
↑ ICP, cerebral irritation/tumour/ metastases	Dexamethasone	Cyclizine Metoclopramide
Abdominal and pelvic tumour	Cyclizine	Add dexamethasone
Gastric stasis	Metoclopramide or domperidone	Reduce gastric secretion ranitidine or octreotide
Chemically or metabolically induced and if beginning opioids	Metoclopramide or haloperidol (other drugs and metabolic causes haloperidol)	Dexamethasone or substitute with levomepremazine
Movement related nausea and vomiting	Cyclizine	Hyoscine hydrobromide (consider transdermal patch)
Unknown cause	Cyclizine	Dexamethasone Levomepremazine Metoclopramide

Related topics

📖 Syringe drivers; 📖 Palliative care in the home.

Further information

📖 Clinical Knowledge Summaries (Prodigy) guidelines palliative care: nausea and vomiting: www.cks.library.nhs.uk

Symptom control in palliative care: breathlessness

Breathlessness = breathing feels uncomfortable and/or difficult. The emotional experience of breathlessness is inextricable from the sensation and biomedical causes. Common in patients with primary lung cancer but 19–64% of patients with cancer have symptoms. Reduces activity, social life and self-esteem, few patients are continuously breathless, bouts triggered by exertion and emotion. Often characterized by:
- Rapid respiration
- Nasal flaring and using accessory muscles to breathe
- Feelings of panic and being unable to get enough breath
- Fears of impending death
- May be accompanied by cough, sputum, haemoptysis, fatigue, insomnia, pain, loss of appetite, anxiety, and depression.

Breathlessness: possible physical causes
- Cancer: airway constriction/obstruction, size and site of tumour, inflammation, involvement of pleura, pericardium, vessel involvement. Neural involvement e.g. phrenic nerve.
- Indirect consequence of cancer: PE, pneumonia, pneumathorax, anaemia (<9.0g/dL), folic and B12 deficiency.
- Respiratory muscle weakness (severe), cachexia-anorexia, drug induced (corticosteroids, benzodiazepines), electrolyte imbalances/abnormalities.
- Surgery: for example, pneumonectomy, lobectomy.
- Radiation-induced pneumonitis or fibrosis, pericarditis.
- Chemotherapy-induced pulmonary and cardiac toxicity, myelosuppression.

Care and management
Evidence for non-pharmacological nursing interventions for breathlessness suggest following help QoL.
- Careful assessment of what relieves or exacerbates symptoms and if symptoms have rapid or gradual onset.
- Exploration of what breathlessness means to patients about their disease and their feelings about the future.
- Advice and support for patients and families on management strategies training in breathing control techniques, progressive muscle relaxation and distraction exercises.
- Goal setting alongside breathing and relaxation techniques.
- Early recognition of problems that need pharmacological/medical intervention.

Treatments: non-pharmacological approaches
Relaxation strategies help 'undo' established reactions to breathlessness: and give patient a sense of control.
- To relax shoulders, upper back and neck, exhale slowly letting shoulders 'drop and flop' into a relaxed position.

[1] Bredin, M. et al. (1999). Multicentre randomized controlled trial of nursing intervention for breathlessness in patients with lung cancer. British Medical Journal, **318**, 901–4.

- If accessory muscles are used for breathing and to encourage slower breathing, rest a hand on the upper back and move slowly in a downward movement.
- To promote improved respiratory muscle function alter positioning so that when sitting lean forward from the hips, with forearms resting above the knees.
- Controlled breathing techniques/breathing retraining e.g. Pursed lip breathing (PLB) and diaphragmatic breathing helps develop slower, relaxed, and more efficient breathing pattern.
- Activity pacing and planning.

Pharmacological approaches and related treatments
(See BNF: Prescribing in palliative care.)
- Opiates/opioids: act by ↓ sensitivity of the respiratory centre to CO_2 altering the sensation of breathlessness and feelings of distress. No evidence for using nebulized morphine.
- Oxygen and air: symptomatic relief of acute breathlessness and panic. Use nasal cannula to ↓ oral dryness and inhibition of conversation. (If SaO_2 within normal range reassure patient O_2 not required). Well ventilated room and small fan can be helpful.
- Benzodiazepines ease the psychological aspects of breathlessness. Opioids with benzodiapines provide a sedative effect for terminal breathlessness during the final hours or days of life. Anxiolytics may help relieve sleeplessness.
- High dose steroids, corticosteroids for inflammatory aetiology, bronchodilators for airway obstruction, antibiotics, anticholinergics, nebulised saline, anticoagulants, and diuretics.

Cancer directed therapies and interventions:
- Hormones, chemotherapy and radiotherapy → some symptomatic relief for patients with treatment sensitive primary and metastatic disease.
- Breathlessness from responsive anaemia, pleural effusions, airway obstruction, ascites and superior vena cava obstruction can improve with targeted interventional treatments. Involve MDT in assessment.

Symptom control in palliative care: fatigue

A common and distressing symptom. Significant fatigue is when it is present every day or nearly every day during the same 2wk period in the past month. Associated with pain, psychological factors (particularly depression), serious viral infection, age, anorexia, and cachexia, life events, genetic factors there is a continuum of fatigue ranging from tiredness to exhaustion characterized by:

* Longer duration than that of someone who is healthy and often all consuming and overwhelming.
* Provides little recuperative effect.
* Unrelated to amount or type of activity performed and remains unrelieved by rest.

Treatment-related causes of cancer-related fatigue

* Surgery: linked to changes in muscle physiology, or may occur as part of a general stress response to surgery.
* Radiotherapy commonly occurs from first day of treatment, intensifying over a course of therapy, plateauing between 2nd and 4th week.
* Chemotherapy: fatigue most frequent and distressing side effect.
* Hormone therapy and biological response modifiers.

Many instruments have been developed to assess cancer-related fatigue[1, 2] including symptom diaries, single-item, and multi-item measures.

Pharmacological approaches to the management of fatigue
(See BNF: prescribing in palliative care.)

Glucocorticoids e.g. prednisolone or dexamethasone: prescribed for effects on appetite, mood and energy levels (BNF 6.3).

Progestational steroids e.g. medroxyprogesterone acetate (MPA) or megestrol acetate (MA): relieves anorexia and cachexia in patients whose fatigue related to cachexia (BNF 6.4).

Erythropoietin therapy: can increase energy levels in anaemic cancer patients receiving chemotherapy (BNF 9.1).

Antidepressants may be particularly useful in managing fatigue that is accompanied by depressive symptoms.

Non-pharmacological approaches to the management of fatigue

* Exercise: evidence to suggest that moderate exercise promotes ↑ functional capacity and improved mood.
* Diet: advise to eat when hungry, frequent small amounts.
* Pacing of activities: prioritize and plan for activities.
* Psychosocial interventions: counselling, progressive muscle relaxation.

[1] Ream, E. and Stone, P. (2004). Clinical Interventions for Fatigue. In J. Armes, M. Krishnasamy, and I. Higginson (eds) *Fatigue in Cancer*. Oxford University Press. Oxford, pp. 255–71.
[2] Wu, H.S. and McSweeney, M. (2001). Measurement of fatigue in people with cancer. *Oncology Nursing Forum*, **28** (9); 1371–84.

Related topics

📖 Palliative care in the home.

Further information for professionals and patients

Tadman, M. and Roberts, D. (2007). *Oxford Handbook of Cancer Nursing*. Oxford University Press,, Oxford

Bereavement, grief, and coping with loss

Grief is a normal reaction to bereavement. Traditional models see it as a process where an individual moves through phases to 'recovery'. Not a linear process, individuals likely to oscillate between loss and restoration, memories of the dead person and getting on with life. Normal manifestations of grief:

- *Physical*: hollowness in the stomach, tightness in throat and chest, SOB, sensitivity to noise, dry mouth, and muscle weakness.
- *Emotional*: initial response often shock and numbness. Also normal are feelings of anger, guilt, anxiety, disorganization, and helplessness. Sadness most common manifestation and may only really be experienced months later. Sense of relief and freedom, can → feelings of guilt.
- *Cognitive*: sense of unreality and disbelief, even denial often present in early bereavement. Short-term memory and concentration can be affected. Not uncommon to have sense of the presence of the deceased.
- *Behaviour*: appetite and sleep disturbed, individual may withdraw socially. Some people contemplate rapid changes in their life e.g. new relationship, moving house, may be a way of avoiding pain of loss but not advisable.

Health consequences of bereavement can include ↑ risk of mortality, mental health problems, alcohol abuse, depression, suicidal thoughts, ↓ immune response, disruption of family and working life, ↓ income.

Where there has been nursing involvement and relationship with the family/carers, appropriate for nurse to visit in the month after the death to see how the bereaved are, allow them express how they are feeling and remember the deceased together. NB Care home staff often act as surrogate family to older people and also experience bereavement and loss.

Bereaved children

Children understand what death is by 8yrs, and even 2–3yrs will have some understanding. If possible prepare children for death with the opportunity to ask questions. Excluding children to protect them can increase the pain and feelings of being isolated. Specialist help may be appropriate (see below).

Complicated/abnormal grief reactions

Recognized patterns of abnormal grief (NB impossible to generalize dependent on individual circumstances):

- Inhibited grief: absent or minimal expression
- Delayed onset
- Prolonged or chronic grief.

Predisposing factors can include: unexpected death, multiple/prior (unresolved) bereavements, ambivalent or dependent relationship with the deceased, poor social support, low self-esteem, history of mental illness.

Warning signs of complicated grief
- Long-term functional impairment
- Exaggerated intense grief reactions
- Significant self-neglect
- Idealization of the deceased.

If abnormal grief is suspected monitor carefully, be a non-judgemental listener and keep in regular contact.
- Consider referral e.g. CRUSE (see below)
- Consider possibility of clinical depression refer to GP.

Bereavement benefits
Bereavement benefits payable to ♂ and ♀ whose spouses have died (does not apply to cohabitation except in Scotland). Bereavement payment made when the deceased spouse has paid enough National Insurance contributions or their death was caused by employment. Applications should be made asap after death.
- Bereavement payment lump sum payable if spouse was not entitled to full basic retirement pension at the time of death.
- Widowed parent's allowance paid to widows, widowers with children, or if pregnant.
- Bereavement allowance paid for 52wks from the date of bereavement for spouses <45yrs not bringing up children and under retirement age.

Other payments
Funeral payments for people on low income paid from social fund does not normally cover the full costs.

War widows. Payable if spouses death due to service. Contact veterans agency ⌨ www.veteransagency.mod.uk

Further information
⌨ Child Bereavement Trust: www.childbereavement.org.uk/
⌨ Support for bereaved partners CRUSE: www.crusebereavementcare.org.uk
⌨ Winstons Wish www.winstonswish.org.uk/

End-of-life issues

End-of-life issues include advanced life directives, euthanasia debate, an individual's right to die and the responsibilities of the practitioner.

Living wills (or advanced directive)

Specifies how much medical intervention a person wants if they are terminally ill. It is provision for a time when a patient may be physically or mentally incapable of making a decision for themselves.

- A living will may also express a wish that a named person be involved in decisions or that a certain person be contacted if death is imminent.
- A living will can be obtained from a solicitor. There are also a variety of organizations from which you can obtain the relevant forms (see below).
- Need to be completed with your name, address, and your GP's contact details. They are then witnessed, and copies lodged with your GP, friends, and family.
- For people under 18, living wills do not have the same legal status as those made by adults. The Children Act (1989) emphasizes that young people's views must be considered in any decisions made about their own treatment.
- A living will is not the same as voluntary euthanasia. A living will asks doctors not to give you certain medical treatments, it can equally request that medical treatment is continued.
- Living wills cannot refuse basic nursing care or ask that nursing staff do not offer food and drink by mouth. Cannot refuse treatment that goes against a court order made because of a medical condition.
- Patients can change their minds.

Euthanasia refers to the act of intentional ending of life.

Focus of great debate, engendering on one hand strong feelings about the right to demand death and, on the other, strong feelings that life is so precious that we have a duty to preserve it at all costs. It is illegal in the UK but the issue may be raised by patients and relatives. The RCN is opposed to the introduction of legislation to support euthanasia. The BMA has adopted a position of neutrality (see below).

Important always to consider the views of patients and act in the best interests of those who are not able to give consent.

Issues to consider when patient or relatives are asking for euthanasia:

- Whether all pain and symptom relief information has been shared and its implementation is effective.
- Whether there is reversible clinical depression.
- Patients who are ill, unable to care for themselves, reliant on others for care may feel a burden and under pressure to die quickly.
- The vulnerable deserve protection especially the frail old, disabled, and those with cognitive impairment.
- Patients' beliefs regarding euthanasia maybe on the basis of inadequate information, since it is impossible to identify accurately when an individual patient will die naturally.

Important to recognize where the primary intention is to prevent suffering it is not normally considered to be euthanasia, this includes the following.

Euthanasia is not:
- Withholding or withdrawing futile, burdensome treatment. This includes nutrition and hydration if the patient is dying and is unable to swallow.
- Giving opioids, or any other medications, to control symptoms including pain, fear, and overwhelming distress.
- Sedating a patient in the terminal stages if all other practical methods of controlling symptoms have failed.
- Issuing a Do Not Resuscitate order.

Adapted from Watson et al. (2005). *Oxford Handbook of Palliative Care.* Oxford University Press, Oxford.

Related topics
📖 Consent; 📖 Mental capacity.

Further information for patients and professionals
🖳 BMA Assisted dying debate: www.bma.org.uk/ap.nsf/Content/AssistedDyingDebate

House of Lords (2004). *Assisted dying for the terminally ill Bill.* The Stationery Office London. (HL Bill 17, session 2003–4) (Chairman Lord Joffe).

🖳 ProLife Collaboration: www.prolife.org.uk

Royal College of Nursing (2004). RCN confirms opposition to Assisted Dying Bill and calls for improved palliative care, RCN London. www.rcn.org.uk

Scottish Parliament (2004). *Dying with dignity.* Scottish Parliament, Edinburgh.

🖳 Voluntary Euthanasia Society: www.ves.org

Injection techniques

Drugs are given via parenteral routes when they need to be absorbed quickly or when they would be altered by ingestion. Some drugs are released over a long period of time and need a parenteral route that will absorb the drug steadily. Complications include abscesses and nerve injury. Local policies will apply.

Key principles

- Ensure an anaphylactic shock kit is easily accessible
- Assess patient's anxiety and if they need reassurance
- Prepare medication according to manufacturer's instructions
- Check local policy for medicine administration
- Ensure dose tallies with accurate prescription
- Wash hands and apply gloves and apron according to local policy
- Avoid sites where there is an inflammation, swelling, or skin lesions
- Ensure prompt disposal of sharps according to local policy
- Document procedure (drug name, dose given, site, batch, expiry date).

Subcutaneous injections

The SC route is used for slow, sustained absorption of medication. Up to 1–2mL may be administered. It is relatively pain free and suitable for frequent injections. Sites include the upper outer arm, abdomen, front and outer aspect of thighs, and buttocks. Absorption is most rapid from the abdomen, slower from the arms, and slowest from the thighs and buttock area. Insulin injections are recommended in the abdomen for fast acting insulin, thighs for intermediate acting insulin or the evening dose of twice daily insulin regimens, and buttocks for intermediate or long acting insulin.

- For frequent injections, rotate sites and check for fat hypertrophy and scarring on a regular basis
- For insulin injections rotate within each day daily
- Cloudy insulin should be adequately mixed before injection
- For insulin injections use a 31–29 gauge needle between 5–8mm
- For other SC injections use a 25 gauge needle between 10–25mm
- Use of alcohol swabs prior to frequent injections will harden the skin
- Pinch skin to lift adipose tissue away from underlying muscle
- Insert needle, bevel side up at a 90 degree angle
- Do not aspirate
- Leave needle in skin for 6–10sec after depressing plunger
- Hold skin fold until needle has been withdrawn.

Intradermal injections

The ID route provides a local, rather than systemic effect and is used for diagnostic purposes such as allergy or tuberculin testing or for local anesthetics. BCG is always given by the ID route. Suitable sites are similar to those for SC injections (see above) but also include ventral forearm and upper back. The preferred site for BCG is at the point of the insertion of the left deltoid muscle.

- Use a 25 gauge, 10mm needle
- Stretch skin taut with thumb and forefinger of free hand

- Insert needle bevel side up at a 10–15 degree angle for about 2mm
- When testing for allergies, label area to monitor an allergic response
- BCG vaccinations should never been covered with a plaster or dressing.

Intramuscular injections

IM injections provide rapid systemic action and allow the administration of relatively large doses. Sites include the deltoid muscle in the upper arm, the dorsogluteal site using the gluteus maximus muscle, the ventro-gluteal site using the gluteus maximus muscle, and the quadriceps muscle on the outer side of the femur. The ventrogluteal site is the optimum choice for adults and children >7mths.

- Discard needle after preparation of medication
- Use a 21 or 23 gauge, 25–38mm needle
- Use a low dose syringe for injections <1mL
- For injections of 5mL or more, divide equally between 2 sites
- For frequent injections rotate sites
- Cleanse skin according to local policy
- Consider ice or freezing spray to numb the skin (e.g. in children)
- If patient has reduced muscle mass 'bunch up' the muscle before injecting
- Pull the skin downwards or to one side of the intended site (moving cutaneous and subcutaneous tissue by 1–2cm)
- Keep the skin taught and insert needle at a 90 degree angle
- Aspirate for several seconds and if blood aspirated withdraw needle
- If no blood appears inject at a rate approx 1mL every 10sec
- Leave needle in skin for 6–10sec after depressing plunger
- On removal release retracted skin
- Do not massage but apply gentle pressure with gauze swab if indicated.

Administration of goserelin implant (Zoladex®)

Goserelin reduces the production of testosterone and oestrogen. It is also used in assisted reproduction. It is produced in ready-mixed sterile syringes and is administered every 28d (3.6mg) or every 12wks (10.8mg).

- Consider application of topical anaesthetic agents
- Position patient sitting or semi-recumbent
- Administer SC in anterior abdominal wall below naval line
- Cleanse proposed site with alcohol swab
- Pinch skin to lift adipose tissue away from underlying muscle
- Insert needle, bevel side up at a 30–45 degree angle, until hub of barrel touches the skin and depress plunger until it depresses no further
- Remove the device and cover site with a sterile plaster.

Further information

📖 Royal College of Paediatrics and Child Health (2002). Position statement on injection technique: www.rcn.org.uk/publications/pdf/injection-technique.pdf

📖 Shire Hall Communications (2001). UK guidance on best practice in vaccine administration: www.rcn.org.uk/publications/pdf/guidelines/rcn_vaccine_uk_guidance.pdf

Peripheral venepuncture

Venepuncture is the introduction of a needle into a vein to obtain a blood sample for haematological, biochemical, or bacteriological analysis. It is one of the most common invasive procedures undertaken in primary care settings. Veins in the arm are usually chosen (basilica, cephalic, or median cubital veins in the antecubital fossa). Risks include arterial puncture and nerve injury. Sampling veins in the dorsal aspect of the hand will subject the patient to discomfort and sampling veins in the foot might result in DVT or tissue necrosis in diabetics. Local policies will apply.

Choosing a vein

Palpate and visually inspect. Choose sizeable veins with wide lumen and thick walls. Suitable veins will feel soft and bouncy and refill when depressed. Vasodilatation might be encouraged by applying a warm pack. Use non-dominant arm where possible.
- Do not use infected areas, oedematous limbs, or limbs affected by CVA
- Do not use limbs adjacent to mastectomy or anxillary node dissection
- Do not use hard, cord-like, sclerosed, firosed, or thrombosed veins
- Do not use same arm as an IV infusion

Preparation
- Determine whether patient has experienced an adverse outcome with venepuncture previously (such as fainting) so that reassurances can be given and further action taken.
- Determine whether patient has allergy to latex or plasters.
- Check when patient last ate or drunk before fasting, samples and time and dose of last medication before drug samples and hormone levels.
- Consider application of topical anaesthetic agents (e.g. in children and anxious adults).
- Cleanse visibly dirty skin with soap and water and dry thoroughly.
- Cleanse proposed puncture site with alcohol swab for 30sec and allow to air dry for 30sec.

Procedure (using vacuum system)
- Wash hands according to local policy.
- Apply tourniquet (preferably single use only) to upper arm (approx 7–10cm above proposed puncture site).
- Apply enough pressure to impede venous circulation but not arterial blood flow (check for an arterial pulse).
- Patient may assist venous filling by clenching and unclenching hand.
- Observe and palpate selected vein.
- Release tourniquet and check vein has decompressed (thrombosed veins will remain firm and palpable).
- Select needle or winged infusion device (winged infusion device in children and other high-risk patients).
- Select smallest possible gauge needle or winged infusion device.
- Screw needle or winged infusion device into open-ended plastic cylinder.
- Wash hands and put on gloves and apron according to local policy.

- Reapply tourniquet.
- With arm in a downward position, align needle with vein.
- Anchor mobile veins with thumb about 2–5cm below proposed puncture site.
- Smoothly insert needle, bevel side up at a 20–40 degree angle.
- Stabilise needle by holding guide sheath firmly.
- Stabilise winged infusion device by flattening wings and securing with hypoallergenic tape.
- Insert collection tube into plastic cylinder (consider order to avoid cross contamination of additives between tubes).
- Allow collection tubes to fill.
- Observe maximum blood volumes to be drawn from children under 14yrs.
- Release tourniquet.
- Slip cotton wool ball over puncture site, do not apply pressure until needle fully removed, once removed apply digital pressure until bleeding stops (patients taking warfarin may need to apply pressure for a longer period).
- Prompt disposal of sharps according to local policy.
- Do not allow patient to bend arm.
- Once puncture site has stopped bleeding, cover with a plaster or cotton wool ball and hypoallergenic tape.
- Make no more than 2 attempts to obtain blood samples (if unsuccessful obtain assistance from more experienced colleagues).
- After procedure children should be praised and rewarded.
- Label collection tubes and check details against request form.
- Discuss arrangements for patients or parents to receive results.
- Ensure safe and timely transport of specimens in appropriate container.
- Document procedure.

Essential reading

Buckbee, K. (1994). Implementing a paediatric phlebotomy protocol. Medical Laboratory Observer, **26** (4), 32–5.

Dougherty, L. and Lister, S. (eds) (2006). *The Royal Marsden Hospital Manual of Clinical Nursing Procedures*, (6th edn). Blackwell Publishing, Oxford.

RCN (2005). Standards for infusion therapy:
www.rcn.org.uk/publications/pdf/standards-infusiontherapy.pdf

Recording a 12 lead electrocardiogram

An electrocardiogram (ECG) is the collection of electrical waveforms produced by the heart. Indications for recording a 12 lead ECG include chest pain, palpitations, and history of syncope. It is often undertaken by practice nurses on the request of the GP.

Procedure

- To help produce a clear, stable trace without interference, make sure the room is warm and try to relax the patient.
- Position the patient in a semi-recumbent comfortable position—adjust the backrest on the couch as appropriate.
- Prepare the skin if necessary.
- Apply the limb electrodes and leads (NB refer also to manufacturer's guidance as colours can vary):
  - Red: inner right wrist
  - Yellow: inner left wrist
  - Black: inner right leg, just above the ankle
  - Green: inner left leg, just above the ankle.
- Apply the chest electrodes and leads (Fig. 10.4):
  - V1: 4th intercostal space, just to the right of the sternum
  - V2: 4th intercostal space, just to the left of the sternum
  - V3: midway between V2 and V4
  - V4: 5th intercostal space, mid-clavicular line
  - V5: on anterior axillary line, on the same horizontal line as V4
  - V6: mid-axillary line, on the same horizontal line as V4 and V5
- Ask the patient to remain still and breathe normally.
- Print out the ECG following the manufacturer's recommendations.
- Correctly label the ECG e.g. patient's name, date of birth, date and time of recording, ECG serial number together with any relevant information e.g. if the patient was pain free or complaining of chest pain during the recording.

Accuracy, quality, and standardization

- Accuracy: ensure all the electrodes and leads are correctly applied.
- Quality: minimize interference e.g. patient movement and electrical interference, as this can produce a 'fuzzy' trace.
- Standardization: e.g. standard calibration (1mV = 10mm), standard paper speed (25mm/second), and standard patient position.

Further information

Jevon, P. (2003). *ECGs for Nurses*. Blackwell Publishing. Oxford.

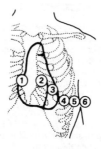

Fig. 10.4 Positioning of chest electrodes and leads. Reproduced with permission from the Oxford Handbook of Clinical Medicine 6e, Longmore, M *et al.* (2004), Oxford University Press.

Tracheostomy care

A tracheostomy: artificial opening in anterior wall of trachea created to:
- Bypass mechanical obstructions e.g. advanced cancer
- Aid prolonged and assisted ventilation e.g. motor neurone disease
- Prevent other matter entering lungs e.g. lost swallow reflex.

Potential complications include displaced tube, blocked tube, site infection, pneumonia, and tracheal damage.

Discharge home

Patients, parents and carers taught care, management, and action in emergency in hospital pre-discharge home. Important for primary care nurses to liaise with hospital staff pre-discharge to understand:
- Tube and any humidification device care
- Patients communication methods
- Advice in emergency.

Patients require electric and foot suction pump (for emergencies), and inform power supplier patient requires continuous supply for medical equipment.

The tracheostomy tube

- Cuffed tubes.
  - Have a balloon on the end to prevent aspiration
  - Have cuff pressure checked x2d (must be between 15–20mmHg).
- Fenestrated tubes.
  - Have hole in upper aspect for passage of air and secretions
  - Have a non-fenestrated inner tube to be inserted prior to tracheal suctioning and if additional respiratory support is required.

Care of stoma

- Usually twice daily but frequency assessed individually
- Two people, according to local policy, aseptic procedure (eye protection required)
- Observe and document signs of infection, irritation, and granulations
- Carefully irrigate area with normal saline
- Do not use cotton wool to cleanse (risk of inhaling small fibres)
- White soft paraffin may be applied to protect the skin after cleansing
- Dressings unnecessary except with silver tubes or when clinically indicated then should be polyurethane type dressing
- Secure tube with clean tracheostomy tapes (tied with a reef knot at the side of the neck) or a Velcro tracheostomy holder (tight enough to allow two fingers to be inserted between the tape and the neck).

Cleaning inner cannula

- Usually twice daily but frequency assessed individually
- Once removed, a clean inner cannula should be inserted immediately
- Clean used inner cannula with warm tap water and air-dry
- Do not use brushes to clean plastic tubes.

Changing outer tube

Tubes without an inner cannula changed every 5–7d. Tubes with an inner cannula every 29d (see also manufacturer's instructions).

- Over 3hrs after meal as coughing may induce vomiting
- Two people (refer to local policy and procedure) to perform procedure aseptic procedure with eye protection
- Position patient sitting upright with neck extended
- Test the cuff (if present) on new tube for leakage prior to insertion
- Pre-oxygenate patient before and after procedure according to local policy (caution to be taken with patients with COPD)
- Perform tracheal and oral suction before procedure if indicated
- Deflate cuff (if present)
- Patient to take several deep breaths and as they breathe out remove old tube following the curvature of the tracheal tract
- Insert clean tube with introducer (if present), remove introducer immediately after insertion
- Inflate cuff (if present), insert inner cannula (if present) and secure with tapes or holder
- Observe patient for at least 15min for signs of respiratory distress (respiratory rate, colour, and chest movements)
- Document type of tube and size inserted
- Dispose of plastic tubes but clean and retain silver tubes.

Suctioning

Suctioning only undertaken when patient is unable to clear own airway. Potential complications include cardiovascular instability, hypoxaemia, bronchospasm, vomiting, infection, and tracheal necrosis.

Procedure

- Ensure a non-fenestrated inner cannula is inserted
- Pre-oxygenate patient before and after procedure according to local policy (caution to be taken with patients with COPD)
- Aseptic procedure according to local policy (eye protection required)
- Suction machine pressure must be maintained below 120mmHg in adults (80–100mmHg in children)
- Connect appropriate size catheter (no more than half the diameter of inner cannula) and gently insert catheter into tracheostomy tube (depth of insertion advised by hospital depending on length of tracheostomy)
- Do not apply suction whilst introducing catheter and withdraw catheter 1–3cm before application of suction
- Apply suction and gently remove catheter from tube
- Do not suction adults for longer than 10sec (children 5sec)
- Document colour, viscosity, and quantity of secretions
- Disconnect and dispose of used catheter
- Observe patient for signs of respiratory distress (see above)
- Flush connection tubing with sterile water and clean suction collection container every 24hrs.

Further information

- Great Ormond Street Fact sheet for parents on going home with a tracheotomy: www.ich.ucl.ac.uk/factsheets/index.html
- NHS Quality Improvement Scotland (2003). *Caring for the Patient with a Tracheostomy, Best Practice Statement:* www.nhshealthquality.org

Ear care

Nurses carrying out ear care should ensure they have the knowledge and skills as taught on a recognized ear care study day:

- Understanding of anatomy and physiology of the ear and be able to apply this to patient education.
- The ability to carry out an ear examination using an otoscope and/or head light.
- The recognition of a normal tympanic membrane.
- Documentation and referral process if abnormalities identified.
- Assessment of wax/debris in the ear canal and removal management.
- Referral process for patients with ear and/or hearing problems.

Routine ear examinations

Ear examination to identify normal or abnormal anatomy should be carried out in the following cases:

- Annual checks on patients >65yrs who wear hearing aids.
- Annual checks on patients who have required wax removal (irrigation, manual removal, microsuction) in the past.
- Patients presenting with ear related symptoms—hearing loss, discharge, pain, vertigo, tinnitus, itching, blocked feeling/fullness in the ear.
- Problems with the hearing aid (i.e. whistling) or patients over the age of 60yrs with an audiology appointment.

Examination aims to identify any abnormalities e.g. infections and wax/debris build up. Nurses undertaking ear examinations should be clear when and where to refer for medical or other assessment.

Cerumen/wax

Cerumen is a mixture of lipids, produced by the sebaceous glands to protect the epithelial lining of the external auditory meatus. It needs only to be removed if it is causing problems. Hard impacted wax causes hearing loss deafness, discomfort, and sometimes tinnitus.

- Assess for colour, consistency, odour, and location. Wax that is dull and dark in colour tends to be harder.
- With otoscopic magnification, wax/debris appears greater and is often difficult to judge how far down the ear canal it is located. Hairs around the wax when visible with a headlight tends to be in the outer part of the canal this should be removed manually with appropriate instrumentation such as a wax hook or Jobson Horne probe.
- Use clinical judgement to consider options for removal assessing both the wax and the patient suitability (see Clinical Knowledge Summaries (Prodigy) guidance below)
  patient preference important.

Removal options

- First line treatment option—softening agent (BNF 12.1.3) with natural migration.
- Manual removal with suitable instrumentation as is commonly carried out in primary care.

- Irrigation—not suitable for:
  - Patients that have not given or are not able to give consent or the patient cannot remain comfortably still for at least 10min.
  - Those having had complications with this procedure in the past.
  - History of a middle ear infection in the last 6wks.
  - The patient has undergone *any* form of ear surgery (apart from grommets that have extruded at least 18mths previously and the patient has been discharged from the ENT dept).
  - History of eardrum perforation or mucous discharge in last year.
  - The patient has a cleft palate (repaired or not).
  - Acute otitis externa with pain and tenderness of the pinna.

Irrigation procedure

- Soften wax prior to removal. Use clinical judgement on need, frequency, and length of treatment to soften wax. Example: olive oil, 1 drop twice daily into the ear(s), 5d prior to the appointment. Explain benefit of oil to patient: as irrigation not taking so long, less discomfort and greater chance of success so compliance will be better.
- Electronic irrigators should be used (not metal syringes) as a safer control of water pressure and direction.
- Jet tip applicator should be firmly attached to tubing.
- Straighten the ear canal by pulling the pinna gently up and back.
- Patient holds kidney dish under ear to catch out-flowing water.
- Direct the water flow backwards along the roof of the ear canal, toward back of patients head. Stop immediately if any pain caused.
- Water softens wax; if the wax remains after 5min of irrigation, move onto the other ear as the introduction of water should soften the wax and you can retry irrigation after about 15min. Excessive soft wax or crumbly wax and debris can often be wiped out with cotton wool wound onto a Jobson Horne probe.

Microsuctioning and other forms or removal are usually only found in 2° care settings.

Hearing loss

(Deafness 📖).

When you are with a patient be sensitive to a hearing loss and appropriate referral will improve their quality of life. Patients over the age of 60yrs can usually be referred directly to the audiology department providing they do not suffer any other ear related problems and there is no wax in their ears.

Further information

- Information on anatomy and physiology of the ear. Patient advice sheets and ear wax removal procedures can be downloaded free of charge from: www.entnursing.com
- A simple effective hearing loss assessment at: www.hartfordign.org
- Ear care information: www.earcarecentre.com and www.earcareservices.com
- Clinical Knowledge Summaries (Prodigy) guidance on ear wax at: www.cks.library.nhs.uk/home

Blood transfusion (adults)

Around 3.4 million blood components are transfused every year in the UK. Blood transfusions are increasingly being carried out in the home and in local treatment centres. Patients suited to out of hospital transfusions include those with haematological disorders or malignant conditions that require regular transfusion therapy. This is usually undertaken as part of a shared care agreement between primary care practitioners and the hospital consultant. Local policies will apply.

Key principles

- Patients being transfused for the first time must have their initial transfusion in hospital in case of transfusion reactions.
- Each patient must have a unique identification (ID) number to be used throughout the process.
- Patients must have an ID wristband (or an ID card).
- A written plan of action to be followed in case of emergency or transfusion reactions.

Pre transfusion blood sampling

- Pre-transfusion sampling is required for cross match purposes.
- Local policy should establish who is permitted to complete the pre transfusion request form.
- Ensure patient has an ID wristband or ID card recording their correct name, address, date of birth, and unique ID number.
- Collect blood sample and immediately label (❶ do not use pre-labelled sample tubes or addressograph labels).
- Sample tube must be signed by person bleeding the patient.
- Check details on sample tube and request form correspond.
- Send to transfusion laboratory.

Prescription

Prescription should state the patient details (name, date of birth, and unique ID number), blood component to be transfused, any special requirements (such as concomitant diuretic therapy), number of units to be transfused, and duration of transfusion.

Transportation of blood component

- Check patient has IV access prior to collecting blood component.
- The person removing the blood component from the hospital blood refrigerator must check the patient details on the blood component label against the prescription chart.
- Transport blood component in validated carrier.
- Do not store blood component outside hospital blood refrigerator for more than 30min.

Pre-administration

- Positively identify patient by name, date of birth, and unique ID number.
- Check patient consent.
- Undertake baseline observations (BP, pulse, and temperature).
- Check access to anaphylaxis drugs and functionality of emergency equipment (including landline telephone).

- Check prescription and any special requirements.
- Check blood component expiry date and visually inspect for discolouration, clumping and leaks.

Administration

- Positively identify patient by name, date of birth, and unique ID number.
- Check prescription.
- Check blood group and donation number on compatibility report are identical to those on the blood component.
- Flush cannula with normal saline.
- Administer blood component through blood administration set with 170–200mcg filter.
- ❶ No therapy with the exception of desferioximine to be infused through same lumen.
- From starting the infusion the blood component should be given within a maximum of 4hrs.
- On completion flush and remove cannula.
- Discard empty bags according to local policy.

Monitoring for allergic and haemolytic reactions

- Monitor for breathlessness, chest or loin pain, flushing, shivering, and rashes.
- Monitor temperature and pulse 15min after beginning transfusion.
- Subsequent observations according to patient condition and local policy.
- Maintain visual and verbal contact with the patient throughout transfusion.
- Maintain accurate records throughout.
- Stop transfusion if reaction suspected and seek medical assistance.
- ❶ Report reactions to the Serious Hazards of Transfusion (SHOT) scheme (☎ 0161 251 4208).

Essential reading

🔲 BCSH Blood Transfusion Task Force (1999). Guidelines for the administration of blood and blood components and the management of transfused patients, *Transfusion Medicine*, 9, 227–38. Available at: www.bcshguidelines.org
🔲 RCN (2004). *Right blood, right patient, right time: RCN guidance for improving transfusion practice.* www.rcn.org.uk
🔲 UK Blood Transfusion Services (2004). *Handbook of Transfusion Medicine.* The Stationary Office, London: www.transfusionguidelines.org.uk/index.asp

Percutaneous endoscopic gastrostomy (PEG) feeds

A PEG is a feeding tube that passes through the abdominal wall into the stomach so that the patient can receive nutrition without swallowing. May be treatment of choice for patients following stroke (📖), for those who have MS (📖), MND (📖), also can be used as part of palliative care. PEG feeds are used if:

- Patient is unable to swallow.
- To provide extra nutrition (supplements) for people who can still eat.
- When long-term artificial feeding is required.

Inserting a PEG feeding tube into the stomach through an insertion in the abdominal wall is a hospital procedure done under local anaesthetic.

Care of patient with a PEG tube

Patients and carers can manage feeds using PEG but this must be their choice and it should only happen with direct access to nursing and dietician support and regular review.

Feeding through the PEG tube

- Patient's head and shoulders should ideally be elevated during feed to ↓ risk of aspiration.
- The length and frequency of feeds varies, can be continuous for 12–18hrs or by syringe (bolus) several times a day for 30–40min.
- Pump to administer continuous feed (often overnight) set up according to manufacturer's instructions. Feeds are provided on prescription (BNF 9.4.2 and Appendix 7).
- Only specially prepared feeds should be administered through the PEG and medicines in liquid form and administered according to dietician instructions.
- Flush the tube with 30–50mL of cooled boiled water before and after each feed and/or administration of medicines.
- Be aware of the danger of bacterial infection from feeds left hanging at room temperature, ideally should not be left up for more than 4hrs.
- Do not crush medication and do not use with a tube: slow release medication and those for use by other routes (e.g. sub lingual, chewable etc.).

Care of PEG tube

- When the skin has healed around the insertion patient can shower and bathe with the PEG tube firmly clamped.
- No need for dressing unless site oozes (this should be checked by nurse).
- Good hand hygiene essential when caring for site and changing feeds.
- Important to ensure that oral hygiene is maintained, suggest sucking ice cubes to keep mouth moist or use swabs moistened with water.

Problems associated with PEG

- Patients may experience bloating, diarrhoea, reflux, or constipation if this occurs: review type and rate of the feed with the dietician.
- Nausea or vomiting can be associated with the feed rate being too fast; monitor closely as danger of dehydration and electrolyte imbalance.
- Inflammation and local infection. The entry site should be kept clean and checked for any signs of infection and good hand hygiene maintained.
- Monitor patient's weight and review regimen if marked ↑ or ↓.
- Tube blockage: irrigate with cool boiled water. NB Some medicines coagulate with feeds so should be given an hour apart and/or with extra dilution.
- It takes 2–3wks for the stoma to form/stabilize. If the tube falls out tell the patient to cover with a dressing to absorb any leakage and contact DN or doctor for a replacement to be fitted.
- If the tube is damaged it should be clamped and patient referred to hospital.

Related topics

Motor neurone disease 🕮; Cystic fibrosis 🕮; Palliative care in the home 🕮.

Further information for health professionals and patients

🖥 Digestive Disorders Foundation: www.digestivedisorders.org.uk

Dougherty, L. and Lister, S. (eds) (2006). *The Royal Marsden Hospital Manual of Clinical Nursing Procedures*, (6th edn). Blackwell Publishing, Oxford.

🖥 NICE (2003). Section on care of enteral feeding in *Infection control: prevention of health care associated infection in primary and secondary care*. www.nice.org.uk

Care of people with long-term conditions

Osteoarthritis (OA)

OA is the biggest cause of joint related pain and mobility problems in adults ♀>♂ with onset in middle age (average 50yrs). Approx 8 million are affected in UK and approx 1 million seek treatment. Very variable condition involves the whole joint → pain, stiffness, and joint instability.

- Knee OA > common than hip OA: together affect 10–20% population >65yrs
- OA of the hands develops gradually with swellings on the back of joints—Herbeden's nodules
- OA of the neck: spondylosis may not present with pain or symptoms.

Causes

- Age: OA is uncommon before 40yrs
- Obesity: especially with knee
- Joint injury or earlier operation
- Hard repetitive activity may injure joints e.g. sport and physical labour
- Hereditary.

Problems associated with OA

(Wide variation of experience.)
- Painful and stiff joints with pain ↑ on exercise
- Joint may give way because of weak muscles
- Symptoms vary with some having periods of remission
- Advanced OA pain is severe and constant
- Compromised mobility and difficulty completing ADL
- Depression.

Support and advice to ↓ pain and progression

- Advise patient about disease and health promotion, healthy diet, smoking cessation.
- Reduce stress on joints by maintaining ideal weight.
- Exercise to strengthen muscles to stabilize and protect joints. Consider referral to physiotherapist for advice and teaching of exercises.
- Pace activities and do physically demanding work intermittently.
- Wear flat heels and footwear with thick soft soles to act as shock absorbers.
- Walking sticks (use on opposite side to OA joint) can ↓ weight and stress on hip and knee.
- Home modifications that avoid trips and falls and ↓ the need to bend and strain. Consider OT referral.
- Psychological support. NB OA does *not* always worsen, symptoms may reach a peak a few years after first onset and plateau or lessen.
- Activities to optimize joint movement and maintain general health, regular aerobic exercise e.g. swimming.

Treatment

- Expert patient, peer support groups (Expert patient 📖).
- Analgesia (BNF 4.7.1): paracetamol first choice or combined analgesia. NSAIDs for inflammation of the joints (NB also refer to local formulary advice for prescribing).
- Glucosamine and chondroitin from health shops and chemists. NB Evidence mixed about their effectiveness.
- Steroid injections (BNF 10.1.2.1) for severe pain.
- Surgery: hip and knee replacement to address severe pain or immobility.

Related topics

📖 Expert patient; 📖 Rheumatoid arthritis; 📖 Healthy ageing.

Further information for professionals and relatives

🖳 Arthritis Care: www.arthritiscare.org.uk
🖳 Arthritis Research Campaign: www.arc.org.uk
🖳 Disabled Living Foundation: www.dlf.org.uk

Rheumatoid arthritis (RA)

Immunological chronic disease of connective tissue with no cure, believed to be triggered by environmental factors in patients that have a genetic predisposition. Characterized by inflammation of peripheral joints and tendons.

>350,000 people in UK have RA occurs at any age most common 40–50yrs, 3x as many ♀ affected as ♂. Variable disease characterized by exacerbations and remissions. For some it is a rapid progressive disease.

Onset and symptoms of RA

Important that treatment for RA is started as soon as possible as this affects the progression of the disease and damage caused by the inflammation process. Any patient with symptoms that might be RA should see GP for onward referral to rheumatology service.

- Often starts slowly: discomfort and intermittent swelling of joints, pain in the morning, often people do not seek help until they experience difficulty in movement.
- For 20% of sufferers onset is very rapid and painful.
- In addition to joint related pain people may experience fatigue, stiffness, and anaemia.
- Eyes may become dry and irritable (use artificial tears B.N.F.11.8.1). Rheumatoid nodules may appear on elbows, hands, and feet.

Care and support to ↓ pain and progression

Difficult to tell a patient how their RA will progress and for many it will be characterized by exacerbation and periods of remission. RA sufferers may experience depression, fatigue a common symptom.

- Encourage exercise to maintain function and muscle strength *but* if joints feel warm, become painful or swollen, rest.
- Devise exercise programme that the patient can do e.g. gentle exercises, gym, swimming is often the best exercise.
- Choose footwear that cushions the foot and acts as shock absorber.
- Mixed evidence about diet and RA, encourage healthy low fat diet.
- Expert patient, peer support groups (Expert patient 📖).
- Medication likely to involve analgesics including paracetamol (BNF 4.7.1), NSAIDs (BNF 10.1.1), disease modifying anti-rheumatics, DSMARDs see ARC website below for more detail (BNF 10.1.3.), and corticosteroids (BNF 10.1.2.1).
- Advise patient about possible SE of medication (see Table 11.1 below for monitoring and SE).
- People with RA may be more at risk of stroke and cardiovascular disease.
- May need referral for surgical review, e.g. to relieve trapped nerve and tendons or full joint replacement.
- Referral to physiotherapist for exercises and possible joint support and strapping. Consider OT referral for home modifications.
- Disabled 'blue' parking badge if mobility affected.

Table 11.1 Specific drugs: side effects and monitoring

Drug	Monitoring	Side effects to monitor
Methotrexate: 7.5–20mg wkly Followed the day after by calcium folinate 15mg every 6h for 24h i.e. wkly as well.	FBC, U&E, Cr, and LFTs before starting treatment, wkly for 6wks then every 2–3mths ❶ Advise patients NOT to self-medicate with OTC aspirin or ibuprofen. Avoid alcohol	Ask patients to report all symptoms/signs of infection, especially sore throat Severe respiratory symptoms in the 1st 6mnth—refer to ED.
Sulfasalazine: 1g bd maintenance	FBC, LFTs + U&E,Cr at 2, 4, 6 & 8wks then every 4wks. for 3mths then 3 mthly. Urgent FBC if intercurrent illness during initiation of treatment	Rash (1%) Nausea/diarrhoea—often transient Bone marrow suppression in 1–2% in the first months.
Intramuscular gold (Myocrisin®): 50mg mthly	FBC, urinalysis, ESR, prior to each injection. LFTs, U&E, Cr3-mthly	Ask patients to report: All symptoms/signs of infection—especially sore throat Bleeding/bruising Breathlessness/cough Mouth ulcers/metallic taste in mouth or Rashes
D penicillamine: Initially 125–250mg/d increased after 4wks to 500–750mg/d, max 1.5g/d	FBC, urinalysis 2 wkly for 8wks & 1wk after any ↑ dosage. then monthly. LFTs and U&E, Cr annually	Altered taste—can be ignored, rash
Azathioprine: up to 2.5mg/kg/d. maintenance	FBC wkly for 6wks then 1x/mth U&E and LFTs 1x/ mth for 3mth then 3-mthly	GI side effects, rash, bone marrow suppression
Ciclosporin: up to 3.5mg/kg/d. maintenance	Cr & BP 2 wkly to stable dose then 1x/mth FBC, U&E, LFTs 1x/mth until stable for 3mth then 3-mthly. Lipids 6-mthly	Rash, gum soreness, hirsitism, ↑ Cr, ↑BP, renal failure
Hydroxychloroquine: 200–400mg/d maintenance	Baseline eye check and periodically on advice of local ophthalmologist	Rash, GI effects, ocular side effects (rare)
Leflunomide 10–20mg/d maintenance	FBC, LFTs, U&E, BP— 2 wkly for 6mths. then mthly	Rash, GI, ↑ BP, ↑ ALT

* GMS contract: national enhanced service funding is available for shared care drug monitoring for: penicillamine, auranofin, sulphasalazine, methotrexate, and sodium aurothiomalate (myocristin).

Adapted with permission from Simon, C., Everitt, H., and Kendrick, T. (2005), *Oxford Handbook of General Practice*, 2nd edn. Oxford University Press, Oxford.

Related topics

📖 Expert patient; 📖 Osteoarthritis (OA); 📖 Healthy ageing.

Further information for professionals and relatives

▤ Arthritis Care: www.arthritiscare.org.uk
▤ Arthritis Research Campaign: www.arc.org.uk
▤ Disabled Living Foundation: www.dlf.org.uk

Osteoporosis

A progressive, systemic, skeletal disease, characterized by low bone mass and micro-architectural deterioration of bone tissues, → ↑ in bone fragility and susceptibility to fracture, significant cause of mortality, pain, and disability particularly in older people and can result in:

- Vertebral deformity
- Loss of height
- Limitations in daily activities.

Prevalence

In the UK, 310,000 osteoporotic fractures occur each year with a cost in excess of £1.7bn. More than $1/3$ of ♀ and $1/12$ ♂ will sustain ≥1 osteoporotic fractures in their lifetime. Often diagnosed after first fracture.

Priority to ↓ osteoporotic fractures.

Risk factors

- Oestrogen deficiency:
  - Premature menopause (<45yrs)
  - Prolonged 2° amenorrhoea (>1yr).
- 1° or 2° hypogonadism in ♂.
- Corticosteroid therapy: prednisolone >7.5mg/day for 6mths or more or repeat courses of steroids or high-dose inhaled steroids.
- Maternal history of hip fracture.
- Low body mass index (<19kg/m^2).
- Other disorders associated with osteoporosis: anorexia nervosa, malabsorption syndromes, 1° hyperparathyroidism, post-transplantation, chronic renal failure, chronic liver disease, hyperthyroidism, prolonged immobilization, Cushing's syndrome.
- Previous fragility fracture, esp. hip, spine, wrist.
- Loss of height, thoracic kyphosis.
- Risk assessment should include use of validated tool, see further information below, GP can refer for bone mineral density (BMD) for definitive diagnosis. NB screening tool forthcoming from NICE.

Prevention of osteoporotic fractures: each primary care organization should have:

- Lead clinician for falls prevention/osteoporosis programme/monitor organization's performance.
- Establish local osteoporosis interest group to facilitate multidisciplinary implementation.
- Use of a selective case finding approach to target treatment of individuals at ↑ risk of osteoporotic fracture.
- Access to adequate levels of diagnostic and specialist services including falls clinics.
- Promotion of care pathways and auditing to standards of care.

Preventive interventions

- Nutrition (Nutrition and healthy eating 📖):
  - Calcium reference nutrient intake 700mg/day for adult men and women, 800–1000mg/day for 11–18yrs, 350–550mg for children, 525mg/day for infants. Found in dairy products and green leafy vegetables, flour products, some fish.
  - Vitamin D helps absorb calcium. Found in dairy products and fish oils, but major source sunlight on skin. Requirement is 15–20mins/day during summer months, but avoid burning. ❶ Elderly people in nursing homes at higher risk of deficiency.
- Exercise and physical activity. Recommendation 30mins/day for 5 or more days/week. Weight-bearing, high impact exercise most beneficial e.g. running, jumping, climbing stairs or exercise referral for frailer and older people (Falls prevention 📖).
- Stop smoking → ↑ toxic effect on bone. Stopping ↓ fracture rate by 25% (Smoking cessation 📖).
- Moderate alcohol intake. 3–4units/day for men, 2–3units/day for women. Alcohol is damaging to bone turnover (Alcohol 📖).
- HRT postpones post-menopausal bone loss and ↓ fractures. *But* concerns around risk of breast cancer → not first choice for prevention (Menopause 📖).
- Hip protector pads although often poorly tolerated.

Further information and resources

- CREST (2002). Guidelines on the prevention and treatment of osteoporosis (includes Royal College of Physicians guidelines): www.crestni.org.uk/publications/osteo.pdf
- National Osteoporosis Society (2002) *Primary Care Strategy for Osteoporosis and Falls*: www.nos.org.uk
- National Osteoporosis Society: www.nos.org.uk
- NICE guidelines on prevention and treatment of osteoporosis: www.nice.org.uk
- NSF for older people (2001). Standard 6 includes prevention of osteoporosis as key intervention (England only). DH, London.

Low back pain

Common complaint; 80% of adult population will experience low back pain sometime in their lives, 50% of these will have recurring symptoms.
• Acute low back pain = new episode of <6wks duration.
• Chronic low back pain = pain lasts >3mths, if >1yr poor outlook.
Some back pain involves irritation of the nerve roots (radicular pain). Sciatica = when pain radiates down buttocks and leg caused by irritation of sciatic nerve.

Causes

• Postural
• Pregnancy
• Prolapsed disc
• Trauma
• Osteoporosis (🕮).
• Degenerative joint disease, osteoarthritis (inc. ankylosing spondylitis).

NB Refer to GP if pain is non-mechanical, involves thoracic pain, previous history of cancer, taking steroids, HIV, also unwell, observable structural deformity, accompanied with weight loss, neurological symptoms and impairment, or muscle weakness in leg and foot.

Care and support for acute back pain

• Regular and effective pain relief: paracetamol, NSAIDs (BNF 4.7.1).
• Hot and cold compresses to affected area (will not benefit everyone).
• Encourage to be as active as possible do not lie flat on back for prolonged periods unless advised by doctor.
• Evidence mixed on manipulation but many find it helpful to consult osteopath/chiropractor.
• If no improvement in 6wks should see physiotherapist for advice on back exercises.

Care and support for patients with chronic back pain

Patient should see GP and possible orthopaedic/rheumatology referral to discount need for surgery and/or possible referral to pain clinic if available locally.
• Overall aim to improve self-management (Expert patient 🕮) and reduce and manage pain.
• Encourage patient to regularly practice back exercises and maintain activity.
• Chronic pain can lead to loss of sleep, depression, and reduced QoL psychosocial support, analgesia should be used when exacerbations and amitriptyline at night can give relief (BNF 4.7.3).
• For chronic pain use painkillers e.g. paracetamol regularly and add NSAID for acute exacerbations.
• TENs can be helpful.

Health promotion and prevention

• Improve posture and overall physical fitness and activity levels.
• Exercise and interventions that improve back strength: cycling and swimming (avoiding breast stroke), yoga, Alexander technique.
• Advice from physiotherapist on back exercises and correct lifting techniques.

- Review household and work furniture: use chairs that support lumbar spine, firm mattresses etc. Workplace assessment by OH dept may determine need for specialist furniture/equipment.
- Reduce weight if BMI >25.

Related topics

📖 Pain assessment and management; 📖 People with depression; 📖 Talking therapies; 📖 Expert patient; 📖 Osteoarthritis (OA).

Further information for professionals, patients, and carers

📓 Clinical Knowledge Summaries (Prodigy) guidelines and PILs: www.cks.library.nhs.uk
📓 Backcare: www.backcare.org.uk
📓 The Pain Relief Foundation: www.painrelieffoundation.org.uk ☎ 0151 523 1486

Measuring lung function

The early identification and management of COPD (📖) requires the use of spirometry. The management of asthma (📖) requires the use of peak flow meters. 80% of GP practices in the UK have spirometers. Practice nurses, with appropriate training (see below), are often the most frequent users of this equipment in practices.

Peak flow

Measures how hard and how quickly a patient can exhale. Peak flow is used to monitor progress of disease and affects of treatment for patients with asthma. (Link with self-management plan.) Peak flow meters are available on NHS prescription. Since 2004, EN 13826/EU standard peak flow meters are supplied. Peak flow charts are available from NHS supplies (Form FP1010) and drug companies.

Measuring peak expiratory flow rate (PEFR)
- Ask the patient to stand up (if possible) and hold the peak flow meter horizontally. Check the indicator is at zero and the track clear.
- Ask the patient to take a deep breath and blow out forcefully into the peak flow meter ensuring lips are sealed firmly around the mouthpiece.
- Read the PEFR off the meter. The best of 3 attempts is recorded.
- Consider using a low range meter if predicted or best peak flow rate (PEFR) is <250L/min.
- Normal values: see Table 11.3.

Spirometry

Measures the volume of air the patient is able to expel from the lungs after a maximal inspiration.
- **FEV_1: (forced expiratory volume in one second):** volume of air the patient is able to exhale in the first second of forced expiration.
- **FVC (forced vital capacity):** total volume of air the patient can forcibly exhale in single breath.
- **FEV_1/FVC:** ratio of FEV_1 to FVC expressed as a %.

Measuring FEV_1 and FVC
- Note patient's sex, age, and (measured) height so that the measurements can be compared against predicted normal values.
- Sit the patient comfortably.
- Ask patient to breathe in as deeply as possible and hold their breath long enough to seal their lips around the mouthpiece.
- Ensure patient does *not* purse their lips and ideally ask them to pinch their nose.
- Patient should then breathe out forcibly as hard and as fast as possible until there is nothing left to expel.
  - Patients with severe COPD—this can take up to 15 seconds.
- Repeat procedure and repeat again → 3 readings of which the best 2 should be within 100ml or 5% of each other.

Readings are interpreted against normal values—see Table 11.3 and Table 11.4 for normal valves. If results are borderline normal then repeat in a few months.

Table 11.2 Interpretation of spirometry results

	Restrictive lung disease e.g. fibrosing alveolitis	Obstructive lung disease e.g. COPD
FEV$_1$ (% of predicted normal)	↓ (<80%)	↓ (<80%)
FVC (% of predicted normal)	↓ (<80%)	Normal or ↓
FEV$_1$/FVC	Normal (>70%)	↓ (<70%)

Reproduced with permission from Simon, C., Everitt, H., and Kendrick, T. (2005). *Oxford Handbook of General Practice*, 2nd edn, Oxford University Press, Oxford.

Essential reading

🖫 British Thoracic Society (2005). *Spirometry in practice: A practical guide to using spirometry in primary care*. Available from www.brit-thoracic.org.uk

Further information on training

ARTP/BTS Certificate in spirometry. Further details and list of approved training centres is available from ☎ 0121 697 8339. email admin@ARTP.org.uk, www.artp.org.uk

🖫 National Respiratory Training Centre: www.educationforhealth.org.uk

🖫 Respiratory Education and Training Centres: www.respiratoryetc.com/

Normal spirometry and peak flow values

Table 11.3 Predicted PEFR measurements in L/min (EU scale)[*]

Children: Height is the only determinant of PEFR in children. With ↑ age, the pattern of adult values takes over.

Height: Ft	3'	3'4"	3'8"	4'	4'4"	4'8"	5'	5'4"	5'8"	6'
M	90cm	1	1.1	1.2	1.3	1.4	1.5	1.6	1.7	1.8
PEFR l/min.	88	105	136	172	220	265	313	371	427	487

Women
Height →

ft	4'10"	4'11"	5'	5'1"	5'2"	5'3"	5'4"	5'5"	5'6"	5'7"	5'8"	5'9"	5'10"
m	1.47	1.5	1.52	1.55	1.57	1.6	1.62	1.65	1.67	1.7	1.72	1.75	1.77
Age													
15yrs	379	382	385	389	391	394	397	400	402	405	407	411	413
20yrs	402	406	409	413	416	419	422	425	428	431	434	437	439
25yrs	415	419	422	426	429	433	435	439	441	445	447	451	453
30yrs	419	424	427	431	433	437	440	444	446	450	452	456	458
35yrs	418	423	425	430	432	436	439	443	445	449	451	454	457
40yrs	413	417	420	424	427	431	433	437	439	443	445	449	451
45yrs	405	409	412	416	418	422	425	428	431	434	436	440	442
50yrs	394	399	401	405	407	411	414	417	419	423	425	428	430
55yrs	383	387	389	393	395	399	401	404	407	410	412	415	417
60yrs	370	373	376	379	382	385	387	391	393	396	398	401	403
65yrs	356	360	362	366	368	371	373	376	378	381	383	386	388
70yrs	343	346	348	351	353	356	358	361	363	366	368	371	372

Men
Height →

ft	5'2"	5'3"	5'4"	5'5"	5'6"	5'7"	5'8"	5'9"	5'10"	5'11"	6'	6'1"	6'2"
m	1.57	1.6	1.62	1.65	1.67	1.7	1.72	1.75	1.77	1.8	1.82	1.85	1.87
Age													
15yrs	479	485	489	494	498	503	506	511	515	520	523	528	531
20yrs	534	540	545	551	555	561	565	571	575	580	584	589	593
25yrs	568	575	580	587	591	598	602	608	612	618	622	628	632
30yrs	587	594	599	606	611	617	622	628	633	639	643	649	653
35yrs	594	601	606	613	618	625	629	636	640	646	650	657	661
40yrs	592	599	604	611	615	622	627	633	637	644	648	654	658
45yrs	582	590	594	601	606	612	617	623	627	634	638	644	647
50yrs	568	575	580	586	591	597	601	608	612	618	622	627	631
55yrs	550	557	561	568	572	578	582	588	592	598	602	607	611
60yrs	529	536	540	546	550	556	560	566	570	575	579	584	588
65yrs	507	513	517	523	527	533	536	542	545	551	554	559	562
70yrs	484	490	493	499	503	508	511	517	520	525	528	533	536

❶ For normal values in age groups/heights not represented on these charts or for conversion from the old Wright scale peak flow meters, see 🖥 www.peakflow.com

[*] Based on values from Gregg, I. and Nunn, AJ. (1989) *BMJ* **298**:1068–70, and from Godfrey, S. *et al.* (1970). *Brit J Dis Chest* **64**:15.

Spirometry normal values reproduced with permission of the British Thoracic Society. Reproduced with permission from Simon, C., Everitt, H., and Kendrick, T. (2005). *Oxford Handbook of General Practice*, 2nd edn, Oxford University Press, Oxford.

Table 11.4 Predicted FEV1 and FVC measurements (in L)
❶ These values apply for Caucasians. ↓ values by 7% for Asians and 13% for people of Afro-Caribbean origin.

Women

Height	ft	4'11"	5'1"	5'3"	5'5"	5'7"	5'9"	5'11"
	m	1.5	1.55	1.6	1.65	1.7	1.75	1.8
Age								
38–41yrs	FEV_1	2.3	2.5	2.7	2.89	3.09	3.29	3.49
	FVC	2.69	2.91	3.13	3.35	3.58	3.80	4.02
42–45yrs	FEV_1	2.2	2.4	2.6	2.79	2.99	3.19	3.39
	FVC	2.59	2.81	3.03	3.25	3.47	3.69	3.91
46–49yrs	FEV_1	2.1	2.3	2.5	2.69	2.89	3.09	3.29
	FVC	2.48	2.7	2.92	3.15	3.37	3.59	3.81
50–53yrs	FEV_1	2	2.2	2.4	2.59	2.79	2.99	3.19
	FVC	2.38	2.6	2.82	3.04	3.26	3.48	3.71
54–57yrs	FEV_1	1.9	2.1	2.3	2.49	2.69	2.89	3.09
	FVC	2.27	2.49	2.72	2.94	3.16	3.38	3.6
58–61yrs	FEV_1	1.8	2	2.2	2.39	2.59	2.79	2.99
	FVC	2.17	2.39	2.61	2.83	3.06	3.28	3.5
62–65yrs	FEV_1	1.7	1.9	2.1	2.29	2.49	2.69	2.89
	FVC	2.07	2.29	2.51	2.73	2.95	3.17	3.39
66–69yrs	FEV_1	1.6	1.8	2	2.19	2.39	2.59	2.79
	FVC	1.96	2.18	2.4	2.63	2.85	3.07	3.29

For women ≥70yrs, use the formulae:
- $FEV_1 = (0.0395 \times \text{height in m.} \times 100) - (0.025 \times \text{age in yrs}) - 2.6$.
- $FVC = (0.0443 \times \text{height in m.} \times 100) - (0.026 \times \text{age in yrs}) - 2.89$.

Men

Height	ft	5'3"	5'5"	5'7"	5'9"	5'11"	6'1"	6'3"
	m	1.6	1.65	1.7	1.75	1.8	1.85	1.9
Age								
38–41yrs	FEV_1	3.2	3.42	3.63	3.85	4.06	4.28	4.49
	FVC	3.81	4.1	4.39	4.67	4.96	5.25	5.54
42–45yrs	FEV_1	3.09	3.3	3.52	3.73	3.95	4.16	4.38
	FVC	3.71	3.99	4.28	4.57	4.86	5.15	5.43
46–49yrs	FEV_1	2.97	3.18	3.4	3.61	3.83	4.04	4.26
	FVC	3.6	3.89	4.18	4.47	4.75	5.04	5.33
50–53yrs	FEV_1	2.85	3.07	3.28	3.5	3.71	3.93	4.14
	FVC	3.5	3.79	4.07	4.36	4.65	4.94	5.23
54–57yrs	FEV_1	2.74	2.95	3.17	3.38	3.6	3.81	4.03
	FVC	3.39	3.68	3.97	4.26	4.55	4.83	5.12
58–61yrs	FEV_1	2.62	2.84	3.05	3.27	3.48	3.7	3.91
	FVC	3.29	3.58	3.87	4.15	4.44	4.73	5.02
62–65yrs	FEV_1	2.51	2.72	2.94	3.15	3.37	3.58	3.8
	FVC	3.19	3.47	3.76	4.05	4.34	4.63	4.91
66–69yrs	FEV_1	2.39	2.6	2.82	3.03	3.25	3.46	3.68
	FVC	3.08	3.37	3.66	3.95	4.23	4.52	4.81

For men ≥70yrs use the formulae:
- $FEV_1 = (0.043 \times \text{height in m.} \times 100) - (0.029 \times \text{age in yrs}) - 2.49$.
- $FVC = (0.0576 \times \text{height in m.} \times 100) - (0.026 \times \text{age in yrs}) - 4.34$.

Reproduced with permission from Simon C., Everitt, H., and Kendrick, T. (2005). *Oxford Handbook of General Practice*, 2nd edn., Oxford University Press, Oxford.

Asthma in adults

Asthma is a lung disease, with intermittent narrowing of the bronchi, causing shortness of breath, wheezing, and cough. During an asthma attack the muscles in the bronchi contract and the lining swells, becomes inflamed, and produces excess mucus. The inflammatory process is reversible, if left unchecked causes irreversible damage to airways. Estimates of 7% of adult population with medically diagnosed asthma, of these 1–2% occupational asthma. Categorized into 2 groups: extrinsic (atopic) e.g. response to allergens and family history and intrinsic (non-atopic) usually middle age onset.

Symptoms

- Wheeze
- Breathlessness
- Cough
- Tightness of chest.

Symptoms are variable, intermittent, worse at night and provoked by triggers which can include:

- Exercise
- Household allergens including house mites, fur and feathered pets
- Emotion
- Weather (fog, cold air, thunderstorms)
- Air pollutants (smoke and dust).

Diagnosis is made on clinical history and using objective lung function tests (Measuring lung function 🕮). Referred for specialist opinion when diagnosis unclear or atypical features.

Aims and principles of management

- To control symptoms
- To restore normal or best possible long-term airway function
- To reduce risk of severe attack
- To minimize absence from work
- To involve patient in active management
- To use lower effective doses of medications, minimizing side effects.

Primary care asthma services

When asthma care is delivered by GPs and nurses trained in asthma management there is evidence it improves diagnosis, prescribing, patient education, monitoring and continuity of care. General practices should:

- Keep a register of asthma patients to ensure adequate follow-up
- Recall asthma patients at least annually for review
- Follow-up any who fail to attend for review.

Practice nurses, with training, often run the register and review programme. Audit materials are available with the national guidelines (see below). High quality performance is recognized in QOF (🕮).

Patients who have had near fatal asthma attacks or brittle asthma i.e. well-controlled but sudden unexpected severe attacks should always be reviewed by specialists.

Review and monitoring

- Check and record symptoms and control since last seen e.g.:
  - Needing more and more reliever treatment

- Unable to sleep because of symptoms
- Exacerbations of symptoms, attacks
- Non-attendance at work because of asthma
- Unable to do usual activities e.g. housework, sports.
- Review PEFR (Normal spirometry and peak flow values 📖).
- Review medication use, problems, inhaler technique.
- Check smoking status and advise to cease.
- Check influenza vaccination up-to-date.
- Identify and address any other health or psycho-social problems that may be impacting on asthma management.
- Address any problems, education needs, and queries.
- Agree management plan and next review date.

Patient self-management

Patients should have:
- Education and information (including written) about asthma tailored to them including:
  - Nature of the disease and treatment
  - Identification of areas where patient most wants improvement
  - Development of self-monitoring/self-assessment skills and when to consult GP
  - Recognition and management of acute exacerbations
  - Appropriate allergen or trigger avoidance.
- Written action plan, negotiated in the light of their asthma goals, including recognizing symptoms of asthma worsening and actions to take.
- Patient-held record of asthma reviews.
- PEFR monitoring, often home monitoring helpful in managing symptoms.

Asthma UK (see below) produces a range of material to support this.

Secondary non-pharmalogical prophylaxis

- In committed families wishing to try house dust mite avoidance, suggest barrier bed covering, removal of carpets, removal of soft toys from beds, high temperature washing of bed linen, dehumidification.
- Smoking cessation by patient and household members reduces symptoms and severity.
- Weight reduction in obese patients to improve asthma control.

Pharmacological treatment

See 📖 Pharmacological treatment of asthma.

Related topics

📖 Measuring lung function; 📖 Expert patient; 📖 Asthma in children.

Essential reading

📰 British Thoracic Society and Scottish Inter-Collegiate Guidelines Network (revised 2004). *British Guideline on Asthma Management*: www. brit-thoracic.org.uk/and 2005 electronic update www.sign.ac.uk/.

Further information for patients and professionals

📱 Asthma UK www.asthma.org.uk/ ☎ Adviceline: 08457 01 02 03, Monday–Friday, 9am–5pm

Pharmacological treatment of asthma

A stepwise approach is used to abolish symptoms and to optimize peak flow. The aim is to achieve early control and to maintain control by stepping up treatment as necessary and down when control is good. Includes short-acting inhaled bronchodilator therapy (relievers) e.g. salbutamol or tetrabutaline and prophylactic therapy (preventers) e.g. regular inhaled steroids (BNF 3.1). Approach is summarized in Fig. 11.1.

Inhalers

The effective inhaler is one that the patient is able to use and this may involve trial and error, for useful overview see Wan.[1]

- Inhalation delivers drug directly to the airways. Pressurized metered-dose inhalers are an effective and convenient method.
- Patients should be advised to inhale slowly and hold breath for 10secs after inhaling.
- Patients should be told explicitly of dose, frequency, and maximum number of inhalations in 24hrs in action plan.
- Advise to seek medical help if prescribed dose failing to relieve symptoms or relieving for <3hrs.
- Inadequate technique may be mistaken for drug failure. Check technique at each review.
- A spacer may improve delivery but adults are often unwilling to use it. Advice on inhalers and spacers includes:
  - Shake inhaler well before fitting to spacer, press inhaler once and without delay take 5 slow breaths in and out of the spacer (tidal breathing).
  - Remove inhaler, shake well, and repeat as prescribed.
  - Spacers should be cleaned monthly in mild detergent as per manufacturers instructions, replace every 12mths (BNF 3.1.5).

Steroids

Patients on oral or high dose inhaled steroids should carry steroid cards for their own information in case of illness etc. and to alert any other practitioner who might prescribe treatment (see BNF 6.3.2 for information and sources).

Related topics

📖 Asthma in adults; 📖 Asthma in children; 📖 Expert patient.

Essential reading

📖 British Thoracic Society and Scottish Inter-Collegiate Guidelines Network (2004). *British Guideline on Asthma Management*: www.brit-thoracic.org.uk/.

Further information for patients and professionals

Asthma UK: www.asthma.org.uk/ ☎ Adviceline: 08457 01 02 03, Monday–Friday, 9am–5pm

---

[1] Wan, Y. (2005). BMJ Clinical review of asthma: methods of delivering drugs *BMJ* **331**: 504–6.

Step 5: Continuous or frequent use of oral steroids:
• Use daily steroid tablet in lowest dose providing adequate control
• Maintain high-dose inhaled steroid at 2000mcg/d*
• Consider other treatments to minimise the use of steroid tablets
• Refer patient for specialist care

Step 4: Persistent poor control
Consider trials of:
— Increasing inhaled steroid to 2000mcg/d*
— Addition of a 4th drug e.g. leukotriene receptor agonist, SR theophylline, β_2 agonist tablet

Step 3: Add-on therrapy
• Add inhaled long-acting β_2 agonist (LABA)
• Assess control of asthma:
— Good response to LABA—continue LABA
— Benefit from LABA but control still inadequate—continue LABA and ↑ inhaled steroid dose to 800mcg/d*
— No response to LABA—stop LABA and i inhaled steroid dose to 800mcg/d*. If control is still inadequate, institute trial of other therapies e.g. leukotriene receptor antagonists or SR theophylline

Step 2: Regular preventer therapy
• Add inhaled steroid 200–800mcg/d*
— 400mcg/d is an appropriate starting point for many patients>12y
— Start at dose of steroid appropriate to severity of disease

Step 1: Mild intermittent asthma
Inhaled short-acting β_2 agonist as required

* Beclometasone dipropionate or equivalent.

Fig. 11.1 Summary of stepwise management in adults (reproduced from the British Thoracic Society/SIGN. British Guidelines on the Management of Asthma (2004) www.brit-thoracic.org.uk. With kind permission of the British Thoracic Society.

Asthma attacks

Primary care nurses in all settings should offer patient and carer education in managing asthma attacks. School staff in particular may need advice and training. Patients diagnosed with asthma should have written guidance in their action plan (Asthma in adults 🕮) on what to do in the event of an acute exacerbation (see below).

Most (88–92%) attacks of asthma, severe enough to require hospital admission, develop relatively slowly over a period of six hours or more. In one study, over 80% of attacks developed over more than 48 hours. Earlier stepwise intervention in the community can prevent hospital admission of many people.

> **Advice to patients** (and parents)
>
> * If asthma symptoms slowly get worse don't ignore them! Quite often, using the reliever is all that is needed to get the asthma under control again.
> * At other times, the symptoms are more severe and more urgent action is needed in the following steps:
>   1. Take your usual dose of reliever straight away, preferably using a spacer.
>   2. Keep calm and try to relax as much as your breathing will let you.
>   3. Sit down, don't lie down, rest your hands on your knees to help support yourself try to slow your breathing down as this will make you less exhausted.
>   4. If the condition is stable or improving wait 5–10mins.
>   5. If the symptoms disappear, you should be able to go back to whatever you were doing.
>   6. If the reliever has no effect, call the doctor or ambulance.
>   7. Continue to take your reliever inhaler every few minutes until help arrives preferably using a spacer. It is safe to keep taking your reliever inhaler until help arrives. It is not possible to overdose on reliever.

Carers, parents, relatives, school staff need to be made aware that signs such as unable to complete sentence in one breath, too breathless to feed or speak, continually coughing in children indicate severe attack and the doctor or ambulance should be called rather than waiting as in step 4 above.

Attending doctor (or nurse with appropriate training), in the home or surgery increases treatment in line with the step-up model but arranges hospital admission if symptoms fail to respond or immediately if signs of life threatening asthma e.g. silent chest, cyanosis, feeble respiratory effort, bradycardia, <33% predicted peak flow.

Risk factors for fatal or near fatal asthma attacks

An enquiry into asthma deaths in the UK revealed that most had chronic severe asthma, poorly treated and monitored, did not have written action plans, failed to return for review often with associated psycho-social problems e.g. psychosis, depression, alcohol or drug abuse, learning difficulties, employment problems, income problems, social isolation, childhood abuse, severe domestic, marital or legal stress. British guidelines (see below) support a well structured asthma management programme in primary care (Asthma in adults 📖).

Related topics

📖 Measuring lung function; 📖 Asthma in adults; 📖 Asthma in children.

Essential reading

📖 British Thoracic Society and Scottish Inter-Collegiate Guidelines Network (revised 2004). *British Guideline on Asthma Management.* www.brit-thoracic.org.uk and 2005 electronic update www.sign.ac.uk.

Further information for patients and professionals

Asthma UK www.asthma.org.uk/ ☎ Adviceline: 08457 01 02 03, Monday–Friday, 9am–5pm

Chronic obstructive pulmonary disease (COPD)

A slowly progressive respiratory disorder, characterized by airflow obstruction that is not fully reversible and does not change markedly over a number of months. COPD is the preferred term for conditions previously called emphysema, bronchitis. Usually caused by smoking. Results in about 30,000 deaths per annum and accounts for about 25% hospital admissions.

Airflow obstruction

- Defined as reduced FEV_1 and reduced FEV_1/FEC ratio (Measuring lung function 🕮) measured by spirometry.
- Caused by inflammation of large and small airways, increased mucus production, damage to alveoli.

Advanced lung destruction causes respiratory failure i.e. disorder of such extent not meeting metabolic requirements. Type 1: hypoxaemia without CO_2 retention, type 2: hypoxaemia and retention of CO_2. Other consequences include cor pulmonale, right sided heart failure, and oedema.

Breathlessness can be very frightening. COPD patients can be very anxious and restrict activities, this sets up a vicious cycle leading to further restrictions. Often also leads to depression.

Indications for a COPD diagnosis to be considered

- >35yrs
- SOB on exertion (see dyspnoea scale below)
- Smoker or ex-smoker
- Chronic cough, producing sputum
- Increased chest problems in winter.

Diagnosis by clinical presentation and spirometry. May also require other investigations e.g. chest X-ray, and referral to specialists if diagnosis uncertain, other problems or poor symptom control.

MRC dyspnoea scale

Grade	Degree of breathlessness related to activities
1	Not troubled by breathlessness except on strenuous exercise.
2	Short of breath when hurrying or walking up a slight hill.
3	Walks slower than contemporaries on level ground because of breathlessness, or has to stop for breath when walking at own pace.
4	Stops for breath after walking about 100 m or after a few minutes on level ground.
5	Too breathless to leave the house, or breathless when dressing or undressing.

NICE (2004). Quick Reference Guide COPD p3 (*reproduced with permission of NICE*)

Severity of airflow limitations
- Mild: FEV_1 50–80% predicted
- Moderate: FEV_1 30–49% predicted
- Severe: FEV_1 <30% predicted.

Key principles in management
- On diagnosis:
  - Coded on GP patient records to be added to practice COPD register
  - Baseline spirometry reading, dyspnoea scale, and BMI recorded.
- Key principles in management:
  - Help patient stop smoking if still a smoker
  - Effective inhaled therapy (including inhaler technique)
  - Annual flu and pneumcoccal vaccination
  - Weight reduction if BMI >25, nutritional supplements if <18.5
  - Pulmonary rehabilitation programme and then maintenance of activity and strength levels
  - Advice on action to take in an exacerbation
  - Provide sources of advice and support in living with breathlessness e.g. British Lung Foundation details, leaflets on travel, sex, and breathlessness etc.
- Follow-up review at least annually in mild/moderate, 6-mthly for severe COPD.

Related topics
 Measurement of lung function; Management in stable COPD; Management of exacerbation COPD.

Essential reading
 British Thoracic Society/NICE Guidance (2004). *Chronic Obstructive Pulmonary Disease. Management in adults in primary and secondary care*: www.nice.org.uk.

Further information and support for patients
 British Lung Foundation www.lunguk.org/index.asp

Management in stable COPD

The lung damage cannot be repaired but the symptoms and their impact can be managed. Key elements are smoking cessation, effective inhalation therapy, pulmonary rehabilitation, optimum BMI (low BMI indicator of poor prognosis), and immunization.

Smoking cessation

A key issue to prevent further lung damage. Offer help to quit at every consultation if patient is still a smoker. (Smoking cessation 📖.)

Effective inhaled therapy

Step wise increase according to COPD severity and frequency of exacerbations:

- Short acting beta2-agonists bronchodilators (BNF 3.1.1.1) prn.
- Long-acting inhaled bronchodilators or anticholinergics (BNF 3.1.2) added for those who continue to experience problems despite short-acting drugs.
- Inhaled corticosteroids (BNF 3.2) added to decrease exacerbation frequency in patients with an FEV_1 less than or equal to 50% or >2 exacerbations requiring antibiotics or oral corticosteroids in 12mths.
- Combination of medications may be used but stopped if ineffective.
- Effective inhaler technique needs to be taught (Pharmacological treatment of asthma 📖).
- Nebulizers may be used to increase drug delivery when maximum therapy ineffective (Pharmacoloical treatment of asthma 📖).
- Oral theophylline (BMF 3.1.3) may be considered.

Other medication

- Prescribed according to other problems e.g. diuretics in cor pulmonale.
- LTOT (Oxygen therapy in the community 📖) in chronically hypoxic COPD.

Immunization

Offered pneumococcal vaccination and an annual influenza vaccination. A QOF indicator (Quality and outcomes framework 📖).

Weight management

BMI >25 or <18.5 may require referral to dietician. ↑ BMI places additional strain on cardiovascular system and mobility. ↓ BMI requires nutritional supplements (Weight management: malnutrition 📖).

Pulmonary rehabilitation

Shown to reduce dyspnoea, improve quality of life, and reduce disability and use of health services irrespective of age, of impairment or smoking status. Usually a 6wk programme led by specialist and therapy services. Includes aerobic exercise, always of lower extremities (brisk walking, cycling) and may include upper extremities. Often includes educational programme and opportunity for tailored advice on smoking cessation, nutrition, minimizing impact on activities of daily living, physical relationships etc.

Table 11.5 Guidance on review and follow-up consultations

Mild/moderate COPD at least annual review	Severe COPD at least 2x yr review
Measurements:	**Measurements:**
• FEV1 and FVC (Measuring lung function 📖)	• FEV1 and FVC
• BMI 📖 Nutrition and healthy eating	• BMI (Nutrition and healthy eating 📖)
• MRC dyspnoea score (COPD 📖)	• MRC dyspnoea score (COPD 📖)
	• O₂ saturation of arterial blood
Assessment of:	**Assessment of:**
• Smoking status and desire to quit	• Smoking status and desire to quit
• Adequacy of symptom control:	• Adequacy of symptom control:
• Breathlessness	• Breathlessness
• Exercise tolerance	• Exercise tolerance
• Estimated exacerbation frequency	• Estimated exacerbation frequency
• Presence of complications	• Presence of cor pulmonale
• Effects of each drug treatment	• Need for LOT
• Inhaler technique	• Patient's nutritional state
• Need for referral to specialist and therapy services	• Presence of depression
• Need for pulmonary rehabilitation	• Effects of each drug treatment
	• Inhaler technique
	• Need for social services and OT input
	• Need for referral to specialist and therapy services
	• Need for pulmonary rehabilitation

Adapted with permission from NICE Guidance (2004). *Quick Reference Guide Chronic Obstructive Pulmonary Disease*, Clinical guideline 12, p.11.

Education
Comprehensive disease education for patient and family to understand nature, symptoms, management, and management of exacerbations.

Advice on exacerbations
See 📖 Management of COPD exacerbation.

Regular review and follow-up
(See Table 11.5.)
GP practice COPD registers aid this, also QOF indicator (Quality and outcomes framework 📖).

Essential reading
📄 British Thoracic Society/NICE Guidance (2004). *Chronic Obstructive Pulmonary Disease. Management in adults in primary and secondary care*: www.nice.org.uk.

Further information and support for patients
📄 British Lung Foundation www.lunguk.org/index.asp

Management of COPD exacerbation

An exacerbation is:
- Acute in onset.
- A sustained worsening of symptoms from stable state:
  - Increased dyspnoea
  - Increased and/or infected sputum.

All patients with COPD diagnosis should be advised on actions to take on identifying an exacerbation.

Self-management of exacerbations

Patients at risk of exacerbations are encouraged to respond quickly. These patients will have been identified at review/follow-up and prescribed antibiotics and oral corticosteroids and advised:
- To start oral corticosteroids if dyspnoea interferes with usual activities
- To start antibiotics if sputum purulent
- How to adjust bronchodilator therapy to control symptoms
- Which health professional/service to contact if symptoms do not improve in a specified timescale.

Initial management of exacerbations

- Increased frequency of bronchodilator use (BNF 3.1) (may use nebulizer, oxygen therapy).
- Oral antibiotics if purulent sputum (BNF 5.1 Table 1).
- Short course of prednisolone for 7–14d (BNF 3.2) for all patients with significant increase in breathlessness unless contraindicated.
- Decision as to whether to manage at home or refer to hospital based on severity, co-morbidity, availability of other services e.g. rapid response team for 24-hr care at home for short periods. Local care pathways inform decision making as well as table opposite.
- If treated at home, may require pulse oximetry to establish blood O_2 saturation levels if severe dyspnoea. Establish on optimum therapy, review and referral to other services/therapies as appropriate.

Related topics

📖 Measurement of lung function; 📖 COPD; 📖 Management in stable COPD.

Essential reading

📑 British Thoracic Society/NICE Guidance (2004). *Chronic Obstructive Pulmonary Disease. Management in adults in primary and secondary care:* www.nice.org.uk.

Further information and support for patients

📑 British Lung Foundation: www.lunguk.org/index.asp

Table 11.6 Factors to consider when managing a COPD patient with acute exacerbation

Factor	Favours treatment in hospital	Favours treatment at home
Able to cope at home	No	Yes
Breathlessness	Severe	Mild
General condition	Poor/deteriorating	Good
Level of activity	Poor/confined to bed	Good
Cyanosis	Yes	No
Worsening peripheral oedema	Yes	No
Level of consciousness	Impaired	Normal
Already receiving LTOT	Yes	No
Social circumstances	Living alone/not coping	Good
Acute confusion	Yes	No
Rapid rate of onset	Yes	No
Significant comorbidity (particularly cardiac disease and insulin-dependent diabetes)	Yes	No
SaO_2 <90%	Yes	No
Changes on the chest radiograph	Present	No
Arterial pH level	<7.35	≥7.35
Arterial PaO_2	<7 kPa	≥7 kPa

Reproduced with kind permission from NHS National Institute for Clinical Excellence (2004). *Quick Reference Guide Chronic Obstructive Pulmonary Disease. Clinical Guideline 12.*, p11. NICE, London.

Oxygen therapy in the community

Oxygen is a prescription-only therapy (BNF 3.6). Oxygen is combustible/explosive near naked flames and cigarettes. Inform patients and carers of risks and strongly advise not to smoke near oxygen supply. Oxygen is used therapeutically in three ways:
- Long-term oxygen therapy (LTOT)
- Ambulatory
- Short burst.

LTOT

In chronically hypoxic COPD (📖) LTOT can:
- Improve life expectancy
- Reduce hospitalization
- Improve QoL.

Clinical signs indicating chronic hypoxia

NB Patients not always excessively breathless.
- New onset or worsening peripheral oedema, extremities become discoloured and skin around mouth.
- Central cyanosis. Blue discolouration of the lips, tongue, and extremities.

Check pulse oximetry when clinical signs noted and routinely when FEV_1 ≤50% predicted.

SaO_2 <92% indicates need for referral for arterial blood gases. Patients referred must be:
- Clinically stable
- On optimal therapy.

LTOT must be:
- Used for ≥15hrs a day
- Given at prescribed flow rate only.

Oxygen on a long-term basis also used in pulmonary fibrosis. High concentrations may be required.

Ambulatory oxygen

Suitable for:
- LTOT patients able and willing to leave their homes
- Patients with exercise induced oxygen desaturation
- Specialist assessment necessary to determine need and flow rate.

Short burst oxygen

Oxygen prn. Frequently prescribed to relieve breathlessness in chronic and end-stage cardiac and respiratory disease. Not supported by research, but some patients benefit subjectively.

Oxygen services

Assessment should be undertaken by specialists. Primary care should refer patients to specialist services (except for use in palliative care).

England and Wales

Independent oxygen contractors provide 'one-stop', integrated oxygen services to NHS. They assess patients' needs and supply suitable equipment. They also maintain equipment and supply disposables.

Prescription made on Home Oxygen Order Form (HOOF) with Home Oxygen Consent Form (HOCF) not FP10 from February 2006.

Scotland and Northern Ireland

Home oxygen supplied on FP10s by pharmacy contractors.

Appropriate oxygen use can prolong and enhance life. Inappropriate use, at best is expensive and, at worst is life threatening.

Further information for professionals

▣ Clinical best practice guidelines for oxygen prescription: www.brit-thoracic.org.uk/c2/ uploads/clinical%20adultoxygenjan06.pdf
▣ Key documents for prescribing home oxygen: www.primarycarecontracting.nhs.uk/120.php
▣ NHS England and Wales background information on home oxygen services: www.primarycarecontracting.nhs.uk/118.php
▣ The British Paediatric Respiratory Society Guide to Ordering Home Oxygen for Children: www.bprs.co.uk/oxygen.html

Further information for patients

▣ British Lung Foundation: www.lunguk.org: Helpline: 08458 50 50 20 Mon–Friday 10am–6pm

Nebulizers

A nebulizer (BNF 3.1.5) converts drug solution into a continuous fine aerosol mist, inhaled by tidal breathing over 5–10mins directly into the lung. Drug solution is POM and patients advised not to use more frequently than prescribed or change dosage.

Indications for use

- Acute exacerbations of acute asthma and COPD.
- Long-term bronchodilator treatment in asthma and COPD to those shown to benefit from higher medication doses (usually after 2wk trial).
- When patient unable to use other inhalation devices.
- Delivery of antibiotics for cystic fibrosis, bronchiectasis.
- To deliver pentamidine for prophylaxis and treatment of pneumo-cytisis pneumonia.

If prescribed for home use, patients and family should have:
- Instruction in use, cleaning, maintenance.
- Regular follow-up by respiratory specialists and their contact details.
- Advised not to treat acute exacerbations at home without also seeking help.
- Details of how to service equipment.

Equipment

Four parts: face mask/mouthpiece, nebulizer chamber for the drug solution, tubing to connect to the compressor or oxygen to drive the nebulizer chamber.

- Jet nebulizers most commonly used as more efficient in drug delivery. Requires an electric compressor.
- Main source of supply through loan from hospital respiratory services. In England and Wales nebulizers and compressors not available on NHS drug tariff. In Scotland some nebulizers available on GP10A. Equipment may be available at local equipment stores depending on local protocols and services.
- Mouthpiece is preferred delivery method as face masks (mostly used with children) inefficient.

Care and maintenance

- Chamber and mouth piece washed in hot soapy water after every use, rinsed well, dried with kitchen towel, and left disassembled to air dry. Changed every 3mths for disposable kits or annually if durable.
- Tubing changed on a regular basis as becomes damp during use, and difficult to dry.
- Compressor left on for a few mins. following disconnection of the nebulizer to blow-out any water droplets.
- Compressor should be serviced yearly, and filters changed according to manufacturers instructions.

Further information

British Thoracic Society: www.brit-thoracic.org.uk

Further information for patients

British Lung Foundation: www.lunguk.org/

Coronary heart disease (CHD)

CHD is one of the main diseases of the heart and circulatory system and the most common cause of premature death in the UK. Approximately 114,000 people die from CHD each year in the UK, approximately 1:5 men and 1:6 women.

Risk factors
- Socio-economic
- Age: risk increases with age
- Family history of CHD, diabetes, hyperlipidaemia, or hypertension
- Low birth weight
- Ethnicity: e.g. Indian subcontinent increased risk
- Gender: higher risk in men <65yrs
- Smoking
- Hypertension
- Hyperlipidaemia
- Diabetes
- Diet
- Obesity (Weight management overweight 📖).

Primary prevention
Attempts to reduce a person's/population's overall risk of developing CHD. Local policies are essential on:
- Smoking cessation
- Promoting healthy eating
- Taking regular exercise
- Controlling weight and/or reducing obesity
- Controlling high blood pressure
- Controlling raised cholesterol
- Controlling blood sugar in diabetes
- Managing stress
- Alcohol within recommended limits
- Identifying those at most risk of CHD by calculating risk score.

Secondary prevention
Attempts to prevent established disease getting worse. 46% of people who die from MI already known to have CHD.

Setting up a practice register of those with diagnosed CHD is essential.

Management and treatment can be jointly managed between nurse and doctor and should focus on:
- Identification of those at risk, registration, and ongoing follow-up
- Providing information on how to modify lifestyle/risk factors
- Best practice according to evidence-based care guidelines
- Stopping smoking.

Medicine management (refer to local protocols for medicines management).
- Management of hypertension (>150/90mmHg) with antihypertensive drugs (BNF 2). See QoF guidelines.
- Anti platelet therapy (BNF 2.9) can reduce cardiovascular morbidity and mortality. Aspirin (75–300mg/d for maintenance treatment), warfarin (BNF 2.8.2), or aspirin if >60yrs and with atrial fibrillation. NB Caution if on anticoagulant therapy, risk of GI bleed.
- Statins (BNF 2.12 Lipid regulatory drugs) and dietary advice.
- If LVF ACE (angiotensin-converting enzyme inhibitors BNF 2.5.5.1) inhibitors.
- Beta blockers (BNF 2.4) if post myocardial infarction.
- Blood sugar control if diabetic.
- Not all people need referral to a cardiologist, depends on previous history and symptoms.

Related topics
📖 Diabetes; 📖 Models and approaches to health promotion; 📖 Exercise; 📖 Cardiac rehabilitation in the community; 📖 QoF.

Further information for relatives and health professionals
🔲 British Heart Foundation: www.bhf.org.uk
🔲 DoH National Service Framework Coronary Heart Disease (2000) www.dh.gov.uk
🔲 Clinical Knowledge Summaries (Prodigy) guidance: www.cks.library.nhs.uk

Angina

Angina pectoris is the classic symptom of chest pain and is due to transient myocardial ischaemia. Typically caused by exertion or emotion, and relieved by rest. 1.2 million in the UK suffer from angina and 300,000 have heart attacks every year. The incidence of angina is higher in ♂ than in ♀ and ↑ with age.

Symptoms

(NB Always consider possibility of myocardial infarct). Some or a combination of:

- Heaviness in central chest
- Squeezing, crushing, or gripping pain
- Radiating pain to neck, jaw, back, or arms (usually the left)
- Breathless on exertion
- Musculo-skeletal pain
- Referred pain from thoracic spine
- Anxiety
- Pain in other sites e.g. pleural pain, acute cholecystitis.

Assessment includes

- What precipitates attack e.g. exertion, cold weather, large meals, stress
- Past medical history and family history
- Lifestyle i.e. smoking, alcohol intake, drug history
- Dietary assessment and the possibility of gastrooesophageal reflux.

Clinical examination

- Blood pressure
- Pulse: rate and rhythm
- Presence of heart murmurs, arrhythmias, and heart failure (joint examination with GP)
- Evidence of anaemia, hyperlipidaemia, and vascular disease (joint examination with GP)
- BMI.

Investigations likely to include

- 12-lead ECG (Recording a 12 lead ECG 📖) and exercise ECG to define risk
- Coronary angiography
- Full blood count, fasting lipid profile, and fasting blood sugar.

Management and treatment

- Advise re: lifestyle factors
- Education about angina and heart attacks
- Patients who drive should inform DVLA
- If job involves heavy work may need to review, some groups need to notify occupational health depts e.g. pilots, seamen.

Medication includes (NB refer to local protocols for medicines management):
- Anti-platelet therapy
- Nitrates GTN or nitrate spray (see box) prn (BNF 2.6.1)
- Beta blockers unless contraindicated
- Calcium channel blockers if beta blockers contra-indicated (BNF 2.6.2)
- Potassium channel openers (BNF 2.6.3)
- Statins (not suitable for people with liver disease, pregnant, or breast feeding) (BNF 2.12).

> ❶ If angina worsens, occurs on minimal exertion or at rest or nocturnal, is more frequent and with persistent pain that lasts longer than 15mins patient is at ↑ risk of MI and needs urgent hospital admission.

Nurse run clinics

(Refer to local protocols for nurse run clinics.)
- Maintain register for call and recall of patients (Quality and outcomes framework 📖)
- Review medication use and compliance, and blood results
- Management of co-existing disease e.g. hypertension and diabetes
- Stop smoking advice and support
- BP control
- Lipid management
- Exercise and dietary advise
- Education about symptoms of heart attack and seeking help.

> *Advice for patients on using GTN or nitrate spray when having an angina attack*
> - Sit down and place GTN tablet or spray under tongue. Leave 5 mins between each dose maximum of 3 doses.
> - Alert someone that you are feeling unwell.
> - If pain is not improved in 15mins then call ambulance and inform GP.
> - If there is no allergy to aspirin chew adult asprin tablet (300mg).
>
> Adapted from British Heart Foundation advice leaflet series no. 6.

Related topics

📖 Hypertenstion; 📖 Cardiac rehabilitation in the community; 📖 Adult basic life support.

Further information for professionals and relatives

- 🖳 British Heart Foundation. *Angina: Heart Information Series 6:* www.bhf.org.uk
- 🖳 NICE guidance: www.nice.org.uk
- 🖳 NSF for CHD (Chapter 4): www.doh.gov.uk
- 🖳 Clinical Knowledge Summaries (Prodigy): cardiovascular disease: www.cks.library.nhs.uk

Hypertension

Hypertension (in people without diabetes) is defined as sustained systolic blood pressure (BP) of >140 mmHg, and/or sustained diastolic BP of >90 mmHg on at least 3 separate occasions. Often symptomless, 40% of adults in England and Wales have raised BP. Hypertension = major risk factor for cardiovascular disease, stroke, and renal failure. People with hypertension:
- ↑ with age
- ↑ in people of Afro-Caribbean origin
- ↑ people of South Asian origin who are commonly insulin resistant and have a high prevalence of type 2 diabetes.

Types of hypertension
- Primary hypertension (aka essential hypertension)–95% unknown cause, alcohol, or obesity may be contributory factors.
- Secondary hypertension—caused by renal, endocrine, or vascular disorder, preganancy, drugs (may need specialist referral).
- Malignant hypertension—rapid ↑ in BP with progressive organ damage. Medical emergency requiring hospital admission.

Assessment
Hypertension produces no symptoms so often picked up at routine screening (see also New patient health check 📖), occasionally patient may c/o headache or visual disturbance.
- Record BP on 3 separate occasions with patient at rest (see Clinical Knowledge Summaries (Prodigy) for guidelines for correct technique and recording of BP, in Further information below).
- Establish significant and family history.
- Examine CVS and fundi (NB only nurses with advanced clinical assessment skills e.g. nurse practitioners).
- Calculate CVD risk (see 🖥 Joint British Risk Prediction Chart www.bhsoc.org.uk).

Investigations
Performed according to practice/local protocols.
- Resting ECG
- CXR
- Urinalysis for proteinuria and haematuria
- Urea and creatinine
- Fasting lipid profile and fasting glucose.
- FBC and LFT

Anti-hypertensive treatment:
(See also NICE 2006 guidelines, below.)
Medication ↓ risk of CVD and death and should be offered to:
- Patients with persistent high BP of 160/100mmHg or more.
- Patients at ↑ cardiovascular risk or existing cardiovascular disease or target organ damage with persistent BP of >140/90mmHg.

Most patients with ↑ BP require 2 or more BP lowering drugs. Principles of medication management should be:

- Patients >55yrs and black patients of any age: first choice should either be a calcium-channel blocker (SE can cause flushing, dizziness and constipation) or a thiazide-type diuretic (BNF 2.2.1).
- Patients <55 the first choice = an angiotensin-converting enzyme (ACE) inhibitor (BNF 2.5.5.1). NB SE can cause dizziness (or an angiotensin-II receptor antagonist if an ACE inhibitor is not tolerated).
- If initial therapy was with a calcium channel blocker or thiazide-type diuretic and a second drug is required, add an ACE inhibitor (or an angiotensin receptor blocker if an ACE inhibitor is not tolerated). If initial therapy was with an ACE inhibitor, add a calcium channel blocker or a thiazide-type diuretic.
- If treatment with 3 drugs needed: combination of ACE inhibitor (or an angiotensin receptor blocker if an ACE inhibitor is not tolerated) calcium channel blocker and thiazide diuretic should be used.
- Beta-blockers (BNF 2.4.) are not a preferred initial therapy for hypertension as evidence indicates they are less effective than other drugs particularly for older people and may increase the risk of type 2 diabetes, CVA, and MI. Their SE include poor sleep, tiredness, and impotence.

General practice nurse run clinic or as part of routine appointments and checks

Aim (Refer to local protocols.)
- To monitor and treat people with hypertension.
- To ↓ the risk of related cardiovascular morbidity and mortality.
- To identify risk factors and offer personalized advice and management.

Achieved by
- Maintaining register for call and recall of patients with hypertension (Quality and outcomes framework 📖).
- General lifestyle advice (stop smoking, reduce hyperlipidaemia, ↓ weight, control alcohol intake, ↓ salt and caffeine intake, initiate regular dynamic exercise (see Cardiac rehabilitation in the community 📖).
- Control BP to less than 140/85mmHg.
- Explain benefits of treatment balanced against possible side effects.
- Once BP controlled regular monitoring at 3–6 monthly and yearly recalculation of CVD risk, BP check, and blood tests and medication review.
- Access and referral to local support initiatives e.g. Support groups, walking groups.

Related topics
📖 Coronary heart disease (CHD); 📖 Expert patient; 📖 Exercise; 📖 Principles of rehabilitation following stroke; 📖 Smoking cessation.

Further information for health professionals and relatives
📓 British Heart Foundation: www.bhf.org.uk
📓 NICE (2006). *Hypertension: management of hypertension in adults in primary care: partial update* NICE guideline 18. www.nice.org.uk
📓 Clinical Knowledge Summaries (Prodigy) for guidelines on treatment and management and PILS: www.cks.library.nhs.uk

Care of a person with high/raised cholesterol (hyperlipidaemia)

UK population has one of the highest average serum cholesterol levels in the world. Two-thirds of people have a serum cholesterol level >5.2 mmol/L. Lowering cholesterol is beneficial in primary and secondary prevention of CVD. Cholesterol is a fatty substance produced mainly by the liver, and has a vital role in cell membrane function. ↑ cholesterol levels or hyperlipidaemia are caused by ↑ serum cholesterol levels of one or more of the lipids: total cholesterol (TC), low-density lipoprotein cholesterol, or triglycerides (TG), or both TC and TG (combined hyperlipidaemia).

Assessment

- Suspected familial hypercholesterolemia e.g. total cholesterol >7.5mmol/l needs specialist referral
- Check for other risk factors e.g. CHD, diabetes, or hypertension
- Calculate 10-year CVD risk (see 🖳 Joint British Society cardiac risk assessment charts: www.bhsoc.org)
- Smoking status
- Review diet and calculate BMI.

Aims

- ↓ total serum cholesterol to <5.0mmol/L or by 20–25%, whichever is lower
- ↓ low-density lipoprotein cholesterol to <3.0mmol/L or by 30%, whichever is lower (see Clinical Knowledge Summaries (Prodigy) guidance ref below.)
- Reinforce all advice with written supporting information and PILs (see below).

Non drug-based interventions and health promotion advice

- ↓ overall dietary fat intake
- ↓ saturated fat intake, use low fat mono/polyunsaturated spreads and oils, 2–3 portions of fish (one oily), lean meat, and low salt food
- Achieve ideal weight and encourage healthy eating
- Lifestyle advice: (as with Cardiac rehabilitation in the community 📖), stop smoking, alcohol within normal limits, exercise promotion

Medication based intervention

Statins (BNF:2.12) most effective if taken in the evening, (contraindications: pregnancy, breast feeding, and active liver disease) appropriate:

- For those with established cardiovascular disease (CVD)
- For those with 20% or greater risk of developing CVD
- For those with familial hypercholesterolaemia
- All people with type 2 diabetes.

Follow-up and review of patients

- Fasting total cholesterol after 6–12wks. If on statins, check LFTs and fasting lipid profile
- If level still raised check thyroid, renal, liver function, and fasting blood sugar checked
- Urinalysis for sugar and protein

- Routine follow-up yearly (Quality and outcomes framework 📖)
- Ask how patient is managing on medication and if there are any SE e.g. unexplained muscle weakness/pain if there is refer for GP review.

Related topics

📖 Coronary heart disease (CHD); 📖 Hypertension; 📖 Exercise; 📖 Smoking cessation; 📖 Nutrition and healthy eating; 📖 Cardiac rehabilititation in the community.

Further information for professionals and relatives

🖾 NICE (2006). Cardiovascular disease: statins guidance: www.nice.org.uk
🖾 *NSF for CHD*. Chapter 2, NICE guidance: www.doh.gov.uk
🖾 Clinical Knowledge Summaries (Clinical knowledge summaries (prodigy)) guidance on hyperlipidaemia and PILs on cholesterol: www.cks.library.nhs.uk

Cardiac rehabilitation in the community

A multidisciplinary approach that almost everyone with CHD can benefit from, regardless of age and condition, that aims to:
- Promote recovery from MI
- Reduce CHD related symptoms (e.g. Angina 🕮) or need for cardiac surgery
- Enable patients to achieve better health
- Reduce risk of death in people with heart disease and provide long-term preventative care, can ↓ morbidity by 25%.

Many of the problems people with heart disease suffer are not physical but are due to anxiety and misunderstanding about their condition ∴ it is important that patients receive adequate, consistent, and accurate advice.

NB On discharge from hospital, patients should have an agreed care plan. Cardiac rehabilitation programmes run out of hospitals provide a mix of exercise promotion sessions, patient education, and psychosocial interventions that lasts between 6–12wks. Uptake is variable and ♀ less likely to receive cardiac rehabilitation than ♂.

❶ A proactive approach to patient participation and monitoring is needed. In some areas primary care nurses run programmes.

Assessment
- Individual risk factors (see CHD 🕮)
- Physical needs e.g. self-caring
- Exercise tolerance testing
- Psychological needs: patients are often anxious, weepy, and depressed following an MI. Should be reassured that this is a normal response
- Social needs e.g. family support systems.

Care and management in liaison with GP and other health professionals
- Patient education and support on medication management and concordance, supported with PILs and review progress.
- Smoking cessation.
- Exercise capacity: misconception that people should reduce or limit their level of activity. Patient should gradually ↑ activity, refer to local advice. Usually: 2wks post MI stroll in garden or street, 4wks walk half a mile a day, 4–6 wks after MI increase to 2 miles per day, and by 6wks increase speed of walking = 2 miles in <30min (Exercise 🕮).
- Returning to work: after an uncomplicated MI: 4–6 wks for sedentary workers, light manual workders 6–8wks, heavy manual workers 3mths.
- No driving for 1mth after MI and inform car insurer; only inform DVLA if HGV and PSV licence holder.
- Dietary advice: low cholesterol, ↑ fruit and vegetables, ↓ salt and caffeine, and review alcohol consumption.

- Sexual activity; resume after 6wks (specific guidance in BHF[1]).
- Psychological aspects: many patients experience depression and anxiety—may benefit from advice on relaxation and talking therapies.
- Educational support including information on basic working of the heart accompanied by PILs and written information.
- Needs of family and carers.
- Patient support and/or self-help groups/use of self-help manuals (see refs below).

Related topics

📖 Coronary heart disease (CHD); 📖 Angina; 📖 Hypertension; 📖 Exercise; 📖 Smoking cessation; 📖 Talking therapies.

Further information for professionals and relatives

🖥 Cardiac rehabilitations useful resource of health professionals: ww.cardiacrehabilitation.org
DH (England) (2000). NSF for Coronary Heart Disease. The Stationary Office, London.
🖥 Clinical Knowledge Summaries (Prodigy) PILs for self-help groups: www.cks.library.nhs.uk

---

1 🖥 British Heart Foundation *Heart Attack and Rehabilitation Guide*, p.39. www.bhf.org.uk

Patients on anticoagulant therapy

Anticoagulants ↓ the formation of new blood clots and the extension of existing clots. Most commonly used with patients with AF, following heart surgery, or at risk of PE and/or DVT. Warfarin antagonizes the effects of vitamin K; and takes 48–72hrs to work. In some areas patients on oral anticoagulants are managed by nurses working to an agreed protocol.

Management: and patient information

(See Tables 11.7 and 11.8 for dose regime and recall periods during maintenace therapy.)

- Check FBC (before and during therapy).
- Check international normalized ratio of prothrombin time [INR] (daily and/or alternate days until therapeutic range achieved, then 4–8 weekly) on a morning sample.
- Check interactions with other prescription drugs (BNF Appendix 1).
- Check urine and stools (if practical) for occult blood regularly.
- Check BP measurement.

Lifestyle advice

Provide oral anticoagulant booklet,[1] specifically:
- Take warfarin at same time each day.
- Carry card with treatment details and/or wear 'medi-alert' band with anticoagulant name clearly written.
- Inform doctor, dentist, or pharmacist about anticoagulant treatment.
- Avoid aspirin or NSAIDs.
- Eat normal diet and avoid sudden changes before blood being taken: make patient aware of high Vitamin K foods affects anti-coagulant effect e.g. leafy vegetables and liver, ↓ INR readings, avoid cranberry juice as it ↑ anticoagulant effect.
- Limit alcohol intake this ↑ INR readings.
- Avoid vigorous nose blowing and teeth cleaning.
- Report bleeding gums, bruises, nosebleeds, joint swelling, increased menstrual loss, abdominal pain, and if pregnant.
- Never stop medication without reference to doctor.

Call 999 if:
- Prolonged bleeding.
- Vomiting with blood.
- Advise about signs and symptoms of PE.

Related topics

📖 Coronary heart disease (CHD); 📖 Cardiac rehabilitation in the community.

Further information for health professionals and relatives

🖥 BNF: www.bnf.org
🖥 Clinical Knowledge Summaries (Prodigy) guidance on atrial fibrillation includes use of warfarin: www.cks.library.nhs.uk

---

[1] 🖥 Chest Heart and Stoke Society for patient information fact sheets: www.chss.org.uk

Table 11.7 Dose regimen for starting warfarin in the community

INR on day 5	Dose days 5–7	INR on day 8	Dose from day 8	Instructions
≤1.7	5mg	≤1.7	6mg	• Give warfarin 5mg od for 4d then check INR
		1.8–2.4	5mg	
		2.5–3	4mg	• Adjust dose as in table
		>3	3mg for 4d	• Recheck INR on day 8 and adjust dose as in table
1.8–2.2	4mg	≤1.7	5mg	
		1.8–2.4	4mg	
		2.5–3	3.5mg	• Thereafter check INR weekly (unless 4d interval stated) and adjust dose accordingly until dose is stable in the target range
		3.1–3.5	3mg for 4d	
		>3.5	2.5mg for 4d	
2.3–2.7	3mg	≤1.7	4mg	
		1.8–2.4	3.5mg	
		2.5–3	3mg	
		3.1–3.5	2.5mg for 4d	
		>3.5	2mg for 4d	
2.8–3.2	2mg	≤1.7	3mg	❶ **High INR**
		1.8–2.4	2.5mg	INR ≥8 (lower if other risk factors for bleeding)—admit to hospital even if not bleeding
		2.5–3	2mg	
		3.1–3.5	1.5mg for 4d.	
		>3.5	1mg for 4d.	
3.3–3.7	1mg	≤1.7	2mg	INR >3.7 and <8—omit warfarin 1–2d and recheck INR. Restart when INR <5 and re-titrate dose
		1.8–2.4	1.5mg	
		2.5–3	1mg	
		3.1–3.5	0.5mg for 4d	
		>3.5	omit for 4d	
>3.7	0mg	<2	1.5mg for 4d	
		2–2.9	1mg for 4d	
		3–3.5	0.5mg for 4d	

Reproduced with permission from Simon, C., Everitt, H., and Kendrick, T. (2005) Oxford Handbook of General Practice, 2nd edn., Oxford University Press, Oxford

Table 11.8 Warfarin therapy: recall periods during maintenance therapy

INR	Recall interval and action
1 INR high ❶ If INR >8 admit	Recall 7–14d. Stop treatment for 1–3d (max 1wk in prosthetic valve patients) and restart at a lower dose
1 INR low	↑ dose and recall in 7–14d
1 therapeutic INR	Recall 4wks
2 therapeutic INRs	Recall 6wks (maximum interval if prosthetic heart valve)
3 therapeutic INRs	Recall 8wks*
4 therapeutic INRs	Recall 10wks*
5 therapeutic INRs	Recall 12wks*

*Except prosthetic heart valves where maximum recall interval is 6wks.
Reproduced with permission from Simon, C., Everitt, H., and Kendrick, T. (2005).
Oxford Handbook of General Pratice, 2nd edn., Oxford University Press, Oxford.

Anaemia

A common problem when the blood fails to produce sufficient red blood cells and haemoglobin (♂ Hb <13g/dL, ♀ Hb 11 <11g/dL), mainly affects ♀ of child bearing age, teenagers, and young children. Also affects 1/6 ♀ >85. Younger people often asymptomatic, should always be considered as a possibility in older people. Anaemia occurs when:

- Decreased red blood cell production
- Increased loss or rate of destruction.

The presence of anaemia may indicate a more serious underlying problem.

Causes

- Iron deficiency anaemia (most common form of anaemia)
- Vitamin deficiency: e.g. B12 or folic acid
- Blood loss either through haemmorhage, menstrual loss, or internal bleeding
- Excessive use: e.g. pregnancy, lactation, cancer
- Defective bone marrow (aplastic anaemia)
- Infection e.g.malaria.

Patients may complain of:

- Tiredness
- Palpitations
- Shortness of breath
- Dizziness
- Recurrent infections
- Appear pale
- Night cramps.

Severe anaemia can cause angina, headaches. Long-term anaemia that arises from iron or B12 deficiency can also create burning sensation in the tongue, oral dryness, and mouth ulcers.

Diagnosis of which kind of anaemia is achieved through a blood test (mean cell volume MCV).

Iron deficiency anaemia

Most common form of anaemia.

Lack of iron prevents bone marrow producing sufficient Hb for red blood cells. May be resolved by diet: good sources of iron include fruit, wholemeal bread, beans, and lean meat. However:

- Malabsorption related problems (e.g. ceoeliac disease) may mean iron is not absorbed.
- Persistent bleeding, arising from problems such as gastritis, peptic ulcer, IBD, haemmorhoids, GI malignancy, and prolonged use of medication e.g. NSAIDs.

Care and management

Oral iron supplements e.g. ferrous sulphate 200mg tds (BNF 9.1.1.). NB Medication can cause constipation and black stools. Hb should improve incrementally by 1g/dL/wk, takes approx 3mths to replenish iron stores. Repeat blood test required. If failure to improve then medically reviewed as cause may be internal bleeding, or failure to absorb iron. If iron not being absorbed a parenteral route or transfusion may be considered or further investigations required.

Vitamin B12 deficiency

B12 found in liver, kidney, fish, meats, and dairy products. Absorption occurs by active and passive mechanisms, latter is dependent on presence of intrinsic factor, a protein produced by gastric cells. Produces anaemia identical to folate deficiency (see below) and potential damage to peripheral and central nervous system.

Care and management

When the cause is inadequate intake, advise on healthy diet (NB vegans may be particularly at risk). If cause is malabsorption e.g. following gastric surgery or pernicious anaemia (see below) treated with vitamin B12 injections IM (BNF 9.1.2). Initially 1mg on alternate days for 1–2wks until blood count is normal, and then, maintenance dose of 1mg/2–3mths.

Pernicious anaemia

Autoimmune disease caused by lack of intrinsic factor due to gastric atrophy, usually develops in people >50yrs. Presence of intrinsic factor antibodies confirm diagnosis. Patient may or may not present with symptoms related to anaemia. Care and management as for vitamin B12 deficiency. NB People with pernicious anaemia have ↑ risk of stomach cancer and should be advised to seek medical advise if they experience dyspepsia (📖) and/or stomach pain.

Folate deficiency

Folates are vitamins essential to the development of the central nervous system. Insufficient folate at conception and early pregnancy leads to neural tube defects in newborns. In adults deficiency causes megaloblastic anaemia, and there is some evidence there are links with arterial disease and dementia. Folate is found in liver, yeast, nuts, spinach and other green vegetables. Causes (as above) often arises from inadequate diet including alcohol misuse, also anticonvulsants.

Care and management

Folate supplements with folic acid (BNF 9.1.2). Treat the cause; 5mg od for 4mths, if malabsorption problems or as a prophylactic in renal disease may need a higher dose; refer to GP.

To prevent neural tube defects ♀ who are planning a pregnancy or are pregnant should take folate supplements up to 12wks gestation 400mcg od (consult with GP if on anticonvulsants or previous medical history). Also see 📖 Pre-conceptual care and advice.

Related topics

📖 Nutrition and healthy eating; 📖 Alcohol.

Further information for health professionals and patients

📄 NHS Clinical Knowledge Summaries (Prodigy) guidelines for anaemia PIL: www.cks.library.nhs.uk

Leukaemias and lymphomas

Acute lymphoblastic leukaemia (ALL)

Cancer that affects the lymphocyte producing cells in the bone marrow. In ALL there is an accumulation of immature lymphocyte precursor cells (blast cells) in the bone marrow. Children: 4:100,000, affects the age range 2–10yrs with median 3–7yrs, responsible for 85% of childhood leukaemia. Adult: 1:100,000 per year with median age 55yrs. Cause largely unknown although exposure to radiation in parent/adult and/or child a factor.

Acute myeloid leukaemia (AML)

Can also be called acute non-lymphocytic leukaemia (ANLL) Most common leukaemia of adulthood affects 10:100,000 incidence ↑ with age, median age at diagnosis 60yrs.

Patients may c/o

- Fatigue and breathlessness because of anaemia: (📖).
- Bruising and bleeding from mucous membranes: gums and gut because of low platelet counts (signs of spontaneous bleeding children need same day referral to paediatric haematology services).
- Persistent infections and fever caused by ↓ white cell counts, high metabolic rate, and ↑ numbers of abnormal cells.

Patients suspected as having ALL or AML will need FBC, blood film, U&E and CXR, referral to GP for investigations and onward referral to specialist oncology/haematology services.

Treatment will include: systemic chemotherapy and possibly bone marrow transplantation. Patients who are immunosuppressed because of treatment should be carefully monitored for signs of infection and referred to 2° care. Also often referred if they are exposed to chickenpox. Prognosis for acute leukaemias in children is >65% survival at 5yrs and for adults 25–30%. Long-term consequences/side effects of treatment can include:

- Heart and lung problems (cardiomyopathy and lung fibrosis)
- Growth delay in children, hypothyroidism, and integrity
- Impaired kidney function
- Psychological problems for patients and family members
- Secondary malignancies may appear after several years.

Lymphoma: cancers of the lymphatic system

Classified according to type of cell involvement, often start in lymph nodes or spleen but can spread to any organ in the body. Patients may initially present with:

- Peripheral lymphadenopathy in neck axilla, groin
- Weight loss
- Night sweats
- Loss of appetite and fatigue
- Pain in the lymph nodes after drinking alcohol (rare)
- Pruritis
- Abdominal swelling and/or pain.

All patients suspected of having lymphoma need urgent referral to haematology.

Once diagnosed, staging of the disease describes size and degree of spread:

- Stage 1: 1 group of lymph nodes affected
- Stage 2: 2 or more lymph node groups affected on the same side of diaphragm
- Stage 3: lymph nodes above and below diaphragm affected
- Stage 4: lymphoma has spread to organs e.g. liver, bones, or lungs.

Treatment involves chemotherapy and radiotherapy. NB Even with extensive spread of the disease good prognosis for many patients: prognosis affected by age and general health.

Non-Hodgkin's lymphoma (NHL): 20 different types and accounts for majority of lymphomas, approx 5000 new cases each year in UK, majority are >50yrs. 80% of patients following treatment have a good outcome: histology and age key factors in prognosis.

Hodgkin's lymphoma: 1400 new cases diagnosed every year, most common in young people 20–30yrs. Risk factors include immunodeficiency also exposure to Epstein–Barr virus that causes glandular fever, may slightly increase risk of developing Hodgkin's.

Related topic

📖 Early signs of cancer.

Further information for health professionals and patients

📟 Leukaemia Research: www.lrf.org.uk
📟 The Lymphoma Association: www.lymphoma.org.uk

Varicose veins, thrombophlebitis, and deep vein thrombosis (DVT)

Varicose veins
Veins (usually in the calf, leg, and/or groin) become visibly swollen, distorted, twisted, or lengthened. Occur because of incompetent valves that allow the blood to flow backwards from the deep to the superficial venous system, causing back pressure and further dilatation. 1: 5 people will have varicose veins and ♀ >♂.

Risk factors:
- Age (unusual in <20yrs)
- Parity
- Occupations that require a lot of standing
- Obesity in ♀
- Family history
- Secondary causes include pregnancy, DVT, pelvic tumour.

Patients may complain of:
- Cosmetic appearance of legs but otherwise be asymptomatic.
- Aching legs, feel heavy and uncomfortable especially in warm weather.
- In severe cases skin can become itchy and thin may develop into varicose eczema and venous ulcers.
- Complications associated with varicose veins include; haemmorhage, oedema, skin pigmentation, white scars and thrombophlebitis.

Care and management
- Prevention: advice on regular exercise, walking helps the circulation, healthy diet, ↓ weight. Avoid standing for long periods and sitting cross legged. If possible raise legs higher than the chest when sitting.
- Support stockings to ↓ swelling.
- Bleeding varicose veins controlled by raising foot about the level of the heart and applying compression, on recovery, advise on compression hosiery and consider referral to GP for possible surgical review.
- Treatment in 2° care: sclerotherapy involves closing off the veins by chemical injection, surgery: vein stripping for recurrent or more severe varicose veins.

COC pill and HRT: ♀ with varicose veins are *not* at ↑ risk of DVT but are at ↑ thrombophlebitis (see below). History of thrombophlebitis a contraindication to the COC pill, stop if using.

Thrombophlebitis
Superficial vein thrombosis or phlebitis involves inflammation and thrombus formation in the superficial veins (often saphenous vein and its linked veins) patients c/o severe pain, erythema, pigmentationa, and hardening of the vein. Cause often linked to presence of varicose veins, occurs because of:
- Damage to the blood vessel because of trauma or infection.
- Stasis of blood flow.
- Hypercoagulability of blood.

- Medication for symptom control and to improve prognosis: ACE inhibitor unless contraindicated (BNF 2.5.5.1) with a diuretic. Once stabilized, a beta blocker (BNF 2.4) prescribed although if symptoms persist patient may be prescribed digoxin or spironalactone (BNF 2.1.1).
- As part of the MDT review patients at least every 6mths. Include physical assessment, medication review, and functional ability.
- Palliative care for people with end-stage heart failure.

Tachycardia/palpitations

Sensation of rapid irregular or forceful heart beats, heart rate >100/min. May or may not be a significant symptom. Potentially serious if pre-existing cardiovascular disease. May have FH of syncope, arrhythmias, sudden death, and/or falls. Other causes include underlying disease, caffeine, alcohol, smoking, and fatigue. Patient may c/o:
- Chest pain, breathlessness, funny turns, sweating, or hyperventilation
- May last seconds, minutes, or longer
- May affect driving or work.

Requires medical assessment and investigation, including blood tests, ECG and related cardiac tests e.g. 24-hr ECG exercise tolerance test. May require specialist assessment and treatment according to cause. Recommend stopping smoking, ↓ alcohol, and caffeine.

Atrial fibrillation (AF)

Fast and erratic heart beat, may be episodic or chronic disturbance of cardiac rhythm 1:20 >65yrs have AF. ❶ Patient with AF has 5x ↑ risk of CVA. 1:6 cases no apparent cause 'lone AF', other causes include hypertension, complication of CHD, hyperthyroidism, PE, cardiomyopathy.

Patients can be asymptomatic but may c/o chest pain, palpitations, dyspnoea and fatigue. Requires medical assessment as above and may be admitted or referred to specialist according to severity or complications. Treatment may include digoxin (BNF 2.1.1), beta blockers (BNF 2.5.5.1), anti-coagulation therapy. Review lifestyle and advise on healthy eating and exercise.

Further information for health professionals and patients

▥ British Heart Foundation Patient information booklet: www.bhf.org.uk
▥ Management of chronic heart failure in adults in primary and secondary care: www.nice.org.uk
▥ Clinical Knowledge Summaries (Prodigy) Guidelines on CHF and AF: www.cks.library.nhs.uk

Diabetes: overview

Diabetes is a common complex disorder affecting >3% of population. Characterized by raised blood sugars and abnormalities of carbohydrate and lipid metabolism due to lack of, or ineffective, endogenous insulin. Inadequate treatment can lead to devastating complications.

Patients have a very high risk of cardiovascular disease and all risk factors should be treated aggressively.

Classification and diagnosis has medico-legal implications. Must be accurate, and in accordance to WHO/IDF 2006 Definition and diagnosis of diabetes mellitus and intermediate hyperglycaemia. www.who.int/diabetes/publications.

Random glucose test: glucose level ≥11.1mmol/l on 2 occasions = diabetes

Fasting glucose test: glucose level ≥7.0mmol/l on two different days

Glucose tolerance test: (see table 11.9) test 2h after glucose drink ≥11.1mmol = diabetes

Impaired fasting glycaemia: ≥6.1 and <7: do GTT to clarify diagnosis

Impaired glucose tolerance: ≥7.8 and <11.1mmol/h

Type 1 diabetes: autoimmune disorder
- 20% of people with DM. More common child to middle-aged adult, most common <30yrs.
- Person has *no* insulin supply and needs insulin injections to survive.

Signs and symptoms
- Sudden onset
- Weight loss
- Thirst
- Blurred vision
- Polyuria
- Urinary ketones may be present.

Management
(See Principles of diabetic care and control 🔲.)
In the first instance referral to specialist services then management in the community. Overall aim to develop flexible regimen for self-management.
- Will need insulin injections for survival.
- Referral to dietician helpful for learning carbohydrate estimation.
- Advise on healthy living, specifically smoking cessation and exercise.
- All drivers must notify the DVLA and their insurance company when starting insulin.
- NB impaired glucose tolerance and impaired fasting glucose = risk factors CVD.

Type 2 diabetes
Insulin produced but not working effectively or insufficient produced or patient becomes insulin resistant. Prevalence is ↑ and accounts for 80% of people with DM. NB Can be asymptomatic. Generally more gradual onset, many people remain undiagnosed. Silent killing disease: life expectancy reduced by 20–40% in the 40–70 age range. Those at risk:
- Older age group >65yrs.
- Family history—strong.

- Obesity: 80% are overweight BMI: >25kg/m^2, (for Asians, >23kg/m^2).
- Ethnicity important (South Asian, Afro Caribbean and Hispanics).
- PMH of gestational diabetes, or if they had big babies >4kg.

Signs and symptoms

- Weight loss
- Thirst
- Polyuria
- Irritability and/or lethargy
- Genital itching/thrush

- Blurred vision
- Recurrent UTIs
- Tingling in the feet
- No urinary ketones present.

Care and management

(See also Type 2 diabetes 📖.)
Aim to ↓ meals glycaemic load and fat and calorie intake, and risk of CHD.
Initially diet control but insulin often needed in later stages of disease.

Diabetes in Pregnancy

(See Common problems in pregnancy 📖.)

Secondary causes of diabetes

- Drugs: steroids and thiazides.
- Pancreatic disease (pancreatitis, surgery, cancer, cystic fibrosis,
  haemochromatosis).
- Endocrine disease (Cushing's disease, thyrotoxicosis, agromegaly).

Acute complications

Diabetic ketoacidosis (DKA), in type 1, due to lack of insulin the body, or
hyperosmolar non-ketotic coma (HONK) in type 2 due in part to dehydration. If blood glucose levels are high, (>12mmol/L) always assess patient for
signs of dehydration, check urinary ketones, drowsiness, infection etc.

Mortality rates are significant, especially in young or older people. If
ketoacidosis suspected, urgent referral for same day specialist assessment or admission to hospital.

Hypoglycaemia/hypoglycaemia unawareness

Emergency management. (See Insulin therapies 📖.) Education about
preventing and treating hypoglycaemia is required. Consider safety
aspects with regards to operating machinery or driving etc. Changing
medication to run blood glucose levels at upper end of normal range for
6–8wks can help regain warning signals in hypoglycaemic unawareness.

Chronic complications

- *Microvascular or small vessel disease* retinopathy can cause blindness,
  neuropathy can lead to amputation, and nephropathy to renal failure.
- *Macrovascular or large vessel disease* causing myocardial infarction,
  strokes, erectile dysfunction, or peripheral vascular disease again
  leading to amputation.

Health promotion and advice for those at risk of DM

Prevention is possible in high-risk groups.

- Daily physical activity (↓ insulin resistance—regularity is important).
- Healthy eating. 5–10% weight loss can improve metabolic profiles for those at risk 📖 Nutrition and healthy eating.
- Goal to maintain as near normal weight/BMI as possible, or at least no weight gain.

Related topics

📖 Principles of diabetic care and control; 📖 Insulin therapies; 📖 Hypertension; 📖 Coronary heart disease; 📖 QoF.

Further information for professionals and patients and carers

▣ Diabetes UK www.diabetes.org.uk ☎ Helpline Phone 0845 120 2960. See DUK *Eating Well* leaflet for the principles for details on medication.
▣ NICE Type 1 diabetes diagnosis and management: www.nice.org.uk

Principles of diabetic care and control

Good diabetic care and control can be managed in the community. Overall aims of diabetic care:

- Alleviation of symptoms
- Minimization of complications
- Regular review
- Open access for patients to advice and support and specialist services e.g. podiatrist, dietician, clinical nurse specialist
- Support and education of the patient and their family/carer
- Regular review.

Each diabetic patient requires at least a 6mth review and this includes a thorough formal annual medical review

- Asking about patient problems e.g. hypoglycaemia
- Medication and side effects
- Skin care and rotation of injection sites
- Self monitored results and discussion of their meaning and level of control
- Diet
- Activity
- Smoking
- Self-management skills
- Foot care
- Other illnesses/problems affecting DM
- In ♀ if contraception required or thinking of starting a family.

Review of possible complications from DM

- **CHD**: ↑ risk of MI and stroke symptoms (2–5x), monitor BP closely, any reduction in BP = reduced risk of cardiovascular complications.
- **Eyes**: blurred vision, and cataracts are more common, DM a risk factor for glaucoma. Referral to optician/optometrist for retinal screening, visual acuity.
- **Renal complications**: UTIs: may exacerbate renal failure. 25% diabetics have renal damage. Ensure annual renal function check. Will need specialist referral if proteinuria or microalbuminuria or raised serum creatinine (>150µmol/L).
- **Neuropathy**: ask about symptoms such as erectile dysfunction, tingling or pain. Can be depressing. Consider referral to GP.
- **Feet**: 5% develop an ulcer in any year arise from peripheral neuropathy and peripheral vascular disease. Should be referred to emergency foot care services if problems. Check pedal pulses and nerves and general condition. High risk if absent pulses, deformity, skin changes, previous ulcer. Consider regular podiatry if poor vision, immobility or poor social conditions/foot hygiene.[1]

Monitoring blood glucose

Good blood glucose (glycaemic) control is achieveable and reduces risk of microvascular complications. (See table below.)

---

[1] NICE (2004). *Diabetic foot care*. NICE, London: www.nice.org.uk

Table 11.9 Indices of control

Measure	Target
Fasting blood glucose (mmol/L)	4–7 (post-prandial <9) mmol/L: adults 4–8 (post-prandial <10) mmol/L: children
Urine	–ve (postprandial sugars <0.5%)
HbA1c (normal 4.0–6.0%): measure every 2–6mths depending on control	<7.5 (≤6.5 if ↑ risk of arterial disease)
Serum cholesterol (mmol/L): 2° prevention, type 2 DM or type 1 DM with risk factors for CVD, metabolic syndrome or microalbuminuria	↓ total cholesterol by 25% or to <4mmol/L, whichever is the lower value or ↓ LDL cholesterol by 30% or to <2.0 mmol/L; whichever is the lower value
BMI (kg/m²)	25–30
BP: without macrovascular disease	<135/85
BP: with macrovascular disease	<130/80

❶ Reference values may vary between laboratories. Aim for glycosylated Hb to be within 1% of the upper limit of normal range.

Reproduced with permission from Simon, C., Everitt, H., and Kendrick, T. (2005). *Oxford Handbook of General Practice*, 2nd edn. Oxford University Press, Oxford.

Urine monitoring: adequate for those who do not require tight control or for those who cannot cope with more complex methods.

Blood monitoring: essential for patients on insulin and desirable for people on oral medication.
- Explain range of monitoring devices available to patient (B.N.F 6.1.6)
- Assess skills and meters if used annually or if problems arise
- Agree targets for pre-meal glucose levels
- Evaluate the reliability of results against HbA1c results.

HbA1c (glcosylated haemoglobin)

Represents a measure of control over previous 6–8wks. Use HBA1c measure at least 2x a year and in conjunction with persons own self-monitoring blood glucose results (see Table 11.9 above).

Documentation: maintain a structured record that the patient holds
- Document agreed main points arising from review
- Agreed targets to next consultations
- Services involved/new referrals
- Changes in treatment/therapy.

Related topics

📖 Diabetes: overview; 📖 Treatment of Type 2 diabetes; 📖 Insulin therapies; 📖 Hypertension; 📖 Coronary heart disease; 📖 Hyperlipidaemia; 📖 Wound care.

Further information for professionals and patients and carers

🖳 Diabetes UK: www.diabetes.org.uk See DUK *Eating Well* leaflet for the principles, and for details on medication. ☎ Helpline: 0845 120 2960

🖳 National Diabetes Support team: Diabetic foot guide: www.diabetes.nhs.uk/downloads/ NDST_Diabetic_Foot_Guide.pdf

🖳 NICE Type 1 Diabetes diagnosis and management: www.nice.org.uk

🖳 NICE (2004). CG10 Type2 Diabetes foot care: www.nice.nhs.uk

Care and management

All care will be with the MDT and in collaboration with specialist neurology services. The range of complications that can arise as a result of MS means much of care involves their identification and management. Patients require long-term coordinated care and emotional support and accurate information and advice about their health, prognosis, entitlement to disability benefits, and access to housing, transport, education, and leisure. Some PCOs have access to MS CNSs for ongoing patient support. MS charities provide guidance and standards for health and social care (see below).

- Supplementing the diet with linoleic acid 17–23g per day (poly unsaturated fats) may help slow progression of disability. Sources include sunflower, cornflower, and safflower oils.
- Influenza vaccination should be offered to all patients.

As there is no cure for MS, modifying therapies are used with the aim of slowing down the effects of the disease. The evidence for these is mixed. Therapies include:

- Beta-interferon and glatiramer acetate (2° care-led treatment)
- Cannabis for pain and spasticity (only through participation in trials)
- Neural therapy (injection of local anaesthetic into key points)
- Reflexology and massage
- Psychotherapy e.g. for depression
- Physiotherapy, speech therapy, and occupational therapy.

Related topics

☐ Urinary catheter care; ☐ Sources of information on benefits and support; ☐ Carers assessment and support.

Further information for health professionals and patients

- Multiple Sclerosis Trust: www.mstrust.org.uk
- Multiple Sclerosis Society: www.mssociety.org.uk ☎ Helpline: 0808 800 8000
- NICE (2003). Diagnosis and management of MS in primary and secondary care: www.nice.org.uk

Motor neurone disease (MND)

MND is a rapidly progressive neurodegenerative disease affecting up to 5000 people in UK. Incidence 1:50,000, prevalence 1:12,000. ♂: ♀ 3:2. Onset usually between 40–70yrs. Causes largely unknown: possible genetic and environmental, familial in 5%.

Three main forms of MND

- Amyotrophic lateral sclerosis (ALS)—most common (65%)
- Progressive muscular atrophy (PMA)—least common (10%)
- Progressive bulbar palsy (PBP)—25% of cases.

Life expectancy varies depending on the form: ALS: 2–5yrs, PMA: 5yrs +, PBP: 6mths–3yrs.

Presentation

Symptoms vary according to form but include:

- Muscle weakness and wasting
- Weight loss
- Weak grip
- Stumbling
- Fasiculation (small involuntary contractions) of skeletal muscles
- Emotional lability
- Dysarthria and dysphagia with nasal speech, poor swallow, and regurgitation if upper motor neurones involved.

> Consciousness and intellect are unaffected.

Aims of care

- Symptomatic relief, maintain for QoL, speed of response essential
- Ensure early referral to MDT and MND Nurse specialist. MDT should have ensured home physio/OT assessment for adaptations/mobility aids
- Full community care assessment process
- Awareness of state benefits for disability and attendance
- Carers assessment and support needs addressed
- Pharmacological: riluzole (BNF 4.9) is only disease-modifying therapy that may prolong life.

Dysphagia

- Control head position with pillows ± collar
- Modify diet and thicken fluids
- Ensure SaLT (Speech and Language Therapist)/dietician assessment
- Initiate discussions of gastrostomy (PEG) early before patient too unwell to tolerate procedure.

Dyspnoea

- Due to poor resp function/anxiety
- Symptom control e.g. O_2 therapy at night, opiods may relieve coughing and choking
- Psychotherapy and relaxation techniques
- Physiotherapy exercises may aid breathing
- Position upright
- Discuss options for ventilation including non-invasive ventilation (NIPPV), consider advantages of prolonging life against prolonging discomfort.

Pain

Due to joint immobility, spasm and cramps, pressure areas, constipation.

- Ensure physio referral, pressure area relief equipment and mattress, drugs e.g. baclofen/quinine for spasm and cramps.
- Dysarthria: early referral to SLT and dietician, provide communication aids.
- Emotional lability (different from depression) treated with amitriptyline (BNF 4.3).

Key issues to consider

- Maintaining emotional, physical, and financial support throughout the course of the disease for patient, family, and carers.
- Ensure there is regular symptom review involving primary health-care team.
- Ensure there are opportunities for discussion about end-of-life and support patient and carer e.g. palliative/respite care/withdrawal of treatment and ventilation.
- Discuss and document patients wishes/advanced directives/preferred place of death.

MND Association can help with information, advice, equipment loan, and financial support (see below).

Related topics

📖 People with depression; 📖 Carers assessment and support; 📖 Talking therapies; 📖 Counselling skills; 📖 Palliative care in the home; 📖 End-of-life issues.

Further information for professionals and relatives

🖥 Motor Neurone Disease Association: www.mndassociation.org
🖥 NICE. Riluzole for motor neurone disease: www.nice.org.uk

Parkinson's disease (PD)

PD is a chronic, incurable progressive, degenerative, neurological disorder. 120,000 PD sufferers in UK. 10,000 are diagnosed each year, 1 in 20 young-onset PD. 15–20% of people with PD have dementia. Causes are largely unknown although environment and genetic susceptibility are possible factors.

Symptoms appear from the age of 50, but in young-onset PD can appear <40yrs.

NB Parkinsonian features seen in other conditions: multi-system atrophy, progressive supranuclear palsy, Lewy body dementia, encephalitis, SE of drugs e.g. haloperidol, chlorpromazine (BNF 4.2.1).

Pathology includes:
- Degeneration of dopaminergic neurones in substantia nigra, part of the basal ganglia (regions in the brain that control voluntary movement).
- 80–90% depletion of dopamine in substantia nigra.
- Presence of Lewy bodies.

Risk factors
- Old age
- Identical twin with early onset PD
- Positive family history
- Exposure to herbicides, pesticides, heavy metals, proximity to industry, rural residence, repeated head trauma.

Presentation
Slow insidious onset:
- Bradykinesia that can include resting tremor, rigidity, disorders of posture—neck and trunk flexion, balance problems
- Gait disturbance: festination, freezing, shuffling
- Loss of facial expression
- Monotonous and hypophonic speech
- Dribbling, dysphagia, micrographia.

Aims of care
Symptomatic relief, maintain QoL, ↓ progression and ↓ SE of medication
- Mainstay of treatment is pharmacological (BNF 4.9). Drugs include levadopa, dopamine agonists, COMT inhibitors, MAO-inhibitors, and anticholinergics.

> NB Rarely achieves complete control of symptoms.

Usually not started till symptoms are disrupting QoL.
- ↑ functional disability → early referral to specialist MDT and nursing support.
- Reduce or delay long-term complications of drug therapy (e.g. on/off effect by delaying start of L-dopa).
- Help come to terms with diagnosis.
- Reduce distress: symptoms worse when stressed.
- Legal obligation patient to inform DVLA and insurers of diagnosis.
- Complementary therapies may help relaxation.

Management in later stages

- Manage drug effects and motor complications—risk of falls.
- Identify and address behavioural/psychological issues: depression, sleep disorders, psychosis. Consider referral to mental health team.
- Monitor BP: risk of orthostatic hypotension → review PD drugs and advise to avoid sitting out in sun, getting up quickly, or sitting in one position for long periods. Sit down immediately if feeling dizzy. Encourage leg exercises that maintain ankle flexion and dorsiflexion.
- Monitor other complications: constipation, urinary incontinence/retention, impotence, poor nutrition.
- MDT should have ensured:
  - Home OT/physiotherapist assessment for home adaptations and mobility aids
  - Full community care assessment process
  - Awareness of state benefits for disability and attendance
  - Carers assessment and support needs addressed.

Related topics

📖 Constipation in adults; 📖 People with depression; 📖 People with dementia; 📖 Falls prevention.

Further information for health professionals and public

📑 NICE (2006). Parkinson's Disease: national clinical guidelines for diagnosis and and management in primary and secondary care. www.nice.org.uk
📑 Parkinson's Disease Society: www.parkinsons.org.uk

Common adult health problems

Bacterial skin infections

Skin infections can range from minor to life threatening conditions.

Impetigo

- A superficial cutaneous infection caused by *Staphylococcus aureus* and/or beta-hemolytic streptococcus.
- Vesicles that rupture easily, producing golden yellow exudates, forms a crust when dry.
- Commonly involved sites: face, neck but can be more extensive.
- Impetigo can occur as a 2° infection on excoriated skin conditions, e.g. eczema, scabies.
- Contagious.
- Children in poor living conditions, overcrowding or with poor hygiene are at greater risk of developing impetigo.

Treatment and advice

- Either topical mupirocin, fusidic acid or 0.3% neomycin (BNF 13.10.1) to the area for up to 10d, tds or if severe or multiple sites then systemic antibiotics (flucloxacillin or erythromycin) for 10d.
- Saline soaks to cleanse area and remove crusts.
- Encourage basic hygiene practice to limit the contact and spread of infection, e.g. not sharing towels, face cloths.
- Exclusion from group child care/school until lesions crust over (Infectious disease exclusion times 📖).
- Bacterial culture for diagnosis if not clearing.

Infection of the hair follicles

There are three types:

Follicullitis

- A superficial active pustular inflammation of hair follicles caused by *Staphylococcus aureus*.
- Triggered by: shaving, waxing, tar ointments, oil based ointments.

Furuncle (boil)

- A deep infection of the hair follicle caused by *Staphylococcus aureus*.
- Characterized by inflammation, nodule with peeling of the overlying skin. The area will be tender.
- The nodule will erupt and discharge the contents.
- Common areas affected are areas affected by sweat and/or friction (nose, face, axilla, buttocks).
- Patients who are immunosuppressed or have diabetes are more prone to boils.

Carbuncle

- Deep infection of a group of hair follicles by *Staphylococcus aureus*.
- Common site—nape of neck.
- Characterized by a dome-shaped area of erythema developing into a deep, painful abscess.
- May rupture spontaneously.

Treatment
- Exclude diabetes.
- Systemic antibiotics (flucloxacillin or erythromycin).
- In recurrences longer courses of 4–6wks of antibiotics may be required and bacterial culture from lesion and carrier sites.
- Large carbuncle or in sensitive area may require incision and drainage.
- OTC antiseptic washes and emollients may help to avoid recurrences.
- Referred to specialists if not responding to primary care treatment and management.

Cellulitis

- Infection of the subcutaneous tissues with *Streptococcus pyrogenes*.
- Most commonly the lower legs are affected, becoming erythematous, oedematous, and painful. Blisters may be noted.
- The patient will become systemically unwell and pyrexial.
- The organism enters the tissue through a fissure caused by eczema, tinea pedis, leg ulceration, although entry port not found.
- It is often a recurrent problem.

Treatment
- Antibiotics (flucloxacillin, penicillin V, BNF 5.1 Table 1) orally or in severe infection benzylpenicillin and flucloxacillin IV.
- May require prophylactic antibiotics if recurrent.
- Analgesia p.r.n.
- Monitor the edges of the cellulitis to assess treatment effectiveness.
- Emollient therapy (BNF 13.2.1) helps prevent fissures in dry skin.

Further information for professionals and patients

▣ Clinical Knowledge Summaries (Prodigy) guidance on impetigo, boils, cellulitis: www.cks.library.nhs.uk Includes leaflets for patients.

Skin cancer

Primary cutaneous cancer is most commonly of the keratinocytes or melanocytes. Caused by genetic factors, exposure to sunlight, sometimes exposure to carcinogens (See also Skin cancer prevention 📖).

Incidence
- 70,000 new cases of skin cancer are reported in the UK each year.
- Over 2000 people die from skin cancer each year.

Types of skin cancer
There are 2 main types of skin cancer:
- Malignant melanoma.
- Non melanoma skin cancer: basal cell carcinoma, squamous cell carcinoma.

ABCDs of melanoma

A useful guide for determining which moles are potential melanomas and teaching patients warning signs:
- **Asymmetry**: an unusual shape or a non-symmetrical shaped mole, should be evaluated further.
- **Border**: a benign mole will usually have a smooth clearly demarcated border. If an ill-defined or irregular border is noted, evaluate further.
- **Colour**: pigment variation indicative of malignancy and should be evaluated.
- **Diameter**: most melanomas are >6mm.

These changes usually take place over a relatively short time from wks to mths.

Other signs can include mole or growth that crusts, bleeds or is itchy, or sore that won't heal.

Malignant melanoma

Malignancy of the melanocytes. The most serious form of skin cancer. Good prognosis depends on early detection and treatment. 4 types:
- Superficial spreading malignant melanoma: an enlarging brown/black macular/popular lesion, may be irregular with colour variation.
- Nodular melanoma: a pigmented papule that enlarges and ulcerates.
- Acral melanoma: brown/black macules on the non-hair bearing skin of the palms, soles, and nail beds.
- Lentigo mailgna melanoma: an irregularly shaped, flat, pigmented lesion on sun damaged skin. Most frequently occurs on the face or other sun exposed sites.

Treatment
- All suspected cases of melanoma referred to 2° care, usually the 'mole' clinic in the dermatology department.
- Surgical removal of the suspected lesion to establish the histological diagnosis. May require further surgery to ensure adequate margins around the excised lesion.
- Patient assessed for the presence of metastatic disease.
- The patient followed up by 2° care for at least 5yrs.

Non melanoma skin cancer

Basal cell carcinoma (BCC)

- Most common type of skin cancer. Also known as rodent ulcer, locally invasive, low grade tumours of the basaloid cells that rarely metastasize. Usually occur on sun exposed skin of older patients but can affect younger patients.
- There are different types of basal cell carcinoma:
  - Nodular BCC: slow growing with a characteristic translucent or pearly surface. Dilated vessels may be visible. The area may ulcerate.
  - Cystic BCC: similar to nodular but there will be more dilated vessels.
  - Superficial spreading BCC: thin lesions that gradually increase in surface area. There may be reddened, slightly raised, with some scaling.
  - Morphoeic BCC: white/yellow morphoeic plaques resembling an enlarging scar. Ulceration and crusting are usual.

Squamous cell carcinoma (SCC)

- An invasive tumour of the keratinocytes that can metastasize.
- There are different types of SCC:
  - Actinic keratosis: these are pre malignant lesions, if left untreated a small percentage will develop into SCC. Appear in sun exposed sites as tiny, palpable lesions.
  - Bowen's disease (SCC *in situ*): may appear on non-sun exposed sites. Appears as a persistent, erythematous, indurated, plaque.
  - Nodular SCC: hard nodule which increases in size rapidly.
  - Ulcerated SCC: Nodular area on the edge of an ulcer or an ulcer on a scar.

Treatment

All suspected BCC and SCC refered to dermatology. Treatment is dependent on the site, type, and size of lesion, but may include: cryosurgery, curettage and electro surgery, fluorouracil topically applied, excision, radiotherapy, surgery, photodynamic therapy.

Patients need to be offered clear information about the diagnosis, prognosis, and any changes required to their lifestyle.

Further information for patients and professionals

- Cancer Research: www.cancerresearchuk.org/sunsmart/skincancer/
- Cancer Bacup: www.cancerbacup.org.uk/Cancertype/Skin/
- MARC'S Line: www.wessexcancer.org/templates/wessexcancer/

Eczema/dermatitis

An acute and/or chronic pruritic inflammation of the skin. Only about 20% seek medical help for these conditions.

Clinical features

Atopic Eczema: usually presents between 3–12mths of age (Eczema in childhood 🕮). There is an inherited predisposition to eczema, and hay fever. It may start on the face and scalp. In older children and adults eczema is often localized to the flexures. Eczema can continue through into adulthood.

Seborrhoeic dermatitis: associated with an overgrowth of pityrosporum ovule yeasts in adults. The distribution is characterized by pink, orange/brown, scaly patches on the scalp, eyebrows, eyelashes, nasolabial folds, external ear, centre of chest, and centre of back.

Discoid (nummular) eczema: characterized by well demarcated, round, scaly plaques. There may be numerous vesicles present that produce exudate and crusting.

Contact dermatitis: eczema can be associated with exposure of the skin to certain irritants or allergens.

Pompholyx: eczema on the hands and feet may present as crops of vesicles with severe itching. There may be peeling and cracking of the skin.

Gravitational (venous, varicose, stasis) eczema: occurs on the lower legs of patients with venous hypertension.

Management

Emollients (BNF 13.2)

Patients with eczema usually have dry skin and therefore should be prescribed an emollient package:

- Bath additive (e.g. balneum, hydromol, oilatum): 10–20ml of the oil should be added to the bath.
- Soap substitute (e.g. aqueous cream, emulsifying ointment): soap has a drying affect on the skin and should not be used.
- Moisturizer (e.g. 50:50 white soft paraffin: liquid paraffin WSP:LP, Oilatum cream, Epaderm): The moisturizing emollient should be applied after the bath and then frequently throughout the day.

Topical steroids (BNF 13.4)

There are different strengths of topical steroids (mild, moderate, potent, and very potent). The weakest steroid that is effective should be the steroid of choice. Usually a mild steroid is sufficient to treat eczema on the face. Many patients are aware of the potential side effects of over use of topical steroids and therefore allow time for advice and questions. It is only applied to the affected areas and not mixed with emollient.

Topical immunomodulators

These are recommended if the eczema has not responded to topical steroids or is severe. Prescribed by dermatology specialists. The treatment acts by blocking the molecular mechanisms of inflammation (BNF 13.5.3). The patient may experience burning or stinging of the skin for about 20min when the treatment is applied.

Antihistamines

Antihistamines e.g. chlorphenamine are useful for short-term use in acute phases of the eczema for their sedative effect. They are used an hour before bed time, daytime use should be avoided.

Infection

- Bacterial: *Staphylococcus aureus*, characterized by pustules, yellow crusting or weeping. Sometimes presents as a flare up not responding to usual medication. Treated with systemic flucloxacillin (BNF 5.1.1) or erythromycin (BNF 5.1.5).
- Viral: herpes simplex, characterized by painful, small umbilicated vesicles. Requires medical assessment as widespread inflection (ezcema herpeticum) may be life threatening. The patient will be unwell and will require systemic aciclovir (BNF 5.3.2) as inpatient.

General advice

- Avoid the use of soaps and detergents on the skin.
- Extremes of temperature, cold winds, or hot environment with a low humidity may exacerbate eczema.
- Cotton clothing should be worn next to the skin.
- Nails should be kept short to reduce damaging the skin if scratching.
- Eczema in a family can cause an increase of stress for other family members.
- Dietary manipulation is indicated if there is a history of specific food allergy. It should be undertaken with medical and dietician advice.

Related topic

📖 Eczema in childhood.

Further information for professionals and patients

- ▣ National Eczema Society www.eczema.org
- ▣ Clinical Knowledge Summaries (Prodigy) Guidance on the management of atopic eczema and seborrhoeic dermatitis www.cks.library.nhs.uk Clinical Knowledge Summaries (Prodigy) guidance patient information leaflets also available

Fungal infections

Fungal infection in humans is largely attributable to 2 groups:
- Dermatophytes—multicellular filaments or hyphae
- Yeasts—unicellular forms replicating by budding.

Infection can occur from direct contact with infected animals, humans, or soil, or contact with a contaminated object for example shared towels.

Dermatophyte (tinea) infection

Superficial infection in keratinized tissue (hair, nails, stratum corneum). 3 types—Trichophyton, microsporum, epidermophyton. Diagnosis usually clinical but can be confirmed by skin scrapings, or nail clippings (depending on site) sent for mycology. General advice on good hygiene.

Tinea corporis (ringworm)
- Single or multiple pink scaly plaques on trunk or limbs, which gradually increase in size. As expands the centre clears to look like a ring.
- Localized area treated with an imidazole cream (BNF 13.10.2) applied bd for 2–4wks or terbinafine cream for 7–10d. Continued 7d after visibly clears.
- Extensive areas need systemic treatment with itraconazole, griseofulvin, or terbinafine (BNF 5.2) for 2–4wks started after confirmation of diagnosis from mycology.

Tinea pedis (athlete's foot)
- There are 5 patterns of tinea on the feet:
  - Itchy, scaling and maceration between the toes usually 4th and 5th.
  - Plaques of tinea similar to tinea corporis on the dorsum of the foot.
  - White itchy scaling on the soles of 1 or both feet.
  - Scaling on the sides of the foot.
  - Vesicles on the instep usually on 1 foot.
- Treated with an imidazole cream bd for 2–4wks or terbinafine for 7d. Continue for 7d after clears. (BNF 13.10.2).
- Oral treatment if widespread, severe, or treatment failed.

Tinea cruris (ringworm in the groin)
- Common in young men, may be associated with tinea pedis.
- Itchy, pink scaly patches with central clearing on insides of thigh, scrotum rarely affected.
- Treated with imidazole cream bd for 2–3wks or until clear.

Tinea manium
Uncommon. Affects hand with powdery scaling. Treatment topical imidazole creams for 2–3wks.

Tinea unguium
- Nail(s) becomes thickened, discolored white or yellow
- Treated if patient requests, or is causing other recurrent infections
- After diagnosis confirmed by mycology, oral, pulsed itraconazole (200mg bd for 7d repeated after 21d for fingernails and 2 more for toes). (BNF 5.2).

Tinea capitis (scalp ringworm)

- Most common in children. Rare in adults. Causes discrete bald areas with short broken off hairs. The underlying skin is scaly and red.
- Treated systemically. Griseofulvin 15–20mg/kg body weight/day od with food for 6 wks. (BNF 5.2).
- Sometimes also a kerion, a red boggy swelling discharging pus. Treated by softening crusts with olive oil. Swab for MSC. Treat with flucloxacillin if *staphylococcus aureus* is present as well as the griseofulvin.

Yeast infections

Candida (thrush) skin infections. Common. Caused by the opportunistic pathogen Candida albicans. Advise good hygiene, allow air to circulate etc. Common in use of broad spectrum antibiotics, poor nappy hygiene but other reasons should be investigated e.g. if immunosuppressed, patient with diabetes. Usually flexures are affected and pattern is symmetrical.

Cheilitis

- Infections causing inflamed and cracked grooves at corner of mouth.
- Common when wear poorly fitted dentures. Advise the patient to clean the dentures after each meal, sterilize at night and see dentist.
- Clotrimazole cream (BNF 13.10.2) bd.

Oral candidiasis (seen as white plaques) requires oral forms of anti-fungal (BNF 12.3.2).

Genital candidiasis ♀ see (Vaginal and vulval problems 📖). ♂: redness, sore glans penis, ± ulceration of foreskin. Not usually transmissable. Treated with 1% clotrimazole (OTC BNF 13.10.2)

Intertrigo

- In skin folds due to heat and humidity. Common if overweight
- The area will be painful, red with red satellite lesions
- Clotrimazole and 1% hydrocortisone cream clears infection reduces symptoms but recurrence is common.

Paronychia

- Infection of nail fold and loss of cuticle. Creates chronic infection.
- To induce growth of new cuticle: advise to keep hands dry by wearing cotton glores inside rubber gloves when washing up, etc. and apply petroleum jelly to affected nail several times a day to protect the area.

Pityrosporum skin infections

Pityriasis versicolor

A scaly rash that occurs most commonly in young adults due to pityrosporum orbiculare. Characterized by pigmentary skin changes, either hypo- or hyperpigmentation and occasionally red patches.

- If localized use clotrimazole cream BD (BNF 13.10.2) for 2wks. Ketoconazole or Selsun (unlicensed use) shampoo can be used as a body wash for 2wks.
- Referred to dermatologist if extensive.
- Reassure patient as pigmentary changes may take 3mths to go.

Further information

📖 British Association of Dermatologists www.bad.org.uk for professional guidelines and patient information leaflets

📖 Clinical Knowledge Summaries (Prodigy) Guidance on candida infections: www.cks.library.nhs.uk

Psoriasis

Psoriasis is a chronic, relapsing, inflammatory, hyperproliferative skin disease. Whilst rarely fatal, it affects psychological, socio-economic, and physical well-being. Affects 2–3% of the population. Appears at any age, most commonly between 20–30yrs. Affects ♀ = ♂. Genetically predetermined but also caused by infection, stress, drugs e.g. lithium, anti-malarials, beta-blocking agents, systemic glucocorticoids, environment e.g. usually worsens in the winter, however a small percentage worsen in the summer.

Clinical features

- Chronic plaque psoriasis: well demarcated, raised pink plaques, dry silver/white scales. Commonly on elbows, knees, and lower back.
- Scalp psoriasis: may be dry and scaly or in more severe cases will be inflamed, with thickened, scaly, well demarcated plaques.
- Guttate psoriasis: multiple red papules and small psoriatic lesions. Usually on the trunk in a 'raindrop' distribution commonly following a streptococcal infection.
- Flexural psoriasis: well demarcated, red, smooth plaques affecting the submammary, axillary and anogenital areas.
- Pustular psoriasis.
  - Localized—multiple small, sterile pustules, with erythema and hyperkeratosis on the palms and soles, As they dry, brown patches develop.
  - Generalized—multiple tiny pustules on generalized erythrodermic skin. The skin is unstable and requires emergency dermatology care.
- Erythrodermic psoriasis—involves entire skin surface. Patient febrile, ↑ white cell count, ankle oedema, and problems controlling their temperature. Requires emergency dermatology care.
- Psoriatic arthropathy—less than 10% of patients with psoriasis will also have psoriatic arthropathy. The most common form seen is characterized by distal interphalangeal involvement.

Symptoms and signs

- The distribution of psoriasis is largely symmetrical.
- Can be itchy although it is often considered not to be. Scratching removes overlying scale, elicits pinpoint bleeding—'Auspitz sign'.
- Often occurs at sites of trauma—'Koebner phenomenon'.

Management

Consider the following:
- The severity and affect on QoL
- Previous therapies, other drug therapies, time available for treatments
- The physical ability of the patient to apply topical treatments.

Treatments for psoriasis fall into 3 groups.

Topical Treatments

Used for mild to moderate psoriasis, or with other therapies.
- Emollients (BNF 13.2.1): regular use reduces scaling, itching and ↑ penetration of other topical medications.

Further information and patient support

⊞ Alopecia Online UK (patient information and support resource): www.alopeciaonline.org.uk/
⊞ British Assocation of Dermatologists guidelines for the treatment of alopecia areata
   www.bad.org.uk/healthcare/guidelines/

Hirsutism or excess hairiness

Additional hair in male pattern on face, torso, and limbs, affects 1 in 100 women. Mostly idiopathic although may be associated with therapies e.g. steroids, or syndromes e.g. polycystic ovary syndrome. Referred to specialist as required, topical treatments available on consultant prescription only. Advice to those with idiopathic hirsutism includes home therapies of cosmetic bleaching, removal by creams, shaving, waxing, electrolysis. Laser therapy available in some areas for those with severe problems.

Hypertrichosis

Excess hairiness in non-male pattern. Often caused by drug therapies e.g. ciclosporin. If idiopathic advised as hirsuitism above.

Further information

⊞ British Association of Dermatologists Information Leaflet on Hirsutism: www.bad.org.uk

Allergies

An allergic reaction is an exaggerated response by the immune system to an allergen. Common allergens are house dust mite excreta, grass and tree pollen, moulds, pet hair, wasp and bee stings, industrial and household chemicals, medicines e.g. pencillin, and foods such as milk and eggs. Less common allergens include latex, nuts, and fruit. The first exposure to the allergen causes the immune system to produce immunoglobulin E (IgE) antibodies which attach to mast cells. In subsequent exposures the allergens attach to the IgE antibodies and the cell releases histamines, causing widened blood vessels, leakage of fluid into tissues and muscle spasms. Particular conditions associated with allergic problems include asthma (📖), eczema (📖), conjunctivitis, rhinitis, hay fever, anaphylaxis.

Signs and symptoms

Common allergic symptoms include itching, watering eyes, sneezing, swelling, urticaria, and wheezing. See also 📖 Anaphylaxis.

Assessment and management

Investigations depends on the type and severity of symptoms and associated conditions e.g. asthma. Referred to specialist allergy clinic if diagnosis in doubt, investigation and management of anaphylaxis, food allergies, occupational allergies.

Management strategy
- Allergen avoidance e.g. exclude pets, documentation of medication allergies especially penicillin, avoid pollen (keep windows shut, avoid grassy areas in pollen release season, wear wraparound sunglasses, wash hair/shower after being out, cover bed during day), check food labels for food allergens.
- Medication for symptoms or condition as required.
- Education and information on allergen avoidance and management.
- In severe allergic reactions, provision and education in the use of pre-loaded syringes of adrenalin for self administration or administration by family, carers, school staff. Also advice on wearing medic alert bracelets.

Hayfever (seasonal)

Most caused by grass pollen (June–August) and silver birch (April) pollen in the UK. Often first starts in teenage years and may improve as gets older. Avoidance of allergen is key strategy as above. Treated with systematic antihistamine (BNF 3.4.1), and/or topical nasal spray (BNF 12.2.1) and/or eye drops (BNF 11.4.2). Most preparations available OTC. Severe symptoms may require a short course of oral steroids.

Bee/wasp sting allergy

About 3 in 100 people who are stung have some kind of allergic reaction, a minority of these have severe reactions. Local or mild generalized reactions are treated with antihistamine. Severe reactions are usually followed up in allergy clinics. These individuals may be given pre-loaded syringes of adrenaline (epinephrine) (BNF 3.4.3) and taught how and when to use them (including all family, carers, others e.g. school staff). May also be considered for a desensitization (to the allergen i.e. insect venom) programme at the specialist clinic.

Food allergies and intolerances

Present in about 5–7% of children but less in adult population. A limited number of foods cause real allergic reactions—nuts (especially peanuts) wheat, eggs, fish, shellfish, and cows' milk. Some such as nut allergies provoke an acute, severe reaction and will be managed as severe reactions to stings as above.

There are a wide range of other types of food intolerances many caused by enzyme deficiencies (e.g. Coeliac disease 📖) or reactions to additives that do not involve an allergic response but cause symptoms such as rashes, abdominal pain, vomiting, diarrhoea, palpitations. Referred to specialist allergy clinic for identification and advice on management. Advice for prevention of food allergy or intolerances developing includes breast feeding, delaying introduction of solid food as per guidelines (see Bottle feeding and weaning 📖), avoid foods with preservatives and additives.

Further information for professionals and the public

- The Allergy UK Information, factsheets and Helpline: www.allergyuk.org/index.html ☎ 01322 619898
- Clinical Knowledge Summaries (Prodigy) guidance on allergic rhinitis and PIL on allergies, and hayfever: www.cks.library.nhs.uk
- UK Food Standards Agency advice on food intolerances: www.eatwell.gov.uk/healthissues/foodintolerance/

Deafness

Nearly 9 million in the UK are deaf or hard of hearing, being deaf can lead to depression and isolation. Categorized as:

- Mild deafness is when a person has difficulty following speech in noisy situations.
- Moderate deafness is when a person has difficulty following speech without a hearing aid.
- Severe deafness is when they use lip-reading to supplement use of hearing aid.
- Profound deafness means that there is so little ability to hear sounds, that BSL will be first language or may prefer lip reading for communication.

There are multiple possible causes:

- Age: >50% of people >60yrs have a hearing loss and 71% of >70yrs will have some hearing loss.
- Noise: prolonged and repeated exposure to loud noise at work/leisure NB young adults particularly vulnerable through personal stereos/ and loud dance music.
- Conduction problems: ear wax, trauma, perforated ear drum, and inflammation/infection.
- Genetic: 1 in every 1000 babies born moderately/profoundly deaf, 50% are thought to be due to genetic causes.

Presentation in adults (see Hearing screening for children 📖)
Slow onset with increasing difficulties understanding people e.g. when there is background noise. Questions to ask as part of assessment:

- Do people seem to be mumbling?
- Are you often saying pardon?
- Do you always hear the phone/door bell?
- Are conversations sometimes difficult to follow?
- Do other family members complain that the TV is on too loud?

Management

Check that problem not caused by ear wax (Ear care 📖), or presence of infection. If there is no obvious cause referral to GP for audiology or specialist ENT assessment to find cause for deafness, qualify hearing loss and assess for possible hearing aid. Principles in working with people with hearing loss:

- Always face the deaf person in a well-lit room when talking to them.
- Write down important information.
- Mark nursing and medical notes with sign/sticker to alert other staff to hearing problems.
- Hearing aids are a significant step for many people and can take time to adjust to. Encourage to wear for short periods (10min) of time to build confidence.
- Loop systems: often available in public places for people with hearing aids helps to cut out background noise.
- Advise on telecommunications products that use both speech and text, which help with media like films and TV.

- Alerting devices are available to help improve deaf person's awareness of things happening around them e.g. flashing light doorbell alert. May be purchased through RNID or supplied as part of Community Care support.
- Hearing dogs (www.hearing-dogs.co.uk) trained to alert owners to significant sounds, have full access to public places under Disability Discrimination Act.

Tinnitis

Ringing or buzzing heard in ear or head, occasional tinnitus common in 15% of population, for minority (2%) severe and can interfere with life and ability to sleep. Cause often unknown. Can be very distressing and depressing. Possible management:
- Mask with background music/radio.
- White noise aid available from ENT depts.
- Surgical sectioning of cochlear nerve: last resort and causes permanent deafness.

Deaf people are eligible for benefits if the disability interferes with ability to work (Benefits for disability and illness 🕮).

Related topic

🕮 Deafness in children.

Further information for health professionals and public

▣ British Deaf Association: www.signcommunity.org.uk
☎ Telephone: 0808 808 0123; Textphone: 0808 808 9000
▣ Hearing dogs for the deaf: www.hearing-dogs.co.uk
▣ Royal National Institute for the Deaf: www.rnid.org.uk and informationline@rnid.org.uk

Mouth, nose, and throat problems

Mouth ulcers

Common problem can make it difficult to eat, drink, and talk. Caused by:

- Trauma e.g. tooth brushing, minor burns from hot drinks: last for approx a week unless trauma recurs/persists e.g. a rough tooth.
- Apthous ulcers: painful white ulcers commonly believed to be associated with stress (but no evidence to support this) and poor health. May first appear at puberty, take longer to heal and likely to recur until there is an improvement in health.
- Ulcers caused by herpes infection, or inflammatory bowel disease usually linked to other symptoms.
- Iron or vitamin B12 deficiency (Anaemia 🕮).

All red or white patches in the mouth and ulcers persisting for >3wks need referral to oral surgeon to exclude possibility of malignancy.

Care and management

- Advise on good dental hygiene and regular dental check-ups.
- Healthy diet avoiding food and drink that may exacerbate symptoms e.g. highly spiced foods.
- ↓ pain: paracetamol, iced water rinses, OTC anaesthetic gels, wafers.
- Adcortyl in Orabase® or Corlan® pellets (BNF 12.3) can be effective in treatment.

Gingivitis

Inflammation of the gums often occurs with a build up of plaque, mild cases patients may only have reddened gums can also be caused by:

- Trauma to gum
- Pregnancy
- DM
- Smoking
- Stress
- SE of medication e.g. phenytoin
- Diet.

Can lead to receding gums, halitosis, infection, abscesses, or loss of teeth.

- Occasionally patient may have acute ulcerative gingivitis (Vincent's angina) this will need antibiotic treatment.

Care and management

As above, see dentist to clean teeth and address any dental problems, also:

- Antiseptic toothpaste and mouth washes
- Smoking cessation (🕮).

Sore throat (including laryngitis and tonsillitis)

70% sore throats have viral cause and 90% resolve in a week, antibiotics unnecessary for most patients. Patients c/o pain on swallowing, fever. Adolescents with persistent sore throat possibility of glandular fever.

Care and management

- Pain relief and antipyretics.
- ↑ fluid intake and try aspirin (not in <16yo) or salt gargles.
- Laryngitis as above, recommend resting voice and steam inhalations.

- NICE 2001 guidelines recommend antibiotics *if* evidence of systemic illness 2° to the sore throat, unilateral peritonsillitis, a history of rheumatic fever or patient is at ↑ risk of acute infection e.g. immunodeficiency or child with DM.
- Patient with tonsillitis may be considered for tonsillectomy if patient has >4–6 episodes of sore throat/tonsillitis per year, effects interfere with normal functioning and schooling.

Sinusitis

This is an acute or chronic inflammation of sinuses >90% of patients with maxillary sinusitis will clear in <1week without antibiotics. Frontal sinusitus is associated with brain absess and cavernous sinus thrombosis, and should ∴ be treated with amoxicillin or erthromycin. It is more common in adults and those with nasal abnormalities, cystic fibrosis, allergic rhinitis, and smokers. Acute sinusitis may follow upper respiratory tract infection, although 10% may come from dental problems. Characterized by:
- Acute headache and facial pain often worse bending or coughing
- Fever
- Blocked nose and/or purulent discharge
- Loss of smell and taste.

Care and management
- Stopping smoking and avoiding smoky environments
- Pain control
- Decongestant nose drops or sprays
- Steam inhalations
- ENT referral for chronic sufferers for surgery to drain sinuses.

Allergic rhinitis (including hayfever)

Characterized by an irritation and inflammation of nose and eyes. Common disorder, often seasonal or perennial triggered by allergens affecting 16% of the UK population. Incidence ↑. Hayfever: is an allergic rhinitis caused by pollen. Sufferers may experience:
- Blocked stuffy nose, like having a permanent cold
- Allergic conjunctivitis/itchy watery red eyes
- Hayfever sufferers may have wheeze
- Headaches and ear ache
- Sleep disturbed and snoring
- Poor concentration
- ↓ sense and smell.

Care and management
- ↓ exposure to possible allergens (hay fever common causes grass pollen and silver birch pollen).
- Steam and inhalations may provide temporary relief.
- Medication: low dose steroid nasal sprays and nose drops but need to be used on a daily basis. Decongestants also helpful but short-term use only (BNF 12.2.1, 12.2.2). Check patient understands how to apply correctly or application will not effective.
- Antihistamine medication e.g. loratidine 10mg od (BNF 3.4.1) is more effective for hay fever, treatment should begin 2–3wks before pollen season: see ⊞ BBC pollen index www.bbc.co.uk/weather/pollen
- Consider referral to allergy clinic for testing and specialist review.

Related topics
📖 Deafness; 📖 Asthma; 📖 Eczema/dermatitis; 📖 Allergies.

Further information for health professionals
🖳 Clinical Knowledge Summaries (Prodigy) guidelines and PILs on all of the above: www.cks.library.nhs.uk

Adrenal disorders

The adrenal gland produces adrenaline and noradrenaline. The steroids have 3 main functions: virilization, conversion of tissue proteins to glucose, and salt and water retention. Adrenocortical disorders include:

Cushing's syndrome

Caused by high levels of adrenocortical hormones. In the majority of cases this is the result of the administration of prednisolone or other corticosteroids. Other rare causes include a pituitary adenoma. Cushing's syndrome has high morbidity and mortality.

Signs and symptoms

- Redistribution of body fat to create a moon face and truncal obesity
- Hypertension
- Hirsuitism
- Acne
- Bruising and striae
- Osteoporosis
- Glycosuria
- Hyperglycaemia.

Management

Steroids are reduced or stopped. If the cause is not due to prescribed steroids then patient should be referred to an endocrinologist.

Addison's disease

Adrenal cortical insufficiency. Most cases due to surgery, cessation of therapeutic steroids, autoimmune disorders. TB is a major cause outside of the UK.

Signs and symptoms

Early symptoms are:
- Languor
- Debility
- Weight loss
- Pigmentation of the skin and mucous membranes

Can present as a crisis in a coma.

Management and treatment

Referred to endocrinology. Treatment usually involves replacing deficient steroids. Treated patients have a normal lifespan. Advise patients to tell any health professional treating them about their condition and to wear a warning bracelet in case of emergency.

Patient advice and support

Addison's Disease Self-help Group: www.adshg.org.uk

Pituitary disorders

The pituitary gland secretes many hormones (ACTH, ADH, growth hormone, MSH, FSH, LH, TSH, oxytocin, and prolactin) and affects the function of most other glands in the endocrine system. Pituitary disorders are relatively rare in the UK.

Hypopituitarism

↓ production of all pituitary hormones. Caused by tumour, surgery, trauma, and necrosis from postpartum haemorrhage.

Signs and symptoms
- Hypogonadism
- Hypothyroidism
- Debility
- Weight loss.

Management
Referred to neurology or endocrinology. Treatment is lifelong hormone-replacement therapy supervised by a specialist.

Pituitary tumours

These are relatively rare, can affect any part of the pituitary and be either malignant or non-malignant. Many pituitary adenomas are tiny and accidental findings on CT scans. These are usually left and watched.

Sign and symptoms
Associated with pressure effects on surrounding structures, e.g. chronic headache and visual disturbances. Also:
- Hypopituitarism (see above)
- Hyperprolactaemia with associated galactorrhoea
- ↓ libido
- Menstrual disturbances
- ↓ fertility
- Impotence.

Management
Referred to neurology. Treatment options include surgery and radiotherapy. Prolactinomas will be treated medically.

Acromegaly

Hypersecretion of the growth hormone. This is a rare condition (40–60 per million) that has an insidious course over many years.

Signs and symptoms
- Intercranial pressure effects, e.g. headaches.
- Changes in appearance:
  - Coarse, oily skin
  - Change in facial appearance with coarsening of features
  - ↑ foot size
  - ↑ teeth spacing.

- Other effects:
  - Deepening of voice
  - Sweating
  - Paraesthesiae
  - Proximal muscle weakness
  - Progressive heart failure
  - Goitre.

Management

Referred to endocrinologist. Treatment options include surgery and radiotherapy.

Diabetes insipidus

Impaired water reabsorption by the kidney caused either by ↓ ADH secretion or by trauma, tumour, or inherited.

Signs and symptoms
- Polydipsia
- Polyuria
- Dilute urine
- Dehydration.

Management

According to cause.

Patient support and information

☎ The Pituitary Foundation: 0845 450 0375

Further information

▣ The Pituitary Foundation GP Fact files: www.pituitary.org.uk

Thyroid

The thyroid concentrates iodine in order to produce the hormones thyroxine (T_4) and triiodothyronine (T_3). Thyroxine controls many body functions, including heart rate, temperature, and metabolism. It also plays a role in the metabolism of calcium in the body. Thryoid disorders present in 4% of the population.

Enlargement or lumps in the pre-tracheal neck region require medical assessment. Solitary thyroid nodules can be benign (~90%) or malignant (~10%). Goitres are enlarged thyroid glands that can be:
- Physiological (associated with teenagers, pregnancy): do not require treatment.
- Nodular: do not require treatment unless thyrotoxic, compressing other structures, or cosmetically unacceptable.
- Toxic or inflammatory: require treatment and referral to an endocrinologist.

Hyperthyroidism

Affects 2% ♀ and 0.2% ♂. Peak age: 20–49yrs. Graves disease is the most common cause of hyperthyroidism. It is an autoimmune disease associated with smoking and stressful life events in which antibodies to the TSH receptor are produced. Other causes include:
- Thyroiditis
- Amiodarone
- Kelp ingestion
- Toxic nodular goitre: older women with past history of goitre.

Signs and symptoms
- Weight loss
- Tremor
- Palpitations
- Hyperactivity
- Eye changes, exophthalmus
- AF
- Emotionally labile
- Infertility.
In older people symptoms may be less obvious and include confusion, dementia, apathy, and depression.

Management
Referred to an endocrinologist (and ophthalmologist if eye problems). Treatment options include beta-blockers to control symptoms, carbimazole (warn patient to immediately stop taking the drug and seek medical help if they develop a sore throat or other infection) and radioactive iodine (may take 4mths for effects to become apparent). Women of childbearing age should avoid pregnancy during and 4mths after radioactive iodine treatment. Surgery is an option for patients with large goitres or who decline radioactive iodine. Long-term monitoring of thyroid function is necessary.

Hypothyroidism (myxodoema)

A deficiency of thyroid hormones resulting in a lowered rate of all metabolic processes. Common: 10% ♀ >60yrs. ♀:♂ ~ratio 8:1.

Causes

Chronic autoimmune thyroiditis, that occurs after treatment with radioactive iodine, thyroidectomy. Onset tends to be insidious and may go undiagnosed for years.

Patients with hypercholesterolaemia, infertility, depression, dementia, obesity, and other autoimmune diseases, Turner's syndrome or congenital hypothyroidism. should be screened using TFTs.

Signs and symptoms

Non-specific symptoms may include:
- Depression
- Fatigue
- Lethargy or general malaise
- Weight gain
- Constipation
- Hoarse voice or dry skin/hair
- Mental dulling.

Management

Lifelong replacement of thyroxine. If <65 and healthy, 100mcg of thyroxine is prescribed and TFTs re-checked after 6wks. Once TSH is within the normal range then TFT is monitored annually. If >65 or pre-existing heart disease, has 25mcg of thyroxine and dose ↑ every 4wks, according to TFTs. Patients taking thyroxine replacement are entitled to apply for free prescriptions (Prescribing 📖).

Related topic

📖 Hyper- and hypocalcaemia

Patient information and advice

🖳 British Thyroid Foundation: www.btf-thyroid.org

Hyper- and hypocalcaemia

Also see 📖 Thyroid; 📖 Common musculo-skeletal problems.

Most of the calcium in the body is in bone and needed for constant renewal. Calcium is important in normal neuro-muscular activity and blood coagulation. Check calcium levels on an *uncuffed* blood sample to avoid falsely high readings (Peripheral venepucture 📖). Assessment of serum calcium concentration includes consideration of serum albumin levels (Biochemical and haematological values 📖).

Hypocalcaemia

↓ level of serum calcium.

Causes

Hypoparathyroidism (may be 2° to thyroid or parathyroid surgery), insensitivity to parathyroid hormone, osteomalacia, overhydration, pancreatitis.

Signs and symptoms

- Tetany
- Neuromuscular excitability
- Carpo-pedal spasm (wrist flexion and fingers drawn together).

Management

Calcium supplements prescribed and referred to specialist for investigation of cause.

Hypercalcaemia

↑ level of serum calcium (>2.6mmol/L).

Prevalence

~ 1:1000.

Causes

1° hyperparathyroidism, malignancy (10% tumours), chronic renal failure. More rarely: familial benign hypercalcaemia, milk alkali syndrome (high use of antacids for indigestion), thyrotoxicosis, vitamin D treatment.

Signs and symptoms

Often very non-specific but can include:

- Lethargy
- Weakness
- Weight loss
- Low mood
- Mild aches and pains
- Nausea.

Management

According to cause.

Anal conditions

Anal itch (pruritis ani) often occurs if anus is moist or soiled, e.g. fissures, incontinence, poor hygiene, contact dermatitis. NB Possibility of thread worm, haemorrhoids (see below).

Care and management: advise on personal hygiene particularly after bowel movement, OTC anaeasthetic cream and avoiding spicy food may help.

NB Any signs of trauma around anus in child should consider possibility of child abuse (Identifying the child in need of protection 📖).

Anal fissure is when anal mucosa is torn, occurs at any age, can be acute or chronic (>6wks), 95% on posterior aspect of anal canal. Patient may complain of severe pain on defaecation, anal spasm, fresh rectal bleeding (noticed on toilet paper). Majority caused by trauma from hard faeces/constipation, other causes include post parturition (anterior fissure), rare causes: include Crohn's disease, anal intercourse, cancer, psoraisis, syphilis, and herpes.

Care and management: aim to ↓ pain, encourage good personal hygiene, treat constipation, high fibre diet, and good fluid intake → soft stools. Warm baths may provide relief. Advise use of topical treatments such as OTC haemorrhoid preparations. Glyceryl trinitrate (GTN) 0.2% ointment: relieves spasm and pain but may cause headaches (BNF 1.7). If no relief refer to GP for specialist surgical opinion.

Haemmorhoids (piles) approx 50% of people in UK will develop a haemmorhoid at some stage in their life. Occurs when the veins in anus distend and swell. Patients c/o discomfort, fresh red bleeding, feeling of incomplete emptying, mucous, pruritis ani. Risk factors: constipation, straining, pregnancy and related FH, portal hypertension. Classified according to severity:

- 1st degree: small swelling inside the anal canal, not visible external to anus or palpable, most common but may enlarge to become 2nd degree.
- 2nd degree: prolapse from anus (often on defaecation) but spontaneously reduce.
- 3rd degree: prolapse from anus, can be felt as small soft lumps, possible to reduce and push back with a finger.
- 4th degree: permanently prolapsed.

Care and management: as with anal fissures (see above). Encourage patients not to wait to open their bowels. For patients >40yrs if feeling incomplete bowel emptying persists or there is persistent blood in stool or change in bowel habit refer to GP for possible proctoscopy/sigmoidoscopy.

Possible complication of 3rd and 4th degree:
- Thrombosis: intensely painful should be treated with ice packs, analgeasia, and bed rest. May need referral to specialist.
- Strangulation: circulation obstructed by anal sphincter: intensely painful may need hospital admission if unrelieved by analgeasia and ice packs.

Perinanal haematoma due to ruptured peri-anal vein, presents with sudden onset of severe pain and visible 'dark blue berry' under skin next to the anus: treated with analgeasia, settles spontaneously over a week.

Pilonidal sinus obstruction of hair follicles between the buttocks (natal cleft) → foreign body reaction that includes pain, swelling abscess, and or fistula formation often with foul smelling discharge. Most common in teenagers and young adults and more common in ♂. Risk factors include:
• Sedentary occupation (especially if involves long hours driving)
• Obesity
• Persistent irritation or trauma in affected area
• FH.

Care and management: surgery to excise and drain sinus tract. NB Can recur. Post operatively encourage personal hygiene. NB Post operative wounds can take weeks to heal. Alginate dressing then a foam dressing *in situ* to prevent premature closure of wound edges (contraindicated if signs of infection). Progressively reduce foam dressing as wound heals and contracts.

Peri-anal abcess Affects people of any age and is an infection in a peri-anal gland, patients may c/o gradual onset of pain becoming more severe, defaecation and sitting very painful. Requires medical assessment for urgent referral for surgery to drain abscess. NB peri-anal abcess can be difficult to diagnose.

Rectal prolapse Relatively common and people may live with it for years before seeking help. Occurs either in the very young or those >60yrs. In adults there are 2 types:
• Mucosal: bowel musculature stays in position but redundant mucosa prolapses out of the anus: occurs in adults with 3rd degree haemmorrhoids.
• Complete: decent of the upper rectum into the anal canal. Often caused by weak pelvic floor muscles following child birth.
Referred for specialist assessment for surgery or where this is not possible a supporting ring may be used.

Skin tags Seldom cause any problems. Cause unknown.

Anal cancer Squamous cell cancer. Associated risk factors: anal sex, syphilis. Patient may present with bleeding pain, anal mass or ulcer, pruritis and change in bowel habit. Refer to GP for specialist treatment.

Related topic
📖 Constipation in adults; 📖 Faecal incontinence; 📖 Pregnancy; 📖 Wound dressings.

Further information
🖥 Clinical Knowledge Summaries (Prodigy) guidelines: anal fissures, haemorrhoids and piles on pilonidal sinus www.cks.library.nhs.uk
🖥 World wide wounds website: pilonidal sinus disease. www.worldwounds.com

Dyspepsia, gastroesophageal reflux disease, and peptic ulceration

Dyspepsia

Very common, characterized by recurrent epigastric pain, heartburn, or acid regurgitation, can include bloating, nausea and vomiting. Cause often unknown but can be due to gastric oesophageal reflux disease (see below), gastric and peptic ulceration, or rarely cancer. Can also be exacerbated by:

- Medication (e.g. Ca^{2+} agonists, nitrates, theophyllines, bisphosphonates, SSRIs, corticosteroids, and NSAIDs).
- Previous gastric surgery or history of ulceration.

NB People presenting with 'indigestion' may in fact have cardiac pain.

Requires urgent medical assessment if any of the following with dyspepsia:
- Bleeding and/or iron deficiency anaemia.
- Dysphagia.
- Recurrent vomiting and/or weight loss.

Helicobacter pylori (major cause of gastric ulceration) present in approx 50% of UK middle aged population so does not always trigger disease. In patients with non-specific symptoms consider referral to GP for tests (e.g. urea breath test, faecal antigen test) and eradication therapy of antibiotics and anti secretory medication according to set regimen.

Care and management
- Review with patient possible triggers to avoid e.g. medication, particular foods or actions such as bending, posture etc.
- Lifestyle advice e.g. weight loss, smoking cessation, alcohol.
- Self care: antacids and alginates for symptomatic treatment (BNF 1.1).
- If *H. pylori* has been excluded then patient may benefit from low dose proton pump inhibitor PPI (e.g. omeprazole BNF 1.3) for a month following by the use of self-care alternatives e.g. antacids/alginates using antacids as the need arises.
- Eating smaller meals, not eating before bed and propping up bed head can help control symptoms.
- Referred to 2° care patients with unresolved/ongoing symptoms.

Gastrooesophageal reflux disease (GORD)

Heartburn common symptom of GORD can also experience reflux of acid in the mouth, nausea and vomiting, nocturnal cough. Symptoms caused by regurgitation of gastric contents irritating oesophagus. Affects approx. 5% population. Can cause oesophagitis, oesophageal strictures, oeasophageal haemmorhage, and anaemia.

Risk factors
- Foods and drink: fatty foods, alcohol, coffee
- Smoking
- Large meals
- Hiatus hernia (see below)
- Barrett's oesophagus (intestinal metaplasia)

- Obesity
- Pregnancy
- Tight-fitting clothes.

Care and management: see 📖 Dyspepsia, gastroesophageal reflex disease, and peptic ulceration.

Hiatus hernia

Common present in 30% of >50yrs, 50% have GORD. Occurs when proximal stomach herniates/protrudes through a tear or weakness in the diaphragm into the thorax. Major risk factor is obesity.

- Sliding hiatus hernia (80% of sufferers)
- Rolling hiatus hernia where a bulge of the stomach herniates into the chest alongside the oesohoagus.

Care and management: as for dyspepsia and GORD.

Gastritis

Inflammation of the stomach mucosa when there is no ulcer present although may lead to subsequent ulceration if *H. pylori* is the cause. Vitamin B12 deficiency can cause symptoms and certain medication e.g. NSAIDs.

Care and management: as above.

Peptic ulceration

i.e. gastric (GU) and duodenal ulceration (DU).

- GU: usually affects middle-aged and older ♂, may be asymptomatic or c/o epigastric pain made worse with food but helped with antacids and/or lying flat.
- DU affects young/middle aged ♂, can affect any adult, maybe asymptomatic or relapse and remit. Epigastric pain typically relieved by food and worse at night.

Complications

- Bleeding
- Perforation requiring emergency admission
- Pyloric stenosis = scarring from chronic DU: unrelieved and copious vomiting of food refer for 2° care and surgery.

Risk factors

- *H. pylori* (main cause in both types of ulcer >90% in DU)
- NSAID use (in GU) high risk if 3–4x day
- Delayed gastric emptying (GU), rapid gastric emptying, gastric hyperacidity (DU)
- Smoking
- Evidence unclear if stress is a risk factor for DU.

Care and management

- Investigation and treatment (esp if *H. pylori* present) as for dyspepsia
- If possible stop NSAIDs or lower dose or safer option e.g. paracetamol
- Medication PPI or H2 receptor agonist (BNF 1.3)
- Lifestyle advice as above, eat little and often, avoid eating 3hrs before bed
- Once symptoms controlled if patient treated with PPI/H$_2$ receptor agonist, review diet, medication, and symptoms annually.
- Referred to 2° care if symptoms persist/unrelieved.

Further information for health-care professionals

📖 NICE guidelines on managing adults with dyspepsia in primary care: www.nice.org.uk

Irritable bowel syndrome (IBS)

Extremely common GI problem. 5–19% of ♀ and up to 12% of ♂ although majority will not seek professional help. A remitting and relapsing condition with no cure or known cause. Stress/food intolerance/infection are often thought to precipitate symptoms that can occur at any age though most commonly first presents between 30–50yrs (NB may have had unrecognized symptoms for many years).

Characterized by abdominal pain and change in bowel habit although can include the following:
- Constipation or diarrhoea
- Feeling bloated
- Flatus
- Mucus
- Urgency to open bowels (incontinence if unable to reach toilet in time)
- Feeling of incomplete emptying of the bowel
- Sharp pain in the lower rectum (often relieved with defaecation)
- Nausea/vomiting.

Socially isolating condition that is often misunderstood and not taken seriously by professionals and/or friends and family. People with IBS have poorer QoL compared to those without symptoms.

> ❶ Patient should see GP for confirmation of diagnosis of IBS and to discount other possible causes e.g. colonic cancer, inflammatory bowel disease (Crohn's disease), infection, pelvic inflammatory disease, endometriosis.

Aim of care
- Reassurance: IBS is not a life-threatening condition, support patient and provide information about condition (see below).
- Reduce incidence and impact of symptoms on patient's life.

Care and management
Information, reassurance, and lifestyle changes are often sufficient for many IBS sufferers.
- Review with patient possible triggers (e.g. particular foods, social situations) and plan how to avoid these. For some exclusion diets are successful e.g. exclude dairy products/citrus/caffeine/alcohol/gluten/eggs.

General advice
- Some patients find small and frequent meals helps reduce symptoms.
- Healthy diet that is rich in fibre. Probiotics often recommended but evidence weak, consider referral to dietician.
- Smoking cessation (📖).
- Exercise (📖).
- Expert patient programme (📖).

For specific symptoms
- For constipation if diet insufficient: consider bulk forming laxatives.
- For abdominal pain: peppermint oil and antispasmodics e.g. mebeverine (BNF 1.2).
- For diarrhoea: loperamide (BNF 1.4). Sometimes possible to anticipate events and situations that precipitate symptoms and take antidiarrhoeals prophylactically.
- Psychological support: talking therapies/counselling (Talking therapies 📖).

Patients will need specialist referral if symptoms are severe, change and/or do not respond to treatments.

Related topics

📖 Faecal incontinence; 📖 Inflammatory bowel disease; 📖 Colorectal cancer.

Further information for health professionals and patients

📱 Irritable bowel syndrome network offers support and patient information:
www.ibsnetwork.org.uk

📱 Irritable Bowel Syndrome: Clinical Knowledge Summaries (Prodigy) guidelines: www.cks.library.nhs.uk

Inflammatory bowel disease

Ulcerative colitis (UC) and Crohn's disease (CD) are chronic, relapsing inflammatory non-infectious conditions of the gut. Cause is unknown although environmental and genetic factors, infections, and possibly foods are thought to adversely affect susceptible individuals.

> NB no evidence to support disease linked with MMR immunization.

All patients with suspected UC or CD referred to specialist gastro-enterology for assessment.

Ulcerative colitis

(See Table 12.1)
- Approx 1:1000 in UK develop UC.
- Usually begins in the rectum, and for some may only affect the rectum.
- Can develop at any age, majority develop symptoms 15–40yrs.
- 50% of sufferers have mild and infrequent symptoms, 20–30% of patients with severe symptoms will require surgery.

Crohn's disease

(See Table 12.1)
- Any part of the gut wall can be affected from mouth to anus: ileum commonest site. Unlike UC there is unaffected bowel between ulcerated patches of inflammation.
- 1:1500 people affected, ♂>♀.
- Onset of symptoms most common between 15–40yrs.
- 50% of sufferers will have surgical intervention within 10yrs of onset.

> ❶ Emergency referral to hospital by GP if any of the following: severe abdominal pain, severe diarrhoea >8/d and bleeding, dramatic weight loss, fever, and signs of systemic disease.

Care and management

Both conditions are lifelong and characterized by flare-ups and periods of remission. Patients can become socially isolated and depressed. Most patients have ongoing hospital follow-up and the MDT always provides care across 1° and 2° care settings.
- UC: most patients will have symptoms controlled by medication to reduce the impact of inflammation and prolong periods of remission. Mainstay of treatment are 5-ASA derivatives, aminosalicylates e.g. mesalazine and steroids e.g. prednisolone (BNF 1.5). CD patients receive similar medication regimen NB NSAIDs can exacerbate symptoms.
- Surgery: for CD to remove damaged part of the colon and/or as for UC when symptoms cannot be managed medically → ilestomy/ileoanal pouch.
- Advise patients on SE of steroid treatment and consider increased risk of osteoporosis (📖).
- Diet: Advise on healthy diet important to maintain fluid intake during bouts of diarrhoea, frequent eating can exacerbate pain and discomfort during acute phases of disease. Patients may need supplements to correct problems of malabsorption. Enteral feeds can be used for people with CD to rest the bowel.

Table 12.1 UC and CD symptoms vary according to extent and severity of inflammation

Ulcerative colitis	Crohn's disease
• At any time 50% will be asymptomatic	• Diarrhoea often with blood and mucous, mouth ulcers
• **Mild**: 30% have mild symptoms, usually limited to rectum (proctitis) with diarrhoea and or rectal bleeding may be mistaken for haemorrhoids	• Abdominal pain, weight loss
	• Fever and general tiredness
	• Peri-anal sores and/or abscess with discharge (may be first indication of CD)
• **Moderate**: symptoms more severe with frequent stools with blood (4–6 liquid stools a day), pain relieved with defaecation. General tiredness, fatigue, weight loss. Other symptoms may occur: skin rashes, uveitis, arthritis, inflammation of the liver	• Can also have related symptoms that included uveitis, pain, arthritis, skin rashes liver inflammation
	• Complications include: strictures caused by scar tissue = impedes the passage of food → pain and vomiting
• **Severe**: profuse diarrhoea, bleeding, high fever, abdominal tenderness and distention, tenesmus (constant desire to defaecate). ↓ appetite and weight, fatigue	• Perforation of the gut wall (potentially life threatening)
• Severe episodes uncommon but can cause serious illness, danger of perforation or haemmorhage (requiring surgical intervention)	• Creation of fistulas (often peri-anal between colon and other organs = leakage). People with CD have a small ↑ risk of cancer
• Patients with UC have an increased risk of developing cancer	

- Smoking cessation (📖).
- For constipation in UC: bulk forming laxatives.
- For diarrhoea: loperamide or codeine phosphate (BNF 1.4).
- Patients who have had ileal resection will need B12 levels checked and possible supplementation.
- Women should be advised on family planning ideally to avoid pregnancy when disease active. NB Oral contraceptive pill weak evidence trigger for CD, non-oral methods should be considered. Mirena® (BNF 7.3.2) contraception of choice.
- Expert patient (📖) programme.
- Psychological support: talking therapies (📖).

Related topics

📖 Faecal incontinence; 📖 Irritable bowel syndrome; 📖 Colorectal cancer; 📖 Constipation in adults.

Further information for health professionals and patients

📖 Crohn's organization: www.crohns.org.uk
📖 Digestive disorders foundation: www.digestivedisorders.org.uk
📖 PILs on ulcerative colitis and Crohn's disease. Clinical Knowledge Summaries (Prodigy) guidelines www.cks.library.nhs.uk

Coeliac disease

Common autoimmune GI disease; UK prevalence approx 1:300 (many undiagnosed). Lifelong inflammatory disease of the upper small intestine triggered by eating gluten: protein found in wheat, rye, and barley (occasionally oats). Occurs at any age, causing villous atrophy → malabsorption problems. Peak occurrence in childhood. Then further peak in mid-adulthood.

Risk factors
- Environmental
- FH (risk increases 1:10 if family member has coeliac disease).

Patients are often either asymptomatic or have non-specific symptoms. The following summarizes how coeliac disease can present:
- *Infants and children*: in babies being weaned may fail to thrive, suffer from diarrhoea and vomiting and be generally pale and irritable with swollen abdomen. Older children may present with loss of appetite, anaemia and vitamin deficiencies, may have steatorrhoea. NB Lack of growth may be most significant symptom.
- *Adults*: majority c/o tiredness and fatigue, weight loss, and bowel symptoms e.g. constipation, diarrhoea, flatus. May have mouth ulcers, sore tongue and mouth. Some patients develop dermatitis herpetiformis (itchy skin condition) and/or osteoporosis related bone pain.

Associated health issues and complications
- Due to of malabsorption of calcium ↑ risk of osteoporosis.
- Link between coeliac disease and type 1 diabetes and hypthyroidism.
- Small ↑ risk of GI malignancy, reduced after gluten free diet for 3–5yrs.
- Lactose intolerance: common in undiagnosed people once inflammation of the intestine subsides then intolerance usually goes.

All people with suspected symptoms of coeliac disease will need referral for specialist assessment and confirmation of diagnosis.

Care and management
Gluten-free diet will give complete remission from symptoms within weeks. Patient will need to remain on a gluten-free diet for life.
- Reassure that there is a wide choice of alternative gluten-free foods and refer to dietician for specialist support and advice.
- Patient may initially need vitamin supplements.
- ♀ planning a family should have folic acid until 12wks gestation.
- Skin symptoms can take up to a year to settle.

Related topics
📖 Irritable bowel syndrome; 📖 Inflammatory bowel disease.

Further information for health professionals and patients
📓 Coeliac UK: www.coeliac.co.uk

Colorectal cancer

Lifetime risk 1:25. Incidence increases with age and 99% occurs in people >40yrs. 2nd biggest cause of cancer death in Scotland.

Risk factors
- Inflammatory bowel disease
- FH
- Previous history of colorectal cancer
- Possibly diet: diets high in animal fat and protein and low in fibre may increase likelihood of colorectal cancer.

Screening
Faecal occult blood testing to detect patients with the early stages of the disease increases survival rates (UK screening programmes 📖).

Patients should receive an urgent referral for specialist hospital assessment if they present with any of the following and especially if a FH.

- Patients >40yrs with rectal bleeding with change in bowel habit involving looser stools and/or increased stool frequency for 6wks or more.
- Patients >60yrs with rectal bleeding for 6wks+ but without change in bowel habit.
- Patients >60yrs with change in bowel habit to looser stools for >6wks without rectal bleeding.
- ♂ of any age c/o anaemia and a Hb of 11g/100mL or below.
- Non-menstruating ♀ with unexplained iron deficiency anaemia and Hb of 10g/100mL or below.
- Patients c/o abdominal or rectal mass.

Care and management
Treatment usually surgical, also radiotherapy and/or chemotherapy. Care provided by MDT.
- Patient education, support, and advice: patients with tumour confined to bowel wall have >90% chance of survival.
- Genetic advice for family members and possible referral for screening e.g. colonoscopy.
- May have stoma postoperatively.
- May benefit from review of diet and referral to dietician.
- Advise on smoking cessation and diet.
- Link to support organizations (see below).
- Consider referral to community palliative care services for patients with advanced disease.

Related topics
📖 Faecal incontinence; 📖 UK screening programme.

Further information for professionals and patients
🖳 British Association of Cancer United Patients: www.bacup.org.uk
🖳 Clinical Knowledge Summaries (Prodigy) guidelines on cancer of the lower bowel: www.cks.library.nhs.uk
🖳 SIGN management of colorectal cancer: www.sign.ac.uk

Appendicitis, diverticulitis, hernias, and intestinal obstruction

Appendicitis

Infection in the appendix. Most common surgical emergency in the UK. Affecting mainly people aged 10–30yrs. Always requires emergency admission (although 50% suspected appendicitis admissions turn out to be something else e.g. UTI, food poisoning, ectopic pregnancy, diverticulitis, or false alarm). Complications can include peritonitis from perforation, abscess and ♀ infertility.

NB Symptoms and signs may be atypical in children, pregnancy, and older people.

Commonly patient will c/o:
- Abdominal colicky pain becoming progressively worse and more constant and localising in right iliac fossa, worse on walking and movement (may walk stooped)
- Tenderness and guarding when palpated
- Dysuria, may be blood or leucocytes in urine
- Nausea and vomiting
- Anorexia
- Fever and generally flushed and unwell
- May have nausea and vomiting

Requires medical assessment and emergency referral.
- ♀ childbearing age consider ectopic pregnancy and test to exclude.

Diverticulosis

A common condition that occurs when colon wall is weaker in some areas than others and small 'pouches' (ie. diverticula) are forced outwards through the outer layer of the colonic wall. Common in >30% of people >60yrs, the majority have no or only mild symptoms. Diagnosis confirmed through endoscopy or barium enema. Predisposing factors include low roughage diet, history of constipation and increasing age. Encourage patients to:
- ↑ fibre and fluid intake (may benefit from bulk forming agents e.g. bran, ispaghula, and methylcellulose)
- ↑ activity will ↓ constipation
- Anti spasmodic medication and peppermint oil can ↓ colicky pain.

Diverticulitis

Occurs when there is infection and inflammation precipitated by faeces trapped in the diverticula and bacterial infection. A complication of diverticulits is peritonitis. Patient c/o:
- Altered bowel habit
- Abdominal colicky pain
- Nausea and flatulence (may be improved with defaecation).

Requires medical assessment. Acute diverticulitis treated with antibiotics (e.g. co-amoxiclav), painkillers, anti spasmodics, laxatives, and diet. In severe cases or patients at higher risk (e.g. older person, someone who is immunosuppressed) may be admitted to hospital. Diverticulitis recurs in up to a third of cases, advise on diet and prevention as above.

Hernias

Occurs when there is an abnormal protrusion of peritoneal contents through a weakness in the abdominal wall. Common problem: inguinal hernia most common, occurs in ♂>♀, and at any age. May be precipitated by a chronic cough, constipation, urinary obstruction, heavy lifting previous abdominal surgery. Patient c/o:

• Lump in the groin which in ♂ can track down into the scrotum
• Discomfort when straining or standing for long periods.

Requires medical assessment. Usually requires surgery, high success rate with little recurrence advised because hernia may enlarge and ↑ discomfort, risk of strangulation → emergency surgery. Small hernias may not require surgery. Trusses are used for patients who are a poor surgical risk or are awaiting surgery. Lifestyle advice: to maintain ideal weight, healthy diet and learn correct lifting and handling procedures.

Hiatus hernia

See 📖 Dyspepsia gastroesophageal reflux disease, and peptic ulceration.

Incisional hernia (post abdominal surgery)

Bulging at the side of operation site occurs when there is a breakdown of the muscle closure at an abdominal wall. Late complication in up to 10% of surgical cases. May have been preceded by wound infection or haematoma. Does not always need surgical intervention. If causing pain, discomfort or risk of obstruction or strangulation then referred to 2° care for surgical review/treatment.

Umbilical hernia

Most common in infants, in adults may present as a bulge next to the umbilicus. Requires medical assessment and referral for surgical assessment, as strangulation or obstruction risk is high.

Intestinal obstruction

Arises from mechanical obstruction or failure of peristalsis, Types:

• Obstruction external to bowel: e.g. adhesions, volvulus, external malignancy, strangulated hernia.
• Obstruction internal to the bowel: e.g. cancer of the bowel, infarction, inflammatory bowel disease, diverticulitis.
• Obstruction in the lumen: constipation/impaction, large polyps, intussusception, swallowed foreign body, gallstone ileus.
• Ileus functional obstruction: e.g. post op, DM, uraemia, anticholinergic drugs.

Patient c/o anorexia, nausea and vomiting, abdominal pain and distention, though no guarding or rebound, uncomfortable, and restless.

Requires urgent medical assessment and referral for surgical intervention.

Related topics

📖 Irritable bowel syndrome; 📖 Inflammatory bowel disease; 📖 Food poisoning.

Further information for health professionals and patients

📖 NHS Clinical Knowledge Summaries (Prodigy) Guidelines for diverticulosis and diverticulitis: www.cks.library.nhs.uk

Problems of the liver, gallbladder, and pancreas

See also 📖 Hepatitis.

Cirrhosis

Characterized by fibrosis/scarring of the liver due to progressive cumulative damage. More common in people >40yrs and in ♂, 3000 deaths a year. Uncertain prognosis: 50% living for >5yrs. Causes can include:

- Excessive alcohol intake (misconception this is the only cause)
- Chronic hepatitis B or C infection
- Autoimmune chronic active hepatitis
- Active hepatitis
- Primary biliary cirrhosis and other chronic diseases of the bile duct e.g. sclerosing cholangits, biliary atresia in children
- Congenital disease
- Prolonged exposure to drugs or toxins
- Vascular disease.

Patients with cirrhosis can be asymptomatic, but they may experience:

- Anorexia
- Lethargy, fatigue, and general feeling of being unwell
- Nausea and vomiting.

In the later stages of the disease:

- Jaundice
- Itching
- Ascites and oedema
- Haematemesis (see below)
- Confusion arising from encephalopathy
- Weight loss
- Hepatomegaly.

Patient requires specialist gastroenterological care. Complications include hypertension, liver cancer, liver and renal failure. Ongoing care:

- Avoid alcohol and advice on diet and nutrition: refer to dietician
- Pruritis (itching) may be relieved by colestyramine (BNF 1.9.2)
- Ensure flu and pneumoccal immunization.

To reduce the risk of developing cirrhosis patients should be advised to:

- Drink alcohol within normal limits
- Safe sex to avoid risk of hepatitis B
- Consider immunization against hepatitis A and B.

Portal hypertension

Consequence of chronic liver disease/cirrhosis. Other rarer causes are parasitic disease (common in middle east), pancreatic disease, and clotting disorders. BP ↑ in portal vein which carries blood from bowel and spleen to liver → collateral circulation. Causes oesophageal varices, that can ooze blood causing anaemia, maleana or hemorrhage and/or haematemesis. Early treatment of varices can be very effective but bleeding is a medical emergency.

Treatment analgesia, calamine lotion, and as other viruses e.g. rest, fluids. May result in postherpetic neuralgia for some time after. Eye involvement requires urgent medical assessment and referral to specialist.

- Herpes simplex HSV 2: genital (Sexually transmitted infections 📖).
- Herpes simplex HSV1: commonly causes cold sores, herpetic stomatitis and keratitis. Prodromal period (<6hrs) of tingling or itching, small vesicles appear, persist for a few days, then dry forming yellowish crust. Healing occurs 8–12d after onset. Remains dormant in nerve ganglia, recurrent eruptions can occur triggered by sunlight, illness, stress or unknown. Cold sores can be treated in prodomal phase by OTC topical aciclovir. Eye involvement requires medical assessment and referral to specialist Can cause severe infections e.g. in patients with eczema or immunosuppression requiring systemic treatment as inpatient.

Glandular fever (infectious mononucleosis)

Caused by Epstein–Barr virus. Most common in teenagers and young adults. Characterized by high temperature, sore throat, malaise, fatigue, and swollen lymph glands. Diagnosis through symptoms and blood test (FBC and Paul Bunnell and/or glandular fever antibodies). Treated with rest, fluids, and paracetamol. May last some months.

Further information

📖 HPA A–Z Seasonal Influenza: www.hpa.org.uk
📖 NICE (2005). *Guidance on the use of Zanamivir (Relenza®), oseltamivir and amantadine in the treatment of influenza.* www.nice.org.uk

Further information for patients

📖 Herpes Virus Association: www.herpes.org.uk

Meticillin-resistant *Staphylococcus aureus* (MRSA)

Staphylococcus aureus is a Gram positive bacterium which is carried as a skin commensal by about 30% of the population, usually in moist sites such as nose (anterior nares), axillae, and perineum. It causes infections such as boils and styes and is the commonest cause of wound infections.

Most strains are resistant to penicillin and some strains are resistant to several classes of antibiotics, including meticillin (flucloxacillin), these are known as MRSA.

> MRSA is not a notifiable disease but MRSA bacteraemias must be reported as part of a national surveillance programme. In England and Wales, the numbers of reported cases of MRSA bacteraemias as a proportion of all *Staphylococcus aureus* bacteraemias are among the highest in Europe, at around 40%.

Some strains of MRSA have a particular ability to spread and cause epidemics; referred to as EMRSA. There are now 17 different types of EMRSA. EMRSA 15 and 16 are the most prevalent in the UK. EMRSA 15 is particularly associated with colonization of chronic wounds and urine whilst EMRSA 16 causes invasive infections such as pneumonia.

MRSA poses therapeutic challenges because some strains are sensitive only to vancomycin. However, strains with intermediate-level resistance to vancomycin (VISA) have now emerged, so the prevention of cross-infection is paramount.

Infection control measures

The spread of MRSA can be prevented by:

* Hand washing, hand washing, and more hand washing (with liquid soap), especially after giving patient care, and after removing protective clothing (gloves and aprons).
* Judicious use of antibiotics (according to local policy).
* Aseptic handling of catheters or any invasive device/procedure.
* Cleaning equipment after use (hot, soapy water is best).
* Covering patients' wounds and pressure sores and skin lesions on staff or patients with an impermeable dressing.
* Controlled handling of contaminated dressings and linen.
* Washing laundry at 65°C.

Patients who are colonized with MRSA can come home from hospital or go to a care home if their general condition allows. PHCT and care home staff should be informed of patient's status.

In the UK 4–7% of older residents in nursing homes are colonized with MRSA but clinical infections in such settings are uncommon. For those who have open lesions, invasive devices, or catheters, a single room, with a wash hand basin is preferable although sharing with another resident who has MRSA would be acceptable.

The Community Infection Control Nurse can help to evaluate the risk to other residents and provide advice on infection control measures. Staff who require treatment for MRSA carriage should follow local policies and be referred to their GP.

Related topics

📖 Personal protective equipment; 📖 Wound assessment; 📖 HIV; 📖 TB.

Further information for health professionals

📖 European Antimicrobial Resistance Surveillance System data. Accessed at: www.earss.rivm.nl/pagina/interwebsite/home_earss

Viral hepatitis

Hepatitis is inflammation of the liver. Viral infection is responsible for around half of all cases of acute hepatitis and is a notifiable disease (Infectious disease notification 📖). Incidence of about 100,000 cases annually in the UK.

Hepatitis A (HAV)

- *Spread*: faecal-oral route. Patients are infectious 2wks before feeling ill.
- *Incubation*: 2–7wks (average 4wks).
- *Risk factors*: travel to high-risk areas, living or working in an institution, poor hand hygiene, poor access to toilet and hand washing facilities, IV drug use, high-risk sexual practices.
- *Signs and symptoms*: may be asymptomatic (especially young children); fever; ↓ appetite; nausea ± vomiting; pale stools ± diarrhoea; fatigue; jaundice; dark urine; abdominal pain.
- *Investigations*: LFTs, hepatitis serology.
- *Management*: supportive. Advised to avoid alcohol until LFTs are normal. Most recover in <2mths. There is no carrier state and hepatitis A does not cause chronic liver disease. After infection immunity is lifelong.

Prevention

Vaccination is indicated for travellers (Travel health care 📖) to high-risk areas, people with chronic liver disease or working in high-risk situations. Hepatitis A vaccine (and combined with typhoid) is a single dose with booster 6–12 months later.

Hepatitis B (HBV)

Common. Endemic in much of Asia and the Far East.

- *Spread*: infected blood, sexual intercourse, mother to newborn; human bite.
- *Incubation*: 6–23wks (average 17wks).
- *Risk factors*: travel to high-risk areas; babies of infected mothers; sexual partners of infected patients or patients with high-risk sexual practices; IV drug users; healthcare workers.
- *Signs and symptoms*: may be asymptomatic or present with fever, malaise, fatigue, arthralgia, urticaria, pale stools, dark urine, and/or jaundice.
- *Investigations*: LFTs, hepatitis serology.
  - HBsAg is present from 1–6mths post-exposure. If present >6mths after the acute episode defines carrier status.
  - HBeAg suggests high infectivity. Present from 6wks–3mths after acute illness.
  - Anti-HBs antibodies appear >10mths after infection. Imply immunity.
- *Management*: advised to avoid alcohol. Refered for specialist advice. Treatment is supportive for acute illness. Chronic hepatitis is treated with interferon and lamivudine with varying success.
- *Prognosis*: ~85% recover fully, 10% develop carrier status, 5–10% develop chronic hepatitis—may lead to cirrhosis and/or liver carcinoma.

Prevention
- Advise patients re: 'safe sex'.
- High-risk groups (including health workers) immunized. MSM offered immunization at first visit to sexual health services (See also Targeted immunization in adults 📖).
- Passive immunization with human immunoglobulin is used to protect non-immune high-risk contacts of infected patients.

Hepatitis C (HCV)

Common—a major cause of liver damage. Most patients unaware. Treatment can clear virus in >50%.
- *Spread*: contact with infected blood; mother → baby. *Not* easily spread through sexual contact. In 10% no source of infection is identified.
- *Incubation*: 2–25wks (average 8wks).
- *Patients at high risk of infection and should be offered HCV test*: unexplained jaundice, ever an IV drug user, blood transfusion pre-1992 or blood products pre-1986, had dental or medical treatments in countries with poor infection control, child of HCV mother, regular sex with HCV+ person, accidental exposure to blood, has had tattoos, piercings, acupuncture etc where infection control poor.
- *Signs and symptoms*: as for HBV often asymptomatic.
- *Screening*: anti-HCV antibody detectable 3–4mths post-infection. Positive antibody results are followed by HCA RNA blood test. Positive antibody test advised not to donate blood or carry organ donor cord. Positive HCA RNA referred to specialist.
- *Treatment*: referred to specialist. Advised to avoid alcohol and how to avoid infecting others.

Hepatitis E (HEV)

- *Spread*: faeco-oral route.
- *Incubation*: 2–9wks (average 40d).
- *Risk factors*: travel to developing countries (especially pregnant women).
- *Symptoms and management*: similar clinical presentation to HAV infection. Diagnosis is made after serological confirmation. Treatment is supportive. There is no chronic state. No vaccine exists. Mortality in pregnancy can be as high as 20%.

Further information

📓 DH: *The Green Book: immunization against infectious disease*. www.dh.gov.uk
📓 Health Protection Agency (HPA) Topics A–Z: Hepatitis A, B, C, E www.hpa.org.uk
📓 NHS Hepatitis C awareness web site: www.hepc.nhs.uk ☎ Information Line on 0800 451451

Pandemic Influenza

Pandemic influenza is different from seasonal influenza. Caused by a novel influenza virus type A spreading rapidly to people, who are unlikely to have any immunity, covers large geographical areas and a significant proportion of the population in each country. Likely to have more severe effects than seasonal flu. e.g. 'Hong Kong flu' of 1968–9 estimated to have caused a million deaths across the globe. Transmission by droplet. Can occur at any time of the year. No vaccine is available until the virus has been identified (and may take 4–6mths to develop), likewise current anti-virals may or may not be effective.

Pandemic threat

Recent pandemic viruses thought to originate in birds through the spread of the highly pathogenic avian flu (A/H5N1) to humans involved in close contact with poultry. Intercontinental virus spread is rapid e.g. severe acute respiratory syndrome (SARS) in 2003 affected 8000 people in 30 countries across 6 continents in 4 mths, and 900 people died. Another pandemic is likely although when can't be predicted, may come in several waves. Estimates that 14.5 million will be affected in UK. UK part of international network of flu surveillance to monitor evolution of flu virus and detect anything unusual. DH England coordinates the pandemic alert status for the UK.

Preparation and action in a pandemic

UK has flu pandemic contingency plans. A key principle is *social distancing* in order to slow down spread and give more time for vaccines and anti-virals to be developed. May include:
- Voluntary home isolation of cases
- Voluntary quarantine of contacts of known cases
- Restrictions of mass gatherings
- Travel restrictions
- School closure.

Each PCO and general practice has local contingency plans. These plans are activated on identification of the new virus in the UK. Each GP practice is advised to have a named flu coordinator in order to plan for:
- Clinical management of patients with influenza
- Management of patient demand, including those without influenza
- Priority vaccination programme as directed by CMO
- Minimizing risk of infection spread.

In the event of a pandemic many primary care nurses are likely to be directed to work specifically on the implementation of local plans.

Key primary care principles

- Those with or likely to have flu should be kept physically apart from those without flu, where possible e.g. telephone triage, separate waiting area in surgeries.
- Avoid working practices and procedures which risk enhancing transmission of flu.

- Plan for reducing patient movements and contacts e.g. telephone triage, prescriptions collected from pharmacy not surgery.
- Sensible barrier precautions to be used in close contact with a flu-infected patient:
  - Fluid repellent surgical face mask (changed when moist or moving to non-infected patient), aprons to reduce transmission of droplets to clothes, gloves if sufficient supply but not strictly necessary.
  - Coughing and sneezing patients should also use mask in consultations.
- Strict adherence to infection control practices in patient contact e.g. regular and effective hand washing, equipment, premises.

Key advice to patients and public

- To reduce transmission:
  - Cover nose and mouth when coughing or sneezing, using a tissue when possible, dispose of dirty tissues promptly and carefully.
  - Avoid non essential travel and large crowds whenever possible.
  - Maintain good basic hygiene, e.g. wash hands frequently with soap and water.
  - Clean hard surfaces (e.g. door handles) frequently using a normal cleaning product.
  - Make sure children follow this advice.
- On symptoms of influenza: stay at home, do not go to GP or hospital, rest, take plenty of fluids and paracetamol.
  - In uncomplicated illness usually resolves in 7d with rest, fluids, and paracetamol but cough, malaise and lassitude can persist for wks.
  - Pre-existing medical conditions may worsen and require further medical treatment.

Further information

- Department of Health: www.dh.gov.uk/pandemicflu includes contingency planning, infection control in a pandemic, pandemic influenza clinical management guidelines
- Royal College of General Practice. *Helping Practices Plan for a Pandemic* www.rcgp.org.uk
- UK Health Protection Agency: www.hpa.org.uk
- World Health Organization: www.who.int

Tuberculosis: bacterial infection

Tuberculosis (TB) is a serious, but treatable infectious disease caused by inhaling *Mycobacterium tuberculosis*. Transmitted in the air by tiny droplets of mucus and saliva produced when an infectious person coughs, sneezes or talks. 7,000 cases a year in Britain, $\frac{1}{2}$ in London, where rates have doubled in the past decade. Anybody can catch tuberculosis but more likely amongst:
- Socially excluded groups in large cities
- People from areas of the world with a high prevalence of TB
- Homeless/hostel dwellers
- People with a history of imprisonment and/or overcrowding
- Problem drug/alcohol users
- People that are HIV positive/immunocompromised.

Key issues
- Need to prevent the emergence of multi-drug resistant (MDR) TB, which is more difficult and more costly to treat.
- TB is still highly stigmatized and patients can feel isolated and find it difficult to communicate their problems.

Prevention
Bacillus Calmette–Gurin (BCG) immunization is now recommended to:
- All infants living in areas where the incidence of TB is equal to or >40/100,00 (Childhood immunization 🕮).
- Infants whose parents or grandparents were born in a country with a TB incidence of 40/100,000 or higher.
- Previously unvaccinated new immigrants from high prevalence countries for TB.
- Those at risk due to:
  - Their occupation e.g. health-care workers, veterinary staff.
  - Contacts of known cases.
  - Intend to live or work in high TB prevalence countries.

Children who would otherwise have been offered BCG through the schools' programme will be screened for above risk factors. Those who have them are tuberculin skin tested and vaccinated as appropriate (Childhood immunization 🕮).

Apart from infants <3mths, tuberculin skin test by intradermal injection of Mantoux (BNF 14.4) for hypersensitivity to TB prior to BCG. +ve results not given BCG and investigated for TB.

Common symptoms
- Persistent cough, night sweats, fever, loss of appetite, weight loss, and fatigue.
- TB of the lymph glands will cause enlargement of the glands.
- TB affecting other parts of the body (most commonly the kidneys, bones, or joints) causes other symptoms. Children may not have such specific symptoms but may be generally unwell.

Patients presenting in general practice will have the following investigations:
- CXR.
- Sputum samples—keep in the fridge and send for culture (tick AFB, acid-fast bacilli on the form). Culture confirms diagnosis and drug sensitivities.
- Bloods to include FBC, renal, liver, ESR, CRP, + urates.
- Tuberculin skin test +ve (may be –ve in immunocompromised).

Management
- Referred to the TB service, often based at Chest Clinic OPD.
- TB is a notifiable disease (Infectious disease notifications 📖) and this initiates contact tracing by TB specialist nurses (see below).
- Medication prescribed by the TB service to monitor compliance:
  - Most people are completely cured by a course of 3–4 antibiotics for the 1st 2mths. then 2 antibiotics for a further 4mths.
  - Antibiotics used are rifampicin, isoniazid, pyrazinamide, and ethambutol.
  - All have potentially serious side effects (including jaundice) and require blood monitoring.
  - Following 2wks Rx or 3 negative sputums most cases are non-infectious.

Concordance, compliance, and DOT
- Concordance and compliance for the whole length of Rx is very important to prevent further transmission and drug resistance.
- Non-compliance is best managed by directly observed therapy (DOT) in which drugs are taken in the presence of a health professional e.g. primary care nurse—usually on a 3 × weekly regimen.

Contact tracing depends on sputum microscopy. 'Close' usually household contacts are screened first. If transmission is found 'casual' contacts—friends, colleagues, school year groups may be screened.

Related topic
📖 Targeted immunization in adults.

Further information
Key reference
Control and prevention of tuberculosis in the UK: Code of Practice. *Thorax* (2000), **55**, 887–901.

📖 British Thoracic Society: www.brit-thoracic.org.uk
📖 British Lung foundation: www.britishlungfoundation.org
📖 Health Protection Agency Topics A–Z: Tuberculosis: www.hpa.org.uk
📖 Health Protection Agency (HPA) TB and BCG: www.hpa.org.uk
📖 www.immunization.nhs.uk

Food poisoning

(NB See also Home food safety and hygiene 📖.)
>35000 recorded food poisoning incidents each year in England and Wales. Incidents are under reported. Food poisoning is defined as:
'Any disease of an infectious or toxic nature caused by or thought to be caused by the consumption of food or water' (WHO).

Factors which most commonly contribute to outbreaks

- Preparation of food > half a day in advance of needs
- Storage at ambient temperature
- Inadequate cooling
- Inadequate reheating
- Use of contaminated processed food
- Undercooking
- Contaminated canned food
- Inadequate thawing
- Cross-contamination from raw to cooked food
- Infected food handlers and poor hygiene. People do not play a significant role in outbreaks except in *Staph. aureus* food poisoning; they tend to be victims, not sources.

NB Meat and poultry account for 75% of outbreaks.

Notification

All cases of suspected food poisoning are statutorily notifiable. GP notification to environmental health dept of the LA. Providing information about food eaten, signs, symptoms, and incubation period (see Table 12.2) may suggest the micro-organism involved (Infectious disease notifications 📖).

Personal care

- Give symptomatic care and treat signs such as dehydration.
- Do not advise antidiarrhoeal drugs (e.g. kaolin, codeine phosphate, loperamide) as **contraindicated** in children, rarely needed in adults. NB Can aggravate nausea and vomiting and occasionally ileus.
- Antibiotics are rarely indicated, may prolong the carrier state.

Infection control measures

- Hand washing before and after contact with patient and vomit/urine/faeces is essential (applies to family members).
- Handling contaminated material wear PPE e.g. gloves, aprons.
- Discard excreta directly into the drainage system.
- Anyone with gastroenteritis should not attend work or school until free from diarrhoea and vomiting, and, if necessary, clearance tests have been completed.
- Obtain faeces for microscopy and culture if the patient has been abroad, is severely ill, comes from an institution or works as a food handler or has symptoms for >1wk.
- Buy eggs with the Lion stamp on them, indicating they come from poultry flocks vaccinated against *Salmonella enteritidis*.

Related topics
📖 Personal protective equipment.

Further information for health professionals and patients
Department of Health (1994). *Management of Outbreaks of Foodborne Illness*. DoH, London.
🖥 Health Protection Agency (HPA) Infections topics A–Z: www.hpa.org.uk

Table 12.2 Causes and characteristic clinical features of food poisoning

Organism	Common source	Incubation period (hrs)	Signs and symptoms					Duration
			Vomiting	Diarrhoea	Abdo pain	Prostration	Pyrexia	Other	
Bacillus cereus (toxin in food)	Inadequately heated rice	1–16hrs	Profuse	Slight	Often present	Moderately severe	Absent		12–24hrs
Campylobacter jejunii (infection)	Undercooked poultry and meat; unpasteurised milk	3–5d	Slight	Often profuse	Often severe	Often severe	Often present	Blood stained faeces often	Days or weeks
Clostridium botulinum (toxin in food)	Contaminated canned food	12–96hrs usually 18–36hrs	Slight	Absent	Absent	Severe	Absent	Nausea, vertigo, aphonia, respiratory paralysis and death can occur	Death in 24hrs to 8d, or slow convalescence over 6–8mths
Clostridium perfringens (toxin in intestine)	Spores on contaminated meat	8–22hrs	Absent	Moderate	Colicky pains often present	Slight	Absent		24–48hrs
Escherichia coli (infection and toxin)	Undercooked beef and beef products, milk and vegetables	12–72hrs	Slight	Moderate	Slight	Slight	Absent	E.coli 0157 bloody diarrhoea	1–7d

Organism	Common source	Incubation period (hrs)	Signs and symptoms						Duration
			Vomiting	Diarrhoea	Abdo pain	Prostration	Pyrexia	Other	
Listeria monocytogenes	Freshly cut salads, paté, soft cheeses	48hrs 3wks	Slight	Slight	Often present		Present	Pregnant women especially vulnerable	Few days
Norovirus	Contaminated water and food, especially shellfish.	24–48hrs	Moderate	Moderate	Not usually		Present	Person-to-person spread common via contact with faeces and vomit	
Salmonella (infection)	Meat, poultry, eggs, dairy products	6–36 usually 12–24hrs	Slight	Moderate	Often present	Possibly in later stages	Often present	Blood stained faeces in up to 25% cases	1–7d
Staphylococcus aureus (toxin in food)	Cooked food (meat, poultry, fish) and dairy products (custards, creams, trifles)	2–6hrs	Profuse	Slight	Often present	Often severe	Absent		6–24hrs
Vibrio parahaemolyticus (infection)	Seafood	2–48hrs usually 12–18hrs	Moderate	Moderate	Often present	Slight	Absent		2–5d
Vibrio cholerae	Water, seafood	24–72hrs	Slight	Profuse	Often present	Often severe	Often present		

NB Cholera and food poisoning are statutorily notifiable diseases, Public Health (Control of Diseases) Act, 1984

Human immunodeficiency virus (HIV)

HIV is a retrovirus that infects immune system cells particularly the CD4 (T-helper cells) and over a number of years the CD4 cells malfunction and die to a point where they jeopardise immunity. Due to the advancement in treatments the term AIDS (acquired immune deficiency syndrome) is no longer used in diagnosis (although still used for epidemiological purposes).

Transmission

Transmitted through body fluids: seminal, vaginal fluids, including menstrual fluids, breast milk, blood. In the UK most people with HIV are either men who have sex with men (MSM) or people of sub-Saharan African origin. Injecting drug users are also at high risk. Transmission from mother to baby and through infected blood products is very rare in the UK.[1]

Prevention

- Safer sex practices e.g. use of male and female condoms and dental dams (latex sheets for covering female genitalia in oral sex).
- ↓ IV drug abuse and ↓ needle sharing.
- All donated blood screened for HIV.
- Risk ↓ of mother to child transmission by zidovudine given antenatally, during delivery, and to the baby 6wks, elective Caesarian delivery, and not breast feeding.
- PEP (post exposure prophylaxis) is a combination of anti-retroviral medicines stared as soon after possible exposure and taken for 4wks. Available through GUM clinics (genitourinary medicine), ED, and some GPs.

Detection

HIV infection is detected by an HIV antibody test. Available through GUM clinics and some general practices. Test 3mths after possible exposure to ensure true negatives. Early detection ensures treatment at the earliest stage. Pre and post-test information and psychological considerations are important, checklist given in Medfash guide.[1]

Disease progression

Normal CD4 count is 500 cells/mcL.
- *Primary HIV infection*: flu-like symptoms also fever, fatigue, diffuse rash, oral ulceration, diarrhoea. Known as seroconversion illness.
- *Asymptomatic HIV*: follows seroconversion, present for some years.
- *Symptomatic HIV*:
  - CD4 count <200cells/mcL risk of serious opportunistic infection e.g. *Pneumocystis carinii* Pneumonia (PCP), TB, toxoplasmosis, candida, herpes simplex, varicella zoster.
  - CD4 count <100cells/mcL ↑ risk of more serious infections e.g. mycobacterium avium intracellulare, cytomegalovirus and aggressive malignancies e.g. Kaposi's sarcoma.
  - Untreated disease progression leads to wasting and malnutrition, multisystem failure and death.

[1] The Medical Foundation for AIDS & Sexual Health (MedFASH) (2005). *HIV in Primary Care.* www.medfash.org.uk/publications/current.html

Management of HIV infection

Undertaken by specialist teams (and community nursing services when specialist services unavailable). Antiretroviral therapy (BNF 5.3.1) has made an enormous impact on morbidity and mortality (in those countries that can afford it). Involves:

- Antiretroviral therapy (ART) limits HIV replication. Three or more antiretrovirals are used in combination. Adherence essential as HIV mutates easily and cross resistance irreversible. Decisions to start ART are based on CD4 counts and viral load. Side effects common and some are serious.
- Prophylactic antibiotics based on CD4 counts.

Living with HIV infection

Specialist teams and services available to help address a wide range of psychological, emotional, social, as well as physical needs arising from the infection, treatments, and progression of the disease. Primary care services work in partnership as in any long-term condition. Also has health promotion role e.g.:

- Health promotion advice e.g. safe sex practices even when both partners have HIV diagnosis as they are at risk of acquiring drug resistant strain.
- Screening e.g. annual cervical smears as more at risk of malignancies.
- Immunization e.g. annual influenza immunization, hepatitis A immunization for MSM.

Palliative care

While ART has meant that death is much less common, there are still patients who progress through the stages and require all aspects of palliative care (Palliative care in the home 📖).

Further information

📖 British HIV Association HIV Treatment Guidelines (2003). www.bhiva.org

Information and support for patients and public

📖 Aidsmap: www.aidsmap.com ☎ 0207 840 0050
📖 Children with AIDS charity (CWAC): www.cwac.org ☎ 020 7247 115
☎ National AIDS Helpline: 0800 567 123 (24hrs. helpline)
📖 Terrence Higgins Trust: www.tht.org.uk ☎ 0845 1221 200

Common musculo-skeletal problems

Sporting related injuries

Often can be avoided with suitable equipment e.g. knowing your limitations, gradual build up of activity, trainers, good warm up routines, proper training and supervision. As a general principle remember 'RICE'.

- **R**est: rest affected part
- **I**ce: use straightaway to deal with injury (e.g. ice in towel, bag of frozen peas) for 10min max, and analgesia
- **C**ompression strapping and bandaging can be used to help reduce swelling and help prevent acute sprains and strains
- **E**levation.

Muscle and ligament injuries may need referral to GP and/or physiotherapist.

Neck problems

Most neck pain acute but self-limiting within days or weeks. Patients with persistent pain should be referred to GP for specialist assessment. Causes can be multifactoral e.g. arthritis, infection.

> NB Any significant neck trauma requires neck immobilization with a hard collar and referral to ED.

- **Torticollis:** relatively common, can be triggered by poor posture, sleeping awkwardly: A sudden onset of pain due to muscle spasm that immobilizes neck. Self-limiting, treat with heat, gentle mobilization and analgesia.
- **Cervical spondylosis:** degenerative disease of the cervical spine, characterized by intermittant pain often related to exercise and decreased movement. Can cause nerve root pain. Will need diagnosis confirmed, usual treatment: analgesia.
- **Whiplash injuries:** often after RTA: sudden extension of neck → stretches or tears cervical muscles. Pain may occur hrs or days after injury, can radiate to head, shoulders, and arms. Medical assessment to exclude other causes. Treatment: analgesia, early mobilization, and a collar initially not long term. Recovery often slow.

Back pain

(Low back pain 🕮.)

> **Shoulder Problems** ❶ Always consider possibility of pain referred from neck, cardiac ischaemia, PE, gallbladder problems, or subphrenic abcess (i.e. pain arising from diaphragmatic irritation).

- **Frozen shoulder:** affects patients often between 40–60yrs, cause unknown, more common in people with diabetes, painful stiff shoulder with very restricted movement, pain often worse at night. Care: NSAIDs, referral to physiotherapist. May benefit from steroid injections. Recovery often slow with uncertain outcome.
- **Dislocated shoulder:** usually because of a fall, refer to ED for reduction. Recurrent dislocation can occur in teenagers with no history of injury but general joint laxity: referral to physiotherapy and/or GP.

Elbow, wrist, and hand problems

- **Pulled elbow:** common in children <5yrs, a traction injury often occurs when child pulled up suddenly by the hand. Child stops using the arm. Refer to GP.

- Golfer's elbow and tennis elbow: characterized by pain and tenderness: tendon inflammation caused by repeated strain, advise patient to avoid trigger movements, take NSAIDs, often resolves with rest. Physiotherapy and/or local steroid injection may help.
- Ganglion: smooth firm painless swelling usually around the wrist, can resolve spontaneously, no treatment needed unless causing problems.
- Repetitive strain injury: work related upper limb pain often in arm and wrist e.g. related to computer keyboard use. Suggest patient review working posture and habits and involve occupational health to review office equipment. Rest from aggravating activities and then gradually reintroduce, may help to have workstation and physiotherapy assessment.
- Carpal tunnel syndrome: pain, numbness, pins and needles in the fingers due to nerve compression, often worse at night. Symptoms are improved by shaking wrist. Can occur with pregnancy, hypothyroidism, obesity, and carpal arthritis. Symptoms can be helped with night splints and steroid injections. Surgery an option in moderate to severe pain.

Growing pains and leg cramps

- Growing pains: term used for non-specific and diffuse pain in children. May involve child waking at night with leg or arm pain, rubbing the affected limb brings rapid relief. Resolves spontaneously.
- Leg cramps: transient involuntary episode of pain lasting for a few minutes (10min max) cause unknown. Care and management: check not on drugs with SE of cramps, reassure benign, advise passive stretching and massaging of affected muscle. If persist refer to GP.

Ankle and foot problems

- Ruptured Achilles tendon: patient c/o sudden pain in back of ankle 'like a kick' during activity. Walks with a limp and cannot raise heel from floor or stand on tiptoe. Urgent orthopaedic referral.
- Plantar fascitis (burstitis) common cause of heel pain. Worst when person gets out of bed. Suggest shoes with soft padding and support, if pain persistent refer to GP for review.
- Flat feet: normal in young children, painless flat foot where arch is restored when standing on tiptoe does not need treatment. Needs referral if painful and/or not restored on tiptoe.
- Hammer and claw toes: if causing pain, foorwear or mobility problems will need surgery.
- Bunion (hallux valgas) lateral deviation of the big toe exacerbated by wearing high heels and tight fitting shoes, arthritis pads can help but severe deformation will need surgery.
- Ingrowing toe nail: most common in big toe caused by ill fitting shoes and poor nail care. Nail grows into the skin causing pain and inflammation. If infected will need antibiotics. Advise to cut nails straight and with edges beyond the flesh and refer to podiatry. Persistent problems may need referral for surgery.

Related topics

📖 Osteoarthritis; 📖 Rheumatoid arthritis; 📖 Nutrition and healthy eating.

Further information for professionals and relatives

📓 Arthritis Research Campaign: www.arc.org.uk
📓 Clinical Knowledge Summaries (Prodigy) guidelines: musculo-skeletal quick reference guide on leg cramps: www.cks.library.nhs.uk

Bone and connective tissue disorders

Pagets disease of bone
Metabolic disorder, unknown cause that can be asymptomatic. Affects bone growth, bone deformity, weakness, and risk of fracture. Present in 1:10 of older people. Patients may experience:
- Pain or dull ache aggravated by weight bearing but can persist at rest.
- Deformity of the bone, bowing of weight bearing bones e.g. femur. Skull may increase in size and spine may curve.
- May have associated symptoms of nerve compression and pain, disturbed vision and dizziness.
- May have fractures as a 2° complication and osteoarthritis.

> NB Only small proportion experience severe symptoms.

Patient need rheumatology referral for treatment and ongoing management, manage pain with analgeasia.

Rickets/osteomalacia
Caused by vit D deficiency (found in diet oil-rich, fish and margarine with D supplements and sunshine). Rickets is the term used for children and osteomalacia for adults. Characterized by:
- Widespread bone pain and muscle weakness and muscle cramps
- Deformity: e.g. bow legs, pigeon chest, and pelvic deformities
- Pathological fractures
- Dental caries and delayed teeth formation
- Impaired growth and short stature (may not be reversible)
- Low calcium → numbness of extremities: hands and feet

People most at risk of rickets/osteomalacia:
- Older people especially >80yrs and those in residential care
- People with deficient diet and/or little access to sunshine
- Immigrants with pigmented skin
- People with Crohn's disease, coeliac disease and other absorption problems.
Care and management: following diagnosis by blood test, majority treated with vitamin supplements.

Osteomyelitis
Infection of the bone requiring urgent referral to 2° care, *Staph. aureus* most common cause (also *E.coli*, proteus, pseudomonas, TB). May follow systemic infection and/or injury, children and people with DM most susceptible. Complications: septic arthritis, chronic osteo-myelitis chronic infection, bone deformity, and pathological fracture. Characterized by:
- Pain and reluctance to move affected limbs
- Warmth and effusion in affected joints
- Fever and malaise.
Treatment with IV and then po antibiotics and surgery to drain abscesses.

Systemic lupus erythramatosis (SLE)

Rare autoimmune connective tissue disease 1:3000 >♀ onset 15–40yrs higher prevalence in Asian, African, and Polynesian populations. No cure. Affects multiple systems, and has multiple variations in how SLE presents. Majority of patients have skin and joint involvement and often c/o severe fatigue.

- Joints: e.g. arthritis, arthralga
- Skin: hypersensitivity, facial 'butterfly rash', vasculitis, hair loss
- Lungs: pleurisy, pneumonitis, alveolitos
- Kidneys: proteinuria, ↑ BP, glomerulonephritis, renal failure
- Heart: pericarditis, endocarditis
- Central nervous system: depression, psychosis, infarction, fits, psychosis.

Patients will need specialist rheumatology treatment and ongoing care. Steroids are used to control acute episodes (advise on SE of steroids)

Care and management

- Advise patients to avoid direct sunlight (can exacerbate rash)
- Avoid exposure to infections
- Limited evidence about diet, some recommend oily fish and foods low in saturated fat
- Women using contraception should use progesterone only or low dose oestrogen pill or barrier methods: oestrogen can exacerbate SLE.

Raynaud's syndrome

Approx 10m sufferers in UK affecting mainly women. Intermittent ischaemia of the fingers, precipitated by cold and/or emotion. Cause unknown. Fingers are very painful, numb, tingle ache and change colour becoming pale then blue and red on being warmed. 5% may go on to develop other rheumatic disease e.g. SLE and scleroderma (rare disease = skin becomes tight shiny and fibrosed can involve other organs).

Care and management

- Smoking cessation
- Patients with mild symptoms should use thermal gloves, avoid cold and draughts
- More severe symptoms consider medication e.g. vasodilators and serotonin re-uptake inhibitors and specialist referral.

Vibration Induced White Finger people who work with machinery that vibrates are prone to Raynauds, condition is permanent = an industrial disease eligible for compensation.

Related topics

📖 Osteoarthritis; 📖 Rheumatoid arthritis; 📖 Smoking cessation.

Further information for professionals and relatives

📠 Arthritis Research Campaign www.arc.org.uk
📠 Arthritis Care www.arthritiscare.org.uk
📠 National Association for the Relief of Paget's Disease www.paget.org.uk
📠 Raynauds and Scleroderma Assoc www.raynauds.org.uk

Seizures and epilepsy

A seizure or fit is when there is a sudden disturbance of neurological function associated with an abnormal neuronal discharge.
(See also Febrile convulsions 📖).

A careful history is important since fits may take many forms and a first fit has enormous consequences. Use the term 'seizure' to avoid the emotive term of epilepsy unless a specialist diagnosis has already been made.

Epilepsy is recurrent seizures other than febrile convulsions. 60% of adult epilepsy starts in childhood. 456,000 people in the UK have a diagnosis of epilspsy. Diagnosis made on history, clinical examination, and EEG (can be a prolonged process).

Causes
Often none is found but of the known causes:
- Genetic: (20%).
- Physical: trauma and injury, space occupying lesions, raised BP, CVA.
- Metabolic: alcohol withdrawal, drug related, hyper/hypoglyecaemia, hypoxia, electrolyte disturbance.
- Infective: e.g. encepahlitis.

Focal epilepsy: involves one part of the body and may progress to other parts becoming generalized (Jacksonian epilepsy).
Grand mal epilepsy: generalised seizure with sudden onset of tonic contraction of the muscles, often associated with a cry or a moan, falling to the ground. The tonic phase gives way to clonic convulsive movements occurring bilaterally and synchronously, slows and stops, followed by a variable period of unconsciousness and gradual recovery.
Myoclonic epilepsy: a variant of petit mal epilepsy characterised by atonic drop attacks.
Petit mal epilepsy: a pause in speech or other activity and patient is unaware of the episode.
Temporal lobe epilepsy: a disorder with seizures originating from the temporal lobe with numerous, bizarre presentations can include altered perception and oral and auditory hallucinations.
Status epilepticus: a generalized convulsion, lasting 30min or longer, or when successive convulsions occur that the patient does not recover consciousness between them.

Management and support
- Structured care plan and review at least annually.
- Controlled by medication (BNF 4.8.1). In 80% of cases fits are controlled with drugs. Monotherapy wherever possible. Combination therapy if seizures continue. The drug chosen is matched to the individual patient and type of epilepsy. (See Table 12.3.)
- Women: information re. contraception, pregnancy, childcare, menopause.
- Inform patient about counselling services, voluntary organizations, expert patient programme.

Migraine

Migraine is a syndrome characterized by periodic headaches with complete resolution between attacks. Most patients can successfully manage the condition. Most common cause of recurrent disabling headache in the population. NB <1% patients with headaches have a brain tumour.

- ♂ 8%, ♀ 25%; 15% ♀ with migraine have attack around menstruation
- 80% people have their 1st attack ≥30yrs age
- Prevalence ↑ until age 40yrs, then ↓
- Average 13 attacks a year but varies
- Common migraine (without aura) is 3x more common than classical migraine (with aura).

Causes

No accepted aetiology of migraine; possible theories include:
- Vascular
- Neuronal
- Hypothalamic trigger.

Trigger factors

- Emotional and/or physical stress
- Diet/food e.g. sugary foods or long breaks without food
- Environmental e.g. bright lights
- Hormonal.

Signs and symptoms

An attack can include all or some of the following stages:
- Prodrome: change in mood or appetite before migraine onset.
- 10% sufferers experience aura before onset of headache: visual disturbance; motor or sensory disturbance.
- Headache (common migraine): often pulsatile and unilateral, lasts 4–72hrs; moderate/severe intensity may be associated with symptoms of nausea and vomiting, photophobia, phonophobia, aggravated by movement.
- Resolution.

Prevention

- Identify and avoid trigger factors.
- Refer to GP to discuss use of prophylactic medications e.g. Beta-blockers, amitriptyline.

Management and health promotion advice

- Explanation and reassurance to patient, treatable but not curable.
- Offer patient information:
  - Avoiding trigger factors can ↓ frequency by up to 50%
  - Regular sleep pattern and dietary pattern
  - ↓ caffeine and alcohol intake and drink 2L water a day
  - Keep a migraine diary to help identify triggers
  - Review possible environmental triggers e.g. ↓ VDU use.
- Foodstuffs trigger in 20% patients.
- Advise on smoking cessation.
- ♀ who have focal aura contraindication for combined oral contraceptive. (Combined hormonal methods 📖).

Management of acute attack

- 1st line treatments should be taken early in an attack e.g. aspirin, ibuprofen, or paracetamol.
- Anti-emetics e.g. metoclopramide, domperidone relieve nausea and efficacy of the oral analgesics.
- Referral to GP. 2nd line treatments are the triptans e.g. sumatriptan.

For patients with persistent symptoms referral (by GP) to migraine clinic may be an option.

Complementary/alternative therapy: Some evidence that accupuncture and feverfew help migraine.

Related topic

📖 Pain assessment and management.

Further information for nurses, patients and carers

- 🖥 Gpnotebook: www.gpnotebook.co.uk
- 🖥 Migraine Action Association: www.MigraineTrust.org
- 🖥 Migraine Trust www.migraine.org.uk

Common problems affecting eyes

Conjunctivitis

Inflammation of the conjunctiva cause can be infective irritant or allergic unilateral (often if infection present) or bilateral eye most common condition seen in primary care. Characterized by:

- Red sore eye
- Discharge
- Swollen eyelids
- Eyes stuck together after sleep
- Linked to seasonal changes (hay fever) or contact with allergen e.g. cats (allergic)
- Close contact with another affected person (infective)
- Presence of upper respiratory infection (infective)
- In neonates <21d old with purulent discharge possibility of STI related infection from mother. Take swabs for M, C & S, chlamydia. If positive for *N. gonorrhoea* treated with topical antibiotics and referred to specialist.

Care and management

- Most symptoms self-limiting and resolve in 2–5d, maintain good eye hygiene (see below). If symptoms persist may benefit from topical antibiotics e.g. chloramphenicol.
- If infective conjunctivitis advise on not sharing towels, pillows, or face-cloths and good hand hygiene. School and group child care exclusion until treated (Infections diseases exclusion times 📖). Avoid contact lens until no symptoms.
- For people with allergic conjunctivitis treat with antihistamines or topical anti inflammatory (BNF 11.4.2).

Blepharitis

4.5% of all opthamological problems seen in primary care, cause unknown, a chronic persistent condition usually bilateral may be characterized by:

- Sore inflamed eyelids, red rimmed eyes
- Eyelids may stick together in the morning (consider possibility of infection)
- Eyes may feel gritty
- May be scales on eyelashes
- Complain of dry eyes, blurred vision
- Unable to tolerate contact lens.

Care and management

- Good eye hygiene may be all that is needed. Use warm compresses to eyelids and around the eyes to loosen the crusting and cleanse the eye. Advise patient to dilute baby shampoo 3–4 drops in half a cup of warm water or sodium bicarbonate (1tsp in boiled water) and use to cleanse eye with soft cloth 2x daily. Once symptoms improve: 1x daily.
- Gentle massage of the eyelids.
- Advise patients to avoid eye makeup or use water soluble eyeliner.
- Do not use contact lens.
- Avoid rubbing eyes.
- If eyes are persistently dry may benefit from artificial tears (BNF11.8).
- If persists may need specialist referral.

Subconjunctival haemorrhage

Common in older people: a painless localized haemorrhage in the eye that occurs spontaneously. Clears in 1–2wks, consider referral to specialist if history of trauma or edges of haemorrhage cannot be seen

❶ Red eye symptoms that are potentially dangerous should have same day referral to doctor/specialist if one or more following are present:
- Moderate-to-severe eye pain (not surface irritation) and/or photophobia
- Reduced visual acuity
- Inability to move eye
- Visibly dilated blood vessels seen between white of eye and iris. Loss and/or affected sight
- Corneal damage (often only visible after fluroscein staining)
- Absent or sluggish pupil response
- Eye involvement when patient has shingles (herpes zoster)
- History of trauma or post-operatively

Related topics

📖 Blindness and partial sight; 📖 Allergies; 📖 Eye trauma.

Further information for health-care professionals

🖳 Clinical Knowledge Summaries (Prodigy) Guidelines: Eyes, Conjunctivitis, and blepharitis. www.cks.library.nhs.uk

Blindness and partial sight

Affects 2:1000 in UK. Blindness is inability to perform any work where sight is essential. **NB Blindness does not always mean total absence of sight.** Blindness: <3/60 vision (although may be >3/60 if severe visual field defect). Partial blindness: no one definition but implies vision in the range 3/60–6/60.

> ❶ Sudden loss of vision is an emergency needing specialist attention.

Risk factors
- DM
- Smoking
- FH
- Age
- Poor diet
- Hypertension
- Steroid treatments
- Alcohol misuse
- Prolonged exposure to sunlight.

Health promotion for people at risk or with partial sight
- Protect eyes from bright sunlight with sunglasses
- Healthy diet rich in fruits and green leafy vegetables
- Monitor blood pressure
- Smoking cessation
- Eye test every 2yrs.

Age related macular degeneration (AMD)
Cause of blindness in 1:2 people registered blind. Bilateral disease affecting one eye more than the other. Characterized by deterioration of central vision affects reading, face recognition, and ability to see colour.
- Most common form of AMD macula cells decay and disintegrate.
- Emphasize that not all sight will be lost, should be possible to maintain independence *but* reading and television and driving will become impossible.

Cataracts
Occurs when the lens of an eye becomes cloudy, develops gradually, affecting 1 in 3 people >65. Patients may report blurred vision or spots or halos around bright lights and dazzled by car lights. Affects distance judgement.
- Advise patients to have regular eye checks.
- Check patient does not have DM.
- Treatment: when interferes with everyday life routine surgery day case operation. Cloudy lens is removed and is replaced with an artificial plastic lens. Patient will need glasses to adjust for refractive changes.

Chronic simple glaucoma (open angle)

An increase in eye pressure causes damage to the optic nerve. The prevalence of glaucoma rises from 1–2% >40s to 5% >75s. African-Caribbean origin 4x the risk as whites. Initially asymptomatic as peripheral vision is the first to be affected, people often present late. Symptoms include visual loss and sausage-shaped blind spots. Patients will need lifelong follow-up, therefore important:

● All adults with a FH are regularly checked.
● All adults >35–40yrs should have regular eye (every 2–4yrs) checks to detect early glaucoma. >50yrs 1–2yrs. Treatment: aims to reduce eye pressure and prevent further damage to optic nerve. Achieved through:
  ● Eye drops: these will either ↓ amount of aqueous humour or ↑ drainage of aqueous humour. Important that treatment maintained (BNF 11.6).
  ● Surgery: trabeculectomy, creating channel between inside of eye to under conjunctiva.

Retinal detachment

Relatively rare condition: painless loss of vision, like a curtain coming across the vision. Often develop in eyes with retinas weakened by a hole or tear so that fluid seeps underneath, weakening retinal attachment.

● 50% have some premonition with flashing lights or spots.
● Important to have urgent treatment to secure retina (laser or freezing).

Diabetic retinopathy

(Diabetes overview 📖.)

Registering as blind

(Includes people with low vision.) Only 50% of those eligible to register actually do so. The majority of people eligible to register are likely to have low vision.

● Referred to consultant ophthalmologist for assessment to determine eligibility and for referral to social services.
● Eligible for support from LA social worker/rehabilitation officer and specific benefits including income support, disabled parking badge, training in Braille or typing, information about further education and leisure activities.
● Access to equipment and aids to support independent living e.g. talking clocks and books, large button telephones.
● A free radio from the Wireless for the Blind 🖬 www.blind.org.uk
● Free directory enquiries from BT.
● Concessionary travel.
● Free NHS sight tests.
● Free postage on items marked 'articles for the blind'.

Related topics

📖 Common problems affecting eyes; 📖 Allergies; 📖 Eye trauma.

Further information for health-care professionals and patients

🖬 Macular Disease Society: www.maculardisease.org
🖬 Clinical Knowledge Summaries (Prodigy) Guidelines: Clincal speciality: Eyes www.cks.library.nhs.uk
🖬 Royal National Institute for the Blind: www.rnib.org.uk

Pneumonia

Inflammation of the lungs, is usually caused by infection, most commonly *Streptococcus*. Community acquired pneumonia (different from hospital acquired) is very common in the UK, annual incidence about 250,000 cases. Can affect any one but more common and usually more serious in the very young, the very old, smokers, anyone with long-term illness, and those immunocompromised (e.g. those with 1° immunodeficiency, receiving chemotherapy, receiving immunosuppressant drugs, HIV +, or other conditions such as hyposplenism, malnutrition, nephrotic syndrome). Those less seriously affected are managed in the community but about 20% need hospital admission, of these between 6–14% die.

Symptoms

Acute illness characterized by:
- Flu-like symptoms e.g. fevers, shivers, aches, raised temperature
- Cough with usually purulent sputum
- Dyspnoea
- Some have pleural chest pain
- Older people may have acute confusion and/or walking difficulties.

Prevention

- Pneumococcal and influenza vaccination
- Smoking cessation.

Treatment and management

Clinical assessment (may include investigations and pulse oximetry increasingly available in primary care), and decision made as to whether hospital admission required based on severity, social circumstances, and concomitant illness. If patient has one or more of following considered for hospital admission, if 3 or more then urgent admission required:
- Confusion
- Respiratory rate ≥30 breaths/min
- Blood pressure: systolic <90 mmHg; diastolic ≤60 mmHg
- Age ≥65yrs.

When managed at home
- Advised
  - No smoking and other smokers in home to cease
  - Get plenty of rest and drink plenty of fluids
  - Simple analgesia as required e.g. paracetamol.
- Commenced on antibiotics e.g. amoxicillin 500mg–1g tds, (BNF 5.1).
- Should improve within 48hrs. Patient should be reviewed at this point and if deteriorating or not improving considered for hospital referral.

Further information

📖 British Lung Foundation www.lunguk.org
📖 British Thoracic Society (2001). *Guidelines for the management of community acquired pneumonia in adults*, and Update (2004). Also children (2002). www.brit-thoracic.org.uk

Government scheme for compensation Under the Pneumoconiosis etc (Workers' Compensation) Act 1979 if unable to get damages from employer (e.g. out of business). See DWP leaflets or TUC Work smart web site below.

Related topic
📖 Health and safety at work.

Further information
☎ Benefit Enquiry Line: 0800 88 22 00: People using a textphone ☎ 0800 24 33 55
📠 British Lung Foundation: www.lunguk.org
📠 Department of Work and Pensions online and printed guides to all benefits: www.dwp.gov.uk
📠 RIDDOR: www.riddor.gov.uk ☎ 0870 1545500 email: hseinformationservices@natbrit.com
📠 TUC guide to work related injuries and personal injury claims: www.worksmart.org.uk

Lung cancer

About 38,000 people in the UK diagnosed annually with lung cancer. Leading cause of cancer death. Affects more men than women, second leading cause of death in men, after CHD. Smoking and passive smoking cause 90% lung cancers.

• Incidence ↑ with age: 85% aged >65yrs and 1% <40yrs at presentation.
• 20% are small cell lung cancer, the rest are non-small cell mainly squamous cell carcinoma or adenocarcinoma.
• 80% of people diagnosed with lung cancer die within the year as at diagnosis the majority have advanced disease.

Prevention

Smoking cessation (🕮).

Signs and symptoms

• Persistent cough
• Dyspnoea
• Haemoptysis
• Chest/shoulder pain
• Finger clubbing
• Unexplained weight and appetite loss.

Referred for urgent X-ray and to specialist. Investigations may include bronchoscopy, lung biopsy, CT, MRI or other scans.

Stages of lung cancer

Non-small cell lung cancer—4 stages:
1. Localized cancer
2. Cancer in lymph nodes at top of lung
3. Cancer spread to chest wall
4. Metastases.

Small cell lung cancer stages—2 stages:
1. Limited (to nearby lymph nodes)
2. Extensive (metastases).

Treatment and management

Depends on type of cancer. May include:
• Surgery—rarely suitable for small cell lung cancer
• Radiotherapy
• Chemotherapy—standard for small cell lung cancer.

If in advanced stage palliative care offered with full involvement of primary care professionals and palliative care services.

Related topics

🕮 Palliative care in the home; 🕮 Symptom control in palliative care: breathlessness and fatigue.

Further information for professionals

🖪 Management of patients with lung cancer: a national clincial guideline SIGN—Scottish Intercollegiate Guidelines Network (February 2005): www.sign.ac.uk

Further information and support for patients

🖪 Cancer Bacup (British Association of Cancer United Patients): www.cancerbacup.org.uk
☎ Helpline: 0808 800 1234

Renal problems

See also 📖 Urinary tract infection.

Glomerulonephritis

Inflammation of both kidneys that can affect all or part of the kidney's glomeruli. Most common in children, young adults, and men. Can be acute or chronic but can cause renal damage with long-term consequences. Patient may be initially asymptomatic or have vague symptoms e.g. tiredness, more acute symptoms include proteinuria, oliguria, haematuria, oedema, anorexia, and hypertension. Suspected cases need urgent hospital referral but if the inflammation is mild no treatment may be necessary apart from monitoring and tests for proteinuria and U&Es.

Nephrotic syndrome

Proteinuria that leads to oedema and hypoalbuminaemia. Patients have ascites, swelling of the face, peripheral oedema. Also fatigue, anorexia. Due to kidney damage arising from:
- Minimal change glomerulonephritis (90% children, 30% adults)
- Nephropathy: caused by thickening of glomeruli
- Glomerulonephritis
- Scarring of glomeruli (focal segmental glomerulopnephritis)
- DM.

Suspected cases referred for specialist renal care. Prognosis depends on cause, children with minimal change disease respond well to treatment.

Renal stones (renal colic)

Passage of a stone in the ureter or kidney or bladder that causes acute, severe pain that comes in waves. Patients may have haematuria and appear pale and sweaty. Occurs in 0.2% of population, ♀>♂. Believed incidence of stones ↑ because of western diet and obesity, often no underlying cause. Severity of pain unrelated to size of stone. Risk factors:
- People with recurrent UTI
- People with neuropathic bladder dysfunction e.g. paraplegia
- People on certain medication e.g. loop diuretics, thiazides, antacids, aspirin, calcium, vit. D, steroids
- People with congenital kidney abnormalities that cause urinary stasis
- Dehydration
- Patient with ileostomy → increased alkali loss from gut
- FH.

Care and management

Stones usually pass spontaneously, priority is good pain control. Patient will need an emergency hospital admission if fever, pain uncontrolled, has not passed urine, lives alone and/or symptoms persist for>24hrs.
- Pain relief: diclofenac IM (BNF 7.4).
- ↑ fluid intake, and encourage high fluid intake to ↓ risk of recurrence.
- Sieve urine to catch stone for future analysis; composition of stone will guide future dietary advice and interventions to prevent recurrence.

Chronic Kidney Disease (CKD)/Chronic renal failure (CRF)

Progressive loss of renal function over time. Treat causes early to prevent CRF. Incidence ↑ with age. Causes (majority treatable/manageable):

- Diabetes
- Hypertension, vascular disease
- Glomerulonephritis
- Chronic infection and recurrent UTIs
- Obstruction, possibly from renal stones
- Polycystic kidneys
- Hyperlipidemia.

CKD programme prevalence ↑ age, ♂, South Asian, and African Caribbean ethnicity.

- Early identification important to ↓ progression and ↑ risk of CVD and other health problems
- 5 stages CKD based on estimated glomerular filtration rate (eGFR). eGFR included with creatine testing
- Minority of people with CKD 1 or 2 develop more advanced disease
- 5% population have stage 3–5
- CKD stages 3–5 (eGFR <60mL/min/1.73m^2 for >3m) have <60% kidney function.

Care and management

- Important all patients have pnemococcal and influenza immunizations.
- All risk factors should be eliminated e.g. smoking.
- Monitor and treat BP and possible UTIs.
- Diet advice to ameliorate CRF specific symptoms e.g. ↓ salt, ↓ protein.
- Depression is common; ensure there is adequate emotional support.
- Eligibility for financial assistance and housing should be considered.
- Stage 3 CKD moderate ↓ GFR with or without evidence of kidney damage.
- Stage 4 severe ↓ GFR.
- Stage 5 established renal failure.

Patients with > stage 3 refer specialist management (see QoF).

End-stage renal failure when kidney function is <5% of normal function and damage is irreversible. Dialysis is needed for the rest of the patient's life or until kidney transplant. Two types: haemodialysis and peritoneal.

Haemodialysis: blood flows through dialysis machine, waste products cleared along a concentration gradient across a semi permeable membrane. Occurs 3x a week in hospital, a session takes 3–5 hours.

Continuous ambulatory peritoneal dialysis (CAPD) a permanent catheter inserted into peritoneum and dialysis fluid is introduced and kept there. Changed for fresh fluid up to 5x a day. Process takes approx 30 min, can be done at home. Automated peritoneal dialysis: uses a machine, and can be performed overnight. Possible problems include: peritonitis, catheter blockage (requires admission to hospital as emergency), weight gain, pleural effusion, leakage and poor diabetic control.

Related topics

📖 Diabetes: overview; 📖 Benefits for disability and illness.

Further information for professionals and relatives

▣ National Kidney Federation: www.kidney.org.uk
▣ National Kidney Research Fund: www.nkrf.org.uk

Urinary tract infection (UTI)

UTI; may be asymptomatic occurring at any site of the urinary tract. *E.coli* is the commonest bacterial cause in the community >70%. Up to $^1/_3$ with symptoms do not have bacteriuria.

Types and symptoms
- Cystitis: infection of bladder, frequency, dysuria, haematuria, suprapubic pain.
- Pyelonephritis: infection of kidney, (acute) fever, rigor, vomiting, loin pain and tenderness, acute renal failure. NB if unwell may need IV antibiotics.
- Prostatitis: infection of prostate: flu-like symptoms, low back pain, few urinary symptoms, swollen tender prostate.
- Urethritis: inflammation of urethra.

Patients who are catherized may c/o suprapubic pain and discomfort and have cloudy and foul smelling urine.

NB Older people who appear confused and disoriented may have UTI.

Risk factors

♀	♀ and ♂
• Sexual intercourse	• Urinary tract obstruction or malformation
• Diaphragm contraceptive	• Dehydration
• Pregnancy	• Delayed micturition (e.g. due to long journeys)
• Menopause (decreased oestrogen)	• Renal stones
	• DM
	• Catheterization

Ascending infection from a UTI can lead to:
- Pyelonephritis, renal failure, and sepsis.
- Undiagnosed bacteriuria in pregnancy can cause pyelonephritis, premature birth, and low birth weight.

Management
Majority of untreated acute uncomplicated cystitis will resolve in three days.

SIGN (see below) advises antibiotics should only be used when evidence that eradicating a bacterial infection will result in health gains e.g. symptom relief. NB bacteriuria common in asymptomatic older patients and treating = more harm than good. Treatment of bacteriuria in pregnancy beneficial.
- In non-pregnant ♀ with multiple signs and symptoms (e.g. dysuria, urgency, frequency with no vaginal irritation or discharge) not necessary to use dipstick, commence empirical antibiotics.
- If diagnosis uncertain and non-pregnant ♀ has <2 symptoms test urine with dipstick to guide management.

Obtain urine culture and consider blood tests i.e. U&Es, Cr, and or PSA if:
- >40yrs and ♂
- UTI in child
- If temperature persists or >38.5°C
- Recurrent UTIs
- Pregnancy
- Suspected pyelonephritis
- Haematuria
- Unclear history
- Patient is catheterized (NB if UTI suspected begin antibiotics before culture results known and consider removing catheter before starting treatment for symptomatic UTI.

Prevention and care
- Pain relief: paracetamol or ibuprofen (BNF 10.1,4.7.1).
- Drink plenty of fluid (especially if patient is catheterized).
- Double voiding: go to the toilet and repeat 5min later.
- Voiding after intercourse (if UTI persist may need prophylactic antibiotics post coitally).
- Wipe from front to back after going to the toilet (♀).
- Limited evidence cranberry juice: some evidence to suggest ↓ 2° bacteruria.
- ♀ with recurrent UTI may need prophylactic antibiotics or have a prescription in readiness for prompt treatment when first have symptoms.
- Menopausal ♀ with recurrent symptoms may benefit from topical or oral HRT (Menopause 📖).
- Pregnant ♀ should be monitored carefully.
Referred to specialist 2° care if symptoms unresolved.

Related topics
📖 Urinary continence in women; 📖 Urinary catheters care; 📖 Sexual health: general issues.

Further information for professionals and relatives
📓 Continence foundation: www.continence-foundation.org.uk
📓 Clinical Knowledge Summaries (Prodigy) guidelines and patient information sheets on lower UTI urology: www.cks.library.nhs.uk
📓 Womens Health Concern Factsheets on cystitis: www.womens-health-concern.org/index.php
📓 SIGN Scottish Intercollegiate Guidelines Network www.sign.ac.uk

Men's urology and renal problems

Benign prostatic hypertrophy (BPH)

(Also known as benign prostatic hyperplasia). Affects 10–30% ♂ >70yrs. Prostrate enlarges with ageing → narrowing of urethra and partially obstruct the flow of urine. Symptoms often initially mild but may interfere with QoL and become more severe, patients may c/o:

- Poor and reduced stream: taking longer to empty their bladder
- Hesitancy: have to wait before urine flows
- Dribbling of urine soon after finishing micturition causing staining and leakage
- Feeling of incomplete emptying
- Frequency, urgency, and nocturia.

Complications
- Recurrent UTI
- Acute urinary retention (1–2% develop urinary retention)
- Chronic obstruction
- Overflow incontinence
- Haematuria
- Affect sexual function (erectile dysfunction, pain on ejaculation).

Care and management
- Patient completing the International Prostate Sympton Score (IPSS)[1] provides an useful baseline measure of severity and impact on QoL.
- Address any concerns patient may have about possibilities of cancer (see below).
- Patients with mild-to-moderate symptoms: strategy of 'watchful waiting', reassurance, education, and advise on reducing caffeine and alcohol intake, avoiding constipation, bladder retraining.
- Planning ahead and reducing fluid intake before important events but important to maintain good fluid intake of min 1.5L per day.
- Control urgency with distraction and relaxation techniques.
- ♂ with mild-to-moderate symptoms and/or who experience ↓ QoL may benefit from drug treatment: alpha blockers 5 alpha reductase inhibitors or combination of both (BNF 2.5).
- Referred for surgery if other treatment failed or there are complications.

Prostatitis

Considered a possibility for all men with UTI (🕮) treated with antibiotics.

Prostate cancer

Sixth most common cancer in the world and kills 9000♂/yr in the UK. Incidence rising. Early cancer is symptomless, ♂ may present with:

- Haematuria
- Urinary retention/obstruction
- Erectile dysfunction
- Lower back pain and or bone pain (from metastases)
- Weight loss.

---

[1] 🖳 www.cks.library.nhs.uk/pk.uk/patient_information/pils/prostate_symptom

Risk factors
- Age: 85% of men that have diagnosis of prostrate cancer >65yrs
- FH
- Ethnic group: highest rates in black men, lowest in Chinese men
- Diet some evidence to suggest low fruit intake and high fat, high meat diet predisposes to prostrate cancer.

Confirmation of diagnosis is by GP (by digital rectal examination (DRE) and test for ↑ prostrate specific antigen PSA) and referral to urology specialist.

Care and management
NB If asymptomatic then opinion divided about treatment options i.e. no intervention vs. aggressive treatment.
- Watchful waiting and careful monitoring PSA: ↑ PSA or DRE or ↑ nodule size then active treatment.
- Radical prostatectomy: potential for cure but risks and complications associated with surgery in older patients as well as impotence and incontinence.
- Radiotherapy: evidence on effectiveness unclear.
- Hormone therapy: evidence on effectiveness unclear in early disease.

For patients with symptoms
Hormone manipulation main treatment approach to help ↓ PSA, bone pain, and incidence of complications such as spinal cord compression.
- Luteinising hormone releasing hormone (LHRH) analogues: a SC injection every 4–12wks to ↓ testosterone levels equivalent to those of a castrated man (BNF 8.3.4.2). (Injection techniques) SE impotence, hot flushes, gynaecomastia, local bruising around injection site.
- Anti androgens either in combination with LHRH or as monotherapy.
- Surgical castration.
- Bony metastases: corticosteroids and radiotherapy.

Related topics
 Incontinence in men; UK screening programmes; Healthy ageing.

Further information for professionals and relatives
 NICE: Improving outcomes in urological cancers: www.nice.org.uk
 Prostrate Research Campaign UK: www.prostate-research.org.uk

Sexual health: general issues

Continued rises in sexual risk behaviours and diagnoses of HIV and acute sexually transmitted infections (STIs) highlight the need to increase access to a range of prevention, diagnostic, and treatment opportunities. Target groups include young people (<25yrs), men who have sex with men (MSM), and black and minority ethnic (BME) groups. Although centralized genitourinary medicine (GUM) clinics, also known as sexual health clinics, have been the traditional provider of STI/HIV care, other primary care services are now being encouraged to assess, screen, diagnose, and manage specific elements of infection, sometimes independently or in partnership with GUM services. If in doubt, refer people with suspected cases of STIs and HIV to local GUM clinic (Sexual health consultations 🔲).

Confidentiality

Concerns over confidentiality can be overcome by developing a non-judgemental and empathetic culture within the service (Anti-discriminatory health care 🔲). Non-discrimination and confidentiality statements should be displayed for patients to see. GUM clinics operate under specific legislation to protect confidentiality. Patient records are kept separate from other medical records and GPs are not informed unless the patient consents.

Client may be concerned about STI testing, confidentiality, and future insurance or mortgage applications. If HIV or STI testing is appropriate, they should be offered (Access to records 🔲). GPs are approached by insurance companies with written consent from patients for medical histories. Positive HIV results are disclosed to insurance companies if requested. Negative HIV tests do not affect future insurance applications.

Confidentiality and <16yrs
See Fraser guidelines, 🔲 Contraception: general.

Partner notification

- Explain to patient that partner notification (PN) is essential (except for candida and BV) to reduce risk of reinfection to self, and to stop the spread of infection to other partners.
- Encourage patient to notify recent sexual partner(s) of their STI, and advise them to seek treatment.
- For complex cases, seek advice or refer to health advisers or other GUM staff. Health advisers can perform provider referral PN, whereby the index patient provides information on partner(s) to a health adviser, who then confidentially traces and notifies the partner(s) directly.

Sexual assault

Disclosure of non-consenting sex should never be ignored. People who have been sexually assaulted or raped can be referred as urgent cases to GUM, or to designated sexual assault referral centres (SARCs) that can provide forensic examination and liaison with the police, as and if requested by the patient. Patients can self refer to SARCs. Non-consenting sex in <16yrs requires local child protection procedures to be followed (Child protection 🔲).

Health promotion

Sexual health should be proactively and positively promoted as an important aspect of an individual's overall health and well-being. Specific health promotion includes:

- Promote consistent condom use for vaginal and anal sex, plus water-based lubricant for anal sex.
- Provide condoms and lube, or suggest where individual can access these.
- Discuss regular contraception and awareness of emergency contraception.
- Awareness of sexually transmitted infection signs and symptoms.
- Provide sexual health leaflets, web-links, and helpline numbers.
- Refer to sexual health services for specialist intervention on ↓ sexual risk-taking.

Related topics

📖 Sexual health consultations; 📖 Sexually transmitted infections; 📖 Contraception: general.

Further information

📟 HIV management guidelines, available at: www.bhiva.org.
📟 National STI/HIV policy in each UK country e.g. England: www.dh.gov.uk
📟 Recommended standards for sexual health and HIV services, including primary care: www.medfash.org.uk
📟 STI/HIV epidemiological data: www.hpa.org.uk
📟 STI management guidelines, available, at: www.bashh.org.

Patient information and support

📟 Comprehensive information about HIV and AIDS: www.aidsmap.com
📟 DH England website on sexual health: www.playingsafely.co.uk and Helpline: ☎ Sexual Health Line 0800 567 123
📟 FPA UK provides online details of GUM clinics, SARCs in UK, and STI infections www.fpa.org.uk also ☎ Helpline: 0845 310 1334
📟 Sexwise advice on sex, relationships, and contraception for <18yrs: www.ruthinking.co.uk
☎ Helpline tel: 0800 28 29 30

Sexual health consultations

See also 📖 Sexual health: general issues.

Practitioners should ensure that the consultation is under taken in a non-judgemental and empathic manner.

Sexual history assessment

Degree of assessment depends on practitioner skill and competence. Good practice suggests:

- Ask about symptoms (location, type, severity, duration, aggravation/alleviating factors, self-treatment).
- Recent sexual partner(s) (gender, type of sex, condom use).
- Contraception use.
- Past STIs, HIV status and testing history, and cervical cancer screening in ♀.

Physical examination

Degree of examination dependent on practitioner competence. Referral to medical colleagues or GUM service (see below) may be required if not competent, equipment not available, or history indicates complex problems. If performing an examination, offer a chaperone (📖). Good practice suggests an examination should include:

- Observe external genital area for ulceration, rashes, warts, and other abnormal lesions/growths, other dermatoses, pubic lice, scabies, palpate for lymphadenopathy.
- ♂: observe for urethral discharge (colour, consistency), palpate testicles for irregularities, pain, epididymal tenderness, other abnormalities.
- ♀: speculum examination for abnormal discharge (colour, consistency, odour, pH), internal warts or ulcers, cervical erosion or contact bleeding. Palpate for lower abdominal tenderness. Bimanual examination for adnexal tenderness and cervical excitation (NB if competent).

STI testing

- Undertaken in primary care according to local policy, availability of skilled staff, equipment, and diagnostic capability.
- Practices and clinics preparing to undertake testing should confirm with local laboratory the testing methods available, required samples, and how soon these should reach the laboratory.
- Local treatment and referral pathways determined by local sexual health clinical networks.
- Opportunistic chlamydia self-taken swab or urine screening becoming widely available for <25yrs in GP, family planning clinics, high street pharmacies, youth centres.
- Other STI tests performed according to signs and symptoms (STIs 📖).
- Genital sites for STI testing dependent on signs and symptoms, and sexual behaviour/orientation.

HIV testing

- All nurses have the communication skills required to engage patients in a pre-HIV test discussion, supported with leaflets and information on local availability of testing.
- Local policies will determine if practice or clinic provides HIV antibody tests and whether nurses can order them.
- Where high risk of HIV infection, the patient may require ↑ support before or after testing, which can be provided in GUM clinics.

Referral to GUM clinics

- Patients referred if equipment and/or diagnostic technology not available, diagnosis unclear, specialist investigation or treatment required, or according to local care pathways.
- Complex partner notification should be managed by GUM specialists.
- Referral letter useful if investigations have already been performed and treatment commenced.
- Patients can self-refer to GUM clinics and SARCs.

Confidentiality and partner notification

See 📖 Sexual health: general issues.

Sexual health promotion

See 📖 Sexual health: general issues.

Related topic

📖 Sexually transmitted infections.

Further information

- STI management guidelines available at: www.bashh.org
- HIV management guidelines available at: www.bhiva.org
- Recommended standards for sexual health and HIV services, including primary care: www.medfash.org.uk

Patient information and support

- FPA UK provides online details of GUM clinics, SARCs in UK, and STI infections www.fpa.org.uk ☎ Helpline: 0845 310 1334.
- DH England website on sexual health: www.playingsafely.co.uk and Helpline: ☎ Sexual Health Line: 0800 567 123
- Sexwise advice on sex, relationships, and contraception for <18yrs: www.ruthinking.co.uk ☎ Helpline tel: 0800 28 29 30.
- Comprehensive information about HIV and AIDS: www.aidsmap.com

Sexually transmitted infections

Bacterial vaginosis (BV) (see vaginal and vulval problems)

Candidiasis (thrush) (see Fungal infections 📖, ♀ see vaginal and vulval problems 📖)

Chlamydia

- ♀: mostly asymptomatic or ↑ vaginal discharge, post-coital or inter-menstrual bleeding, dysuria, lower abdominal pain, dyspareunia.
- ♂: often asymptomatic or mild to moderate clear or whitish urethral discharge, dysuria.
- Rectal: ↑ MSM. Mucopurulent blood stained rectal discharge, rectal pain and tenesmus. GUM referral essential for management of potential lymphogranuloma venereum (see below).
- Pharyngeal: ↑ MSM, although incidence and natural history not known.

Investigations

The testing methods available should be confirmed with local laboratory.
- ♀: endocervical, vaginal self-swab or urine for nucleic acid amplification test (NAAT). Endocervical swab for culture or EIA.
- ♂: urethral swab or urine for NAAT. Urethral swab for culture or EIA.

Treatment

- Doxycycline 100mg/12h po for 7d (contra-indicated in pregnancy) (BNF 5.1.3).
- Azithromycin 1g po as a single dose (BNF 5.1.5).
- Erythromycin 500mg/12h po for 14d (BNF 5.1.5).

Genital herpes

Blistering and ulceration, usually painful, multiple, and clustered. Systemic flu-like symptoms may be present during primary episode. Recurrences usually less painful, but can be variable. ❶ Specialist advice required if in third trimester pregnancy.

Investigations

Usually swab lesions, placed in viral transport medium and stored in fridge until transported. Culture result can take 10–14d.

Treatment

Treated on symptoms. Advise saline bathing and analgesia for symptom relief. Aciclovir, famciclovir or valaciclovir (BNF 5.3.2).

Genital warts

External anogenital skin lesions. Also found on vagina, cervix, urethral meatus, and anal canal. Soft and fleshy, or firm and irregular growths. Single or multiple, raised or flat. Usually non-painful, sometimes itchy.

Diagnosis

Clinical observation in most cases. Referred to GUM if doubt.

Treatment

Podophyllotoxin solution or cream (BNF 13.7) suitable for home treatment. Other treatments available in GUM clinics.

Gonorrhea

- ♀: ~80% asymptomatic or ↑ vaginal discharge, dysuria, intermenstrual bleeding.
- ♂: almost always yellow/green purulent discharge, dysuria within 2–5d of sexual contact.
- Rectal: ↑ MSM. Often asymptomatic. Mucopurulent discharge, pain, tenesmus, bleeding, constipation, anal pruritus.
- Pharyngeal: ↑ MSM. Usually asymptomatic, occasionally pharyngitis.

Investigations

Usually exposed sites (endocervical, urethral, pharyngeal, rectal) swabbed and sent for culture where available. Rapid diagnosis available in GUM.

Treatment

- Ceftriaxone 1g IM as a single dose (BNF 5.1.2).
- Cefixime 400mg po as a single dose (BNF 5.1.2).

HIV

(Human immunodeficiency virus 📖.)

Hepatitis A/B/C

(Viral hepatitis 📖.)

Lymphogranuloma venereum (LGV)

UK outbreaks in MSM since 2004. Ano-rectal syndrome presents with anal discharge, pain, and tenesmus. Inguinal syndrome presents with genital ulceration, painful inguinal adenopathy.

Investigation and treatment

All MSM with ano-rectal symptoms referred to GUM for management.

Non-gonococcal urethritis (NGU)

♂ only: mild to moderate clear or whitish urethral discharge ± dysuria. Chlamydia (see above) is the cause of 30–50% of cases.

Investigations

Diagnosis relies on microscopy, usually only available in GUM clinics. Urethral swab for gonorrhea and chlamydia. Can be treated on clinical signs and symptoms if other STIs excluded.

Treatment

- Doxycycline 100mg/12h po for 7d (BNF 5.1.3).
- Azithromycin 1g stat po (BNF 5.1.5).

Pubic lice

See also (Insects and infestations 📖). Treated with permethrin, phenothrin or malathion (BNF13.10.4).

Syphilis

Resurgence in UK since 1999; substantial increases in MSM. Incubation 9–90d. Referred to GUM for investigation, treatment, and partner notification. Presents in 1 of 4 stages:

- Primary syphilis: usually a solitary, painless, indurated ulcer (chancre) at point of sexual contact (genital, oral, rectal).

- Secondary syphilis: 2–4wks after chancre. Non-itchy, macular or papular rash, may affect palms and soles. Systemic symptoms: fever, malaise, generalized lymphadenopathy.
- Latent syphilis: asymptomatic period between untreated secondary and tertiary stages.
- Tertiary syphilis: very rare in UK. Cardiovascular or neurological manifestations up to 30yrs after untreated infection.

Treatment

Dependent on stage. Referred to GUM for management.

Trichomonas vaginalis (TV)

- ♀: ↑ vaginal discharge (discoloured, offensive, frothy), vulval soreness, dyspareunia, dysuria. Can be asymptomatic.
- ♂: rarely diagnosed in men but should always treat if a sexual contact.

Investigations

Usually swab from posterior vaginal fornix sent in transport media (e.g. Amies, Stuarts) to laboratory within 6hrs. Refrigerate while awaiting transportation. Rapid diagnosis available in GUM clinics.

Treatment

- Metronidazole 2g po as a single dose (BNF 5.1.11).
- Metronidazole 400mg/12h po for 5d (preferred in pregnant women).

Further information

🖳 British Association for Sexual Health and HIV guidelines available at: www.bashh.org

Patient information and support

🖳 DH England sexual health: www.playingsafely.co.uk and Helpline: Sexual Health Line ☎ 0800 567 123

🖳 FPA for details of local GUM clinics: www.fpa.org.uk ☎ 0845 310 1334

🖳 Sexwise advice on sex, relationships, and contraception for <18yrs 🖳 www.ruthinking.co.uk free Helpline: ☎: 0800 28 29 30

Sexual problems

Sexual problems can be physical or psychogenic in origin, or a mix of both. Careful, non-judgemental history taking (see below) can ascertain whether referral to practitioners specializing in psychosexual counselling or pharmacotherapy is warranted. General counselling (Counselling skills 📖; Talking therapies 📖) can help resolve hidden conflicts, deal with various emotions, and explore relationship issues. Psychosexual therapy provides more specialist intervention. Local GUM, urology, and contraception services offer various degrees of assessment and management. In all problems it is useful to provide patient with accurate and relevant information. Various self-help books and videos are available (see below for link sites).

History taking

Define the exact nature of the problem and consider key clues as to its origin. Explore associated factors:
- Why is the patient seeking treatment now?
- What does the patient think is the cause?
- What has the patient tried?
- Does the patient's partner know?
- What is the partner's attitude?
- What does the patient hope to gain?
- Past/current medical and psychiatric history.
- Social and relationship history including life events associated with problem.

Loss of libido

Poorly understood and often difficult to treat. May be a result of physical illness, hormonal changes, medication side effects, psychological problems, relationship difficulties, partner attraction issues, or life changes. Identify and treat physical cause and/or refer for counselling.

Dyspareunia

Dyspareunia is recurrent genital or pelvic pain associated with sexual activity. Repeated sexual pain can set up a cycle, in which fear of pain leads to avoidance of the sexual activity that produces it, in turn leading to lack of arousal, failure to achieve orgasm, and loss of sexual desire.
- ♂ may be anatomical problem e.g. phimosis, or infection.
- ♀ may be physical causes, e.g. scarring from childbirth, genital circumcision, lack of lubrication or psychosexual problems.

Abdominal and vaginal examination ± STI screening and treatment as required excludes physical causes. Referred to GUM as necessary. Psychosexual: similar treatment approaches used for vaginismus can be effective.

Vaginismus

Vaginismus is an involuntary reflex spasm of the muscles surrounding the entrance to the vagina that may be severe enough to prevent any form of vaginal penetration. Vaginal examination may exclude physical cause. A penetration desensitization programme may be helpful, in which patient is encouraged to insert 1 finger, then 2, then 3 into her vagina, while relaxing the lower vaginal muscles. Clear instructions and regular follow-up are vital for success. If problems persist, refer to psychosexual therapist or sexual problems clinic. Partner involvement may be helpful.

Erectile dysfunction

Failure to achieve or maintain satisfactory erection. History may denote physical or psychogenic cause. ↑ association with CVD or diabetes. May be adverse-effect of medication (e.g. some antidepressants, anti-hypertensives). Hormonal evaluation is often requested, although erectile dysfunction is seldom due to hormonal problems. Mainstay of treatment includes oral pharmacological agents taken prior to sex (e.g. sildenafil). Counselling may be of benefit for psychogenic causes.

Premature ejaculation

Ejaculation with minimal sexual stimulation before the person or partner wishes. Clinical and psychosocial history may identify cause (e.g. anxiety/depression, relationship difficulties). Squeeze/stop-start technique common approach to controlling ejaculation—intercourse is halted and penis is firmly squeezed at base of glans when man feels close to ejaculation/orgasm. Sex can then resume until point of ejaculation is reached again, squeeze/stop-start repeated, and so on. Other treatments include formal psychosexual counselling and pharmacotherapy prescribed by sexual dysfunction specialist.

Further information

▢ Sexual dysfunction management guidelines at: www.bashh.org
▢ The Sexual Dysfunction Association provides public and professionals with information about sexual problems: www.sda.uk.net

Patient information and support

▢ British Association for Sexual and Relationship Therapy provides a list of UK therapists: www.basrt.org.uk
▢ PACE provides sexual and relationship counselling for lesbians and gay men: www.pacehealth.org.uk
▢ Relate provides therapy for sex problems: www.relate.org.uk

Sexual health and adults with a learning disability/difficulty (LD)

2% general population have a LD. In a GP list of 7600 there will be approx 150 people with a LD, and 30 will be severely learning disabled.[1] All people with LD must be registered with a GP.

- Most people with are seen in a primary care setting at least once per year due to concomitant health needs.
- Annual health screening is good practice.

Those with mild to moderate LD may have sexual health and other needs not catered for through inappropriate, or absence of appropriate service provision

Learning disability/difficulty defined as:
- Onset before adulthood.
- Sub-average intellectual functioning with an IQ of 70 or less.
- Deficits or impairments in present adaptive functioning in at least 2 of the following: communication, self care, home living, social interpersonal skills, use of community resources, self direction, functional skills, work, leisure, health, safety.

Registration of people that are learning disabled is now a QoF indicator for general practice.

NB Health professionals may hold discriminatory attitudes to people with learning disability which affects provision of sexual health services. Professsionals need to consider the following:

Sexual health needs
Sexual health needs of people with LDs will vary but frequently include the following:
- Relationship guidance and counselling (boundary setting, giving and withholding consent, keeping safe, emotional health and issues such as love, friendship etc.).
- Bodily awareness and information on sexual functioning and management e.g. menstruation, erection, sexual intercourse etc.
- Contraception and family planning, e.g. the use and application of barrier and chemical contraceptives.
- Pregnancy and childbirth.
- Information on and access to screening services e.g. cervical and breast screening.
- Information on and access to GU services when needed.

Fundamental elements in service provision
- Liaise with the community learning disability team to acquire background knowledge.
- Involve family and carers when appropriate ❶ *But* maintain confidentiality wherever possible.
- Communicate directly with the client.

[1] Department of Health (2001). *Valuing People. A new strategy for learning disability for the 21st Century* TSO, London.

Communication

48% of people with a LD has impairment in one sensory domain and 18% are doubly impaired ∴ informed consent is hard to achieve. Assess on an individual basis, check understanding regularly in ways that can be checked, e.g. asking client to outline what has just been explained to them.

• Speak clearly and directly to the client.
• Treat clients with the same dignity and respect given to any other client.
• Use pictures, signs, and large clear print to get your message across. For resources contact the local community LD team.
• Use models to demonstrate techniques where appropriate, and allow return demonstration and follow-up when necessary.
• People with LD may be limited in terms of conceptual thinking, where possible try to demonstrate on life like equipment.

NB Some women with LD may have been sexually abused. Studies show this often starts at an early age, and is unrelated to the severity of LD.

• Many women smoke cigarettes, combined with unprotected sexual intercourse ↑ vulnerable to cervical cancer, (Cervical cancer screening 📖).

Attitudes of professionals and carers

Many people with LD are sexually active, and their carers may not know or acknowledge this.

• Assumptions regarding health need and negative attitudes are related to the degree of physical evidence of a disability, but may bear little resemblance to reality.
• Be extra vigilant for signs of abuse and look out for warning signs and listen to the client.

Consent versus cooperation

Ethical dilemmas arise when client cannot give verbal consent, and the difficulty is in determining whether the treatment is in the client's best interest. Where verbal consent is not possible, and there is reason to believe that the client is sexually active or has been exposed involuntarily to sexual activity:

• Co-operation may be all that is achievable.[2] Consider the consequences to the client of withholding the treatment/service when making a decision.

Time and place

People with LDs will need more time: plan visit/try to allocate a double appointment accordingly.

• Try to allocate the first or last appointment.
• Try to avoid crowded rushed or noisy situations.
• Ensure that access to your service is physically possible, some people with LD are also physically disabled.

Related topics

📖 Models and approaches to health promotion; 📖 Contraception: general; 📖 Mental capacity.

[2] National Health Service Cancer Screening Programmes (2000). *Good Practice in Breast and Cervical Screening for Women With Learning Disabilities*. NHSBSP Publication no 46, NHSCSP Publication no 13, Sheffield, NHSBSP/CSP

Breast problems

❶ Women should be referred to GP and then onto breast specialist if they report:
• Lump: new, discrete lump; breast abscess; cyst persistently refilling/recurrent cyst
• Pain: associated with a lump; persistent pain
• Nipple discharge
• Nipple retraction, distortion, or nipple eczema
• Change in skin contour
• FH: request by any woman with a strong FH

Breast cysts: firm, rounded lump of any size, single or multiple, occurs pre-menopause, not associated with skin changes. Refer to GP for assessment.

Fibroadenoma: majority of all benign breast neoplasms. Common in women <35yrs. Giant fibroadenomas may occur in older women. Presents with painless, hard, extremely mobile lump. Usually removed.

Breast problems associated with breast feeding: e.g. mastitis, breast abcess, see 📖 Breast feeding

Breast pain (mastalgia)

Many ♀ experience breast pain. Most common in in ♀ 30–50yrs. Cause unknown. In many women it is mild, but in some women it becomes more severe and can affect day-to-day life. Can be cyclical pain associated with menstruation or non-cyclical. For some it is also associated with a lump or diffuse lumpiness that change size through the cycle (known as benign mammary dysplasia). Refer to GP for assessment.

Management of mastalgia (once other serious problems ruled out) includes:
• Mild: no treatment, simple, analgesics, advise on well supporting bra.
• More severe:
  • Wear a well supporting bra 24hrs especially approaching period.
  • Some ♀ find caffeine ↑ pain so stop tea, coffee, and cola, although evidence limited to support this.
  • Some ♀ find low fat, high carbohydrate diet helps.
  • Take painkillers such as ibuprofen regularly on the days when the breasts are painful.
  • COC or HRT can make pain worse in some ♀. Review by GP.
  • RCT shows topical NSAIDs e.g. ibuprofen (BNF 10.1.1) are effective and well tolerated, available OTC.
  • Oestrogen reducing medication (e.g danazol BNF 6.7.2) used for severe, cyclical, persistent pain but side effects e.g. weight gain, menorrhagia. Effective in about 80% ♀.
NB In the UK, the Committee for Safety of Medicines has withdrawn the prescription license from evening primrose oil because of lack of efficacy, but it is still available OTC.

Related topics

📖 Breast awareness and cancer prevention; 📖 Breast cancer.

Further Information for professionals and women

▣ BMJ Clinical Evidence Breast Pain: www.clinicalevidence.com
▣ Womens Health Information Leaflets: www.womenshealthlondon.org.uk

Breast cancer

Most common cancer in the UK. Accounts for 18% of all female cancers—British women have a 1:9 lifetime risk of developing the disease. Although mortality is falling, breast cancer is the 3rd most common cause of cancer death in the UK accounting for ~13,000 deaths/yr.

Risk factors

- *Age:* ↑ with age—80% in women >50yrs.
- *Reproductive history:* ↑ risk if early menarche or late menopause; late age at 1st birth ↑ risk; ↑ parity → ↓ risk; breast feeding ↓ risk.
- *Hormones:* slight ↑ risk in current and recent users of combined oral contraceptives—excess risk disappears >10yrs after stopping; in users of combined HRT risk ↑ by 6 cases/1000 after 5y and 19 cases/1000 after 10yrs use.
- *Lifestyle:* obesity ↑ risk post menopause; 30% ↓ risk if taking regular physical activity; high fat diet is probably associated with ↑ risk; alcohol ↑ risk by 7%/unit consumed/d.
- *Physical characteristics:* taller women have ↑ risk; women with denser breasts have 2–6x ↑ risk.
- *Ionizing radiation:* exposure ↑ risk.
- *Previous breast disease:* past history of either benign or malignant breast disease ↑ risk.
- *Family history:* 1 first degree relative with breast cancer (mother or sister) ↑ risk x 2—but 85% of women with breast cancer have no FH. If several family members with early onset breast cancer refered for genetic screening—BRCA1 and BRCA2 genes account for 2–5% all breast cancers.

Prevention

- Lifestyle measures: ↓ alcohol intake; ↓ weight; avoid exogenous sex hormones (e.g. HRT); breast feed.
- Chemoprophylaxis: Tamoxifen ↓ risk of breast cancer by 40% in high-risk women but limited by side effects (thromboembolism and endometrial carcinoma)—other drug trials in progress.
- Prophylactic surgery: ↓ risk by 90% in very high-risk women.

Presentation

- Found at breast screening (Breast awareness and cancer prevention 📖).
- Clinical presentation: breast lump (90%); breast pain (21% present with painful lump; pain alone <1%); nipple skin change (10%—see below); FH (6%); skin contour change (5%); nipple discharge (3%). In the older people breast cancer may grow slowly and present with extensive local lesions.
- *Paget's disease of the breast:* intra-epidermal, intraductal cancer. Any red, scaly lesion or eczema around the nipple suggests Paget's disease.

Management

Referred for urgent assessment to a breast surgeon. Specialist investigation includes USS; mammography ± fine needle aspiration or biopsy; investigations to evaluate spread (e.g. CT, liver USS, bone scan).

Classification

Virtually all breast cancers are adenocarcinomas.

- *In situ* (non-invasive) *Stage I:* ≤2cm diameter; no LNs (lymph nodes) affected; no spread beyond breast.

- *Stage II and III:* 2–5cm or >5cm diameter and/or LNs armpit affected; no evidence of spread beyond armpit.
- *Stage IV:* any sized tumour; LNs armpit affected; spread to other parts of the body.

Treatment

Includes surgery (lumpectomy ± axillary clearance, mastectomy), endocrine therapy, radiotherapy, and/or chemotherapy. Tamoxifen ↑ survival of patients with oestrogen receptor +ve tumours (60% tumours) of any age but rare risk of endometrial carcinoma—warn to report any untoward vaginal bleeding. Tamoxifen for ≥5yrs (BNF 8.3.4.1). Anastrozole blocks oestrogen synthesis. Higher efficacy than tamoxifen in hormone sensitive early cancer in post-menopausal ♀ and first choice for post-menopausal ♀ with advanced cancer. Used for ≥5yrs. In ♀ who are HER2 positive (i.e. the 1.5 ♀ whose breast cancer cells have a large number of the HER2 receptors on surface), Trastuzumab (Herceptin®) is used when at high risk of recurrence or at advanced stage. Given IV 3 weekly for 1yr.

Lymphoedema

All patients who have breast surgery are at risk. Injury to the arm on the surgery side may precipitate/worsen lymphoedema. *Do not* take blood from that limb or BP measurement, use it for IV access or vaccination. (See Lymphoedema 📖).

Post surgery

- Pain: some women find that their breast and arm are sore for up to a year after the treatment, encourage appropriate pain relief.
- Arm and shoulder stiffness, tingling: encourage exercises.
- Pins and needles, burning, numbness or darting sensations in the chest area and down the arm quite common. Can go on for weeks.
- Cording feels like a tight cord running from armpit, down arm through to the back of hand. Can appear 6–8wks after surgery. Thought to be hardening of lymph vessels. May resolve or may need physiotherapy.
- A lightweight foam prosthesis (sometimes called a cumfie or softie), given to be worn inside bra post-surgery. When wound healed (6–8wks), can be fitted with a silicone prosthesis. Breast care nurse (usually linked to local acute hospital) provides advice on type and care. Several types available from the NHS.
- Possibilities of reconstructive surgery discussed with specialists.

Psychological impact of breast cancer

Depression, anxiety, marital, and sexual problems are common. Psychological support should be offered.

Related topics

📖 Breast awareness and cancer prevention; 📖 Palliative care in the home; 📖 Post-operative wound care.

Further information and support for women

📓 Breast Cancer Care: www.breastcancercare.org.uk ☎ 0808 800 6000.
📓 Cancer Research UK: www.cancerresearchuk.org
📓 BACUP (British Association of Cancer United Patients): www.cancerbacup.org.uk ☎ Helpline: 0808 800 1234

Page 772 reproduced with permission from Simon, C., Everitt, H., and Kendrick, T. (2005) Oxford Handbook of General Practice 2nd edn, Oxford University Press, Oxford

Gynaecological cancers

The possibility, as well as the diagnosis of cancer provokes fear and anxiety in everyone. Most women feel shocked and upset by the idea of having treatment to the most intimate and private parts of their body. Psychological support is important as well as clear information about investigations, treatments, effects including on sex life. Treatment may involve surgical removal of part or whole organs that many women feel are important parts of their female identity. This is often an important area of grieving and loss to address.

The most common cancers are ovarian (4th most common cancer in ♀), cervical, and uterine.

Cervical cancer

Incidence dropping due to screening programme (Cervical cancer screening 📖).

Symptoms: abnormal smear test, postcoital bleeding, vaginal bleeding and/or discharge. Referred to gynaecologist. Diagnosed by colposcopy or cone biopsy.

Treatment: dependent on stage. Localized early cancerous changes destroyed by electrocoagulation, diathermy, laser treatment or cryosurgery, cone biopsy. Later stage cancer requires surgery and radiotherapy (if cancer confined to cervix 5yrs survival rate >90%).

Ovarian cancer

Most common cancer affecting pelvic organs. 5000 ♀ diagnosed in UK each yr. Average age 63yrs.

Risk factors: increasing age, family history, nulliparity.

Symptoms: vaginal bleeding, abdominal discomfort and bloating, ascites.

Treatment surgery (Hysterectomy 📖) and sometimes adjuvant chemotherapy. May also have chemotherapy prior to surgery. If disease is confined to the ovaries/pelvis 5yr survival is 50–90%.

Uterine cancer

Endometrial is the most common form. Peak incidence 55–70yrs.

Risk factors: age, obesity, nulliparity, late menopause, DM, family history of breast, ovary, or colon cancer.

Symptoms: abnormal vaginal bleeding, dysparunia, post-menopausal bleeding.

Treatment: surgery, usually Hysterectomy (📖), radiotherapy, progesterone treatment and/or chemotherapy. Radiotherapy in pelvic area can cause diarrhoea and cystitis.

Vaginal cancer

Rare, <300 ♀ diagnosed/yr in UK. More common as 2° cancer. Squamous cell cancer most common, develops in ♀ 60–80yrs. Adenocarcinoma rare, mainly in ♀ <20yrs.

Symptoms: Vaginal bleeding, dysparunia, problems with micturition.

Treatment
- Surgery. Type depends position and size of cancer. May be part (remaining tissue stretched so vagina intact) or whole vagina (vaginectomy). Sometimes possible for vaginal reconstruction using tissue from other parts of the body. May also need hysterectomy (📖).
- Radiotherapy, may be external or internal. In pre-menopausal ♀, radiotherapy likely to produce menopause about 3mths after treatment, also can cause diarrhoea and cystitis. Radiotherapy causes shortening and narrowing of the vagina, and to prevent this advised to use a vaginal dilator each day during and for some time after the treatment.
- Chemotherapy.

Affect on sex life depends on the type of surgery as well as woman's emotional response to the experience. Clitoris not affected by surgery and orgasms achieved through clitoral stimulation. Vaginal orgasm not possible with vaginal reconstruction.

Vulval cancer

Rare. 90% squamous cells carcinoma, usually grow very slowly. 4% melanoma. $^2/_3$ develop in ♀ who have vulval intraepithelial neoplasia linked to some types of HPV.

Symptoms: skin colour or texture change, itching, burning, lump, or swelling.

Treatment: surgery, extent depends on size and position of cancer—may involve removal of labia and clitoris (vulvectomy), radiotherapy, and chemotherapy. Radiotherapy in pelvic area can cause diarrhoea and cystitis. Vulvectomy alters the outward appearance of the body. It is a change that shocks many and they find hard to accept. Often has a profound effect on attitude to sex. Orgasms still achievable but may need to explore different ways of achieving them.

Related topics

📖 Hysterectomy.

Further information for professionals and patients

🖥 CancerBACUP: www.cancerbacup.org.uk ☎ Helpline: 0808 800 1234
🖥 Cancer Research UK: www.cancerresearchuk.org

Menstrual problems

Menstruation

This is the periodic shedding of the endometrium. Day 1 of bleeding is the start of the menstrual cycle. FSH stimulates the egg follicle to mature, secreting oestrogen which thickens the endometrium. LH causes egg release (ovulation). Some ♀ feel a pain (known as mittelschmerz). Egg viable for about 2d in the fallopian tube. Empty egg follicle produces progesterone. If egg not fertilized, oestrogen and progesterone production stops. Causes endometrium lining to shed, about 14d after ovulation. Normal cycle length 21–40d, average 28d. Normal bleeding 2–8d, average 4–5d. In cycle, changes in consistency of cervical mucus, cervix position, body temperature, breasts, abdominal pain and mood (see below).

Menstrual loss is about 80mL a month. ♀ use internal tampons or external pads for containment. Mooncup (see below) is a reusable silicone menstrual cup used internally. It addresses environmental concerns, financial issues and concerns about bleaches etc in internal tampons.

Toxic shock syndrome

Very rare, acute illness caused by toxins from staphylococci or streptococci. Association with tampons unclear but tampon absorbency thought to be a factor. Preventative advice includes frequent changes, occasional use of pads, not to use 2 tampons at once.

Premenstrual tension (PMT) and syndrome (PMS)

A collection of symptoms and bodily changes that occur on a regular basis anything from a few days to weeks before a woman's period and cease with its arrival. >95% women have some symptoms—debilitating symptoms occur in 5%. Commonest are nervous tension, mood swings, irritability, ↑ weight and abdominal bloating, breast tenderness and headache, cramping and pain. Advice:
- Keep diary of symptoms to establish cyclical symptoms.
- Beneficial effect of good nutrition, weight management, and ↑ exercise.
- Treatment may be by trial and error as poorly understood condition, much conflicting evidence and variety in symptoms experienced.

Treatments
- Conflicting evidence on Oil of Evening Primrose, vit. B6 and magnesium supplements, relaxation, reflexology but may help some ♀.
- Calcium supplements improve breast tenderness, headaches, and abdominal cramps.
- Cognitive therapy improves severe symptoms.
- NSAIDs (BNF 10.1.1) for cramping and pain.
- Effective medical treatments according to symptoms include COC, danazol (BNF 6.7.2), SSRIs (BNF 4.3.3), anxiolytics (BNF 4.1.2).

Menorrhagia/heavy periods

Bleeding >7d and >80mL. In 50% cause unexplained. Other causes: IUD, fibroids, endometriosis, cancer, blood clotting disorder. Following examination and investigations, if does not require or wish hormonal contraception treated with mefenamic acid (BNF 10.1.1) or tranexamic acid (BNF 2.11). If requires contraception as well offered COC or long acting progesterone or IUS. If has IUD changed to IUS. Referred to gynecologist if symptoms indicate or treatment failure.

Dysmenorrhoea/painful periods

Tends to start 6–12mths after menarche when ovulatory cycles are established. Tend to improve after adolescence and after child birth. Uterine hypercontractility (associated with prostaglandin production) and ischaemia of the uterine wall causes pain. Occurs in the first 1–2d of each period. Lower abdominal cramps ± back ache. May be associated gastrointestinal disturbance (e.g. constipation, diarrhoea/vomiting). In about 15% ♀ interferes with ability to go about daily life, attend school, work.

Self-help advice

- OTC painkillers paracetamol, ibuprofen.
- Exercise relieves cramps.
- Hot water bottles or self heating patches or pack (microwaved) comforting.

If pain still a problem may need POM medicines to address pain e.g. mefenamic acid. TENS machines may helps some ♀. Can be treated by COC, IUS insertion. Some ♀ report acupuncture helps.

Pain that still doesn't respond may have underlying pathology (Gynaecological cancer 📖) and requires investigation.

Amenorrhea

Primary amenorrhea: menstruation delayed (Growth 12–18yrs 📖)

Secondary amenorrhea: absence of menses ≥6mths in a previously menstruating woman. Causes may be pregnancy, menopause, stress, low nutritional intake (e.g. anorexia), high levels of exercise, disease of the brain, thyroid, adrenal glands, ovaries. Treatment or action based on cause.

Further information for professionals

📖 National Prescribing Centre (2003). McREC Bulletin. *Tackling Premenstrual Syndrome*: www.npc.co.uk
📖 RCOG (1998). *The initial management of menorrhagia*: www.rcog.org.uk

Further information for women

📖 National Association for Premenstrual Syndrome: www.pms.org.uk/
📖 Information on mooncups: www.mooncup.co.uk/
📖 Women's Health Information Leaflets: www.womenshealthlondon.org.uk

Problems of the ovaries and uterus

Ovarian problems

Ovarian cysts

A growth on, or inside, the ovary. Very common. Functional cysts are the most common type. Many ♀ experience no symptoms. Dependent on size and position may cause discomfort and pain. If <5cm diameter usually resolve spontaneously. >5cm referred to gynaecologist. Acute severe pain and vomiting caused by bleeding into the cyst, rupture or torsion and needs medical assessment urgently.

Treatment: depends on size, position, and possibility of rupture. Laparoscopic fenestration can be used to drain contents, or laporotomy for removal.

Polycystic ovary syndrome

A polycystic ovary is larger than normal with multiple cysts around the edge, disrupting hormonal cycle and inhibiting release eggs. Common in 5–20% pre-menopausal women. Cause unknown. Associated with ↑ risk of cardiovascular disease and endometrial cancer. Women may be asymptomatic or have any or all symptoms of: acne, obesity, infertility, irregular periods, insulin resistance, hirsutism (because excess testosterone produced). Diagnosed on history, pelvic USS, and blood tests.

Treatment: dependent on symptoms, encouraged to maintain weight in BMI range 19–25. Oligomenorrhoea may be treated with progestogens. Clomifene may be used to induce ovulation. Hirsutism may be treated with COC and anti-androgen.

Uterine problems

Endometriosis

Fragments of the endometrium (lining of the uterus) located in other areas of the body, usually pelvic cavity. Fragments under hormonal control so breaks down and bleeds each month. Leads to inflammation, pain, and scar tissue. Most common in ♀ 25–40yrs, Cause unclear. May cause infertility.

Symptoms: vary. May cause heavy menstrual bleeding, severe abdominal pain, dyspareunia, bowel and bladder symptoms. Referred to gynaecologist and diagnosis confirmed on laparoscopy.

Treatment: either hormonal treatment to stop ovulation and allow the endometrial deposits to regress or surgical e.g. local ablation using laser during laparoscopy, or more radical surgery dependent on symptoms.

Fibroids

Benign tumours of the uterus. Affect ~20% women. Often multiple. Oestrogen dependent so more common in pre-menopausal women and shrink post-menopause.

Symptoms: usually asymptomatic but may cause heavy periods (in turn cause anaemia), pelvic discomfort, back ache, pressure on bladder. Diagnosed by pelvic USS. Referred to gynecologist if symptomatic.

Medical treatment: GnRH analogues—tranexamic acid, mefanamic acid may shrink up to 50% can only be used for 6 mths, or insertion of IUS.

Surgical treatment: myomectomy (removing fibroids individually), hysterectomy, or uterine artery embolisation (blocking blood supply).

Pelvic organ prolapse

Very common, particularly in older women. Caused by poor pelvic muscle tone and weakness of pelvic ligaments.

Risk factors: childbirth, menopause. Aggravated by obesity.

Prevention: includes pelvic floor exercises weight maintenance in normal BMI range (Nutrition and healthy eating 🕮) and avoiding constipation.

Types of prolapse:

• Bladder and anterior vaginal wall (cystocele)
• Urethra (urethrocele)
• Rectum and posterior vaginal wall (rectocele)
• Herniation of the top of the vagina (enterocele)
• Uterine prolapse.

Treatment: according to severity and symptoms.

Uterine prolapse

Most common type. Uterus descends into the vagina. Classified by degree:

• 1st degree: cervix remains in the vagina
• 2nd degree: cervix protrudes from vagina on coughing/straining
• 3rd degree (procidentia): uterus lies outside the vagina and may ulcerate).

Signs and symptoms dragging sensation. Often gets worse if standing for a long time, coughing or straining. May be associated with bowel and bladder problems e.g. stress incontinence.

Treatment: depends on severity. In primary care, pelvic floor exercises (Urinary incontinence in women 🕮) and weight reduction encouraged plus treatment of co-existing problems e.g. constipation. Referred to gynecologist. Sometimes HRT prescribed to help, 2nd and 3rd degree prolapse may be treated with surgical repair or hysterectomy.

Vaginal ring pessaries: used to hold uterus in place while waiting for surgery or if surgery not appropriate. Made of latex or PVC, similar to a diaphragm, measured in mm. Fits under pubic bone at the front and to the posterior fornix at the back so the cervix lies within the ring. Ring softens when immersed in warm water to aid fitting. ♀ asked to bear down after fitting to check not expelled. Should not feel it. Oestrogen cream may be used 1 or 2x wk. At 3mths ring removed and cervix and vaginal vault checked, ring washed in soapy water before re-inserted. Checked and replaced every 6mths thereafter. Complications include ulceration of vaginal walls, vaginitis, and discharge.

Related topics

🕮 Menstrual problems; 🕮 Vaginal and vulval problems; 🕮 Urinary incontinence in women, 🕮 Problems with fertility.

Further information for professionals and women

🖳 The National Endometriosis Society: www.endo.org.uk/ ☎ Helpline: 0808 808 222
🖳 Royal College of Obstetricians and Gynecology information sheets: www.rcog.org.uk
🖳 Verity for women with polycystic ovary syndrome: www.verity-pcos.org.uk
🖳 Womens Health Information Leaflets: www.womenshealthlondon.org.uk/index.html

Hysterectomy

One of the most common operations for women. Over 60,000 hysterectomies are carried out in the UK annually. Majority are in ♀ 40–50yrs. Most commonly undertaken for:
- Cancer of the uterus, ovaries, fallopian tube/s or cervix (Gynaecological cancers 📖).
- Electively for painful menorrhagia, endometriosis, fibroids causing pain and bleeding, prolapsed uterus, or pelvic inflammatory disease (PID) or adhesions which cause pain that is not controlled by other means.

Also in emergencies such as rupture/puncture of the uterus during other surgery.

In elective situations, women should have counselling to help make informed choice, based on understanding alternatives, benefits, risks, long-term consequences including:
- Loss of menstruation and ability to have a child.
- Immediate menopause if surgery also removes ovaries regardless of age. 50% who have ovaries intact post surgery experience menopause within 5yrs of operation regardless of age.
- Some women have strong emotional response to the loss of this organ, and experience mourning, loss, and an altered sense of self but others feel liberated and relieved after years of severe pain and heavy bleeding.

Medical alternatives: see 📖 Gynaecological cancers.

Endometrial ablation and resection is a surgical alternative with less consequences used to treat heavy bleeding and remove fibroids and polyps. Techniques include lasers, microwaves, electricity, balloons filled with hot water, freezing, and heated loops.

Types of hysterectomy
- Subtotal hysterectomy removes the uterus leaving the cervix in place, (cervical smears still required see Cervical cancer screening 📖).
- Total hysterectomy (most common) removes uterus and cervix.
- Total hysterectomy with bilateral or unilateral salpingo-oophorectomy removes body of uterus, cervix, fallopian tube(s), and ovary(ies).
- A 'wertheims hysterectomy' removes the uterus, cervix, part of the vagina, fallopian tubes, peritoneum, the lymph glands and fatty tissue of the pelvis, and possibly one or both ovaries.

Performed either through an incision in the lower abdomen (clips or stitches removed after 5d), or through an incision in the top of the vagina, or vaginal surgery with laporoscope (key hole surgery). Decisions about type of surgery influenced by individual circumstances, abdominal surgery is the most common method.

Post hysterectomy
- Takes about 6wks for abdominal muscles and tissues to heal. Advice to remain off work for this period, avoid strenuous exercise or lifting.
- Vaginal discharge for up to 4wks. Sanitary pads rather than tampons used to reduce risk of infection.

- Sex can be resumed after 6wks, post surgery check. Many have no problems with sex but some find the surgery has shortened their vagina and slightly changed its angle. They experience different sensations and responses during sex. This can be very distressing and take time to come to terms with. May also find their vagina is dry and would benefit from a lubricant.
- HRT often prescribed for those whose ovaries removed (Menopause 📖).
- More general advice:
  - Avoid any lifting or housework for the first few weeks.
  - Avoid heavy lifting for about 3mths.
  - Avoid standing for long periods.
  - Do some form of gentle exercise every day, e.g. walking a short distance, slowly increasing.
  - Do the exercises recommended by hospital physiotherapist for Pelvic floor and abdominal muscle strengthening (Stress urinary incontinence 📖).
  - After vaginal discharge has disappeared exercise like swimming is beneficial.
  - Ensure a balanced diet and fluids to help avoid constipation.
  - Feeling low after an anesthetic is common but should recede.

Further information for professionals and women

📖 The Hysterectomy Association: www.hysterectomy-association.org.uk ☎ Helpline: 0871 7811141

Problems with fertility

Many couples trying to conceive are aided by additional information on the most fertile time in the menstrual cycle but should be encouraged to have sex 2 or 3 times a week throughout the cycle. Timing of intercourse using temperature charts or hormone detection kits causes stress and does not improve conception rates, so not recommended. Couple should also be given lifestyle advice on alcohol intake, weight management, smoking as well as preconceptual care. Female fertility declines significantly after 35yrs. Sperm function also declines past 55yrs but less markedly.

Infertility

Affects ~1:7couples and is a cause of considerable psychological distress. Defined as absence of pregnancy after 1yr of regular unprotected intercourse. Infertility is classed as 1° in couples who have never conceived and 2° in couples who have previously conceived. Investigated earlier if other factors present e.g. woman's age, previous surgery, or irregular menstrual cycles. Usually health consultations and investigations dealt with as a couple. This may be in 1° care by GP or referred to specialists. Investigations follow the same pathway:
- Checking ♀ partner is ovulating normally
- Checking ♂ partner has a normal semen analysis
- Confirming normality of the female genital tract.

Infertility may be unexplained (30%), or 2° to ovulatory failure (27%), male factors (19%), tubal factors (14%), or endometriosis (5%).

Treatment

Types of treatment dependent on problems identified:
- Medical e.g. assist with ovulation e.g. clomifene.
- Surgical treatment e.g. tubal surgery to remove obstruction.
- Assisted conception:
  - Intra-uterine insemination (IUI) sperm placed in woman's uterus.
  - Donor insemination (DI) insemination of sperm from a donor into a woman, via her vagina (IUI).
  - In vitro fertilization (IVF) retrieval of the egg(s), mixed with sperm and incubated for 2–3d; the resultant embryo(s) then injected into the uterus via the cervix.
  - Intracytoplasmic sperm injection (ICSI) an individual sperm injected directly into the egg.
  - Oocyte donation stimulation of the donor's ovaries and collection of eggs, then fertilized by the recipient's partner's sperm, embryos transferred to the uterus of the recipient following hormonal preparation of the endometrium.
  - Embryo donation. Couples who have had successful IVF or ICSI decide to donate their spare embryos to help other infertile couples.

Many 2° care centres carry out a range of infertility treatments, but usually only specialist infertility clinics offer IVF, ICSI, and DI. DoH recommends that each PCO offers all women aged 23–39yrs who meet the NICE clinical criteria (have an identified cause for their fertility problems, such as azoospermia) a minimum of 1 full cycle of IVF.

Atrophic vaginitis

Post-menopausal changes create dryness that presents as vaginal soreness and dyspareunia. Treated short term with topical oestrogen as pessaries or vaginal ring (BNF 7.2.1) and advise on lubricants during sexual intercourse.

Bartholins gland swellings

2 glands with ducts opening into vulva, in sexual arousal these secrete lubricant. Obstruction of the ducts leads to vulval swelling and cyst formation. Cysts resolve spontaneously. If infected an abcess results that may respond to antibioitics or need surgical drainage.

Genital warts and herpes

See 📖 Sexually transmitted infections.

Vulval swelling

Can be due to venous or lymphatic obstruction, causes include:
• Secondary to malignancy in the pelvis (Gynaecological cancers 📖)
• Dependent oedema with prolonged sitting in bed, addressing positioning and movement
• Pregnancy, where varicosities may appear, resolves at end of pregnancy
• With bruising may be trauma of a sexual nature (Crime and victims of crime 📖).

Vulval itching (pruritis)

May be caused by infection, infestations, vulval atrophy, dystrophy, carcinoma, allergic response to perfumed soaps etc. Aim of care is to identify cause and treat.

Vulval dystrophy

Changes in appearance of the skin, sometimes with white plaques, and itching, sometimes dysparunia. Occurs mostly in post-menopausal women. Correct term: squamous cell hyperplasia. **Lichen sclerosus** is uncommon. Skin appears thin, white, and crinkly. **Squamous cell hyperplasia** is uncommon, found in older women. There are thickened, asymmetrical, white or grey areas. Treated with clobetasol propionate 0.05% ointment (BNF 13.4).

Psychosexual problems

Women who have any chronic genital disorders may lose interest in sexual activity and have psychosexual problems. Important to give patients the opportunity to express concerns on their sexual function and to offer referral or information on psychosexual counselling (often via community family planning service, sexual health services or Relate see below).

Related topics

📖 Gynaecological cancers; 📖 Dermatology.

Further information

📖 Relate relationship and psychosexual counselling: www.relate.org.uk
📖 Royal College of Obstetricians and Gynecology Information sheets: www.rcog.org.uk/
📖 Womens Health Information Leaflets: www.womenshealthlondon.org.uk

Termination of pregnancy (TOP)

UK Law

England, Wales, and Scotland

The 1967 Abortion Act and 1990 Human Fertilization/Embryology Acts govern TOP. TOP allowed up to 24wks of pregnancy if 2 doctors give their consent and confirm that it is necessary because of one or more of the following:

- Continuation of pregnancy involves ↑ risk to the life of the woman.
- Continuation would cause injury to the mother's physical or mental health (90% TOPs are carried out under this clause).
- Continuation would cause injury to the physical or mental health of the mother's existing children.
- The baby is at substantial risk of being physically or mentally handicapped.

NB Upper gestation limit does not apply if mother's life threatened or serious injury or fetal handicap.

Northern Ireland

TOP illegal (consultation period finishes in April).

Consultations in primary care

Women with an unplanned and unwanted pregnancy

These women need to talk through with partners, and/or relatives and/or close friends, their emotions and choices. Primary care and contraceptive services are often the first health services consulted to confirm pregnancy and advise on options and processes for TOP.

Prenatal diagnosis of abnormality

♀ undergoing routine antenatal screening (Antenatal care and screening 📖) may also be told that their baby has a serious risk of physical and mental impairment and TOP could be considered. Requires specialist support in counselling on options (see below).

Role of health professionals

All health professionals should ensure ♀ are treated non-judgementally and has access to full information, irrespective of their own personal views (Professional conduct 📖). This may mean offering another professional for that consultation or referring the woman elsewhere to receive counselling of options and full information to make an informed choice.

Main areas of information

- ♀ has right to confidentiality irrespective of age (Confidentiality 📖).
- ♀ alone gives consent, does not need agreement of partner or parents (informed Consent (📖) and <16yrs).
- TOPs safer earlier in pregnancy.
- TOPs available through the NHS (local services may have eligibility criteria, medical referral or self-referral process) and private organizations (self-referral and payment). All carried out in NHS hospitals or special licensed clinics.

- Process in all organizations ensures a counselling/assessment visit to help ♀ reach the decision right for her and then time before the TOP visit to change mind.
- Types of TOP.
  - <9wks pregnancy early medical abortion. Involves 2 appointments. Oral mifepristone given at first followed 2d later by oral or vaginal prostaglandin to expel pregnancy in next 4–6hrs.
  - >7–12 or 15wks vacuum aspiration usually under sedation and local anesthetic.
  - >15wks surgical dilation and evacuation under general anesthetic.
- Risks of procedures include: haemorrhage, failure and on-going pregnancy, infection, psychological impact. No association between TOP and subsequent infertility or miscarriage.
- All TOP have a follow-up visit to clinic or GP 2wks later.
- ♀ experience a range of emotions afterwards from relief to sadness and loss, depending on circumstances, reasons for TOP, and decision making process.
- After TOP menstrual cycle returns to normal, can conceive again within 2wks. Contraception options to be considered before TOP (Contraception: general 🕮).

Referral processes for NHS TOP

These vary according to local areas. Primary care professionals may need to confirm pregnancy by test and confirm gestation. May need to refer to doctor in community clinics or GP if gestation uncertain or local referral procedures require it.

♀ following prenatal diagnosis of abnormality referred within NHS hospital.

Further information

🖥 FPA UK www.fpa.org.uk ☎ 0845 310 1334
FPA Scotland ☎ 0141 576 5088
FPA Northern Ireland ☎ 028 9032 5488

Organizations offering TOP services

🖥 British Pregnancy Advisory Service (England, Wales, Scotland): www.bpas.org/ ☎ 08457 30 40 30
🖥 Marie Stopes UK: www.mariestopes.org.uk/uk ☎ 0845 300 8090

Patient information and support for prenatal diagnosis of abnormalities

🖥 Antenatal results and choices (ARC): supports parents faced with prenatal diagnosis of foetal abnormality and those that have had terminations www.arc-uk.org ☎ 0207 631 0285

Minor injuries and emergencies

Adult basic life support (BLS)

Basic life support implies that no special equipment is used by the rescuer other than a protective device.

Chest compression and reducing the number and duration of pauses: key to improving victim's chance of survival.

Cardiac arrest: diagnosis

If the victim is unresponsive, not breathing normally make a diagnosis of cardiac arrest. See Fig. 13.1.

Adult basic life support sequence of actions

1 Make sure the victim, bystanders, and you are safe

2 Check the victim for a response. Gently shake shoulders and ask loudly, 'Are you all right?'.

3a If there is a response:

- If no further danger leave in the position found
- Try to find out what is wrong, obtain help, offer reassurance.

3b If there is <u>no</u> response:

- Shout for help
- Turn the victim onto their back
- Place your hand on his forehead and gently tilt their head back
- With your fingertips under the point of the victim's chin, lift the chin to open the airway.

4 Keeping the airway open, look, listen, and feel for normal breathing.

- Look for chest movement
- Listen at the victim's mouth for breath sounds
- Feel for air on your cheek.

First few minutes after cardiac arrest, victim may be barely breathing, or taking infrequent, noisy gasps. Do not confuse with normal breathing. Look, listen, and feel for **no more than 10 seconds** to determine if breathing normally. If in doubt act as if it is **not** normal.

5a If they *are* breathing normally:

- Turn them into the recovery position (see below)
- Send or go for help, or summon an ambulance
- Check for continued breathing.

5b If they are <u>not</u> breathing normally:

- Ask someone to call an ambulance, if alone, do this yourself. You may need to leave the victim temporarily.

Start chest compression:

- Kneel by the side of the victim
- Place the heel of one hand in the centre of the victim's chest
- Place the heel of your other hand on top of the first hand
- Interlock the fingers of your hands and ensure that pressure is not applied over the victim's ribs
- Do not apply any pressure over the upper abdomen or the bottom end of the bony sternum (breastbone)

The recovery position

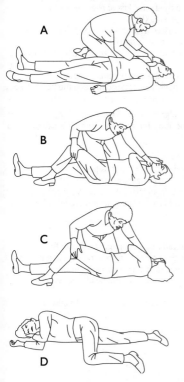

Fig. 13.2 The recovery position. Reproduced with kind permission from Dr. Chantal Simon, Series editor, Oxford General Practice Library.

When circulation and breathing have been restored, it is important to:
• Maintain a good airway
• Ensure the tongue does not cause obstruction
• Minimize the risk of inhalation of gastric contents
For this reason the victim should be placed in the recovery position. This allows the tongue to fall forward, keeping the airway clear.

Putting a patient in the recovery position
• Remove the patient's glasses
• Kneel beside the patient and make sure that both legs are straight (A)
• Place the arm nearest to you out at right angles to the body, elbow bent with the hand palm uppermost (A)

- Bring the far arm across the chest, and hold the back of the hand against the patient's cheek nearest to you (B)
- With your other hand, grasp the far leg just above the knee and pull it up, keeping the foot on the ground (B)
- Keeping the patient's hand pressed against his cheek, pull on the leg to roll the patient towards you onto his side (C)
- Adjust the upper leg so that both the hip and knee are bent at right angles (D)
- Tilt the head back to make sure the airway remains open (D)
- Adjust the hand under the cheek, if necessary, to keep the head tilted
- Check breathing regularly

⚠ Monitor the peripheral circulation of the lower arm. If the patient has to be kept in the recovery position for > 30min., turn the patient onto the opposite side.

The unconcious child
- The child should be in as near a true lateral position as possible with his mouth dependent to allow free drainage of fluid
- The position should be stable. In an infant this may require the support of a small pillow or rolled up blanket placed behind the infant's back to maintain the position.

Cervical spine injury
- If spinal cord injury is suspected (for example if the victim has sustained a fall, been struck on the head or neck, or has been rescued after diving into shallow water) take particular care during handling and resuscitation to maintain alignment of the head, neck and chest in the neutral position
- A spinal board and/or cervical collar should be used if available.

Child BLS

(See Adult basic life support 📖.)

Check responsiveness

1 Ensure safety of both rescuer and child
2 Check responsiveness ask loudly are you alright, stimulate child
3 If child responsive; reassure, if safe, leave in position found, and seek help
4 Unconscious child whose airway is clear and who is breathing spontaneously place in recovery position.

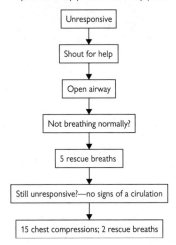

Unresponsive

↓

Shout for help

↓

Open airway

↓

Not breathing normally?

↓

5 rescue breaths

↓

Still unresponsive?—no signs of a cirulation

↓

15 chest compressions; 2 rescue breaths

Fig. 13.3 Child basic life support algorithm (reproduced with permission of the Resuscitation Council UK)

If *no* response

- Shout for help
- Open the child's airway by gently tilting the head and lifting the chin (Fig. 13.4) avoiding pushing on soft tissue under chin as this may block airway.

Start infant and child BLS sequence

- Give 5 initial **rescue breaths** (see below)
- Take no more than 10 seconds to check response before starting **chest compression** (see below)
- If you are on your own, perform **CPR** 30 chest compressions (see below) to 2 rescue breaths for one minute before seeking help.

Fig. 13.4 Lifting the chin

Rescue breaths for a child >1yr:
- Ensure head tilt and chin lift
- Pinch closed the soft part of the child's nose with the index finger and thumb of your hand placed on his forehead
- Open mouth a little but maintain the chin upwards
- Take a breath and place your lips around his mouth, ensuring a good seal
- Blow steadily into the child's mouth for about 1–1.5 seconds, watching for the chest to rise then take your mouth away watch for their chest to fall as air comes out
- Take another breath and repeat sequence 5x
- If appears to be airway obstruction open the child's mouth and remove any visible obstruction. Do not do blind finger sweep of mouth.

Rescue breaths for an infant
- As for >1yr only ensure a neutral position of the head and apply the chin lift and cover the mouth and nose of the infant with your mouth, ensuring you have a good seal.

Checking response to rescue breaths in <10 seconds

Look for signs of circulation: movement, coughing breathing. Check pulse: child >1yr, feel for carotid pulse in the neck. Infant, feel for brachial pulse on the inner aspect of the upper arm.

- If signs of a circulation within 10 seconds continue rescue breathing, until the child starts breathing on their own
- If no signs of a circulation or no pulse, or uncertainty **Start chest compression and combine with rescue breathing.**

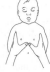

Fig. 13.5 Encircling technique

Chest compressions
- For all children, compress the lower third of the sternum: locate the xiphisternum by finding where the lowest ribs join in the middle, compress the sternum one finger's breadth above this
- Compress the chest by approximately $^1/_3$ of its depth
- Use tips of 2 fingers for an infant or encircling technique (see Fig. 13.5) and 2 hands for a child >1yr
- Repeat at a rate of 100 compressions a minute
- After 15 (30 if alone) compressions, give two effective breaths.

Continue resuscitation until:
The child shows signs of life (spontaneous respiration, pulse, movement); or further qualified help arrives and takes over.

Vital for rescuers to get help quickly when a child collapses
If alone and **witness sudden collapse** in child, likely to be a cardiac arrest through arryhthmia and the child may need defibrillation. Seek help immediately rather than perform 1 minute CPR.

Automated external defibrillators (AEDs)
An unmodified AED may be used in children >1yr. Insufficient evidence to support a recommendation for or against the use of AEDs in infants <1yr.

Further information for health professionals

🖳 Resuscitation Council: www.resus.org.uk

Anaphylaxis

No universally accepted definitions of anaphylactic and anaphylactoid reactions. Anaphylaxis is a severe systemic hypersensitivity/allergic reaction typically mediated by immunoglobulin E (IgE).

Common causes
(See also Allergies 🔲.)
- Foods: nuts, shellfish, sesame seeds and oil, milk eggs, pulses, strawberries
- Stings: wasp or bee
- Drugs: antibiotics especially penicillins, muscle relaxants, contrast media asprin, and other NSAIDs
- Complement mediated: (human proteins e.g. γ-globulin, blood products)
- Latex
- Unknown ('idiopathic')
- Vaccines
- Anaesthetic agents (important causes of anaphylactoid reactions).

Clinical features
Reactions vary in severity, according to the nature and amount of the stimulus, progress may be rapid, slow, or (unusually) biphasic. Onset is usually within min or hrs. Clinical presentations may include:

Respiratory system: respiratory difficulty dyspnoea, swelling of the lips, tongue, larynx, pharxnx, and epiglottis may lead to complete upper airway occlusion. Lower airway involvement—dyspnoea, wheeze, chest tightness, hypoxia, hypercapnoea, stridor. Patients can die from acute, irreversible asthma or laryngeal oedema.

Cardiovascular system: hypotension can present as fainting and loss of consciousness. Cardiovascular collapse is a common manifestation, especially in response to IV drugs or stings, and any cardiac dysfunction is due primarily to hypotension. Arrythmias, ischaemic chest pain, and ECG changes may be present. Beta blockers may increase the severity of an allergic reaction and antagonise the response to adrenaline.

Skin: the skin colour usually changes and the patient may appear either flushed or pale. Urticaria and rhinitis, conjunctivitis, pruritus, erythema, urticaria, and angio-oedema may occur.

GI tract: abdominal pain, nausea, vomiting, diarrhoea.
Often reported that patients have a sense of impending doom.

> All nurses involved in the administration of injections and other procedures in the home and/or clinics should carry/have direct access to an emergency adrenaline pack and be aware of local policy guidelines on the treatment of anaphylaxis.

Treatment (See treatment algorithms for children, Fig. 13.6, and adults, Fig. 13.7.)
- If anaphylaxis suspected call for emergency help immediately.
- Make patient comfortable. If having difficulty breathing sit up, if hypotensive lie flat and elevate legs.

- Ask if the patient has had similar reaction before and if they have an epipen. If yes, use it.
- If O_2 available give at high flow rates 10–15L/min.

Epinephrine (adrenaline) available for use by UK community nurses. It reverses peripheral vasodilatation and ↓ oedema, dilates the airways, ↑ the force of myocardial contraction and suppresses histamine and leukotriene release. IM adrenaline (epinephrine) should be given to all patients with clinical signs of shock airway swelling or breathing difficulty. Preferable injection site—midpoint anterolateral thigh.

Care and management

- Warn patients of possibility of recurrence.
- Advise sufferers to wear a medic alert or equivalent (☎ 0207 833 3034).
- Refer to GP to consider prescribing epipen and training on its use.
- Encourage patients with known allergies to minimize risk e.g. vigilance for hidden allergens in foods e.g. peanuts = groundnuts = arachis oil.
- Emphasize to patients that they should not be afraid of administering adrenaline and should not delay administration.
- Write out a crisis plan and ensure training available for friends, family, and school on how to handle an emergency and, if appropriate, where to locate adrenaline.

Related topics

📖 Adult basic life support; 📖 Child BLS; 📖 Allergies.

Further information for professionals and carers

📟 Anaphylaxis campaign: www.anaphylaxis.org.uk
📟 BBC online and interactive tests for first aid: www.bbc.co.uk/health/first_aid
Wyatt, J. et al. (2006). *Oxford Handbook of Emergency Medicine*. (3rd edn.) Oxford University Press, Oxford.

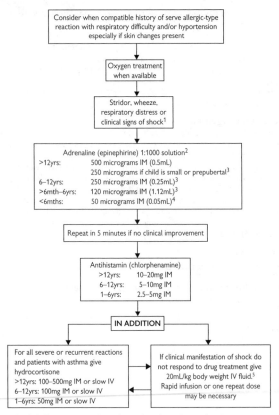

Consider when compatible history of serve allergic-type reaction with respiratory difficulty and/or hypotension especially if skin changes present

Oxygen treatment when available

Stridor, wheeze, respiratory distress or clinical signs of shock[1]

Adrenaline (epinephrine) 1:1000 solution[2]
>12yrs: 500 micrograms IM (0.5mL)
                      250 micrograms if child is small or prepubertal[3]
6–12yrs: 250 micrograms IM (0.25mL)[3]
>6mth–6yrs: 120 micrograms IM (1.12mL)[3]
<6mths: 50 micrograms IM (0.05mL)[4]

Repeat in 5 minutes if no clinical improvement

Antihistamin (chlorphenamine)
>12yrs: 10–20mg IM
6–12yrs: 5–10mg IM
1–6yrs: 2.5–5mg IM

IN ADDITION

For all severe or recurrent reactions and patients with asthma give hydrocortisone
>12yrs: 100–500mg IM or slow IV
6–12yrs: 100mg IM or slow IV
1–6yrs: 50mg IM or slow IV

If clinical manifestation of shock do not respond to drug treatment give 20mL/kg body weight IV fluid.[5] Rapid infusion or one repeat dose may be necessary

1. An inhaled beta$_2$-agonist such as salbutamol may be used as an adjunctive measure if bronchospasm is severe and does not respond rapidly to other treatment.

2. If profound shock judged **immediately** life threatening give CPR/ALS if necessary. Consider **slow** intravenous (IV) adrenaline (epinephrine) 1:10,000 solution. This is **hazardous** and is recommended only for an experienced practitioner who can also obtain IV access without delay. Note the different strength of adrenaline (epinephrine) that may be required for IV use.

3. For children who have been prescribed an adrenaline auto-injector, 150 micrograms can be given instead of 120 micrograms, and 300 micrograms can be given instead of 250 micrograms or 500 micrograms.

4. Absolute accuracy of the small does is not essential.

5. A crystalloid may be safer than a colloid.

Fig. 13.6 Anaphylactic reactions: treatment algorithm for children by first medical responders (reproduced by permission from the Resuscitation Council (UK). Updated May 2005)

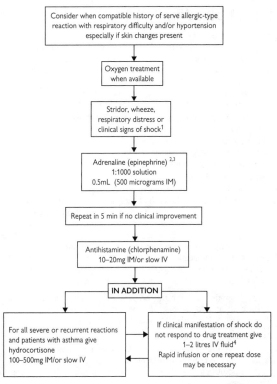

Consider when compatible history of serve allergic-type reaction with respiratory difficulty and/or hypotension especially if skin changes present

Oxygen treatment when available

Stridor, wheeze, respiratory distress or clinical signs of shock[1]

Adrenaline (epinephrine)[2,3] 1:1000 solution 0.5mL (500 micrograms IM)

Repeat in 5 min if no clinical improvement

Antihistamine (chlorphenamine) 10–20mg IM/or slow IV

IN ADDITION

For all severe or recurrent reactions and patients with asthma give hydrocortisone 100–500mg IM/or slow IV

If clinical manifestation of shock do not respond to drug treatment give 1–2 litres IV fluid[4] Rapid infusion or one repeat dose may be necessary

1. An inhaled beta$_2$-agonist such as salbutamol may be used as an adjunctive measure if bronchospasm is severe and does not respond rapidly to other treatment.

2. If profound shock judged **immediately** life threatening give CPR/ALS if necessary. Consider **slow** IV adrenaline (epinephrine) 1:10,000 solution. This is **hazardous** and is recommended only for an experienced practitioner who can also obtain IV access without delay. Note the different strength of adrenaline (epinephrine) that may be required for IV use.

3. If adults are treated with an adrenaline auto-injector, the 300 micrograms will usually be sufficient. A second dose may be required. Half doses of adrenaline (epinephrine) may be safer for patients on amitriptyline, imipramine, or beta blocker.

4. A crystalloid may be safer than a colloid.

Fig. 13.7 Anaphylactic reactions: treatment algorithm for adults by first medical responders (reproduced by permission from the Resuscitation council (UK). Updated May 2005)

External bleeding

There are three types of external bleeding:
- Capillary: most common type of external bleeding when blood oozes from capillaries. Usually not serious and easiest to control.
- Venous: occurs when a vein severed and blood flows steadily. Most veins collapse when cut = aids control of this type of bleeding.
- Arterial: is the most severe type of external bleeding requiring urgent attention. Blood spurts with each heartbeat, often hard to control.

First aid for external bleeding—key principles
- Stop the bleeding using pressure
- Preserve the existing blood volume
- Prevent infection using dressings
- Prevent shock by reassurance and careful patient positioning.

Controlling blood loss
- Stay calm and reassure the victim.
- Apply direct pressure to the wound with thumb and/or fingers over a dressing if available. If a dressing unavailable, use a clean handkerchief, towel, piece of clothing, or your hand alone. If the wound is large, squeeze the sides of the wound together gently but firmly. Patients are often able to apply direct pressure to their own wounds.
- Place a sterile, unmedicated dressing over the wound, ensuring that it fully covers the injury, and secure it with bandage applied firmly enough to control bleeding but not to impede the circulation.

If bleeding continues through the original dressing, apply further dressings on top and bandage firmly. Do not remove the original dressing as this may disturb clots and restart the bleeding.

- If bleeding continues, and you have no reason to suspect a fracture, elevate the wound above the level of the heart if possible.
- As a last resort to control arterial bleeding. Apply indirect pressure at a pressure point (e.g. brachial or femoral arteries), for timed periods of 15min only.
- Superficial wounds: wash with soap and warm water, remove any obvious loose debris or dirt, dry, and apply a sterile dressing.
- Lay the victim down if fainting is a possibility.
- If a foreign body such a knife, arrow, bullet, or stick becomes embedded in the body, **do not remove it**. Place pads and bandages around the foreign body and use tape to stabilise it, seek emergency medical attention immediately.

General precautions
Some diseases such as AIDS and hepatitis B are transmitted through the exchange of body fluids. To minimize the risk of infection, wear disposable gloves and plastic goggles and, where appropriate, a surgical mask (Personal protective equipment 🕮).

Internal bleeding
Signs and symptoms of internal bleeding are:
- Deteriorating conscious level
- Cool, moist skin

- Abnormal pulse and breathing difficulties
- Slow capillary refill time (following cutaneous pressure on a digit, or preferably on the centre of the sternum for 5sec, capillary refill should occur within 2sec. A slower refill time indicates poor skin perfusion)
- Haemoptysis and haematemesis
- Bruises on chest or signs of fractured ribs
- Penetrating wounds to the chest or abdomen
- Bruised, swollen, tender, or rigid abdomen
- Bleeding from the vagina or rectum.

First aid for internal bleeding is limited

- For simple bruising, apply cold compresses to slow bleeding, relieve pain, and reduce swelling
- Monitor the patient and be prepared to administer CPR if required.
- Referred to hospital/ED for specialist investigations and treatment.

Bleeding disorders

Suspect a bleeding disorder if:
- Spontaneous or excess haemorrhage occurs from multiple or uninjured sites into deep tissues
- Delayed bleeding occurs after hours or days.

Ask about previous history of bleeding following trauma, surgery etc., current medication, and recent medical history.

Congenital disorders most adults with a congenital disorder carry a National Haemophilia card or a Medic-Alert bracelet. Many haemophiliacs are the experts about required treatment and will be registered at a haemophilia centre which should be contacted for advice.

Acquired disorders

May be due to liver disease, uraemia, drug use (specifically aspirin, NSAIDs, warfarin/anticoagulants, alcohol (🕮)) or unrecognized conditions such as haematological malignancy.

Routine wound management of patients with bleeding disorders follows standard procedures as above accompanied by prior or simultaneous administration of factor concentrates and platelets under haematological advice.

Related topics

🕮 Child BLS; 🕮 Adult basic life support; 🕮 HIV; 🕮 Viral hepatitis; 🕮 Sickle cell disorders; 🕮 Patients on anticoagulant therapies.

Further information for professionals

🖳 Resuscitation Council (UK) Resuscitation guidelines: www.resus.org.uk

Burns

In England and Wales, approx 50,000 burnt or scalded children attend EDs annually, and 10% require hospital admission. 70% are pre-school children, most common age group 1–2yrs. Highest rates occur in children <5 and in people >75yrs.

Most fatal burns occur in house fires where smoke inhalation is the usual cause of death.

- All flame burns involve high temperatures → most serious injuries.
- Scalds commonly caused by hot drinks, bath water, or cooking oil. Scalds generally involve water below boiling point and contact for <4secs, those involving hot fat or steam at much higher temperatures, → more serious injury.
- Strong association between burns to children and low socio-economic status which contribute to family stress, poor housing, and overcrowding.

Classification of burns

Patients are divided into:
- High risk (children <10yrs and adults >50yrs)
- Low risk (aged 10–50yrs).

Pathophysiology

Two main factors determine the severity of burns and scalds:
- Temperature of the heat source
- Duration of contact.

Epidermal injury occurs after 30sec at 54°C and within 1sec at 70°C.

Types of burn

- Thermal
- Chemical
- Electrical
- Radiation.

NB Asking about the detailed circumstances of the burn will alert to the possibility of other injury (e.g. blast injuries, injuries from escaping fire, inhalation of poisonous fumes, etc).

Assessing depth and extent

- *Superficial burns* involve epidermis (e.g. sunburn) with the skin red, painful and tender but with no blister formation, require only symptomatic relief.
- *Partial thickness burns* involve the epidermis and the dermis (papillary layer) but not the deeper layers of the dermis, hair follicles, and sebaceous glands, very painful to the touch. The skin is blistered, pink, or mottled. These heal within 2–3wks with minimal scarring and full return of function.
- *Full thickness burns* damage epidermis and the dermis and may cause injury to deeper structures as well including hair follicles, sweat, and sebaceous glands. The skin looks white or charred and is painless and leathery to touch. Healing takes between 3–8wks with scarring common. These injuries may need surgical debridement and skin grafting.

Minor burns

Partial thickness burns involving <15% body surface area (BSA) in low-risk patients *or* 10% high-risk patients *or* full thickness burns of <2% without other injuries. Often treated in OP clinics/surgery.

For minor burns, limited to an area no larger than 2–3 inches in diameter:

- **Cool the burn.** Hold burnt area under cold, running water for 15min (timed). If impractical, immerse the burn in cold water or cool with cold compresses. Cooling the burn ↓ swelling. Do not put ice directly onto burn—it may cause tissue damage. If water unavailable, use any cold, harmless liquid such as beer, lemonade, milk, or bag of frozen peas.
- **Remove gently any potential constrictions** (e.g. rings, watches, belts, shoes) before the injured area begins to swell.
- **Dress the burn** with a clean, preferably sterile, non-fluffy material, and bandage. (this restricts air to the injured area, ↓ pain and protects blistered skin). Cling film ideal **for the immediate treatment** of superficial and partial thickness burns if there are low levels of exudate.
- Offer pain relief.
- Do not use adhesive dressings.
- Do not break blisters (which protect against infection).
- Do not apply lotions, ointments, or fat to the injury.

Healing
- Minor burns usually heal in 1–2wks without further treatment.
- Monitor burns for signs of infection.
- Advise patients to use high factor sunscreens for one year.

Moderate burns
Partial thickness burns of 15–25% BSA in low risk *or* 10–20% in high-risk patients, *or* full thickness burns of 3–10% BSA.

Major *burns*
Partial thickness burns >25% BSA in low-risk patients *or* >20% BSA in high-risk patients *or* full thickness burns >10% BSA in anyone. Also includes burns involving hands, face, feet, perineum, or crossing major joints or circumferential of an extremity, plus burns complicated by fractures, other trauma, inhalation injury, or electrical burns in those in poor risk groups and infants and older people.

Common causes
- Clothing on fire
- Hot water immersion
- Contact with flames, hot objects, electricity
- Corrosive chemicals.

All third degree burns require urgent treatment in hospital and possibly referral to a specialist burns unit.

First aid for flame burns
Clothing on fire
- Lay the casualty down immediately to prevent flames burning the face.
- Douse the flames with water or other non-flammable liquid.
- Smother the flames with a blanket or jacket while rolling the casualty on the ground.
- Remove jewellery and tight clothing from the burnt area.
- Do not remove clothing adherent to the burn.
- Do not apply ice, lotion, ointments, or home remedies.
- Immerse the burnt area in cold water or apply cold compresses briefly.

- Children should never be transported with cold soaks in place.
- Wrap patient loosely in clean sheet and transport to hospital.
- If the patient is conscious, not vomiting, and if medical help is more than 2hrs away, give small sips of water.
- Treat for shock.

Chemical burns

- Remove the harmful chemical as quickly as possible.
- Flood the affected area with slowly running cold water for at least 10min to prevent further damage to the burnt tissue.
- Gently remove contaminated clothing and jewellery while flooding the injured area, ensuring you do not contaminate yourself.
- Dress the burn with a clean, sterile, non-fluffy material, and bandage.
- Remove to hospital immediately.
- Alert the hospital to ensure containment of any chemical hazard and safe disposal of contaminated materials.
- Follow-up for health professional staff may require occupational health department and the Health Protection Agency.

Electrical burns

- The first priority in electrical injuries is to SWITCH OFF the current.
- The management of electrocution should follow ABCDE (Airway, Breathing, Circulation, Disability, and Exposure assessment) principles.
- Almost all injuries can be associated with electrocution.
- Entry and exit wounds should be sought to anticipate the pattern of possible internal injury.
- Cardiac arrythmias may occur for some considerable time after electrocution.

Radiation burns

- In the UK, 24-hr advice and assistance is available via NAIR (National Arrangements for Incidents involving Radioactivity) on ☎ telephone 0800 834153 or via the police.
- In an emergency, patients may be taken to any ED for radioactive decontamination treatment.
- Advice and help should be sought urgently from the duty ED consultant and a radiation physicist (from the medical physics or radiotherapy department).
- Treatment of contaminated patients must take place in a designated decontamination room.
- All staff must be decontaminated and checked before leaving this area.

Related topics

📖 Wound assessment; 📖 Wound dressings.

Further information for health professionals

Advanced Life Support Group (2005). The burned or scalded child. In *Advanced Paediatric Life Support*, Mackway-Jones K. *et al* (eds). pp. 199–204, BMJ Books, Blackwell Publishing, Oxford.

📖 Mayo Clinic Tools for healthier lives. http://mayoclinic.com/health/first-aid-burns

📖 NAIR: www.nrpt.org/radiation_incidents/nair.htm

📖 PatientPlus Burns—assessment and management: www.patient.co.uk/showdoc/400011971

Wyatt, J.P., *et al* (2006). Environmental emergencies, pp 256–8. In *Oxford Handbook of Emergency Medicine*. Oxford University Press, Oxford.

Adult choking

Choking usually results from airway obstruction by a foreign body. Early recognition is key to successful outcome, important not to confuse this emergency with fainting, heart attack, stroke, or other conditions which may cause sudden respiratory distress, cyanosis, or loss of consciousness.

General signs of choking
- Attack occurs while eating
- Victim may clutch his neck.

Foreign bodies may cause either mild or severe airway obstruction.
Vital to ask the conscious victim, 'Are you choking?'

Table 13.1 Signs of airway obstruction

Signs of mild airway obstruction	Signs of severe airway obstruction
Response to the question, 'Are you choking?'	*Response to the question, 'Are you choking?'*
- Victim speaks and answers, 'yes'	- Victim unable to speak - Victim may respond by nodding
Other signs	Other signs
- Victim unable to speak, cough, and breathe	- Victim is unable to breathe - Breathing sounds wheezy - Attempts at coughing are silent - Victim may be unconscious

Adult choking sequence
(Fig. 13.8.)

If the victim shows signs of mild airway obstruction
Encourage them to continue coughing, but do nothing else.

If the victim shows signs of severe airway obstruction and is conscious
- Stand to the side and slightly behind the victim.
- Support the chest with one hand and lean the victim well forwards so that head is lower than the chest so that when the obstruction is dislodged it comes out of the mouth and not further down the airway.
- Give **up to** 5 sharp blows between the shoulder blades with the heel of your other hand.
- Check to see if each back blow has relieved the airway obstruction, aim is to relieve the obstruction with each blow rather than necessarily to give all 5.
- If this fails, give up to 5 abdominal thrusts.
- Stand behind the victim and put both arms round the upper part of their abdomen.
- Lean the victim forwards.
- Clench your fist and place it between the umbilicus (navel) and the bottom end of the sternum (breastbone).
- Grasp this hand with your other hand and pull sharply inwards and upwards.

- Repeat up to 5 times.
- If the obstruction is still not relieved, continue alternating 5 back blows with 5 abdominal thrusts.

If the victim becomes unconscious

- Support the victim carefully to the ground.
- Call an ambulance immediately.
- Begin CPR (Adult basic life support 📖). Initiate chest compressions even if a pulse is present in the unconscious, choking victim.

❶ Following successful treatment for choking, foreign material may remain in the upper or lower respiratory tract causing complications later.

- Victims with a persistent cough, swallowing difficulties or with a sensation of an object still lodged in the throat must be referred for an expert medical opinion.
- Abdominal thrusts may cause serious internal injuries and all victims receiving abdominal thrusts must be examined for injury by a doctor.

Further information

📖 BBCFirst aid web site: www.bbc.co.uk/health/first_aid_action
Wyatt, J. et al. (2006). *Oxford Handbook of Emergency Medicine*. Oxford University Press, Oxford.

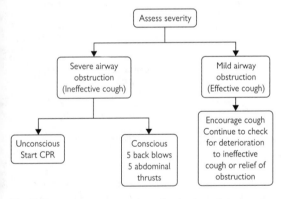

Fig. 13.8 Adult choking treatment (reproduced with permission from the Resuscitation Council UK Resuscitation Guidelines 2005)

Child choking

About 16,000 cases of choking every year; if a blockage completely prevents airflow then this can → permanent brain damage in 2min and death in 3min (see also Adult choking 📖).

Babies and toddlers frequently put objects in their mouths. Majority of choking events in children occur either during play or while eating with carer.

Recognition of foreign body airway obstruction (FBAO)

When a foreign body enters airway, a child will react immediately by coughing. A spontaneous cough is likely to be more effective and safer than any manoeuvre a rescuer might perform. If coughing is absent or ineffective, and object obstructs the airway, the child will rapidly become asphyxiated.

FBAO is characterized by:
- Coughing or choking gagging or stridor (high pitched, noisy respirations like the blowing of the wind).
- Sudden onset.
- Recent history of playing with or eating small objects.

Suspect FBAO if:
- There are no other signs of illness.
- There are clues, e.g. history of eating or playing with small items immediately prior to the onset of symptoms.

Similar signs and symptoms may also be associated with other causes of airway obstruction, such as laryngitis or epiglottitis, which require different management.

Ineffective cough	Effective cough
• Unable to vocalize	• Crying or verbal response to questions
• Quiet or silent cough	• Loud cough
• Unable to breathe	• Able to take a breath before coughing
• Cyanosis	• Fully responsive
• Decreasing level of consciousness	

Relief of FBAO

Fig. 13.9.
- If the child is coughing effectively, no external manoeuvre is necessary. Encourage the child to cough and monitor continuously.
- If the child's cough is, or is becoming ineffective, **shout for help immediately**, and determine the child's conscious level.

Conscious child with FBAO with absent or ineffective coughing.

Back blows in an infant
- Support the infant in a head-downwards, prone position, to enable gravity to assist removal of the foreign body.
- A seated or kneeling rescuer should be able to support the infant safely across their lap.
- Support the infant's head by placing the thumb of 1 hand at the angle of the lower jaw, and 1 or 2 fingers from the same hand at the same point on the other side of the jaw.

- Do not compress the soft tissues under the infant's jaw as this will exacerbate the airway obstruction.
- Deliver up to 5 sharp back blows with the heel of 1 hand in the middle of the back between the shoulder blades.
- Aim is to relieve the obstruction with each blow rather than to give all five.

In a child over one year
- Back blows are more effective if the child is positioned head down.
- A small child may be placed across the rescuer's lap as with an infant.
- If this is not possible, support the child in a forward-leaning position and deliver the back blows from behind.

If back blows fail to dislodge the object, and the child is still conscious, use chest thrusts for infants or abdominal thrusts for children. Do not use abdominal thrusts (Heimlich manoeuvre) for infants.

Chest thrusts for infants
- Turn the infant into a head-downwards supine position. This is achieved safely by placing your free arm along the infant's back and encircling the occiput with your hand.
- Support the infant down your arm, which is placed down (or across) your thigh.
- Identify the landmark for chest compression (lower sternum approximately one finger's breadth above the xiphisternum).
- Deliver five chest thrusts. These are similar to chest compressions, but sharper in nature, and delivered at a slower rate.

Abdominal thrusts for children over one year
- Stand or kneel behind the child. Place your arms under the child's arms and encircle his torso.
- Clench your fist and place it between the umbilicus and xiphisternum.
- Grasp this hand with your other hand and pull sharply inwards and upwards.
- Repeat up to 5 times.
- Ensure that pressure is not applied to the xiphoid process or the lower rib cage as this may cause abdominal trauma.

Following chest or abdominal thrusts, reassess the child
- If the object has not been expelled and the child is still conscious, continue the sequence of back blows and chest (for infant) or abdominal (for children) thrusts.
- Call out or send for help if it is still not available.
- Do not leave the child at this stage.

If the object is expelled successfully, assess the child's clinical condition. Any doubt that part of the object may remain in the respiratory tract seek medical assistance. Abdominal thrusts may cause internal injuries. Children should be examined by a medical practitioner.

Unconscious child with FBAO
- If the child with FBAO is, or becomes unconscious, place them on a firm, flat surface.
- Call out or send for help if it is still not available.
- Do not leave the child at this stage.

Airway opening
- Open the mouth and look for any obvious object.
- If one is seen, make an attempt to remove it with a single finger sweep. Do not attempt blind or repeated finger sweeps in children because these can impact the object more deeply into the pharynx and cause injury.

Rescue breaths
- Open the airway and attempt 5 rescue breaths.
- Assess the effectiveness of each breath: if a breath does not make the chest rise, reposition the head before making the next attempt.

Chest compression and CPR
- Attempt 5 rescue breaths and if no response, proceed immediately to chest compression.
- Follow the sequence for single rescuer approx. 1min before summoning the emergency medical services (if not done already by someone else).
- If the child regains consciousness and is breathing effectively, place in a safe side-lying (recovery) position and monitor till help arrives.

Related topics
📖 Adult BLS; 📖 Child BLS; 📖 Accident prevention.

Further information for professionals and carers
📺 BBC online and interactive tests for first aid: www.bbc.co.uk/health/first_aid_action/
Wyatt, J.P., *et al.* (2006). *Oxford Handbook of Emergency Medicine*. Oxford University Press, Oxford.

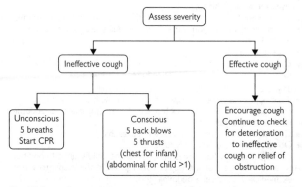

Fig. 13.9 Paediatric FBAO treatment algorithm (reproduced with permission from the Resuscitation council Guidelines 2005)

Eye trauma

There are more than >120,000 accidents in England involving eye injuries every year.

Assessment

- Time and mode of injury: physical/chemical, superficial blunt or penetrating trauma, speed of impact size of object.
- Were glasses or goggles worn?
- Possibility of foreign body.
- Previous and current acuity. Tenderness, bruising, conjunctival haemmorhage.
- Abnormal pupil reactivity, size, or shape (refer for medical assessment immediately),
- Examine the eye in a well-lit area. To find the object, ask person look up and down, then side-to-side.

Prevention of injury and/or further damage

- Wear protective goggles e.g. during construction work and high-risk sports e.g. squash.
- UV protection glasses for sailing, skiing and sunbed use.
- Tell patient not to rub eyes if trauma suspected.
- Stop wearing contact lens until symptom free.
- If in need of further care to reduce eye movement and risk of further infection cover with sterile dressing.

Common injuries

- **Corneal abrasion**: often caused by small sharp objects e.g. finger nail, characterized by intense pain, irritation, and photophibia. Drops of local anaesthetic (e.g. amethocaine BNF 11.7)and fluroscein used (if not available refer to ED) to check no foreign objects in eye, abrasion should heal within 48hrs. Antibiotic drops for healing and dressing only needed to protect eye following anaesthetic.
- **Foreign bodies** in the eye: e.g. small pieces of grit, eyelashes and usually move to lower part of eye, can be washed out or lifted out with a sterile cotton bud tip. If irritant not obvious, grasp the lower eyelid and gently pull down on it to look under the lower eyelid. To look under the upper lid, place a cotton-tipped swab on the outside of the upper lid and gently flip the lid over the cotton swab. If the object is embedded **do not** try to remove or apply any pressure. To reduce eye movement and risk of further infection cover with sterile dressing and refer for immediate specialist care.
- **Chemical injuries**: treat chemical burns **immediately**; hold eyelids open and bathe eyes with copious amounts of water (may be painful to keep eyes open so use anaesthetic drops). Chemical burns often have serious consequences refer urgently to specialist.
- **Arc eye**: welders, skiers, and sunbed users with no eye protection against UV light may damage corneal epithelium. Severe eye pain, watering, and blepharospasm. Give oral analgesic (paracetamol, ibuprofen (BNF 4.7.1)) and pad eye, should recover in 24hrs, if not refer to specialist. Advise on eye protection in the future.

Hypothermia first aid

- Move the patient out of the cold. If not feasible, protect the patient from the wind and rain, cover his head and insulate him from cold ground.
- Handle the patient gently.
- Remove wet clothing and replace with a warm, dry covering.
- Call 999 for emergency medical assistance.
- If breathing ceases or seems dangerously slow or shallow, begin CPR immediately.
- Do not apply direct heat to warm the victim. Apply warm compresses to the neck, chest wall and groin.
- Do not attempt to warm the arms and legs.
- Do not offer conscious patient alcohol. Give warm drinks unless vomiting.
- Treat the patient in a warm room (>21°C).
- Do not massage or rub the patient and treat very gently.

Rewarming methods

External rewarming is usually sufficient if the core temperature is >32°C. Endogenous metabolism and shivering generate heat allowing spontaneous rewarming. Easy, non-invasive process involving:

- Removing cold, wet clothing
- Wrap in warm blankets

In hospital

- Infrared radiant lamps and heating blankets may be used for children
- Aim to rewarm adults at a rate of 0.5–2°C/hr, but do not rewarm older people with prolonged hypothermia too rapidly (>0.6°C/hr) danger of cerebral/pulmonary oedema.

Active rewarming and core rewarming are available in hospital and may include

- Water bath at 37–41°C
- Hot air blanket
- Warm intravenous fluids to 39°C
- Gastric or bladder lavage with normal saline at 42°C
- Airway warming in self-ventilating patients
- Peritoneal lavage
- Extracorporeal: cardiopulmonary bypass maintains brain and vital organ perfusion, in patients with severe hypothermia or those in cardiac arrest.

Related topics

📖 Adult basic life support; 📖 Child BLS.

Further information

📶 BBC First aid action: www.bbc.co.uk/health/first_aid_action

Wyatt, J.P., et al. (2006). *Oxford Handbook of Emergency Medicine.* Oxford University Press, Oxford.

Poisoning and overdoses in adults

Deliberate self-poisoning

Commonest form of self-harm in adults and one of the top 5 causes of acute medical admissions. Estimate UK self-harm is around 400 per 100,000 population per annum, which is higher than most recorded in Europe. Self-harm is now only slightly more common among ♂ than ♀.

Most commonly ingested overdose substances are analgesics, particularly paracetamol. Drugs or poisons may often be taken impulsively. About a quarter of all suicides attend a general hospital after a non-fatal act of self-harm within the year before they die.

Unintentional or 'accidental' poisoning

- Approx 30,000 poisoning incidents a year involve infants and toddlers involving household substances or medicines. Peak incidence is 2yrs (NB many plants are poisonous e.g. privet, laburnum seeds, laurel and yew berries).
- Adult poisoning may result from miscalculation or confusion of doses or by taking the same medications under different names.
- Drug smugglers, who ingest multiple packages of drugs, are at serious risk of poisoning.

Overdoses

- Account for 15% of acute medical admissions
- 65% of drugs involved belong to the patient, a relative or friend
- 30% of self-poisonings involve multiple drugs
- 50% of patients will have consumed alcohol as well
- The history may be unreliable.

Priorities

- Resuscitate the patient
- Reduce absorption of the poison if possible
- Give a specific antidote if available.

Emergency treatment

- Clear and maintain the airway
- If breathing appears inadequate, ventilate with O_2 using a bag and mask or ET tube (NB not mouth to mouth in poisoned patients) if available
- Check pulse: if unconscious and pulseless start CPR
- Monitor vital signs
- If breathing place in recovery position in case of vomiting
- Call 999 for transport to hospital for specialist care.

Note down any information about the exposure to give to specialist services

- Product name
- Time of the incident
- Duration of exposure
- Route of exposure swallowed inhaled injected etc.

Information about poisons

☎ UK Poisons Information Centres Telephone advice is available at all times and a single telephone number 0870-600-6266 for the UK National Poisons Information Service directs the call automatically to the relevant centre. Centres can be contacted directly823on the following numbers:

- Belfast   028 9024 0503
- Birmingham   0121 507 5588 or 0121 507 5589
- Cardiff   029 2070 9901
- Edinburgh   0131 536 2300
- London   020 7653 9191
- Newcastle   0191 282 0300

- Ireland National Poisons Information Centre, Dublin 018092566

Information and advice about chemicals which might be released deliberately in a terrorist attack are available on ⊟ TOXBASE (www.spib.axl.co.uk)

Related topics

📖 Adult basic life support; 📖 Child BLS; 📖 Accident prevention.

Further information for professionals and carers

Wyatt, J.P. (2006). *Oxford Handbook of Emergency Medicine*. Oxford University Press, Oxford.
⊟ BBC online and interactive tests for first aid: www.bbc.co.uk/health/first_aid

Fractures

A fracture is a broken or cracked bone, most common are classified as:
- **Closed fracture**: there is no open wound associated with this fracture.
- **Open fracture**: there is an open wound associated with this fracture.
- **Complicated fracture**: the end of the fractured bone penetrates adjacent organs or causes damage to nerves or blood vessels.
- **Stress fracture**: occurs in the foot and toes can occur following prolonged or excessive exercise.
- **Greenstick fracture**: a type of incomplete fracture occurring in children where one cortical surface of a bone breaks and the other side bends.
- **Torus ('buckle') fracture**: incomplete fracture in childhood characrerised by buckling of the cortex.

All fractures are associated with soft tissue injury with consequent bleeding and tissue swelling. Bony fragments may penetrate adjacent organs causing additional bleeding and occasionally major blood vessels and nerve damage. Open fractures communicate with the skin and open air and may become infected. Fractures are usually painful because of the extensive sensory nerve supply to the periosteum.

Fractures: signs and symptoms

- Pain at or near the site of injury exacerbated by movement.
- Tenderness at fracture site on the application of gentle pressure, with subsequent swelling and bruising.
- Restricted movement, immobility or deformity (shortening, angulation, or rotation) of the affected limb.
- The patient may report the sound of a breaking bone.
- Limb movement may cause crepitus.
- If the fracture involves a large bone or multiple bones, blood loss may be severe and may be life threatening.
- An open fracture causes twice the blood loss of a corresponding closed fracture e.g. a single, open, femoral shaft fracture in a child may result in 40% loss of circulating volume, this could be life threatening.
- Trauma may also lead to partial loss (subluxation) or complete loss (dislocation) of congruity between the articulating surfaces of a joint and may also be associated with fractures of one or more bones.

General management of fractures

All patients with suspected fractures should be referred for X-ray and specialist assessment in ED

- Ensure personal safety and assess patient's airway, breathing and circulation.
- Recognize and treat life-threatening injuries **before** assessing and managing skeletal trauma.
- Haemorrhage must be controlled in the first instance.
- Apply sterile dressings to all open wounds.
- Unless absolutely necessary casualties with fractures should not be moved until skilled help arrives.
- Treat all fractures in the position in which the casualty is found unless there is further immediate danger to life.
- Place soft padding around the broken bones and splint the injury with something rigid such as rolled up newspapers or magazines to prevent the bones from moving.
- Splints should be long enough to extend beyond joints above and below the fracture (see below).
- If there is an open fracture, cover with sterile gauze pad and apply pressure to control bleeding. Under no circumstances, neither attempt to push the bone back into the wound nor clean it.
- Check frequently perfusion including pulses, skin colour, and temperature. If appropriate record, an extremity assessment based on the five Ps: Pain, Pallor, Pulses, Paraesthesia, Paralysis.
- Monitor and treat for shock.
- Do not give patients anything to eat or drink in case surgery is required.

Alignment

Severely angulated fractures aligned only by emergency medical services before transport to hospital, requires analgesia.

Immobilization

Fractures (or suspected fractures) should be immobilized to control pain and further injury using splintage. Emergency splinting techniques are summarized below:

- Hand. This should be elevated and kept comfortable.
- Forearm and wrist. Splinted flat on padded pillows or splints.
- Elbow. Immobilize in a flexed position with a sling which may be strapped to the body.
- Arm and shoulder. Immobilize by sling, secured for additional support, across the patient's chest. Circumferential bandages should be avoided as they may cause constriction, particularly when swelling occurs.
- Femoral fractures should be treated in traction splints, but avoided in patients with suspected pelvic fractures.
- Tibia and ankle fractures immobilized in padded box splints and foot perfusion assessed before and after application.

Traumatic amputation

Traumatic amputation of an extremity may be partial or complete, the former is the greater initial threat to life as completely transected blood vessels go into spasm. Exsanguinating hemorrhage must be controlled with sterile dressings, elasticated compression bandaging and elevation wherever possible.

- Retain the amputated part for possible urgent reimplantation at a specialist centre, particularly if a child is involved.
- Amputated parts viable for 8hrs at room temp, 18hrs if cooled.
- The amputated tissue should be wrapped in a moist, sterile towel, Emergency services place in sterile, bag in an insulated box filled with crushed ice and water. and in same vehicle as patient.

Avoid, at all costs, direct contact between ice and the severed tissue.

Related topics

📖 Bleeding; 📖 Adult basic life support; 📖 Child BLS; 📖 Accident prevention.

Further information for professionals and carers

Wyatt, J.P., et al. (2006). *Oxford Handbook of Emergency Medicine*. Oxford University Press, Oxford.
🖥 BBC online interactive tests for first aid including treatment of fractures: www.bbc.co.uk/health/first_aid

Useful information

Aids and equipment: general

Disability equipment, home adaptations, and aids to nursing are provided through various public services (NHS, social services, housing, education, employment), the private, and voluntary sectors. The system for public provision and public funding is complex and grey areas exist. Individuals may be eligible for direct payment (Social services 📖) to purchase their own equipment. Publicly funded provision may not cover all types of equipment, or there may be a financial ceiling. Some charities provide individual grants, usually on application from a professional (see sources of information below).

Public funding

Authorities divide up responsibilities by:
- Purpose for which equipment is required (e.g. health need = NHS; social care need = LA).
- By type of equipment (e.g. incontinence equipment as health care = NHS responsibility).

LA responsibilities

Aids, adaptations, and equipment provided following an assessment that includes financial assessment. Many LAs will have charges.

NHS responsibilities

Medical, nursing, or therapy equipment are usually free but there exist variable and changing eligibility criteria for some items, e.g. continence pads and nebulizers. Some can be charged for, e.g. spinal supports. Equipment on the medical or nursing drug tariff, e.g. catheters, attracts prescription charges, except for those exempt (Prescribing 📖).

Therapists and specialists

Professionals most commonly involved in provision and advice on aids and equipment are:
- Occupational therapists (OTs): assess and find for problems with daily living activities. Community OTs are part of social service departments or in specialist teams, e.g. rehabilitation teams or special needs children teams.
- Rehabilitation officers for blind and partially sighted people.
- Social workers for deaf people.
- Speech and language therapists: help with communication aids and eating/drinking.
- Physiotherapists assess for mobility aids.
- Orthotists, who make and fit orthoses (externally applied devices, e.g. calipers, collars, splints, footwear, trusses); usually working to the prescription of consultants.
- Podiatrists/chiropodists make and supply orthotic footwear.
- Specialist nurses, e.g. continence advisers, stoma care specialist.
- Disability employment advisors in local Job Centres identify equipment and adaptations required by disabled people for the workplace.

Table 14.1 (Contd.)

Biochemisty

Substance		Reference interval
Adrenocorticotrophic hormone	P	<80ng/L
Alanine aminotransferase (ALT)	P	5–35IU/L
Albumin	P	35–50g/L
Alkaline phosphatase	P	30–150U/L
	P	0–180U/dL
Aspartate transaminase (AST)	P	5–35IU/L
Bicarbonate	P	24–30mmol/L
Bilirubin	P	3–17µmol/L
Calcium (total)	P	2.12–265mmol/L
Creatinine kinase (CK)	P	Men: 25–195IU/L
		Women: 25–170 IU/L
Creatinine	P	70–≤150µmol/L
Ferritin	P	12–200µg/L
Folate	S	2.1µg/L
Follicle stimulating hormone (FSH)	P/S	2–8u/L >25U/L post menopause
Gamma-glutamyl transpeptidase	P	Men: 11–51IU/L
		Women: 7–33IU/L
Glucose (fasting)	P	3.5–5.5mmol/L
Iron	S	Men: 14–31µmol/L
		Women: 11–30µmol/L
Luteinizing hormone (LH)	P	3–16U/L
Osmolality	P	278–305mosmol/kg
Phosphate (inorganic)	P	0.8–1.45mmol/L
Potassium	P	3.5–5.0mmol/L
Prolactin	P	Men: <450U/L
		Women: <600U/L
Prostate specific antigen (PSA)	P	0–4ngms/mL
Protein (total)	P	60–80g/L
Sodium	P	135–145mmol/L
Thyroxine (T₄)	P	70–140nmol/L
Total iron binding capacity	S	54–75µmol/L
Triglyceride	P	0.55–1.90mmol/L
Urate	P	Men: 210–480µmol/L
		Women: 150–390µmol/L
Urea	P	2.5–6.7mmol/L
Vitamin B₁₂	S	0.13–0.68nmol/L
		(>150ng/L)

P = plasma (e.g. heparin bottle); S = serum (clotted—no anticoagulant)

Adapted with permission from Simon, C., Everitt, H., and Kendrick, T. (2005). *Oxford Handbook of General Practice*, 2nd edn. Oxford University Press, Oxford.

Complementary therapies

Acupuncture

Use of needles to alleviate symptoms or cure disease. The mechanism of action remains unclear. Broadly, 2 forms exist – Chinese and Western. Acupuncture is most commonly used to treat musculoskeletal problems and chronic disease. There is some evidence of effectiveness in dental pain, low back pain, migraine and headache, nausea and vomiting, neck pain, substance abuse, and stroke. Reflexology is similar – a representation of the body is found on the foot. Treatment consists of massaging points on the foot or applying acupressure to relieve symptoms. There is no evidence of effectiveness, but unlikely to do harm. *Contacts*: **The British Medical Acupuncture Society**: www.medical-acupuncture.co.uk; **The British Acupuncture Council**: www.acupuncture.org.uk; **Association of Reflexologists**: www.reflexology.org

Herbal Medicine

Use of plants for medicinal purposes. Some herbal compounds of proven effectiveness are: St John's Wort (depression), Oil of evening primrose (mastalgia), Echinacea (common cold), Feverfew (migraine prophylaxis), Serenoa repens (prostatism), Gingko biloba (intermittent claudication/dementia), Chinese herbal medicine (eczema). Herbal remedies may have potent side effects and interactions with other drugs. *Contacts*: **National Institute of Medical Herbalists**: www.nimh.org.uk; **International Register of Consultant Herbalists and Homeopaths**: www.irch.org; **The Register of Chinese Herbal Medicine**: www.rchm.co.uk

Aromatherapy

Inhaling aromatic plant oils or applying them to the skin for physical or emotional benefit. No evidence of effectiveness. Aromatherapy oils are very strong, may cause skin irritation, and can be poisonous if ingested. They are volatile oils readily absorbed through mucus membranes and may be as potent as any other drug. Their safety and interactions with other medications are unknown. *Contact*: **International Federation of Professional Aromatherapists**: www.ifparoma.org

Faith healing

There are many types of 'healers' and mixed evidence of effectiveness. *Contact*: **National Federation of Spiritual Healers**: www.nfsh.org.uk

Dietary manipulation and supplementation

- *Healing foods*: e.g. ginger – anti-nausea effect; cranberry juice – prevention of UTI; garlic and fish oil – cardioprotective.
- *Nutritional medicine*: involves prescribing vitamins, minerals, amino acids and essential fatty acids. Some evidence of effectiveness e.g. vitamins A, C, and E (anti-oxidants) – prevention of heart disease and cancer, help wound healing; calcium supplements + vitamin D – decrease hip fracture in the elderly; folic acid taken preconceptually decreases incidence of neural tube defect.

- *Environmental medicine:* Based on the premise that individuals develop adverse responses to environmental substances, most commonly foods, which manifest as disease. There is evidence it can help some conditions e.g. irritable bowel syndrome, migraine, childhood eczema (<10%).

Contacts: **British Naturopathic Association:** www.naturopaths.org.uk; **The General Council and Register of Naturopathy:** www.naturopathy.org.uk.

Hypnotherapy

Consists of training the patient to relax very deeply. It is useful in pain control – the patient is trained to put the pain out of their mind and relax easing symptoms. In the same way, it can be used to help break addictions and is advocated for smoking cessation. *Contacts:* **The Association for Professional Hypnosis and Psychotherapy:** www.aphp.co.uk.

Homeopathy

Mechanism of action is unclear. Involves treating like with like (i.e. a treatment capable of triggering a smiliar reaction) and using extremely dilute solutions. Homeopathic treatment is slow and most suited to chronic conditions. Meta-analysis pooled all studies comparing homeopathy to placebo and concluded overall that homeopathy works but insufficient evidence about homeopathy for clinical decision making although side effects are rare[1]. *Contacts:* **British Homeopathy Society:** www.trusthomeopathy.org **International Register of Consultant Herbalists and Homeopaths:** www.irch.org.

Osteopathy and chiropractic

Physical treatments aimed at restoring alignment of the joints and improving functioning of the body. In the UK, both are distinguished from other complementary therapies by being under statutory regulation. All osteopaths and chiropractors have to undergo training and after that time are registered with their governing body who enforce a code of standards and discipline. They must have professional indemnity insurance. They are best known for treating musculoskeletal problems, particularly bad backs. Other conditions (e.g. headaches, stress) can respond well too. There is good evidence of effectiveness for back pain. *Contacts:* **The General Osteopathic Council:** www.osteopathy.org.uk; **The British Chiropractic Association:** www.chiropractic-uk.co.uk.

---

1 Linde *et al.* (1997) Lancet **350:** 834-43.

Death confirmation and certification

One-quarter of deaths occur at home. The GP is often the first to be contacted. A doctor is not required to verify death or view the body of a deceased person or report a death has occurred. The doctor who attended the deceased during the last illness is required to issue a certificate detailing the cause of death.

Confirmation of the fact of death

Expected deaths

In many PCOs there are protocols and agreements for registered nurses, with specific training, to verify expected and inevitable deaths of patients to whom they have provided palliative care. The GP and nursing team, in discussion with the family, will have made a prior agreement that the nurse verifies death and informs the GP, who then issues a medical certificate of death for collection by relatives (see below). The recognized clinical signs when verifying death are:

- Absence:
  - Of a carotid pulse over 1min
  - Of heart sounds over 1min
  - Of respiratory movements and breath sounds over 1min.
- Fixed, dilated pupils (unresponsive to bright lights).
- No response to painful stimuli (e.g. sternal rub).

Unexpected and/or sudden deaths

Practitioners visiting in the home finding someone unexpectedly dead should:

- Initiate life support, if appropriate, including calling 999 (Adult basic life support 🕮).
- In unequivocal death, e.g. hypostasis, rigor mortis, massive cranial damage, decomposition, either call 999 or the GP, depending on the circumstances and knowledge of the deceased person.

Some PCOs have developed protocols for first-contact practitioners, working in OOH services, to verify unexpected deaths at home.

Certification of death

This is the process of completing the 'Medical Certificate of Cause of Death'. By law, this must be completed by a medical practitioner who attended the deceased person during the last illness. The certificate is usually issued in a sealed envelope, addressed to the registrar (Registration of deaths 🕮), and given to the next of kin to take to register the death.

Medical practitioners report the death to the coroner (procurator fiscal in Scotland) if:

- A doctor had not seen the patient in the preceding 14 days (28 in Northern Ireland)
- Within 24hrs of admission to hospital
- The death was sudden, violent, unnatural, or suspicious in any way
- The cause is unknown or uncertain

- The death occurred during surgery or recovery from anaesthetic
- The death occurred in prison or policy custody
- The cause was an industrial disease.

The coroner will decide whether a post-mortem and further investigation are required in order to determine the cause of death.

It is good practice for general practices and primary care nurses to inform other care services (e.g. hospitals, social services involved with the deceased person) of their death to avoid ongoing appointments etc. Some general practices keep registers of deaths.

Related topic
📖 Bereavement, grief, and coping with loss.

Further information
RCN (1996). *Verification of deaths by registered nurses.* Royal College of Nursing, London.
💻 The Home Office (2003). *Death Certification and in England, Wales and NI. A fundamental review Cm 5831*: www.homeoffice.gov.uk

Registration of births, marriages, and deaths

It has been a legal requirement since the mid 1800s for UK residents to register births, marriages, and deaths with the civil authorities. It is a criminal offence not to register births and deaths within specified time periods. Birth, marriage, and death certificates are copies of the entries made in the register for that district. The Registrar of births, marriages, and deaths is an official position in each LA responsible for the registers for that district. Details of how to find the Registrar are on every council website, in libraries, and the telephone book.

Births

All births (including stillbirths) must be registered within 42d in the district in which the birth occurred. This can be done by either parent, or together if married. A father not married to the mother can register the birth jointly with her to ensure parental responsibility (NB in the case of unmarried parents only the mother has automatic right of parental responsibility). If neither the mother nor the father can register the birth, someone present at the birth, or with responsibility for the child, can do so. See also 📖 Postnatal care; 📖 New birth visits.

Marriages

A man and a woman may marry if both are aged 16yrs or over and single, widowed, or divorced. Those aged 16 and 17 need parental consent. A transsexual person with a full gender recognition certificate can marry someone of the opposite sex. Details of prohibited marriages of relatives are available through the Citizens Advice Bureau (see below). It can be a civil or religious ceremony. The legal requirements for a marriage are that it is conducted by, or in the presence of, someone authorized to register it, and it is entered into the marriage register.

Civil partnerships

From the end of 2005 same-sex couples have been able to register a civil partnership.

Deaths

A death must be registered within 5 days, but can be delayed for another 9 days if the registrar knows that a medical certificate of death has been issued. Deaths reported to coroners cannot be registered until investigations are completed. If the death was at home, the registration is in that district. If the death was in hospital or care home, then registration is in the district of the institution. Death can only be registered by:

• A relative, present at the death or last illness or living in the district where death took place.
• Anyone present at the death.
• The owner/occupier of the building where the death occurred who is aware of the death.
• The person arranging the funeral.

The registrar will require the medical certificate of death and, if possible, certificates of birth and marriage, and an NHS medical card. See also 📖 Bereavement, grief, and coping with loss; 📖 Sudden unexpected death of an infant.

Further information

📖 Citizens Advice Bureau: www.adviceguide.org.uk

Time off work post surgery

General guidance on expected recuperation time and time off work for uncomplicated procedures.

Table 14.2 Guidance on time off work for uncomplicated procedures

Operation	Minimum expected (wks)	Maximum expected if no complications (wks)
Angiography/angioplasty	<1	4
Appendicectomy	1–2 (laparoscopic)	2–3 (open)
Arthroscopy	<1	<1
Cataract surgery	2	4
Cholecystectomy	2–3 (laparoscopic)	3–5 (open)
Colposcopy ± cautery	<1	<1
CABG or valve surgery	4	8
Cystoscopy	<1	<1
D&C, ERPC, or TOP	<1	<1
Femoro-popliteal grafts	4	12
Haemorrhoid banding	<1	<1
Haemorrhoidectomy	1	4
Hysterectomy	3 (laparoscopic assisted vaginal)	7 (abdominal)
Inguinal or femoral hernia—unilateral	1–2 (laparoscopic)	2–3 (open)
Inguinal hernia—bilateral	1–2 (laparoscopic)	6
Laparoscopy ± sterilization	<1	<1
Laparotomy	6	12
Mastectomy	2	6
Pacemaker insertion	<1	<1
Pilonidal sinus	<1	<1
Retinal detachment	<1	Avoid heavy work lifelong
Total hip or knee replacement	12	26
TURP	2	5
Vasectomy	<1	<1

Adapted from Simon, C., Everitt, H., and Kendrick, T. (2005). *Oxford Handbook of General Practice*, 2nd edn. By permission of Oxford University Press, Oxford.

Sources of information on benefits and support

Millions of pounds of state benefits go unclaimed every year in the UK. Low income is one of the factors affecting health and well-being (UK health profile 🕮). Increasingly, welfare rights advisors are working closely with primary care services to help increase the uptake. This is a general guide (Table 14.3) to help practitioners understand:

- What is available.
- Where information and help can be found to assist in what is often a complicated eligibility and claim process.

❶ 0800 numbers are free; 0845 numbers are charged at local rate.

> ❶ Benefit fraud: the DWP provides a freefone number which members of the public can telephone in confidence to give information about benefit fraud. ☎ 0800 85 44 40.

Further information for professionals

- 🖫 Child Poverty Action Group *Annual Welfare Benefits & Tax Credits Handbook*: www.cpag.org.uk/
- 🖫 Department of Work and Pensions (DWP): www.dwp.gov.uk
- 🖫 DWP Corporate Medical Group provide a guide (IB204) for medical practitioners in England, Scotland, and Wales about providing medical certificates (e.g MED 3, 4, 5) in relation to social security benefits and statutory sick pay: www.dwp.gov.uk/medical/index.asp

Further information for the public

- 🖫 Age Concern: ☎ 0800 00 99 66 www.ageconcern.org.uk
- 🖫 Citizens Advice Bureau: local offices and www.adviceguide.org.uk
- 🖫 Counsel and Care: ☎ 0845 300 7585 www.counselandcare.org.uk
- 🖫 Government information and services: www.direct.gov.uk

	Eligibility	How to apply	Benefits gained
Working tax credit (WTC)	• Age ≥16yrs, working ≥16hrs/wk and responsible for a child (<16yrs or 16–19yrs in full-time education). • Age ≥16yrs, working ≥16hrs/wk and has a disability • Age ≥50yrs, working ≥16hrs/wk and has started work after ≥6mths of receiving 1 of certain benefits • Age ≥25yrs and working ≥30hrs/wk	Apply to inland revenue ☎ 0845 300 3900 🖥 www.inlandrevenue. gov.uk	*Tax credits*: depends on adding together elements: • Basic element: paid to everyone entitled to WTC • Second adult element • Lone parent element • Working >30hrs/wk (can combine both parents if have children) • Disability (if working >16hrs/wk) • Severe disability (if working >16hrs/wk) • Aged ≥50yrs and in receipt of certain benefits before resuming work • Childcare: up to 70% childcare costs
Children's tax credit (CTC)	• Age ≥16yrs and • Responsible for ≥1 child (<16yrs or 16–19yrs and in full-time education) • Family income <£50,000 pa	Apply to inland revenue ☎ 0845 300 3900 🖥 www.inlandrevenue. gov.uk	*Tax credits*: • Family element: credit for any family eligible—↑ if there is a child <1yr old in the family • Child element: credit for each individual child in the family—↑ if the child is disabled/severely disabled
Health benefits	**Automatic entitlement:** • Age >60yrs or <16yrs (19yrs if in full-time education) • Claiming IS or income-based JSA • Pregnant or within 1yr of child birth **By application:** • Low income and • Savings <£8000	If automatic exemption, no need to claim. If not, claim on form HC1 from pharmacies, GP surgeries and JobCentre Plus offices. Pregnancy: see also 📖 Maternity rights, and benefits Free prescriptions: 📖 Prescribing	**Free:** • Prescriptions • NHS dentistry • NHS eye tests and glasses • NHS wigs and fabric supports • Travel to hospital • Milk and vitamins for pregnant and breast-feeding women, and children <5yrs

Table 14.4 (Contd.)

	Eligibility	How to apply	Benefits gained
Housing benefit	Low income, living in rented housing *Exclusions*: full-time students without dependants, people in residential care or with savings >£16,000	Via LA	Pays rent for up to 60wks. Then need to reapply.
Council tax benefit and second adult rebate	• **Council tax benefit**: low income. Exclusions as for housing benefit • **Second adult rebate**: payable if someone who lives with you is aged >18yrs, does not pay rent or council tax, and has low income • **Council tax reduction**: if single occupier or disabled • **Disregarded occupants**: certain people including students, carers, and children, are not counted in calculating the number of people living at a property	Via LA	**Council tax benefit**: pays council tax **Council tax reductions**: • Single occupier: 25% discount • All disregarded occupants: 50% • Disabled: reduction to next lowest council tax band
The 6 Social Fund payments	• **Crisis loan**: anyone except students and people in residential care can apply • **Budgeting loan**: for large purchases. Must receive IS, pension credit, or income-based JSA • **Funeral payments**: Must receive low income benefit and be responsible for the funeral • **Cold weather payments**: average temperature <0°C for ≥7d. Must receive IS, pension credit, or income-based JSA and live with a pensioner, child <5yrs, or disabled person • **Maternity grant**: 🔲 Benefits for mothers, parents, and children • **Community care grant**: 🔲 Benefits for disability and illness	Cold weather payments—should be automatic. All others claim via local JobCentre Plus offices or 🔲 www.dwp.gov.uk	• **Crisis loan**: up to £1000 interest free loan repayable when crisis finished over 78wks • **Budgeting loan**: as crisis loan • **Funeral expenses**: sum towards cost of funeral: usually does not cover full expenses • **Cold weather payments**: £8.50/wk

Adapted with permission from Simon, C., Everitt, H, Kendrick, T. (2005) *Oxford Handbook of General Practice*, 2nd edn. By permission of Oxford University Press.

Benefits for mothers, parents, and children

Table 14.5 Benefits for mothers, parents, and children (NB financial figures given for 2006 may be subject to change)

	Eligibility	How to apply	Benefits gained
Child benefit	• Anyone responsible for the upbringing of a child aged <16yrs or 19yrs in full-time non-higher education • NB Person receiving child benefit automatically qualifies for Home Responsibilities Protection Scheme to protect Basic State Pension (see also 🕮 Pensions)	Application asap after birth or adoption on form CH₂ from local social security office or 🖥 www.directgov/parents/	*Oldest child: £17.00/wks* *Other children: £11.40/wks*
Child Trust Fund	• Born after 1.9.2002 • Receiving child benefit • Living in UK • Asylum seekers (🕮 Asylum seekers and refugees) not eligible	CTF helpline ☎ 0845 302 1470 or textphone on 0845 366 7870 🖥 www.childtrustfund.gov.uk/	Voucher for £250 to invest in special child trust fund account at banks, building societies, friendly societies
Child Tax Credit	• All families with children <16yrs or <19yrs if in full-time non-higher education and • Income < £58,000 a year (£66,000 if child<1yr)	Application form from the Tax Credits helpline on 0845 300 3900, textphone 0845 300 3909, HM Revenue and Customs (HMRC) Tax Credits 🖥 www.hmrc.gov.uk/taxcredits/downtime.htm	Variable dependant on income. Max £2235 (tax year 2005–6)
Welfare foods schemes	• Pregnant and/or children <5yrs • Not living in Devon or Cornwall (see Healthy Start Scheme) and • Receive income support or jobseekers allowance or child tax credit (🕮 Benefits for people with a low income)	Leaflet 'Free milk for pregnant women' countersigned by GP or midwife. 🖥 www.directgov/parents/ If already getting milk tokens when pregnant, call the Token Distribution Unit ☎ 0845 850 1032, textphone 0845 601 7698 when baby is born to tell them infant tokens needed. Automatic if receive child tax credit	Tokens for 4L of cows' milk a week if pregnant, and for each child >1yr and <5yrs Tokens for 900 grams of infant formula a week for each child <1yr Free vitamins (available from child health clinics)

	Eligibility	How to apply	Benefits gained
Healthy start scheme	• Currently in Devon and Cornwall only but may extend • Same eligibility as welfare food schemes above or pregnant and <18yrs	Healthy start application form by calling 08701 555 455 (local rate) or www.healthystart.nhs.uk/index.asp Countersigned by midwife, HV, or GP	• Vouchers worth £2.80 for milk, fresh fruit and vegetables, or infant formula • Pregnant women and children >1yr <5yrs get one voucher a week, <1yr—two vouchers a week • Free vitamins
Statutory maternity pay (SMP)*	• Worked for the same employer for ≥26wks into the 15th week before the baby is due • Pregnant at (or have had the baby by) the 11th week before the baby is due • Earning ≥ NI lower earnings limit in the relevant period	• Inform employer at least 28d before starting leave • MATB1 form: see also Maternity rights and benefits	• Paid for up to 39wks can start from 11th week before EDD • 1st 6wks 90% usual average earnings • 6–33wks 90% of usual earnings or £109/wk whichever is lower
Maternity allowance (MA)*	• Employed/self-employed for ≥26wks in the 66wks preceding the baby's due date (test period). • Average weekly earnings of ≥£30/wk for at least 13wks of the test period • Do not qualify for SMP (e.g. changed jobs).	Apply >26/40 and within 3mths of date MA due to start. Need: • Form MA1 (from social security offices, employer, or DWP) www.dwp.gov.uk • MATB; and, if employed • Form SMP1 from employer	• Paid for 39wks can start any time from 11th week EDD • 90% of usual earnings or £109/wk whichever is lower
Sure start maternity grant	• From 11wks before baby is due to <3mths after birth/adoption • Claiming IS or income based JSA; CTC at a higher rate than the maximum family element or working tax credit with a disability or severe disability element	Form SF100 from social security offices or www.directgov/parents/	£500 payment

 Free prescriptions/dentistry are available to all children <16yrs, mothers while pregnant, and <1yr after birth, and families with low income.

* Incapacity benefit and income support may be available for women unable to claim SMP or MA.

Adapted with permission from Simon, C., Everitt, H., Kendrick, T. (2005) Oxford Handbook of General Practice. By permission of Oxford University Press.

Benefits for disability and illness

Table 14.6 Benefits for disability and illness (NB financial figures given for 2006 may be subject to change)

	Eligibility	How to apply	Amount
Statutory sick pay (SSP)	• Employee age ≥16yrs and <65yrs • Incapable of work due to sickness or disability • Earning ≥National Insurance lower earnings limit (£82wk) • Unable to work ≥4d and <28wks (inc. days when would not normally work) • Those ineligible may be eligible for incapacity benefit or maternity allowance	Notify employer of illness: self-certification first 7d. >7d requires Med 3 certificate signed by GP	£65.20/wk. Some employers have more generous arrangements. Paid through normal pay mechanisms
Incapacity benefit	• Not entitled to statutory sick pay (includes self-employed) or sick unable to work >28wks • Unable to work (Med 3 certification signed by GP until Personal Capability Assessment is applied for, then certificate Med 4 completed by GP may be required • < Pensionable age • Sufficient National insurance contributions (unless aged <20yrs)	Form SC1 available at local JobCentre Plus to claim or at ⌨ www.direct.gov.uk/	1–28wks: £57.65/wks 29–52wks: £68.20/wks >52wks: £76.45/wks Plus additions for dependants
Community care grant (part of Social Fund)	Receiving IS or income-based JSA and: • Want to re-establish or help the applicant or a family member stay in the community • Ease exceptional pressure on the applicant or a family member • To help with certain travel costs	Administered by local JobCentre Plus. Form SF300 from local social security offices or ⌨ www.direct.gov.uk	One off payment—minimum £30. No maximum amount but local JobCentre Plus has an annual budget and decisions made within that allocation
Disabled facilities grant	For work essential to help a disabled person live an independent life. Means tested	Apply via local housing department	Any reasonable application for funds is considered

	Eligibility	How to apply	Amount
Disability living allowance (DLA)[v]	• Disability >3mths and expected to live >6mths* • <65 yrs at time of application **Mobility component:** help needed to get about outdoors • *Higher rate:* unable/virtually unable to walk (age >3yrs) • *Lower rate:* help to find way in unfamiliar places (age >5yrs) **Care Component:** Help needed with personal care • *Lower rate:* attention/supervision needed for a significant proportion of the day or unable to prepare a cooked meal • *Middle rate:* attention/supervision throughout the day or repeated prolonged attention or watching over at night	Leaflet DS704 available from Post Offices or Using claim packs available at CAB and local social security offices or JobCentre Plus 💻 www.dwp.gov.uk	Mobility Component: *Higher rate:* £42.30/wk *Lower rate:* £16.05/wk Care Component: *Higher rate:* £60.60/wk *Middle rate:* £40.55/wk *Lower rate:* £16.05/wk
Attendance allowance (AA)[v]	• Needed help with bodily functions frequently or frequent supervision to avoid substantial danger to self or others for at least 6mths and expected to continue* • Aged ≥65yrs. • Not permanently in hospital or accommodation funded by the LA (but can be in sheltered accommodation). • Higher rate if 24-hour care required/terminal illness* • Or on frequent renal dialysis and require supervision	☎ 0800 882200 (0800 220674 in Northern Ireland) or Leaflet DS704 available from Post Offices or 💻 www.dwp.gov.uk	*Lower rate* £40.55/wk *Higher rate* £60.60/wk (for people who need day *and* night care *or* are terminally ill) Receipt can mean entitlement to pension credit, council tax benefit, housing benefit
Carer's allowance	• Aged ≥16yrs and • Spends ≥35hrs/wk caring for a person with a disability who is getting AA or constant attendance allowance or middle or higher rate care component of DLA; *and* • Earning ≤£82/wk After allowable expenses. • Not in full time education.	Complete form in leaflet DS700 available from local social security offices or 💻 www.dwp.gov.uk	£45.70/wk Plus additions for dependants (❶ No new claims for dependent children have been accepted since April 2003)

[v] Not means tested.

*Terminal illness (not expected to live >6mths): claim under Special Rules. Claims are processed much faster and the highest care rate is automatically awarded. GP or hospital specialist fills in form DS1500 to provide clinical information to support application (fee can be claimed).

❶ People who need someone's help to get out of the house are entitled to free prescriptions

• *Severe disablement allowance* is still paid to those who applied prior to April 2001

Reproduced from Simon, C., Everitt, H., Kendrick, T. (2005). *Oxford Handbook of General Practice*. By permission of Oxford University Press

Mobility for disabled and older people

Table opposite shows an overview of mobility for disabled and elderly people.

Table 14.7 Mobility for disabled and older people

	Eligibility	How to apply	Benefits gained
Blue badge parking scheme	Age >2yrs and has one or more of the following: • War Pensioner's mobility supplement • Higher rate of the mobility component of Disability Living Allowance (DLA) • Motor vehicle supplied by a government health department • Registered blind • Severe disability in both upper limbs preventing turning of a steering wheel • Permanent and substantial difficulty walking	Apply through local social services department ❶ In most circumstances the disabled person does not have to be the driver. The badge should not be used if the disabled person is not in the car 🖥 www.direct.gov.uk/DisabledPeople	Entitles holder to park: • In specified disabled spaces • Free of charge or time limit at parking meters or other places where waiting is limited • On single yellow lines for up to 3hrs (no time limit in Scotland)
Motability scheme	• Higher rate mobility component of DLA or • War Pension Mobility Supplement ❶ Driver may be someone else	Contact Motability. Application guide available at 🖥 www.motability.co.uk	Registered charity. Mobility payments can be used to lease or hire-purchase a car, powered scooter, or wheelchair. Grants may also be available for advance payments, adaptations or driving lessons
Road tax exemption	• Higher rate mobility component of DLA or • War Pension Mobility Supplement or • Person nominated as someone who regularly drives for a disabled person or • Certain types of powered invalid carriages	Usually received automatically. If not and claiming DLA ☎ 0845 712345 6. If claiming War Pension ☎ 0800 1692277 www.direct.gov.uk/DisabledPeople	Exemption from Road Tax.
Seatbelt exemption	Certain medical conditions e.g. colostomy	Medical practitioner must complete DH supplied exemption certificate. Driver Safety Division/Department for Transport tel 02077 9442046	Exemption from wearing seatbelt

❶ Local public transport schemes also exist

Adapted with permission from Simon, C., Everitt, H., and Kendrick, T. (2005). *Oxford Handbook of General Practice*, 2nd edn., Oxford University Press, Oxford.

Pensions

Table 14.8 Pensions

	Eligibility	How to apply	Amount
State retirement pension	• Based on sufficient yrs of National Insurance contributions paid through working life, normally 39yrs but ↑ 44yrs in 2020. ❷ ♀ may be at risk of low contributions but may have home responsibilities protection, or have bought additional voluntary contributions **and** • Men aged ≥65yrs and women aged ≥60yrs if born before 05/04/1950 • At 65 if born after 06/04/1955 (a woman born between 6/04/1950 and 5/04/1955, gets State Pension when reaches State Pension age. This will be between 60 and 65, depending on DOB) Even if still working	Claim forms should be received automatically. If not request one through the local Jobseeker Plus office or local Pension Centre. 🖳 www.thepensionservice. gov.uk ☎ 0845 60 60 265	Full basic state pension £82.05/wk but individual circumstances affect amount (minimum £21.51/wk) ❷ Pensions are taxable. ❷ Pensioners on low income may be eligible for pensions (Benefits for people with a low income 🕮) ❷ If hospitalized, retirement pension is payable for 1yr at full rate. After 12mths, basic pension is ↓ but second state pension stays the same
Non-contributory state pension	• Not eligible for state pension • >80yrs		£49.15 a week
Second state pension	From 2002 replaced State Earnings-Related Pension Scheme (SERPS). Applies to some low and moderate earners, some carers and people with long-term illness or disability. Entitlement calculated when claim state retirement pension (see above)	🖳 www.direct.gov.uk With claim for state pension see above	Individually calculated
Other benefits to pensioners	Free colour TV licence: All pensioners >75yrs	TV licence reminder notification Helpline ☎ 0845 603 6999	

	Eligibility	How to apply	Amount
	• Winter fuel payment: annual payment to all >60yrs plus receiving state pension or IS in qualifying week in September of that year	Automatic or Winter fuel payment advice service ☎ 0800 22 44 88	£100–£200 dependent on circumstances
	• Cold weather payment if receiving pension credit	Automatic on very severe weather	£8.50
	• Concessions on cost of bus travel (bus pass) to people >60yrs	Through the LA	Varies by LA area
Christmas bonus	One-off payment made to people receiving a retirement pension or income support	Automatic	£10.00
War pensions	For people injured whilst serving in the armed forces and their dependants (if injury caused or hastened death)	Administered by the Veterans Agency, Ministry of Defence (MoD). No time limit for claims	**Basic benefits:** • If <20% disabled: lump sum • If >20% disabled: weekly sum (pension) **Other benefits:** Allowances if severely disabled. Some medical costs paid for by Veterans Agency
War widows and widowers' pensions	Paid to widows or widowers and children of someone killed in the Armed Forces or who died later as a result of injury in the Armed Forces	Administered by the Veterans Agency, MoD	

Adapted with permission from Simon, C., Everitt, H., and Kendrick, T. (2005). *Oxford Handbook of General Practice*, 2nd edn., Oxford University Press, Oxford.

Useful websites

National Health Service Organizations

www.nhs.uk	NHS
www.doh.gov.uk	Department of Health, England
www.show.scot.nhs.uk/sehd	The Health Department, Scotland
www.wales.gov.uk/subihealth	Health and Social Care Department, Wales
www.dhsspsni.gov.uk	Department of Health, Social Services and Public Safety, Northern Ireland

Professional and Trade Union Organizations

www.nmc-uk.org	Nursing and Midwifery Council
www.rcn.org.uk	Royal College of Nursing includes country specific web pages
www.msfcphva.org	Community Practitioner and Health Visitors Association (part of Amicus). Includes country specific websites
www.cdna.tvu.ac.uk	Community and District Nursing Association
www.unison.org.uk	Unison (Health Staff Trade Union)
www.amicustheunion.org	Amicus (Health Staff Trade Union)

Evidence-based health care

www.nelh.nhs.uk	National Electronic Library for Health (includes evidence based databases, specialist libraries, protocol, and guideline finder)
www.phel.gov.uk/	Public Health Electronic Library
www.nice.org.uk	National Institute for Health and Clinical Excellence includes public health
www.sign.ac.uk	Scottish Intercollegiate Guidelines Network
www.clinicalanswers.nhs.uk/	NHS National Library for Health question answering service for primary care
www.phru.nhs.uk/casp/casp.htm	NHS Critical Appraisal Skills Programme (includes electronic resources)

Evidence-based prescribing

www.cks.library.nhs.uk	Clinical Knowledge Summaries (Prodigy)
www.bnf.org	British National Formulary
www.bnfc.nhs.uk/bnfc/	British National Formulary for Children
www.npc.co.uk	NHS National Prescribing Centre

UK Primary and Community Nursing Electronic Discussion/Network Groups (active in 2006)

http://health.groups.yahoo.com/group/practicenurse/	Practice nurses discussion group
www.mailbase.org.uk/lists/hv-sn-forum/	Health visitor/school nurse forum
http://health.groups.yahoo.com/group/SENATE-HVSN/	SENATE for health visiting and school nursing
http://health.groups.yahoo.com/group/PrimaryCareNursingResearchNetwork/	Primary Care Nursing Research Network

Other sources of information on UK Primary and Community Nursing

The Directory of Community Nursing is published annually by Professional, Managerial and Health Care Publications Ltd.
Email: admin@pmh.co.uk

Health Advice and Information Services to the Public

www.nhsdirect.nhs.uk	NHS Direct England ☎ 0845 46 47
www.nhsdirect.wales.nhs.uk/	NHS Direct Wales ☎ 0845 46 47
www.nhs24.com	NHS24 Scotland ☎ 08454 24 24 24

Useful general information sites

www.adviceguide.org.uk	Citizen's Advice Bureau
www.direct.gov.uk	UK government information on all public services
http://search.yahoo.com	Search tools
www.google.com	
www.thephonebook.bt.com	Telephone directories
www.yell.com	
www.streetmap.co.uk	Maps
www.multimap.com	

NB Many other websites and sources of information are given at the end of each topic

Index

VICTORIA INFIRMARY MEDICAL STAFF LIBRARY